PRINCIPLES OF
Pharmacology
for Athletic Trainers
········· **Third Edition**

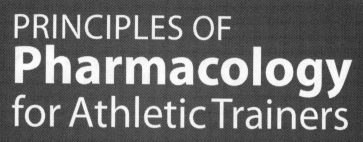

PRINCIPLES OF
Pharmacology
for Athletic Trainers
Third Edition

Joel E. Houglum, PhD
Professor of Pharmaceutical Sciences
Assistant Dean Emeritus
College of Pharmacy
South Dakota State University
Brookings, South Dakota

Gary L. Harrelson, EdD, ATC
Director, Organizational Development and Education
DCH Health System
Tuscaloosa, Alabama

Teresa M. Seefeldt, PharmD, PhD
Associate Professor
Department of Pharmaceutical Sciences, College of Pharmacy
South Dakota State University
Brookings, South Dakota

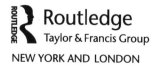

Routledge
Taylor & Francis Group

NEW YORK AND LONDON

First published in 2016 by SLACK Incorporated

Published 2024 by Routledge
605 Third Avenue, New York, NY 10158

and by Routledge
4 Park Square, Milton Park, Abingdon, Oxon OX14 4RN

Routledge is an imprint of the Taylor & Francis Group, an informa business

Library of Congress Cataloging-in-Publication Data

Names: Houglum, Joel E., author. | Harrelson, Gary L., author. | Seefeldt,
    Teresa M., author.
Title: Principles of pharmacology for athletic trainers / Joel E. Houglum,
    Gary L. Harrelson, Teresa M. Seefeldt.
Description: Third edition. | Thorofare, NJ : SLACK Incorporated, [2016] |
    Includes bibliographical references and index.
Identifiers: LCCN 2015037162 | ISBN 9781617119293 (alk. paper)
Subjects: | MESH: Sports Medicine--methods. | Drug Therapy--methods. |
    Pharmaceutical Preparations. | Pharmacology--methods.
Classification: LCC RM300 | NLM QT 261 | DDC 615/.1--dc23 LC record available at http://lccn.loc.gov/2015037162

ISBN: 9781617119293 (pbk)
ISBN: 9781003525936 (ebk)

DOI: 10.4324/9781003525936

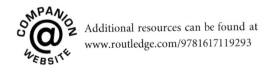

Additional resources can be found at
www.routledge.com/9781617119293

Dedication

To Rita, Dan & Becki, Andrew & Michelle, Cate, Sam, Ella, Nate, Tyler, Violet, and William, who are at the center of my earthly universe. And to our loving Heavenly Father, who has blessed each of us through Christ Jesus.

JEH

To my mother, who modeled love, sacrifice, and service. Not until adulthood could I truly appreciate these characteristics and understand how scarce they are in the world today and what a blessing they were for me. By God's grace may these traits be seen in me.

Love is patient, love is kind. It does not envy, it does not boast, it is not proud.[5] It does not dishonor others, it is not self-seeking, it is not easily angered, it keeps no record of wrongs.[6] Love does not delight in evil but rejoices with the truth.[7] It always protects, always trusts, always hopes, always perseveres....[13] And now these three remain: faith, hope and love. But the greatest of these is love. (1Corinthians 13:4-7, 13)

GLH

Contents

About the Authors

Joel E. Houglum, PhD, received a BS in Pharmacy from the University of Minnesota and a PhD in Pharmaceutical Biochemistry from the University of Wisconsin. He was Assistant Dean and Professor of Pharmaceutical Sciences in the College of Pharmacy at SDSU, where he taught courses in pharmacology and pharmaceutical biochemistry for 28 years. He was recognized by SDSU for his teaching excellence and selected the Pharmacy College Teacher of the Year 10 times. His other publications have been in the areas of leukotrienes, analytical chemistry, curriculum planning and evaluation, and pharmacology for athletic trainers, with publications in the *Journal of Athletic Training* and *Athletic Therapy Today.* He has given presentations at the NATA Annual Meeting & Clinical Symposia and at other professional meetings.

Gary L. Harrelson, EdD, ATC, received a BS in Athletic Training, an MS in Exercise Physiology, and an EdD in Administration and Teaching from the University of Southern Mississippi. He is the Director of Organizational Development and Education (ODE) for the DCH Health System in Tuscaloosa, Alabama. Since his certification as an athletic trainer in 1985, Gary has worked as an athletic trainer in multiple settings, which include high school, clinic, collegiate, and professional sports. Gary has taught in the athletic training curriculums at the University of Alabama and the University of Southern Mississippi. He was an Associate Editor for the *Journal of Athletic Training* and *Athletic Therapy Today.* Additionally, he is the coauthor of the book *Physical Rehabilitation of the Injured Athlete,* 4th edition; *Administrative Topics in Athletic Training: Concepts to Practice;* and a CD-ROM on *Joint Mobilization* and an 8-video series on evaluation. He has written numerous articles and made many professional presentations at the state, regional, and national levels, as well as internationally.

Teresa M. Seefeldt, PharmD, PhD, received a BS in Pharmaceutical Sciences, PharmD, and PhD in Pharmaceutical Sciences from South Dakota State University. She is an Associate Professor in the Department of Pharmaceutical Sciences, College of Pharmacy at South Dakota State University (SDSU) and teaches courses in the areas of pharmacology and toxicology. Teresa has been recognized as the College of Pharmacy Teacher of the Year and received the Edward Patrick Hogan Award for Teaching Excellence from SDSU. Her research interests involve oxidative stress in cardiovascular diseases and cancer.

Contributing Authors

Nathan Burns, MS, ATC, is the Credentialing Service Coordinator for the Board of Certification, Inc. He has over 15 years of experience in collegiate athletic training, academics, and athletic administration. Nathan received a BS from Buena Vista University and an MS in Physical Education with a specialization in Sport Leadership from Southwest Minnesota State University. Prior to his appointment at The National Center for Drug Free Sport, Inc, Nathan was the Director for Athletic Academic Resources and an Assistant Athletic Trainer for Southwest Minnesota State University. He served as Associate Director of Collector Development and Training for The National Center for Drug Free Sport, Inc, before he joined the Board of Certification as a Credentialing Services Coordinator.

Alan D. Freedman, MEd, ATC, has 25 years of experience as a certified athletic trainer in clinical, medical, and academic settings. He received a BS from Appalachian State University and an MEd from the University of Virginia. He is currently an Accreditation Tracking Specialist in the Office of Continuing Medical Education in the medical school at Wayne State University. He also serves as an athletic trainer for the United States Fencing Association. He serves on the Reinstatement Panel for the Board of Certification, Inc. He is a member of the International Ombudsman Association and has a keen interest in bringing awareness and solutions to workplace bullying.

Michael Powers, PhD, ATC, CSCS, EMT, is an Associate Professor and the Athletic Training Department Chair and Program Director at Marist College. Dr. Powers received a BS and an MS in Athletic Training from Northeastern University and the University of Florida, respectively, and went on receive a PhD in Sports Medicine from the University of Virginia.He is a certified athletic trainer through the National Athletic Trainers' Association, a certified strength and conditioning specialist through the National Strength and Conditioning Association, and a certified emergency medical technician. His primary research interests include the safety and efficacy of performance-enhancing supplements and drugs. In addition to his academic duties, Dr. Powers continues to volunteer his services as an athletic trainer for events such as the Boston Marathon, New York City Marathon, state games, and Special Olympics.

Cindy Thomas, MS, AT-R, has over 33 years of experience in collegiate athletic training, academics, and athletic administration. As an active member in the National Athletic Trainers' Association for over 35 years, Cindy received a BS from Longwood University and a MS in Physical Education with a specialization in Athletic Training from Indiana State University. She served as NCAA Assistant Director of Sports Sciences, administering the organization's drug-testing programs, before joining The National Center for Drug Free Sport, Inc, where she is currently Senior Director of External Operations.

Preface

A more drug-using and drug-aware society requires that athletic trainers have an appropriate understanding of pharmacology, especially related to drugs being used by the athlete. This textbook provides the basic principles of pharmacology specifically aimed at the needs of the athletic trainer. Consequently, the drug categories that are included are primarily those that may be pertinent to the treatment of athletic injuries or that may affect athletic performance. A discussion of pharmacological principles of other drug categories, as well as detailed and methodical listings of all available drugs, can be obtained from other references, examples of which are discussed at the end of the first chapter.

The athletic trainer cares for the physically active, but the employment opportunities for the athletic trainer are broad and require the treatment of patients across a wide age range. Athletic trainers not only provide care for a young, physically healthy population, but also for aging yet physically active individuals who have diseases that are being treated with physical activity as well as drug therapy. For example, an athletic trainer may be treating an older patient for a musculoskeletal injury but must be aware that the patient is also taking a beta-blocker medication that reduces cardiac output; thus, the athletic trainer may need to adjust the exercise prescription accordingly. This text addresses the diseases and drug treatment options for the physically active population treated by athletic trainers.

The challenge of writing a textbook such as this is identifying the "need to know" information for the targeted audience. Pharmacology is based in biochemistry, and, knowing that most athletic trainers' backgrounds in biochemistry are limited, we have attempted to present the information as best we can for the athletic trainer. We have used several strategies to help in this quest, which include the following:

- Summaries are not at the end of the chapter, but after each major topic within the chapter. This is to manage cognitive overload and help the reader understand what was just read.

- Advance organizers are used at the beginning of each chapter for the reader to see what the chapter contains and get a sense of how the chapter is structured, which may also manage cognitive overload.

- Key words are in italics and are defined in the glossary.

- Concept maps present important, yet complex, processes in a concise, graphical way.

- Text boxes (shaded) throughout the text either add additional information to the topic or help the reader to recall a key concept or process that was addressed in an earlier chapter.

- Very specific learning objectives are stated at the beginning of each chapter.

The content in all chapters of this edition has been updated. Additionally, Chapter 4, regarding medication management, has been rewritten, fitness supplements have been added to the herbal chapter, and case studies are included. Ancillary materials are available to facilitate the teaching and learning process and include PowerPoint slides and new test questions for each chapter.

Although this textbook provides drug information that will be useful for the athletic trainer in professional practice, caution is also warranted: the athletic trainer will not be transformed into a drug expert by studying this textbook. The athletic trainer should have sufficient knowledge about drugs to provide basic information, to improve adherence with therapy, and to identify drug-related problems in the athlete. Just as important, however, is the ability to realize one's limitations and to appropriately identify the need to refer the athlete. The expertise of the physician and pharmacist regarding drug information should be among the resources used by the athletic trainer. Frequent contact with the athlete provides the opportunity for the athletic trainer to assist the athlete with drug-related issues; this textbook will help provide the knowledge to do it.

Chapter 1: Advance Organizer

Foundational Concepts

What Is a Drug?

Drug Names

Classification of Drugs

- Nonprescription Drugs
- Prescription Drugs
- Scheduled Drugs

The Food and Drug Administration and New Drug Development

Drug Information Sources

Chapter Summary

Introduction to Pharmacology

Chapter Objectives

At the end of this chapter, the reader will be able to:

- Define what a drug is
- Differentiate between a drug's chemical, generic, and trade names
- Explain the difference between a generic name and a generic drug
- List the differences between generic and trade-name drugs
- List and explain the four ways drugs are classified
- Explain the US Food and Drug Administration's (FDA's) role in new drug development and the recall of drugs
- Locate drug information sources for prescription and nonprescription medications
- Use drug information sources to locate specific drugs

The availability and use of drugs for therapeutic purposes continues to increase. The number of prescriptions dispensed increases each year. In 2012, there were over 4 billion prescriptions dispensed. New drugs have been developed in the past several years to treat diabetes mellitus, cancer, infections, cardiovascular disorders, and rheu-

ABBREVIATIONS USED IN THIS CHAPTER	
CDER. Center for Drug Evaluation and Research	**NIH.** National Institutes of Health
FDA. Food and Drug Administration	**NSAID.** nonsteroidal anti-inflammatory drug
IND. investigational new drug	**OTC.** over-the-counter
IOC. International Olympic Committee	**PDR.** Physicians' Desk Reference
NCAA. National Collegiate Athletic Association	**Rx.** prescription
NDA. new drug application	**USP/NF.** United States Pharmacopeia/National Formulary

matoid arthritis, to name a few. In recent years, the number of drugs and therapeutic categories available without a prescription has also increased, and thus, the retail sales of over-the-counter (OTC) drug products continue to increase. Society, including athletes, has many more options for self-therapy, which complicates the task for athletic trainers to monitor the drugs being used by the athlete.

Houglum JE, Harrelson GL, Seefeldt TM.
Principles of Pharmacology for Athletic Trainers, Third Edition (pp 3-15).
© 2016 Taylor & Francis Group.

TABLE 1-1	
DIFFERENT NAMES FOR CHEMICAL STRUCTURE	
TYPE	**EXAMPLE(S)**
Chemical name	4-(dimethyl-amino)-1,4,4a,5,5a,6,11,12a-octahydro-3,5,10,12,12a-pentahydroxy-6-methyl-1,11-dioxo-2-naphthacenecarboxamide
Generic name	Doxycycline
Trade names	Vibramycin Doryx Periostat Vibra-Tabs Monodox

FOUNDATIONAL CONCEPTS

A good starting point for foundational concepts is to define *pharmacology*. Simply put, human pharmacology is the effect of drugs on the body and the effect of the body on drugs. Drugs interact with the cells and extracellular components on a molecular level to produce beneficial and detrimental responses. At the same time, other molecular interactions between the drug and body components will determine how, when, and where the action of the drug will be terminated. Consequently, pharmacology encompasses the therapeutic responses and adverse effects of drugs as well as the absorption, distribution, metabolism, and excretion of drugs.

Subdivisions of pharmacology include pharmacokinetics and pharmacodynamics. A study of the factors that affect the time course of drug events is called *pharmacokinetics*. The rate at which drugs begin to take effect, the duration of the effect, and factors that affect the rate of change in concentration of drugs at the site of action are included in pharmacokinetics. These parameters affect the optimal dosing schedule and route of administration for the drug and will be discussed in Chapter 2. *Pharmacodynamics* is the study of the mechanism of action of drugs. Some drugs, for example, combine with an enzyme to inhibit the enzymatic process, whereas others combine with receptors to either initiate or inhibit a particular effect. A more detailed discussion of pharmacodynamics is the focus of Chapter 3.

WHAT IS A DRUG?

Asking the question "what is a drug?" can spark a philosophical discussion. All drugs are chemicals. Cyanotoxins (toxins produced by bacteria) are chemicals but are very toxic with no therapeutic application; are they drugs? In the realm of therapeutics, drugs are chemicals that are used to treat or prevent disease. Table sugar (sucrose) is typically not considered a drug, but what if a diabetic is experienc-ing the sweating, tachycardia, and jittery feeling associated with hypoglycemia and uses table sugar as treatment; is the sucrose a drug? What about vitamin supplements being used by a person in whom there is no evidence of dietary deficiency? Herbal products are chemicals, many of which have unproven claims of effectiveness in preventing or treating disease; is a chemical a drug if it has no therapeutic benefit but is used for a perceived benefit? Legal, ethical, and therapeutic issues all enter the discussion to obtain an all-encompassing definition. For the purpose of this text, a suitable definition of a *drug* is a chemical that has been demonstrated to be effective for preventing or treating a disease.

DRUG NAMES

Because drugs are chemicals, they each have a chemical name that specifies the chemical structure. The chemical name is often much too cumbersome for common use, and thus a shorter generic name is also assigned to each drug entity (ie, each chemical compound). For example, 4-(dimethyl-amino)-1,4,4a,5,5a,6,11,12a-octahydro-3,5,10,12,12a-penta-hydroxy-6-methyl-1,11-dioxo-2-naphthacenecarboxamide is the chemical name for the generic name doxycycline (a broad-spectrum antibiotic). The generic name is also known as the nonproprietary name because the name is not the property of any company. The proprietary name, more commonly known as the trade name or brand name, is selected by the company that markets the drug. There is only one generic name for each drug, but there may be more than one trade name if the drug is marketed by more than one company (Table 1-1). Doxycycline has more than 10 trade names and is marketed under the generic name by a few other companies.

There is a difference between the generic name and a generic drug. Although every drug has a generic name, not all drugs are marketed as generics. When the patent for the drug expires, companies other than the owner of the patent can market the drug, but these other companies cannot use the trade name owned by the original manufacturer.

	TABLE 1-2	
CONTENTS OF SELECTED PRODUCT COMBINATIONS		
TRADE NAME	**CONTENTS**	**CLASSIFICATION**
Excedrin Migraine	65 mg caffeine 250 mg acetaminophen 250 mg aspirin	OTC
Excedrin P.M.	38 mg diphenhydramine citrate 500 mg acetaminophen	OTC
Tylenol P.M.	25 mg diphenhydramine 500 mg acetaminophen	OTC
Hyzaar	50 mg losartan potassium 12.5 mg hydrochlorothiazide	Prescription
Ziac	2.5 mg bisoprolol fumarate 6.25 mg hydrochlorothiazide	Prescription
Percocet Tablets	5 mg oxycodone HCl 325 mg acetaminophen	Controlled Substance C-II
Vicodin Tablets	5 mg hydrocodone bitartrate 300 mg acetaminophen	Controlled Substance C-II
C = category, referring to category of the controlled substance; HCl = hydrochloride; OTC = over the counter. See Tables 7-2, 7-3, and 10-2 for additional examples of products that contain multiple components.		

Consequently, most of these drugs are marketed by one or more companies using the generic name. These generic drugs are typically less expensive than the corresponding trade-name drug because they bring price competition to the marketplace and because the companies marketing them have not invested the initial research and development costs necessary to obtain FDA approval to market the drug. Similarly, drugs with expired patents can be marketed by other companies under new trade names owned by these companies. For example, because the patent is expired for ibuprofen (generic name), this drug is now marketed by several companies under this generic name and by other companies under various trade names (ie, Advil, Medipren, Motrin, Nuprin, Rufen).

Besides cost, there are other notable differences between using a generic vs a trade-name product. Typically, trade names are shorter and easier to pronounce than the generic name. However, because there can be multiple trade names, it is more difficult to remember all of them. In addition, unlike the generic name, which refers to one chemical entity, the trade name refers to the entire product contents, which may include more than one active ingredient. For example, Vanquish is the trade name for a product that contains the drugs acetaminophen, aspirin, and caffeine. As evident in Table 1-2, there is no way of knowing from the trade name the number of drugs contained in the product.

Patents last for 20 years, but it takes about 8.5 years for an experimental drug to move through the FDA approval process, leaving about 11.5 years for the marketing of the drug to be protected by the patent.

When generic or trade name products contain the same quantities of the same drug(s), they usually do not differ significantly in the observed therapeutic response. Companies that market generic drugs must obtain FDA approval through an abbreviated new drug application (NDA) process. The abbreviated process does not require the company to repeat all of the clinical trials that were conducted by the company that first obtained FDA approval to market the drug. Rather, the approval process focuses on demonstrating that the generic product is *bioequivalent* to the trade-name product.

This approval can be obtained while the trade-name drug is still under patent, thus allowing the generic product to be marketed immediately after the patent expires. As more trade-name drugs go off patent, the number of generic drugs increases. Although the cost of generic drugs is significantly less than trade-name drugs, companies that market generic drugs have the potential to gain significant profits because they do not have to recoup costs associated with research, development, and a lengthy approval process. Consequently,

TABLE 1-3

DIFFERENCE BETWEEN TRADE-NAME AND GENERIC-NAME DRUGS

TRADE-NAME DRUG	GENERIC-NAME DRUG
Can have multiple trade names	Only one generic name
Names are shorter and easier to pronounce	Refers to one chemical entity
Trade name refers to the entire product, which may include more than one active ingredient	Less expensive
	Not all drugs are marketed as a generic drug
	Generic drugs can be marketed by one or more companies
	Must obtain FDA approval, but through an abbreviated process
	Must be bioequivalent to the trade-name drug

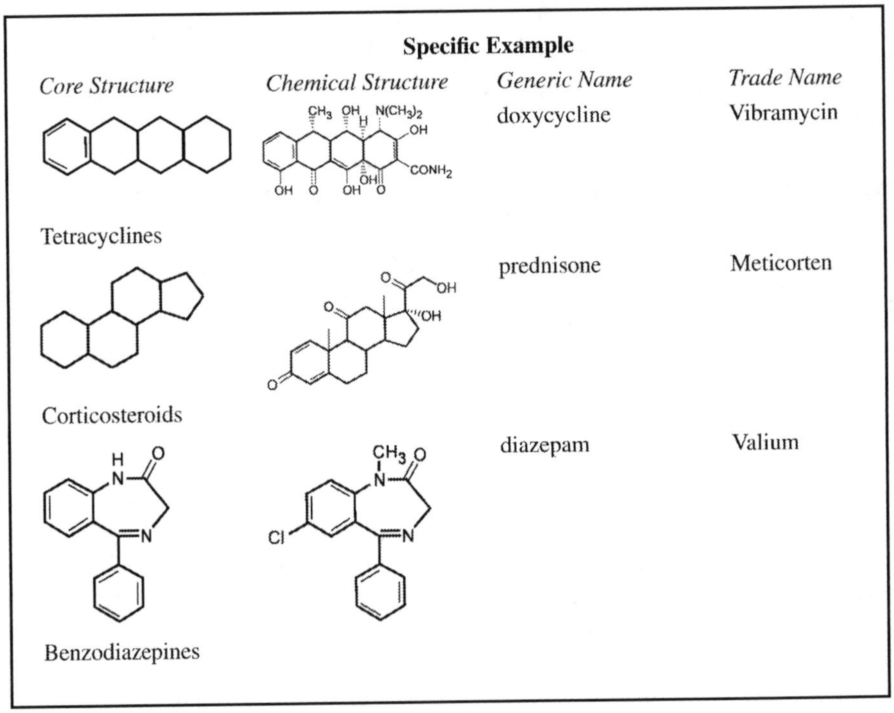

Figure 1-1. Examples of groups of drugs based on chemical structure. The drugs in these 3 chemical categories (tetracyclines, corticosteroids, benzodiazepines) have the core chemical structure shown, but each specific drug also has additional smaller chemical groups attached at various places on the core structure.

profit margin and availability of off-patent drugs are among the driving forces that will continue to increase the number of generic drugs. Table 1-3 provides a summary of the difference between trade name and generic name drugs.

Bioequivalence is discussed in the next chapter. Two drug formulations are bioequivalent if the amount and rate of the drug entering the bloodstream are approximately the same.

CLASSIFICATION OF DRUGS

Drugs may be classified in a variety of ways. Because all drugs are chemicals, they can be grouped based on their chemistry (Figure 1-1). For example, the tetracyclines are a group of antibiotics; each tetracycline contains the chemical structure of 4 rings linked together. Although each of the individual tetracycline compounds, such as doxycycline (Vibramycin), has some unique chemical characteristics, they all have a 4-ring core structure. Other examples of drug categories based on chemical structure shown in Figure 1-1 are benzodiazepines and corticosteroids.

Sometimes drug categories are based on the mechanism of action (ie, the molecular process by which the drug acts). Examples of drug categories based on mechanisms of action are protein synthesis inhibitors, beta (β)-blockers, proton pump inhibitors, H_2-blockers, and β-adrenergic agonists.

- *Protein synthesis inhibitor* is a term used to describe the mechanism of action of several antibiotics,

TABLE 1-4		
EXAMPLES OF THERAPEUTIC CATEGORIES AND SUBCATEGORIES		
THERAPEUTIC CATEGORY	**EXAMPLES OF SUBCATEGORIES**	**CHAPTER REFERENCE**
Analgesics	NSAIDs	7
	Opioids	
Antibiotics	Tetracyclines	5
	Penicillins	
	Cephalosporins	
Antihypertensives	β_1-blockers	12
	Diuretics	
	ACE inhibitors	
Anti-inflammatory drugs	NSAIDs	6
	Corticosteroids	
Asthma drugs	β_2-agonists	9
	Corticosteroids	
	Leukotriene modifiers	
ACE = angiotensin-converting enzyme; NSAIDs = nonsteroidal anti-inflammatory drugs.		

including the tetracyclines and macrolides, as discussed in Chapter 5.

- *β-blockers* comprise a group of drugs used to treat hypertension and certain heart diseases, as discussed in Chapter 12.

- *Proton-pump inhibitors and H_2-blockers* comprise groups of drugs used to treat gastrointestinal disorders as discussed in Chapter 11.

- *β-adrenergic agonists* are drugs used to treat asthma and are discussed in Chapter 9.

Compared with using the chemistry or the mechanism of action to categorize drugs, a broader means of categorization is by therapeutic effect (ie, the condition being treated: pain, infection, hypertension). As shown in Table 1-4, there are generally several subcategories within the therapeutic category.

Yet another means of categorizing drugs is by their legal classification. Several federal laws have created three classifications: OTC drugs, prescription drugs, and controlled substances (Table 1-5). The federal laws that led to these classifications are summarized in Table 1-6 (see Table 4-1 for other federal acts related to the control and distribution of drugs).

Nonprescription Drugs

Drugs that do not require a prescription are also referred to as *OTC drugs*. There are an estimated 1000 active ingredients used in over 100,000 OTC products on the market. Some of these products contain a single drug as the active ingredient, whereas many others contain combinations of active ingredients. Table 1-2 lists a few OTC products and their active ingredients.

Several OTC drugs were originally available only by prescription but were later approved for use in nonprescription products, usually at a lower amount of drug per dosage unit. For example, Motrin (400, 600, or 800 mg ibuprofen per tablet) is a prescription nonsteroidal anti-inflammatory drug (NSAID) that is also available as an OTC medication at a maximum of 200 mg per tablet. It is the responsibility of the FDA to approve a drug in the OTC classification. Many factors are considered, including evidence that there is a relatively low frequency of toxic and other adverse effects, no need for periodic medical examination or laboratory work to monitor the effectiveness or toxicity, and demonstration of effectiveness in a significant proportion of patients at the dosage recommended on the OTC product label.

Prescription Drugs

Compared with OTC drugs, prescription drugs generally have a greater potential for adverse effects, require monitoring for interactions with other medications, should only be used for a restricted time, and have other problems that necessitate the enhanced restrictions associated with prescription drugs. Medical supervision is mandated through the physician writing the prescription and the pharmacist

	TABLE 1-5
CLASSIFICATION OF DRUGS	
CLASSIFICATION	**CHARACTERISTICS**
OTC drugs	• Do not require a prescription • Usually contain a lower amount of drug per dosage unit compared with the corresponding prescription drug • Often contain multiple active ingredients in the same dosage form
Prescription drugs	• Generally have a greater potential for adverse effects than OTC drugs, require monitoring for interactions with other medications, should only be used for a restricted time, or have other problems that necessitate the enhanced restrictions associated with prescription drugs • Medical supervision is mandated through the physician writing the prescription and the pharmacist filling it
Controlled substances	• Also referred to as scheduled drugs; they have an abuse potential and thus have more restrictive requirements regarding distribution, storage, and recordkeeping compared with prescription drugs • Schedule I controlled substances (or C-I drugs) have the greatest potential for abuse, whereas Schedule V (C-V) drugs have the lowest abuse potential

filling it. Refilling the prescription is allowed only if it is specifically authorized by the prescriber.

These drugs are also referred to as *legend drugs* because the Durham-Humphrey Amendment required the label of the prescription drug container prior to dispensing (typically from the manufacturer) to contain the legend, "Caution: Federal law prohibits dispensing without a prescription." The FDA Modernization Act of 1997 changed this labeling requirement so that the drug container now must bear, at a minimum, "Rx only" (Figure 1-2).

Scheduled Drugs

Scheduled drugs have an abuse potential and thus have more restrictive requirements regarding distribution, storage, and recordkeeping compared with other prescription drugs. Table 1-7 provides some examples in each schedule and differentiates the characteristics of the five schedules based on their potential for abuse. Schedule I controlled substances (or C-I drugs) have the greatest potential for abuse, whereas Schedule V (C-V) drugs have the lowest abuse potential. Anabolic steroids are C-III drugs. Individual states can move drugs to a more restrictive schedule. Some state laws permit a limited amount of certain Schedule V controlled substances to be distributed without a prescription, usually only by a pharmacist, as long as certain recordkeeping requirements are followed; codeine-containing cough medication is an example.

THE FOOD AND DRUG ADMINISTRATION AND NEW DRUG DEVELOPMENT

In 1930, the Food, Drug, and Insecticide Administration was changed to the FDA and is now a component of the Department of Health and Human Services. The FDA is responsible for the review and approval of all new drugs before they are available to the public. New drugs proceed through a rigorous process of testing before they can be marketed. Figure 1-3 is a flowchart of this process. Safety and effectiveness must be demonstrated in clinical trials before approval is granted. Prior to the clinical trials, it often takes testing of hundreds of compounds before one emerges with the potential of therapeutic effectiveness. After sufficient data are obtained in animal studies regarding the use, dosage, and toxic effects and adequate safety and effectiveness have been demonstrated, the FDA grants Investigational New Drug (IND) status. Clinical trials (ie, human studies) can only begin after IND status is granted. Alternatively, clinical trials may also begin if the FDA does not reject the IND application within 30 days of it being submitted.

Clinical trials include 3 phases before an NDA is submitted (see Figure 1-3). Phase 1 includes tests on a small number (20 to 80) of healthy volunteers who are not taking other medications. The intent is to assess drug toxicity, absorption, metabolism, excretion, and dosage. Phase 2

TABLE 1-6

FEDERAL LAWS LEADING TO THE THREE CLASSIFICATIONS OF DRUGS

ACT	PURPOSE	COMMENT
Federal Pure Food and Drug Act of 1906	Prohibited adulteration and misbranding of medications	• The label had to accurately reflect the strength, quality, and purity of the contents. However, the Act did not require the drug to be safe or effective. • The United States Pharmacopeia/The National Formulary were also established by this act as the official standards for drug quality. • Drugs that meet the standard can have "USP" placed on the label after the name of the drug.
Food, Drug, and Cosmetic Act of 1938	Required that the safety of new drugs be reviewed and approved by the FDA before the drug could be marketed for interstate commerce	This Act was the beginning of the NDA process. However, efficacy was not addressed.
1952 Durham-Humphrey Amendment of the 1938 Act	Differentiated between prescription and nonprescription drugs	• Drugs that were determined to be unsafe without medical supervision required a prescription. • The amendment also prohibited certain drugs, such as opioids and hypnotics, to be refilled without a new prescription.
1962 Kefauver-Harris Amendment of the 1938 Act	Required that the effectiveness of new drugs, whether prescription or nonprescription, be reviewed and approved by the FDA prior to the drug being marketed	Drugs marketed between 1938 and 1962 were included in this amendment. Consequently, drugs now had to be approved as safe and effective before becoming available to the public.
Comprehensive Drug Abuse Prevention and Control Act of 1970	Established categories designated C-I to C-V (see Table 1-7), for drugs with an abuse potential	• Drugs in schedule C-I have the highest abuse potential and greatest restriction for use. This portion of the Act is referred to as the Controlled Substances Act and thus these drugs are referred to as controlled substances. • The Act regulates the manufacture, distribution, and dispensing of controlled substances. The Drug Enforcement Administration (DEA), a part of the Department of Justice, was designated the responsibility of enforcing the Act.

USP = United States Pharmacopeia.

uses a larger number of volunteers (100 to 300) who have the disease. The intent of Phase 2 is to study the drug's effectiveness and short-term safety, usually by comparing the patients with a control group. Phase 3 involves 1000 to 3000 patients at various clinics and hospitals. These patients are monitored closely for effectiveness and adverse effects of the drug compared with existing treatments for the same disease. Some patients in this phase may be receiving additional treatment for other diseases. The NDA is granted if the studies demonstrate adequate safety and effectiveness. The drug is then available for physicians to prescribe. Phase 4 includes the collection of postmarketing

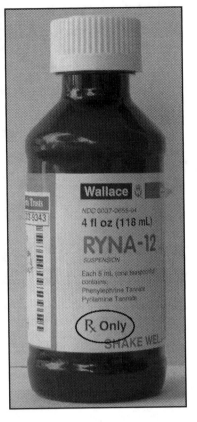

Figure 1-2. Example of "Rx only" labeling that must appear on the label of the prescription drug container prior to dispensing.

data regarding the effects of the drug on the general population, as reported by physicians who prescribe the drug. Some studies may include a comparison with other drugs in the same therapeutic category.

The FDA also reviews drugs that were on the market prior to 1962, including OTC drugs and drug combinations, in an attempt to determine effectiveness of drugs that were already on the market prior to the 1962 Kefauver-Harris Amendment.

Another important responsibility of the FDA is to recall drugs and drug products from the marketplace that are unsafe. Drug recalls are divided into 3 classes:

1. Class I recalls are those in which there is a reasonable possibility that there is a serious threat to the health of the consumer. For example, the need to add additional cautionary labeling on the manufacturer's packaging because of a life-threatening adverse effect that has been discovered in selected patients, or the color-coded oral contraceptive tablets are in the wrong sequence in the packaging.

2. Class II recalls are those in which the use of or exposure to the product in violation may cause a temporary health problem that is reversible or the probability of serious health effects is remote. For example, microbial contamination is discovered in certain lots of an oral dosage form, or an oral suspension antibiotic is found to contain less than the labeled amount of antibiotic.

3. Class III recalls are those in which the use of or exposure to a product that is in violation is not likely to cause a health hazard. For example, the manufacturer's packaging does not contain the "Rx only" labeling, or the manufacturer mislabels the package indicating the drug to be a C-IV instead of a C-III scheduled drug.

Occasionally there is a need to withdraw from the market all dosage forms that contain a certain drug because postmarketing data or additional research information indicates a serious threat to the consumer. Most recalls, however, are to remove certain products (ie, specific formulations produced by a specific manufacturer) or batches of the product. A list of recalls for the previous 60 days is available at www.fda.gov by selecting *Recalls*. The *FDA Enforcement Report Index* is also available through this website, which provides a weekly listing of recalls. Information regarding recalls is also distributed to physicians, pharmacists, and patients by the manufacturer through letters, faxes, e-mails, listings in professional publications, and announcements through the general news media.

DRUG INFORMATION SOURCES

The public is better informed about the names and actions of drugs than ever before. Advertisements of prescription and nonprescription drugs are commonplace in newspapers and magazines and on television and radio. The widespread use of the Internet has provided pharmaceutical companies with another avenue to provide information about their products to the public. Physicians and pharmacists also provide verbal information regarding the appropriate use and storage of drugs, and pharmacies provide product information sheets when new prescriptions are filled. Clearly, the philosophy of the medical community is that the public should be educated regarding the drugs they are taking.

There are many sources of drug information available to the health care professional, examples of which are discussed here and summarized in Table 1-8. These include books that provide a listing of drugs along with their respective uses, adverse effects, and other pharmacological information. As an example, the *Physician's Desk Reference* (PDR) contains information about drugs listed alphabetically by trade name according to manufacturer. The information includes chemical properties of the drug; a physical description of the trade-name product; pharmacology and clinical data; and information about precautions, adverse effects, indications, dosage, and routes of administration. Diagrams are sometimes included to serve as special instructions for administration. An example of this would be a diagram describing the use of an inhaler or the application of transdermal medication. The information in the PDR is provided by the manufacturer and contains information from the official FDA-approved package insert.

\	TABLE 1-7	
\	**CLASSIFICATION OF CONTROLLED SUBSTANCES**	
SCHEDULE	**CHARACTERISTICS**	**EXAMPLES (TRADE NAME)**
I	• High abuse potential • No accepted medical use in the United States • May be used for research purposes	• Heroin • Lysergic acid diethylamide (LSD) • Marijuana • Mescaline • Peyote • Tetrahydrocannabinol (THC)
II	• High abuse potential • Accepted medical use in the United States • Broad range of drugs	• Amobarbital (Amytal) • Cocaine • Codeine • Dextroamphetamine (Dexedrine) • Hydromorphone (Dilaudid) • Meperidine (Demerol) • Methadone • Methamphetamine (Desoxyn) • Methylphenidate (Ritalin) • Morphine • Opium tincture • Oxycodone with acetaminophen (Percocet) • Hydrocodone with acetaminophen (Vicodin, Lortab, Norco)
III	• Lower abuse potential than C-II • Accepted medical use in the United States	• Anabolic steroids • Buprenorphine (Buprenex) • Codeine with acetaminophen or aspirin • Dronabinol (Marinol) • Thiopental (Pentothal)
IV	• Lower abuse potential than C-III • Accepted medical use	• Alprazolam (Xanax) • Chlordiazepoxide (Librium) • Diazepam (Valium) • Flurazepam (Dalmane) • Lorazepam (Ativan) • Phenobarbital (Luminal) • Zolpidem (Ambien)
V	• Lowest abuse potential of controlled substances • Preparations contain smaller quantity of controlled substance • Some products are nonprescription in some states	• Cough mixtures containing codeine (Robitussin A-C) • Antidiarrheal mixtures with opium (Kapectolin PG)

APPROXIMATE YEARS	PHASE	PURPOSE
3 to 6	Preclinical Testing ↓ File IND ↓	Laboratory and animal tests. Determine biological activity. Obtain FDA approval for clinical trials.
1 to 2	Clinical Trials • Phase I ↓	20 to 80 healthy volunteers. Check pharmacokinetic parameters and safe dosages.
2 to 3	• Phase II ↓	100 to 300 patients. Determine effectiveness and short-term adverse effects.
3 to 4	• Phase III ↓	1000 to 3000 patients. Determine effectiveness and adverse effects compared to other therapy.
1.5 to 2.5	FDA Review/ Approval for NDA ↓ Postmarketing Monitoring • Phase IV	Obtain FDA approval for physicians to prescribe. General population of patients. Monitor for adverse effects; long-term effects. Compare with other therapy.

Figure 1-3. FDA new drug approval process.

The PDR also includes indices by manufacturer, trade name/generic name, and product category, which are helpful as a means to locate a drug. For example, if the generic name is known, the trade-name/generic-name index can be used. Doxycycline, for example, can be found under "doxycycline" or under "Monodox" (or any of the other trade names). Alternatively, the page for the doxycycline information can also be found by using the product category index, under the "Tetracyclines" group of the "Antibiotics" section. The PDR also includes color pictures of many products listed in a sepa-

rate section by manufacturer. A picture of Monodox capsules is among those included, and therefore, regardless of which index is used to locate Monodox, the page for the color picture is included with the page for the product information. The PDR is over 3500 pages long and is approximately 9 × 11 inches—too large to conveniently carry as a reference. The information is presented in much greater detail than needed for a quick reference.

There is an array of pharmacology textbooks specifically tailored for pharmacy, nursing, and medical students. These

TABLE 1-8

SELECTED REFERENCES AND DESCRIPTION OF CONTENTS

REFERENCE	TYPE OF INFORMATION
American Society of Health-System Pharmacists. *AHFS Drug Handbook*. Springhouse, PA: Lippincott Williams & Wilkins.	Alphabetical listing of drugs by generic name. Provides quick view of trade names, pharmacologic classification, therapeutic classification, pregnancy category, OTC/prescription classification, and dosage units supplied for each drug. Also includes summary of pharmacokinetics, mechanism of action, uses, dosages, adverse effects, and patient counseling.
DiPiro JT, Talbert RL, Yee GC, Matzke GR, Wells BG, Posey LM, eds. *Pharmacotherapy: A Pathophysiologic Approach*. New York, NY: McGraw-Hill.	Extensive and detailed discussion of drug therapy by disease state with discussion of pharmacologic drug categories. Includes extensive discussion of pathophysiology and clinical presentation for each disease. Extensive references for each chapter.
Drug Facts and Comparisons. St. Louis, MO: Facts and Comparisons.	Comprehensive source of drug information. Generic name of drugs listed alphabetically by therapeutic category. Includes uses, pharmacology, adverse effects, pregnancy risk category, and dosages. Each trade name and corresponding dosage form is listed. Some comparison of uses and effects of drugs within the category are provided at the beginning of sections. Available as loose leaf and bound.
Fetrow CW, Avila JR. *Professional's Handbook of Complementary & Alternative Medicines*. Springhouse, PA: Lippincott Williams & Wilkins.	Alphabetical listing of herbal compounds. Provides results of scientific studies, common names, chemical components, actions, uses, and dosages.
Handbook of Nonprescription Drugs. Washington, DC: American Pharmacists Association.	Textbook-like reference with chapters by disease state that includes discussion of pathophysiology, epidemiology, symptoms, and pharmacology of OTC. Provides examples of drugs but not comprehensive lists.
Hardman JG, Limbird LE, eds. *The Pharmacological Basis of Therapeutics*. New York, NY: McGraw-Hill.	Comprehensive and detailed explanation of the pharmacological effects by drug category followed by discussion of individual drugs for each category. Extensive bibliography for each chapter. Includes history and chemistry for many drugs. Includes chapters on general principles.
Lance LL, Lacy CF, Armstrong LL, Goldman MP, eds. *Drug Information Handbook*. Hudson, OH: Lexi-Comp Inc.	Alphabetical listing of drugs by generic and trade name. Includes summary of uses, pronunciation, pregnancy risk factor, effects, dosages, adverse effects, and patient information in 1 to 2 pages for each drug. Includes an index by therapeutic category and key word.
PDR for Nonprescription Drugs and Dietary Supplements. Montvale, NJ: Medical Economics Co, Inc.	Contains FDA-approved description of OTC products. Includes ingredients, uses, drug interactions, and color photographs of many OTC products. Also information on vitamins, nutritional supplements, and herbal products.
Physicians' Desk Reference. Montvale, NJ: Medical Economics Company.	The PDR. Trade names of drugs listed alphabetically by manufacturer. Contains FDA-approved labeling (package insert) information, including pharmacology, uses, warnings, adverse effects, pregnancy risk category, dosage, dosage forms, and some chemical structures. Drugs indexed by manufacturer, trade name, generic name, and product category. Includes many colored product identification photos. Information regarding some OTC drugs and contents of some combination products.
Skidmore-Roth L, ed. *Nursing Drug Reference*. St. Louis, MO: Mosby, Inc.	Contains section of general pharmacological information regarding major drug categories. Drugs listed alphabetically by generic name. Includes pronunciation of generic names, trade names, actions, dosages, adverse effects, pharmacokinetics, uses, and nursing considerations.

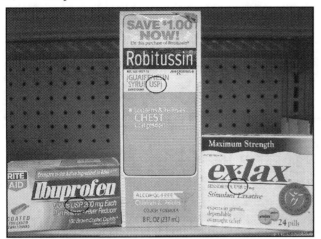

Figure 1-4. Example of "USP" denoted on label. This means that the medicine has met the official standards for purity, strength, and quality set forth by the USP/NF.

texts typically address general pharmacology principles along with a systematic discussion of every therapeutic drug category with relevance to the respective professional practice. The long-standing authority in the arena of pharmacology textbooks is Goodman and Gilman's *The Pharmacological Basis of Therapeutics*. This reference provides an in-depth presentation of the principles of pharmacology and discussion of drugs by pharmacological category. It also includes a broad base of pharmacological information in each category, followed by a discussion of individual drugs in the respective pharmacological category. History, chemistry, and toxicology are provided for many drugs, and each chapter ends with an extensive bibliography of original research and review articles. Textbooks of therapeutics usually discuss drugs by disease category along with a discussion of the pathophysiology, clinical presentation of the patient, and means of diagnosis. The focus is the drug therapy for treating the disease rather than a study of each drug by pharmacological category. A highly regarded comprehensive therapeutics textbook is *Pharmacotherapy: A Pathophysiologic Approach* (see Table 1-8).

Drug Facts and Comparisons is a reference that lists drugs alphabetically by therapeutic category. Each section discusses and compares therapeutic uses, pharmacology, contraindications, adverse effects, and patient information regarding the drugs in that category. All available trade names and dosage forms are listed, along with the name of the manufacturer. Many nonprescription products are also included, as well as a section of color photographs of tablets and capsules. *Drug Facts and Comparisons* is available in a bound format or in loose-leaf form so that monthly supplements can be included throughout the year.

The official pharmacopeia in the United States is the *United States Pharmacopeia/National Formulary* (USP/NF). This reference provides the official standards for the purity, strength, quality, and analysis of drugs. The only

drugs included in this reference are those for which standards have been developed and approved by the USP Convention. It is not a reference routinely useful for the athletic trainer, but it is noteworthy that products that have met these standards, including OTC products, have "USP" on the label (Figure 1-4) after the name of the drug (eg, aspirin, USP).

There are sources of information that focus exclusively on OTC products and their uses. Some OTC medications are also available as prescription drugs and are typically discussed in pharmacology texts, but many OTC medications and combination products are exclusively OTC. *The Handbook of Nonprescription Drugs* contains a comprehensive discussion of OTC products by disease state, pathophysiology, symptom, and pharmacological effects.

All of the references mentioned previously extensively discuss drugs from one aspect or another, but none are convenient reference guides that are easily carried around. However, there are many drug handbooks available (see Table 1-8). These handbooks typically contain a comprehensive alphabetical listing of drugs along with a summary of pharmacological information, uses, adverse effects, description of the dosage forms, trade names, and instructions to the patient. These handbooks provide a quick reference for succinct information but do not typically include explanation of drug action principles, pathophysiology, or basis for specific therapeutic uses. In general, drug handbooks are designed with the assumption that the reader has foundational knowledge regarding pharmacology. Similar handbooks are also available regarding herbal products.

An even more compact source of drug information involves the use of hand-held mobile devices. Several drug references are now available for use with mobile devices (eg, apps for smartphones and tablets), including drug handbooks and a version of the PDR. The use of mobile devices has become popular because they provide a convenient means of carrying and accessing drug information. The Internet is another electronic source of a seemingly unlimited amount of drug information. For example, the National Institutes of Health website (www.nih.gov) provides health topics by disease and organ systems, including information regarding pathophysiology, symptoms, and drug therapy. In addition, the FDA Center for Drug Evaluation and Research provides information on regulatory issues, newly approved prescription drugs, lists of approved drugs, and OTC drug information, and can be accessed at www.fda.gov/Drugs/default.htm. Both the National Institutes of Health and FDA websites have search capability. RxList (www.rxlist.com) is another online resource for drug information. This website has a search tool to find specific medications as well as an alphabetical listing of medications included in the database. Several print drug information resources have developed online versions and/or mobile apps. Examples include the American Hospital Formulary Service, Lexi-Comp, and the PDR. Many of these products operate using a subscription service where purchasers receive periodic updates of drug information.

In addition to information regarding the pharmacology of drugs, it is also important for the athletic trainer to have access to laws that regulate the handling of drugs by an athletic trainer and the policies regulating drug use and drug testing as established by the International Olympic Committee, National Collegiate Athletic Association, and other groups regulating competitive athletics. Chapters 4 and 17 discuss these issues and provide practical information for the athletic trainer. The current policies of the International Olympic Committee and National Collegiate Athletic Association regarding banned substances and anti-doping are available at www.usada.org and www.ncaa.org/health-safety, respectively. Athletic trainers should check with their respective state high school athletic association and their local school board regarding drug use and drug testing in their respective state regarding the policies regulating drug use in high school students.

CHAPTER SUMMARY

Pharmacology is the study of how drugs affect the body and how the body affects the drug. Because the therapeutic use of drugs (or lack of use) can affect athletic performance, it is important for the athletic trainer to have knowledge of pharmacology that will be useful in the professional practice setting; an understanding of the terminology and classifications of drug names is a starting point for this knowledge. The trade name (or brand name) is a name that is owned by a pharmaceutical company, whereas a generic name is not owned by anyone and refers to one specific chemical compound. Drugs can be categorized by the mechanism of action (eg, β-agonists combine with β-receptors), by their chemical structure (eg, all corticosteroids have a similar chemistry), or therapeutic category (eg, all asthma drugs are used to treat asthma, but they are not all β-agonists or corticosteroids). Drugs can also be grouped as to their legal classification of OTC, prescription, or scheduled drugs. The laws regarding the purchase, storage, and distribution differ for these three categories of drugs.

Regardless of the classification of a drug, all drugs must obtain FDA approval to be marketed. New compounds must go through a rigorous process of animal testing followed by three phases of clinical (human) tests before they can be approved for general use. A drug that goes off patent protection can be marketed by other companies after demonstrating that their products are bioequivalent to the original product. This abbreviated approval process helps expedite the marketing of drugs (generic drugs) by companies other than the initial patent holder.

This textbook includes basic pharmacology of drug categories pertinent to the certified and/or licensed athletic trainer and the athletic training student but does not supply a comprehensive list of drugs. However, there are numerous drug handbooks available that are convenient to use as a quick reference regarding specific drugs. Comprehensive textbooks and references are also readily available if a more intensive study of the effects and uses of drugs is desired. Programs are available for use with mobile devices, and an immense amount of information is available via the Internet. All of these sources of information, along with the availability of pharmacists and physicians for individualized assistance, provide excellent resources for the athletic trainer who has a foundational understanding of basic pharmacology.

CASE STUDY

As a third-year athletic training student, Deanna realizes how important it is to know about medications. In her short time as an athletic training student, Deanna has already witnessed her clinical preceptor provide counseling and answer questions for a number of athletes on the various drugs they take. One of the student-athletes, Joan, just asked her a question about what the difference is between Motrin that you can buy OTC and Motrin that requires a prescription. How would you respond to Joan's question?

BIBLIOGRAPHY

Abood RR. *Pharmacy Practice and the Law.* 7th ed. Burlington, MA: Jones and Bartlett Learning; 2012.

Pandit NK, Soltis RP. *Introduction to the Pharmaceutical Sciences: An Integrated Approach.* 2nd ed. Philadelphia, PA: Lippincott Wolters Kluwer; 2012.

Chapter 2: Advance Organizer

Foundational Concepts

- Site of Action
- Onset and Duration of Action
- Half-Life and Clearance Rate
- Bioavailability and Bioequivalence
- Volume of Distribution and
    Protein Binding
- Section Summary

Impact of Chemical Structure

- Solubility of Drugs
- Section Summary

Drugs Crossing Membranes

- Passive Diffusion
- Active Transport
- Facilitated Diffusion
- Section Summary

Routes of Administration, Dosage Form, and Absorption of Drugs

- Oral
  - Oral Absorption
- Sublingual and Buccal
- Rectal
- Parenteral
  - Parenteral Absorption
- Topical
- Inhalation
- Section Summary

Distribution

- Section Summary

Metabolism

- Section Summary

Excretion

- Renal Excretion
- Biliary Excretion
- Section Summary

Effects of Exercise

2

Pharmacokinetic Principles

Processes That Affect Drugs From Entry to Exit

CHAPTER OBJECTIVES

At the end of this chapter, the reader will be able to:

- Apply the concepts of site of action, onset and duration of action, half-life, clearance rate, bioavailability, bioequivalence, volume of distribution, and protein binding to the pharmacokinetic action of drugs
- Apply the concepts of bioavailability and bioequivalence to the biological effect of drugs
- List and explain the variables that affect the volume of distribution of a drug
- Explain how a drug's chemical structure determines its biological effects
- Explain how the solubility of a drug affects the ability of the drug to cross cell and tissue membranes
- Describe 3 primary mechanisms by which drugs cross membranes to reach their site of action
- List and describe the major routes through which drugs can be administered
- Explain what factors affect the distribution of drugs throughout the body
- Describe the primary ways drugs are metabolized through oxidation, conjugation, hydrolysis, and reduction

- List the ways drugs are excreted from the body
- Describe how drugs are excreted from the body by the kidneys
- Explain the potential impact of exercise on the pharmacokinetics of drugs

ABBREVIATIONS USED IN THIS CHAPTER	
CNS. central nervous system	**NSAID.** nonsteroidal anti-inflammatory drug
CYP. cytochrome P450	**OTC.** over-the-counter
GI. gastrointestinal	**t½.** half-life

Pharmacokinetics is the study of the effect of the body on a drug. The primary focus of pharmacokinetics is on the rate and extent to which the drug is absorbed into the bloodstream, distributed throughout the body, metabolized, and finally excreted. These processes will affect the magnitude and duration of the biological responses, the therapeutic (desirable) effects, and adverse (undesirable) effects. The chemical structure of the drug will determine how the body will interact with the drug to dictate the absorption, distribution, metabolism, and excretion.

Houglum JE, Harrelson GL, Seefeldt TM.
Principles of Pharmacology for Athletic Trainers, Third Edition (pp 17-34).
© 2016 Taylor & Francis Group.

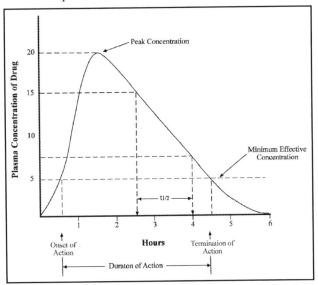

Figure 2-1. Concentration-time curve following a single oral dose of a drug. The onset of action occurs when the concentration is above the level needed to produce an effect (minimum effective concentration). Duration of action (4 hours in this example) is the time between onset and termination of action. The half-life (t½) is the time it takes for the concentration of the drug to be reduced by one-half after it has reached peak concentration. In this example, t½ = 1½ hours (the time it takes for the concentration of drug to decrease from 15 to 7.5).

Pharmacodynamics is the study of the effect of drugs on the body. This includes the study of the therapeutic effects of medications, their adverse effects, and the mechanisms by which those effects are produced. A detailed discussion of pharmacodynamics is contained in Chapter 3. However, it should be noted that pharmacokinetics and pharmacodynamics are closely connected, and both aspects need to be considered when studying pharmacology.

FOUNDATIONAL CONCEPTS

It is necessary to understand some foundational concepts and terminology to fully grasp the discussion of pharmacokinetics. These concepts and terminology include site of action, onset and duration of action, half-life, clearance rate, bioavailability, bioequivalence, volume of distribution, and protein binding. Some of these concepts and terms will not necessarily be used frequently by the athletic trainer, but they are used throughout this textbook and are useful for understanding other drug-related literature.

Site of Action

For any drug to have an effect, it must reach its *site of action*. This is the molecular site where the drug has a significant chemical interaction to produce a biological effect. The site of action for most drugs is either a receptor (usually a protein) on the cell surface or inside a specific cell type or an enzyme within a cell. For example, the site of action may be

receptors on the surface of smooth muscle, enzymes within nerve fibers, or receptors on the surface of platelets. The receptor theory of drug action will be discussed in the next chapter.

Onset and Duration of Action

The *onset of action* (Figure 2-1) is the time it takes for the concentration of drug molecules at the site of action to become large enough to cause a noticeable biological response. This response will continue as long as the minimum effective concentration of drug is maintained at the site of action. The minimum effective concentration varies from one drug to the next. As the drug is metabolized and excreted, the drug molecules dissipate from the site of action. This process continues until an insufficient number of drug molecules are present to cause an observable response and action is therefore terminated. The *duration of action* is the time between onset and termination of action and represents the length of time the drug produces its effect.

Half-Life and Clearance Rate

The *half-life* (t½) of a drug is the time required for the amount of drug in the blood to be reduced by one-half. The mechanisms that clear the drug from the body are metabolism and excretion. The *clearance rate* is a measure of the efficiency of these mechanisms. When drugs are metabolized, they are considered to be cleared from the body in the sense that they are chemically modified to form a different compound.

An accurate assumption for most drugs is that the drug in the blood is in equilibrium with the drug at the site of action. Therefore, the concentration of drug in the blood is a direct reflection of the concentration at the site of action. The t½ can be determined by measuring the blood (or plasma) concentration of the drug at time intervals after it has reached the peak level and no additional doses of drug are given (see Figure 2-1). For example, if the t½ of a drug is 2 hours and the concentration in the blood is 100 μg/mL, it will decrease by 50 μg/mL in 2 hours; if the same drug exists at 10 μg/mL, it will decrease by only 5 μg/mL (ie, 50%) in 2 hours. The rate of decrease is a percentage, not an amount, because the mechanisms by which drugs are removed from the blood are usually not working at their maximum. Thus, the rates at which these mechanisms function are a linear relationship to blood concentration in that they function twice as fast if the concentration is twice as much. Using the example above and assuming no additional drug is given, the 100 μg/mL concentration will be at 25 μg/mL after 4 hours, 12.5 μg/mL after 6 hours, and 6.25 μg/mL after 8 hours.

Drugs with a longer t½ have a longer duration of action. A significantly longer duration of action provides an advantage to the patient in that the drug does not have to be administered as often each day, thus making it easier for patients to remember to take the medication at the appropriate time. For example, naproxen, a nonsteroidal anti-inflammatory drug (NSAID), has a t½ of about 14 hours and is recommended

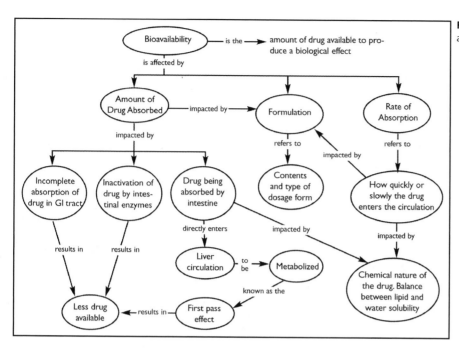

Figure 2-2. Factors affecting the bioavailability of a drug.

as twice-per-day dosing. In comparison, ibuprofen, another NSAID, has a t½ of 2 hours and, therefore, has a more frequent dosing interval of 3 to 4 times per day.

Bioavailability and Bioequivalence

The amount of drug administered has no therapeutic relevance if the drug does not reach the general circulation and have the opportunity to reach the site of action. To be bioavailable, the drug must reach the systemic circulation. There are 2 components to *bioavailability*: the amount of drug absorbed and the rate of absorption. Bioavailability will be reduced if a tablet or capsule incompletely dissolves in the gastrointestinal (GI) tract or if the drug is inactivated by intestinal enzymes (Figure 2-2). Bioavailability is also diminished if the drug is absorbed from the intestine and directly enters the portal (liver) circulation where it first passes through the liver. The liver is the major organ for drug metabolism and may inactivate a portion of the drug before it enters the systemic circulation. This is referred to as the *first-pass effect* and has a significant impact on the bioavailability of some, but not all, drugs. Enzymes in the intestinal cells may also participate in drug metabolism, which contributes to the first-pass effect and thus diminished bioavailability. For drugs that have a first-pass effect, the manufacturer's recommended dose compensates for this characteristic. Calcium-channel blockers used to treat angina and hypertension (see Chapter 12) are examples. In addition, nitroglycerin sublingual tablets (discussed later in this chapter) undergo significant first-pass effect and thus are not effective if swallowed. Because of the first-pass effect, less than half of orally administered morphine is bioavailable. To compensate for the first-pass effect, the oral dosage range of morphine is increased from the normal adult dose of 2 to 10 mg intravenously to 5 to 30 mg orally.

The other component of bioavailability is the rate at which the drug enters the general circulation (see Figure 2-2). As shown in Figure 2-3, if 100% of orally administered drug A and drug B enter the general circulation but drug A is absorbed quickly and drug B is absorbed gradually over a longer time, the peak blood concentration will be greater for drug A. This also means that the biological effect is greater for drug A. The peak blood concentration for drug B will be lower because, as it enters the blood more slowly, it does not have as much of a chance to accumulate before the clearance rate exceeds the absorption rate. Therefore, the bioavailability of these 2 drugs is not equivalent. The formulation can have a significant impact on bioavailability (see Figure 2-2). The *formulation* is also called the *product* and refers to the total contents of the dosage form (active and inert ingredients) and the type of dosage form (eg, tablet, capsule, suspension). Other factors that affect the absorption of drugs are discussed in this chapter.

Bioequivalence is similar to bioavailability but refers to a comparison of the amount and rate of drug entering the general circulation for 2 or more similar formulations of the same drug. This concept is used when a company wants to demonstrate that its generic product is equivalent to a trade-name product. In other words, 2 products (ie, different formulations of the same drug) are bioequivalent if the bioavailability of the 2 products is equivalent. Figure 2-3 illustrates the bioavailability of 2 formulations (A and C) of the same drug. The total amount of drug absorbed is approximately the same, but the absorption of the drug from formulation C is so slow that the minimum effective blood concentration is not attained; the bioavailability of drugs A and C are significantly different, and thus they are not bioequivalent.

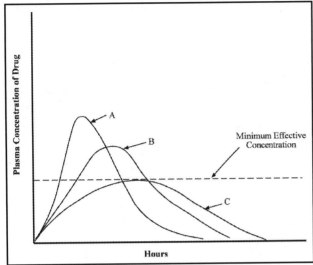

Figure 2-3. Bioavailability and bioequivalence. Concentration time curves for 2 drugs, A and B, illustrate a difference in bioavailability. Bioavailability of drugs can differ because of differences in the rates at which they dissolve in the GI tract, extent of the first-pass effect, extent to which they are affected by the presence of food, and other factors. Lack of bioequivalence is illustrated in the comparison of 2 formulations, A and C, of the same drug. In this case, formulation C is absorbed more slowly than formulation A, and thus C never reaches minimum effective concentration although approximately the same amount of drug is absorbed.

Volume of Distribution and Protein Binding

After a drug is absorbed into the blood, it distributes throughout the body. The extent of distribution in various fluids and tissues depends largely upon the drug's lipid solubility and protein-binding characteristics. The *volume of distribution* is the apparent space in the body that is available to the drug; the more extensive distribution, the larger the volume of distribution. For example, drugs that distribute well into adipose tissue will have a larger volume of distribution. As drugs distribute into these tissue sites, there is less drug available in the blood circulation and thus less drug available to reach the site of action. The extent to which a drug binds to tissue and plasma protein is documented prior to its entry into the market, and the normal dosage range is established based on this information. As the volume of distribution increases, the dose needed to get a sufficient concentration of drug to the site of action also increases.

Another factor affecting the volume of distribution is the physical size of the patient. Body weight is the most common indicator, although body surface area is also used. Obviously, a larger patient has more body tissue into which the drug can distribute. Obese patients have a larger percentage of total body weight in adipose tissue and thus have more tissue into which lipid-soluble drugs can distribute. If the drug resides in body fat, the concentration of drug available to reach the site of action is diminished. Volume of distribution increases with body weight and is the basis for adjustment of drug dos-

TABLE 2-1		
EXAMPLES OF DRUGS THAT EXHIBIT >90% PROTEIN BINDING		
GENERIC NAME	**TRADE NAME**	**DRUG CLASSIFICATION**
atorvastatin	Lipitor	antilipidemic
celecoxib	Celebrex	NSAID
diazepam	Valium	muscle relaxant
diclofenac	Voltaren	NSAID
flurbiprofen	Ansaid	NSAID
fluvastatin	Lescol	antilipidemic
glipizide	Glucotrol	antidiabetic
glyburide	DiaBeta	antidiabetic
ibuprofen	Motrin	NSAID
indomethacin	Indocin	NSAID
lovastatin	Mevacor	antilipidemic
montelukast	Singulair	asthma therapy
naproxen	Naprosyn	NSAID
phenytoin	Dilantin	anticonvulsant
pioglitazone	Actos	antidiabetic
rosiglitazone	Avandia	antidiabetic
simvastatin	Zocor	antilipidemic
tolbutamide	Orinase	antidiabetic
valproic acid	Depakene	anticonvulsant
warfarin	Coumadin	oral anticoagulant
zafirlukast	Accolate	asthma therapy
zileuton	Zyflo	asthma therapy
NSAID = nonsteroidal anti-inflammatory drug.		

age according to weight. See Chapter 3 for additional discussion regarding dose calculations.

Many drugs have the capability of binding to plasma proteins. Albumin is the plasma protein with the largest concentration in the blood (39 to 50 g/L). The percentage of drug that binds to albumin is a constant for any given drug. Some drugs do not bind significantly to albumin, but for many drugs, the percentage of the protein-bound drug is quite significant, >99% in some cases. Examples of drugs that are ≥90% bound to protein are shown in Table 2-1. Because albumin is a protein, it is much larger than drug molecules, and it does not penetrate through the capillaries. Therefore, drugs bound to albumin also do not leave the capillary and thus are not available to bind at the site of action in the tissue (Figure 2-4). Unlike binding to a receptor site, binding to albumin is

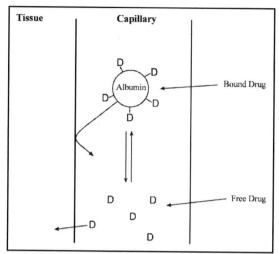

Figure 2-4. Drug binding to plasma protein. Albumin is the most abundant protein in the plasma and many drugs bind to this protein. Drug molecules that are bound to albumin cannot penetrate through the capillary because the albumin is too large. Only unbound (free) drug can leave the capillary circulation, enter the tissue, and reach the site of action.

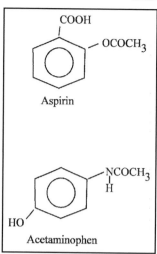

Figure 2-5. Chemical structure of aspirin and acetaminophen, 2 different analgesic drugs with some similar characteristics. The chemical structure determines all aspects of the drug activity.

nonselective in that many drugs with similar chemical characteristics will bind at the same site on albumin. The extent and strength of the binding to albumin depends on the chemical structure of the drug. Usually, the binding forces are weak bonds, and, consequently, protein binding is reversible (ie, the drug binds and then releases from the albumin back and forth). When the drug is not bound to albumin, it is called *unbound drug* or *free drug*; only free drug can bind to the receptor and cause a biological effect. The ratio of free drug to bound drug is a constant for that drug and is determined by the drug's chemical characteristics.

Although bound drug cannot reach the site of action, the extent of protein binding is of little consequence with respect to attaining the therapeutic effect because the protein binding is taken into account when the recommended dosage regimen is established before the drug is marketed. However, protein binding is involved in certain drug interactions and can impact the therapeutic effect in those situations. These drug interactions will be discussed in Chapter 3.

Section Summary

The study of the effects of the body on drugs is pharmacokinetics. The purpose of giving a drug is for the drug to reach the site of action where it can produce the desired response. As the drug enters the blood, the concentration of drug at the site of action becomes high enough to cause a noticeable biological response; the time it takes for this to occur is the onset of action. The action of the drug is diminished as the drug is cleared (removed) by metabolism and excretion processes. The clearance rate will determine how quickly the drug is removed from the blood. As long as the rate of absorption of the drug is faster than the rate of clear-

ance, the blood level will continue to increase. The time it takes for half the drug to be cleared is the half-life of the drug. As the drug is cleared, eventually the concentration at the site of action is not sufficient to cause a noticeable biological effect and the action of the drug is terminated.

The entire dose of a drug will not necessarily reach the general circulation. If the drug is administered orally, the liver may metabolize some of the drug as it first passes to the liver from the GI tract (first-pass effect), and thus a portion of the drug dose never reaches the site of action. The more body fluids and tissues that the drug distributes into (volume of distribution), the lower the concentration of drug that will exist at the site of action. If a portion of the drug molecules bind to plasma proteins (albumin), those molecules are not free to reach the site of action.

IMPACT OF CHEMICAL STRUCTURE

To understand the principles of drug action, it is important to realize that the chemical structure of the drug determines its characteristics. Although acetaminophen and aspirin are both over-the-counter analgesics, they are not the same drug because they have unique chemical structures (Figure 2-5). The chemical structure of the drug is the factor that determines the chemical binding forces between the drug and all of the extracellular and intracellular structures with which it interacts. Consequently, the chemical structure determines the biological effects of a drug, whether good or bad, as well as the absorption, distribution, metabolism, and excretion of the drug (pharmacokinetics).

Small changes in chemical structure can produce significant changes in the biological effects. This is the principal reason there is such an array of drugs in some drug categories. Many drugs have been developed through slight modifications of the prototype drug known to produce significant therapeutic effects. The prototype drug often is a naturally occurring compound produced by plants or microorganisms

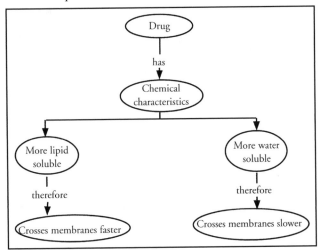

Figure 2-6. Solubility characteristics: water soluble vs lipid soluble.

or is *endogenous* in humans. For example, numerous modifications have been made to the endogenous neurotransmitter epinephrine in an effort to produce drugs that mimic one or more actions of epinephrine. Relatively slight changes in chemical structure can affect not only pharmacokinetic parameters but also therapeutic uses. Modifications of the epinephrine structure have resulted in drugs that are useful as bronchodilators, nasal decongestants, and central nervous system (CNS) stimulants. In a similar manner, a microorganism produces penicillin G, which was the first penicillin for clinical use. It was the prototype for penicillins, and now there are several other drugs available that are modifications of penicillin G. The chemical modifications to penicillin G were made in anticipation of improving its characteristics (eg, to prevent stomach acid from destroying the molecule, to improve effectiveness against various microorganisms, or to increase the duration of action). Other examples of naturally occurring prototypes are morphine as an opiate analgesic, testosterone as an anabolic steroid, and cortisone as a steroidal anti-inflammatory drug.

The chemical structure obviously determines the size and chemical shape of each drug molecule. With the exception of drugs that are polypeptides and proteins (eg, insulin and glucagon), most drugs have a molecular weight of <1000 and are regarded as small compounds. For these small-molecular-weight compounds, size itself does not have a direct bearing on the site of action or ability to penetrate membranes, but for most drugs the solubility of the drug plays the most important role.

Solubility of Drugs

The *solubility* of drugs is important because it affects how quickly a drug is dissolved in the GI tract, how quickly it is absorbed into the bloodstream, the rate and location of distribution throughout the body, the rate of excretion, and the type of liquid dosage form in which it is available.

The two categories of solubility are *water solubility* and *lipid solubility*. Drugs that are water soluble are referred to as *hydrophilic* ("love water"). Drugs that are lipid soluble are referred to as *hydrophobic* ("fear water") or *lipophilic* ("love lipid"). In reality, most drugs have some water solubility characteristics and some lipid solubility characteristics. The more water soluble the drug, the more readily it will dissolve in the GI tract (a necessity for absorption into the blood). However, lipid solubility is also important for absorption because the more lipid soluble the drug, the more readily the drug will cross membranes to move from the GI tract into the blood. Drugs that are more lipid soluble will penetrate the CNS more readily; drugs that are more water soluble will be excreted by the kidney faster. It is evident that a combination of these characteristics, water solubility and lipid solubility, play a significant role in the pharmacokinetic and pharmacodynamic parameters of drugs (Figure 2-6).

Section Summary

Every characteristic of a drug molecule is determined by its chemical structure. The chemical structure will determine the biological activity at the site of action as well as the absorption, distribution, metabolism, and excretion of the medication. An important aspect of the chemical characteristics is the relative degree of water solubility and lipid solubility. Drugs that have a greater degree of water solubility will dissolve more readily in the GI tract; drugs with a greater degree of lipid solubility will cross membranes faster.

DRUGS CROSSING MEMBRANES

Regardless of the chemical structure, every drug must reach the site of action to produce the therapeutic effect. To reach the site of action, drugs must pass through one or more membranes: GI, vascular, cellular, or intracellular. Factors that affect the transport of drugs across membranes will also influence the absorption, distribution, metabolism, and excretion rates of the drugs. Therefore, the ability of a drug to cross membranes has a very important impact on the pharmacokinetics and pharmacodynamics (see Chapter 3) of the drug.

Lipids, primarily phospholipids, and cholesterol are the major constituents of cell membranes. The amount of specific phospholipids and cholesterol varies among the various vascular, cellular, and organelle membranes. Lipids provide the structural integrity of the membrane and affect the ease with which drugs pass through it. Proteins, which are embedded in the sea of lipid, comprise the second-most abundant membrane component. These proteins serve numerous functions such as receptors, transport mechanisms, enzymes, and cell surface recognition sites. Some proteins transverse the entire membrane, whereas others protrude only on one side or the other. Typically, there are multiple copies of each protein within the membrane. Another characteristic of the membrane is that it is a dynamic structure; the proteins are in constant motion within the sea of lipid due to its fluidity. This movement increases the likelihood for drugs and endogenous compounds to contact the proper protein (eg, receptor) so that the appropriate biological action can be initiated.

There are 3 main mechanisms for transport of drugs across membranes: passive diffusion, active transport, and facilitated diffusion. In addition, pores in the membranes allow small polar molecules to penetrate. Ion channels are also present in membranes, and these transport inorganic ions such as calcium. Although their ability to transport ions may be affected by some drugs (eg, calcium channel blockers), ion channels likely have little impact on the transfer of drugs across membranes.

Passive Diffusion

Passive diffusion refers to the drug penetrating through the membrane due to the solubility of the drug in the membrane (Box 2-1). This transport mechanism has the greatest impact on the pharmacokinetics and pharmacodynamics for most drugs. Because membranes are primarily lipids, drugs that are more lipid soluble will diffuse across the membrane quicker than less lipid-soluble drugs. The other driving force for the net transfer of drugs from one side of the membrane to the other is the *concentration gradient* (ie, the difference in concentration of the drug on the 2 sides of the membrane) (Figure 2-7). Molecules in solution are in random motion. Thus, the likelihood of a drug encountering the membrane is directly proportional to the concentration of the drug on that side of the membrane. Drugs that diffuse in one direction can also diffuse in the other direction at a rate dependent upon the concentration of the drug on that side of the membrane. Therefore, the net movement of drug will be in the direction of higher concentration to

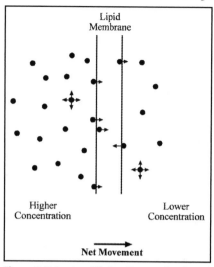

Figure 2-7. Passive diffusion. Drug molecules are in random motion; thus the probability of drug encountering the cellular membrane is based on the concentration of the drug and solubility in the membrane. Net movement of drug will be down the concentration gradient from the side of higher concentration to the side of lower concentration.

lower concentration (see Figure 2-7). When the concentration of drug is equal on both sides, a concentration gradient no longer exists and the rate of diffusion of drug in one direction is equivalent to the rate in the opposite direction.

Active Transport

Active transport mechanisms have a protein with a binding site to which the compound being transported attaches. The transport mechanism facilitates the movement of the compound across the membrane. Active transport mechanisms have the characteristics listed in Box 2-2.

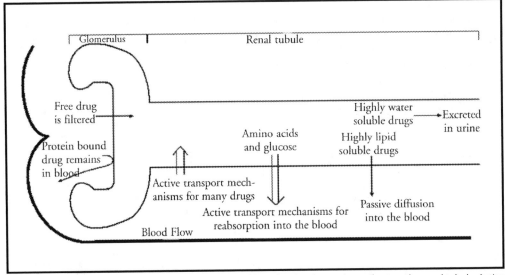

Figure 2-8. Excretion of drugs by the kidney. Free drug is filtered at the glomerulus and enters the renal tubule. Active transport systems (secretion transporters) also facilitate drugs entering the tubule. Reabsorption from the renal tubule into the blood occurs primarily by passive diffusion. Consequently, drugs that are more lipid soluble will be reabsorbed to a greater extent than drugs that are more water soluble.

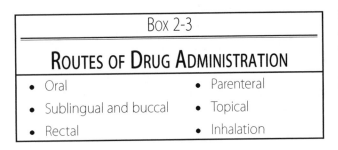

The advantages of the active transport system are selectivity, which will allow only some compounds across the membrane, and the ability to move the compound against a concentration gradient (from a position of lower concentration on one side of the membrane to a higher concentration on the other side of the membrane). Active transport plays an important role for the transport of some drugs into the urine (Figure 2-8) or secretion into the bile.

Facilitated Diffusion

Facilitated diffusion combines the characteristics of passive diffusion and active transport. It requires a carrier protein, and thus selectivity and system saturation are possible, but it does not use energy. Therefore, drugs or other compounds cannot be moved against a concentration gradient by facilitated diffusion, and a high-to-low concentration gradient must be present for net diffusion to occur.

Section Summary

Drugs must cross membranes to reach the site of action. The main mechanisms that allow molecules to cross mem-

branes are passive diffusion, active transport, and facilitated diffusion. Passive diffusion occurs when the drug becomes dissolved in the membrane and passes through to the other side of the membrane. Because membranes are composed primarily of lipid, the concentration of drug and its lipid solubility combine to dictate the rate of passive diffusion. Active transport and facilitated diffusion require a protein carrier on the membrane that has specific binding characteristics for the drug and will then facilitate the movement of the drug across the membrane. In contrast to passive and facilitated diffusion, active transport uses energy for the transport and can move drugs from a side of low concentration to a side of higher concentration. The predominant transport mechanism for drugs is passive diffusion, and, therefore, drugs with a higher degree of lipid solubility will cross membranes faster and drugs with a higher degree of water solubility will cross membranes slower by passive diffusion.

ROUTES OF ADMINISTRATION, DOSAGE FORMS, AND ABSORPTION OF DRUGS

Routes of administration describe the means by which drugs are put in contact with the body for reaching the site of action (Box 2-3). There are advantages and disadvantages to each route. The *dosage form* refers to the physical form in which the drug exists for administration. Oral is a route; tablet is a dosage form. Not all drugs administered by the oral route are tablets, and not all tablets are administered by the oral route. In some cases, the physical or chemical characteristics of the drug dictate the route of administration and may limit the type of dosage form options available. For example, insulin is a protein that is destroyed by digestive enzymes. Because insulin is therefore not effective orally, injectable dosage forms are used. On the other hand, many drugs are available in several dosage forms and selection is based on many factors, including the personal preference of the patient, age (oral liquids are swallowed more readily than solids by infants), cost, and desired speed of onset of action.

Absorption refers to getting the drug into the bloodstream. There is no absorption phase for the intravenous route because the drug is injected directly into the blood. Some factors that affect the rate of absorption by all other routes of administration are lipid solubility of the drug, blood flow to the site of drug administration, and surface area from which the drug can be absorbed. Regardless of the route of administration, drugs must cross membranes for absorption, and drugs that are more lipid soluble will diffuse through membranes faster. When the tissue has a rich capillary blood supply, the distance will be shorter for the drug to travel in the extravascular space before contact with a capillary, and thus absorption rate will be increased. Faster blood flow also carries the drug from the absorption site quicker for distribution to the site of action. Exercise increases blood flow to muscle and skin and increases the absorption of drugs administered by intramuscular and topical routes. Obviously, the greater the tissue surface area with which the drug is in contact, the greater the chance for it to contact the membrane and ultimately reach the site of action.

Oral

The oral route is the most common means of drug administration. The drug is swallowed to obtain a systemic effect, or in some cases, to stay in the GI tract for a local effect. Aspirin can be used orally to obtain the systemic effect of pain relief; laxatives (see Chapter 11) are used orally for a local effect in the GI tract.

There are several reasons why the oral route is the most common route of administration. It is certainly the cheapest and most convenient because technical assistance or instruction is typically not needed for the patient to self-administer the drug. It is also the safest route because no special equipment or devices are needed, and for at least a short time after administration, the drug can be retrieved or the absorption can be inhibited by methods such as gastric lavage or administration of activated charcoal.

There are also several limitations to the oral route. First, not all drugs are effective when given orally. The stomach acid inactivates some drugs, and some drug molecules are physically too large to be absorbed. Proteins such as insulin, erythropoietin, and glucagon are inactivated by intestinal enzymes and are too large to be absorbed from the GI tract. Other drugs, such as aminoglycoside antibiotics, do not

TABLE 2-2	
SUMMARY OF DOSAGE FORMS FOR ORAL ADMINISTRATION	
DOSAGE FORM	**DESCRIPTION**
Tablets	Solid dosage forms, most of which are prepared by compressing the powders into the desired shape and usually combined with "inactive" ingredients
Capsules	Two-piece gelatin containers that are oblong or bullet shaped. The drug and inactive ingredients are placed in one piece of the container and the second piece acts as the cap.
Syrups	Sweetened and flavored aqueous solutions containing one or more drugs and little or no alcohol
Elixirs	Sweetened and flavored solutions of ethanol and water containing one or more drugs
Suspensions	Liquids consisting of a 2-phase system in which a solid is dispersed throughout a liquid.
Emulsions	Liquids usually consisting of small droplets of oil dispersed in water.

penetrate the intestinal cell membranes efficiently and are thus incompletely or erratically absorbed. Patients who are nauseous or unconscious cannot be given oral dosage forms. NSAIDs are examples of drugs noted for their GI irritation and potential for causing GI ulcers. Compared with parenteral routes (intravenous, subcutaneous, intramuscular), it takes longer for drug absorption by the oral route.

Several dosage forms are available for use by the oral route (Table 2-2), and drugs often are available in more than one oral dosage form. For example, ibuprofen is available in tablets, capsules, and chewable tablets; as an oral suspension; and as oral drops.

Tablets are solid dosage forms, most of which are prepared by compressing the powders into the desired shape (Figure 2-9A-C). The drug usually is combined with inactive ingredients that do not have therapeutic activity, but they may affect the effectiveness of the drug by altering the amount of drug absorbed or altering the duration of action. Additives such as lactose or starch may also pose a concern for patients with special dietary restrictions. To some extent, therefore, it is a misnomer to refer to these additives as inactive or inert ingredients. Nonetheless, these additives are

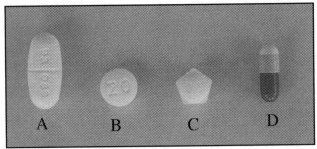

Figure 2-9. Tablets can come in various shapes (A to C); capsules (D) are oblong. Tablets and capsules are the most common solid oral dosage forms.

relatively inert compared with the drug and are essential in the formulation for one or more of the purposes listed in Box 2-4.

Capsules are two-piece gelatin containers that are oblong or bullet shaped (Figure 2-9D). The drug and inactive ingredients are placed in one piece of the container and the second piece acts as the cap. Gelatin is made from chemically processed animal bone and skin to obtain an aqueous soluble, but suitably durable, product. Capsule sizes for human dosage forms range from 000 (the largest), which can hold approximately 600 mg, to 5 (the smallest), which can hold approximately 30 mg. Some patients believe it is easier to swallow capsules rather than tablets and thus prefer capsules. As with tablets, capsules can be manufactured in such a way to give a controlled release of the drug.

Syrups are sweetened and flavored aqueous solutions containing one or more drugs. They contain little or no alcohol and thus are particularly suitable for children, as well as for adults who have difficulty swallowing tablets or capsules. Syrups are effective in masking the taste of water-soluble drugs. Because of the high sugar content, syrups may not be useful for patients who require a calorie-restricted diet, especially if the drug is required for daily, long-term use. Syrups may contain preservatives to prevent growth of microorganisms.

Elixirs are sweetened and flavored solutions of ethanol and water containing one or more drugs. The alcohol is added to dissolve the drug and may contain anywhere from a few percent to more than 70% ethanol. Elixirs are less viscous than syrups and are clear in appearance.

Suspensions are liquids consisting of a 2-phase system in which a solid is dispersed throughout a liquid. When the solid drug cannot be dissolved in water, use of a suspension is an option. Some drugs that are unstable in water are more suitable when formulated for use as a suspension. Additionally, the unpleasant taste of some drugs is diminished when in suspension form. As with other oral liquid dosage forms, suspensions typically have sweetening and flavoring agents added. Viscosity-enhancing agents are added to diminish the rate at which the particles settle to the bottom, but suspensions should be shaken before

use to ensure a more homogenous mixture. Table 2-3 lists some examples of drugs that are available as solutions, suspensions, syrups, and elixirs. Most of these drugs are also available as tablets or capsules.

Emulsions are liquids usually consisting of small droplets of oil dispersed in water. The oil may be the drug or may be used to dissolve a lipid-soluble drug. Dispersing the oil in water masks the unpleasant taste of the oil, and sweetening or flavoring agents may also be added to the aqueous phase. Emulsifying agents have a degree of attraction for the oil as well as for the water and thus are used to keep the droplets of oil evenly dispersed throughout the aqueous phase. Viscosity-enhancing agents may also be added to prevent oil droplets from coalescing. To ensure a homogenous distribution of drug, all emulsions should be shaken before use. Oral emulsions are not used much anymore because suspensions are more efficiently produced and are generally more palatable.

Oral Absorption

The rate and extent to which drugs are absorbed from the GI tract depend on many factors, including rate of solubility, rate that it passes from the stomach into the GI tract, lipid solubility, and stability with other GI contents.

For a drug to be absorbed by the oral route, it must be in solution. The quicker the drug dissolves, the quicker it can be absorbed. Consequently, a drug administered in solution is absorbed faster than if in a solid dosage form. The bioavailability can also be significantly altered by the formulation. Tablets and capsules must break apart for the drug to readily dissolve. The formulation of the product plays an important role in determining how quickly the tablet falls apart and dissolves; 2 products from different manufacturers, but containing the same amount of drug, can differ in bioavailability (see Figure 2-3).

Once the drug is dissolved in the aqueous environment of the GI tract, it must pass through the intestinal

	TABLE 2-3		
EXAMPLES OF DRUGS AVAILABLE AS ORAL LIQUID DOSAGE FORMS			
GENERIC NAME	**TRADE NAME**	**THERAPEUTIC CATEGORY**	**DOSAGE FORM**
cefaclor	Ceclor	antibiotic	suspension
clindamycin	Cleocin	antibiotic	solution
codeine phosphate	generic	analgesic, antitussive	solution
dexamethasone	generic	anti-inflammatory	elixir, solution
dextromethorphan	generic	antitussive	syrup
doxycycline	Vibramycin	antibiotic	suspension
dyphylline	Lufyllin	bronchodilator	elixir
erythromycin	EryPed	antibiotic	suspension
ibuprofen	Children's Advil	NSAID	suspension
loratadine	Claritin	antihistamine	syrup
naproxen	Naprosyn	NSAID	suspension
oxycodone	Roxicodone	analgesic	solution

cell membrane to be absorbed into the blood. The small surface area of the stomach and structure of the stomach membrane prevent effective absorption of drugs. However, the villi and microvilli of the small intestine results in a tremendous surface area compared with the stomach and thus almost all drug absorption occurs from the small intestine. Consequently, drug absorption can be expedited by fast movement of the drug from the stomach to the small intestine (stomach emptying time). Most drugs are absorbed from the GI tract by passive diffusion. Therefore, lipid solubility is a major factor affecting rate and extent of drug absorption. Considering that drugs must be dissolved to be absorbed and that most drug absorption occurs from the small intestine, it is easy to understand why the use of a glass of liquid with oral drug administration is generally recommended. The liquid moves the drug more quickly from the stomach to the small intestine and expedites the rate at which the drug dissolves. On the other hand, because solid food takes longer to move into the small intestine, the administration of a drug with food will generally delay its absorption. Slower absorption can significantly reduce the peak blood concentration because as the rate of absorption becomes similar to the rate of clearance, less drug accumulates in the blood. Gastric emptying time can range from 10 minutes on an empty stomach to hours following a heavy meal. Depending on the amount of food in the stomach, the change in absorption rate can be similar to the change shown for A to that shown for B in Figure 2-3. It is noteworthy that in some instances, the presence of food in the GI tract is an advantage as a protectant from drugs, such as NSAIDs, that have a local irritation effect on the gastric mucosa. Exercise can also affect gastric empty-

ing time; strenuous physical activity can increase gastric emptying time whereas light exercise, compared with no exercise, can decrease gastric emptying time.

Other contents of the stomach and GI tract can also influence absorption. Some drugs are not stable in stomach acid or are degraded by intestinal enzymes. Some foods may also interact with a drug to prevent absorption. For example, calcium ions can bind to the tetracycline antibiotics and prevent the absorption of the tetracycline. Thus, the use of dairy products should be avoided for 1 to 2 hours before and after the oral administration of these antibiotics.

Sometimes the rate of dissolution and absorption is intentionally delayed to give a slower but longer duration of effect. These are often referred to as *sustained-release, prolonged-release,* or *controlled-release* tablets or capsules. These dosage forms contain coatings that increase the time necessary for the tablet to disintegrate or layers of coatings that dissolve at different rates. In these formulations, the dosage form contains a larger amount of drug to compensate for delayed absorption and allow a blood concentration above the minimum effective concentration to be obtained. Some dosage forms contain an enteric coating (Figure 2-10) that does not dissolve in the acidity of the stomach and is intended to delay the release of the drug until it reaches the small intestine. The purpose of the delay is to either protect an acid-sensitive drug from the effects of stomach acid or to protect the gastric mucosa from the irritating effects of the drug. In these situations, delayed dissolution becomes an advantage.

Because absorption rate depends on blood flow to the site of absorption, exercise decreases drug absorption from the GI tract as blood is shunted away from this area to increase supply to the muscles. The extent to which exercise

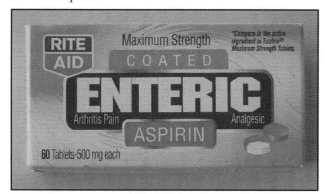

Figure 2-10. Example of packaging indicating enteric coating.

will affect oral drug absorption depends in part on the lipid solubility; drugs that are more lipid soluble are likely to be affected to a greater extent because blood flow is the more limiting factor compared with membrane permeability. In other words, blood flow is the rate-limiting step for oral absorption of drugs that readily cross membranes; therefore, reduced blood flow reduces the absorption rate.

Sublingual and Buccal

Drugs administered *sublingually* or *buccally* are placed under the tongue or against the cheek, respectively. Typically, the dosage form is tablet triturates, which are small tablets usually produced by placing moistened powdered formulation in a mold and allowing it to dry. These tablets are less durable than compressed tablets and thus will dissolve more rapidly when placed under the tongue or against the cheek. A rich supply of blood vessels in these areas facilitates the absorption of the drug into the bloodstream despite the small surface area. Drugs administered by these routes must be relatively potent so that only a small amount of drug needs be absorbed to produce the therapeutic effect. Organic nitrates such as nitroglycerin may be administered by these routes to treat angina pectoris. Nitroglycerin is available in dosages as little as 0.3 mg/tablet and provides a peak response in 3 to 5 minutes. This rapid therapeutic effect is a major advantage of these routes, but the drug must be readily soluble in the mouth if administered in tablet form, yet sufficiently lipid soluble to pass quickly through membranes. In other words, a balance between lipid solubility and water solubility is advantageous. The sublingual and buccal routes also protect the drug from the first-pass effect, which would render sublingual nitroglycerin tablets ineffective if swallowed.

Rectal

The rectal route of drug administration is advantageous in patients who are unconscious, vomiting, or too young to easily swallow oral dosage forms during illness. With this route, the drug is administered as a suppository that is made of a substance such as cocoa butter or polyethylene glycol, which melt at body temperature. The drug dissolves in the rectum and is absorbed into the bloodstream by the hemorrhoidal veins. A disadvantage to this route is that the extent of absorption into the bloodstream is often variable and incomplete. Some drugs in the opiate analgesic and antiemetic categories are available as suppositories for use when either pain or nausea make it difficult for the patient to take these drugs orally.

Parenteral

The primary *parenteral* routes are intravenous, intramuscular, and subcutaneous. Some drugs, such as proteins administered for a systemic effect, are limited to parenteral routes because they are inactivated or poorly absorbed by the GI tract. The parenteral routes produce the most rapid therapeutic response and are advantageous for drug administration to patients who are unable or unwilling to take drugs orally. However, the disadvantages are that more skill is needed to administer drugs by these routes and the dosage forms, syringes, and needles must be handled carefully to prevent contamination.

Intravenous injections require aqueous solutions (ie, no particles visible). Intramuscularly injected dosage forms include aqueous solutions, suspensions, and emulsions. Drugs that are irritating to tissue may cause pain or necrosis at the site of subcutaneous injections but may be suitable as intramuscular injections.

Parenteral Absorption

Because *absorption* refers to entry of the drug into the bloodstream, there is no absorption component associated with intravenous injection. The rate only depends on the time it takes to administer the drug. This is the preferred route for emergency administration of drugs.

Intramuscular injection provides more rapid absorption of drug than the subcutaneous route. In both routes, the drug must cross membranes, and therefore lipid solubility of the drug will affect its rate of absorption. As with the oral route, if the intramuscular drug is not administered in solution form, it must dissolve at the site of injection. Consequently, drugs given as suspensions or emulsions will have a slower onset of action. These dosage forms can also be used for providing a longer duration of action. This type of long-acting injectable medication is referred to as a *depot injection* and can decrease the frequency of medication administration. For example, the antipsychotic medication risperidone is given once or twice daily if taken orally; however, the long-acting injectable product is administered once every 2 weeks.

As mentioned previously, blood flow plays a significant role in determining the rate of absorption. Intramuscular sites generally have better blood flow than subcutaneous sites and thus absorption can be noticeably quicker by the intramuscular route. Exercise increases blood flow to skeletal muscle and skin, which will increase drug absorption from these sites. Vasoconstriction, from use of an ice pack at the injection site for example, will reduce the absorption rate of drugs. This principle is used to an advantage for local anesthetics in which vasoconstrictors are coadministered to delay the anesthetic from being carried from the local site of action; epinephrine added to lidocaine for use in dentistry is an example.

Surface area can play some role in subcutaneous and intramuscular injection. As with other routes of administration, increasing the surface area for the drug to contact tissue will increase the absorption rate. Massaging the site of injection spreads the dose of drug over a larger area to increase the absorption rate. Movement of the muscle after intramuscular injection can accomplish a spreading effect as well as increase blood flow. The site of an intramuscular injection depends on the availability and size of the muscle mass, volume to be injected, degree of discomfort expected from the injection, and patient's preference.

Topical

Drugs administered by topical routes (eg, skin, eyes, nose, throat) are applied to the surface for obtaining either a systemic or a local effect. Drugs applied topically for a localized effect include anti-inflammatory agents, antimicrobial agents, skin moisturizers, sunscreens, and various other drugs for specific dermatological uses. Topically applied drugs for a systemic effect must be relatively potent so that small amounts absorbed through the skin will elicit the therapeutic effect. Drugs used in this fashion are available for estrogen replacement, angina pectoris, hypertension, motion sickness, and analgesia. The rate at which drugs are absorbed depends on the surface area over which they are applied and on their lipid solubility; the more lipid soluble, the more readily the drug will penetrate the epidermis. Using a *lipophilic* vehicle (eg, an ointment) will also increase the rate of absorption for drugs that are not very lipid soluble. The permeability of drugs through the skin is increased if the skin is moist or if the blood flow is increased at the site of application such as near areas of skin that are inflamed, abraded, or burned.

Whether intended for a local or systemic effect, drugs applied to mucous membranes are absorbed readily because there is no epidermal barrier and blood supply is typically rich. Drugs applied to the eye are usually intended for a local effect, although a systemic effect may occur. For example, ophthalmic application of timolol (Timoptic), a drug used for treatment of glaucoma, has caused significant bronchial constriction with difficult breathing for patients who also have asthma.

There are many dosage forms used for topical application. The characteristics of emulsions, suspensions, and solutions have been previously discussed, although sweetening

TABLE 2-4		
EXAMPLES OF DRUGS AVAILABLE BY TRANSDERMAL DELIVERY		
GENERIC NAME	**TRADE NAME**	**PURPOSE**
clonidine	Catapres-TTS	Hypertension
estradiol	Estraderm	Estrogen replacement therapy
nicotine	Nicoderm	Smoking cessation aid
nitroglycerin	Transderm-Nitro	Treatment of angina
scopolamine	Transderm Scop	Motion sickness

and flavoring agents are obviously not needed for topical use. However, other ingredients are added as preservatives, stabilizers, and skin protectants. In addition, lotions, creams, and ointments are common. Lotions and creams are water-washable preparations for external use only; lotions have more of a liquid consistency. Ointments are semisolid preparations for external use only, and although some ointments are water washable, most have an oil base. Ointments also act as excellent emollients (ie, moisturizers that soften skin by increasing moisture content).

When drugs are applied to the skin for a systemic effect, it is referred to as *transdermal delivery*. Ointments and creams for this purpose are somewhat messy, and it is difficult to determine the amount of drug that will be delivered to the bloodstream. Transdermal patches use various thin layers of adhesives, polymer matrices, membranes, and drug reservoirs to control the rate of drug released for contact with the skin. Examples of drugs available by transdermal delivery are listed in Table 2-4.

Inhalation

The inhalation route is actually a topical route of administration because the drug is being applied to the surface of the membrane, but it is also considered separately because of the unique characteristics and specialized delivery mechanisms. Except for gases as general anesthetics, drugs are generally not administered by inhalation for the purpose of obtaining a systemic effect because the amount of drug delivered to the lungs by inhalation and the amount absorbed into the bloodstream are too variable.

Inhalation is the route of choice for the administration of some drugs used to treat asthma. The inhalation dosage forms most frequently used are aerosols and dry powders, which are administered using metered-dose inhalers and dry powder inhalers. Good inhalation technique is required to optimize the delivery of the drug to the lung. The use of metered-dose inhalers and dry powder inhalers, along with other treatments for asthma, will be discussed more thoroughly in Chapter 9.

The rich blood supply to the lungs, permeability of the membranes, and large surface area provide for rapid absorption of drugs by inhalation. For some drugs, the onset of action is less than 5 minutes. The challenge with self-administered inhalation therapy, such as the routine treatment of asthma, is to get an adequate and consistent dose into the lungs.

Section Summary

Absorption is the process of the drug moving into the bloodstream, route of administration is the entry mechanism used to get the drug into the blood, and dosage form is the physical form of the drug used for administration. The oral route is the most common method of administering drugs, and thus many solid and liquid dosage forms (eg, tablets, capsules, syrups, suspensions) are available for oral use. Parenteral routes (eg, intravenous, intramuscular, subcutaneous) can produce a more rapid response, but they also require more skill to inject the drug. In some cases, the condition of the patient or the type of drug used will necessitate a parenteral route. Drugs administered by sublingual, buccal, and inhalation routes are absorbed quickly because of the rich blood supply at these sites. In contrast, absorption of drug from the surface of the skin for a systemic effect (transdermal) is relatively slow because the drug must penetrate the epidermis. Nonetheless, transdermal patches are a convenient means of providing slow but continuous delivery of potent drugs.

Absorption by the oral route occurs primarily from the small intestine. The drug must be dissolved in the aqueous GI tract and then penetrate the GI membrane to enter the blood. A balance between water solubility and lipid solubility facilitates absorption, but drugs have varying degrees of these characteristics, and thus the rate of absorption varies among drugs. Food in the stomach will decrease the absorption rate because it takes longer for the drug to move into the small intestine. Strenuous physical exercise will also delay stomach emptying whereas light exercise will stimulate it.

DISTRIBUTION

Distribution refers to the movement of the drug throughout the body to the various compartments. Aside from blood, these compartments include the CNS, cells (eg, muscle, adipose, liver, kidney), excretory fluids (eg, urine, bile, sweat), and plasma proteins (primarily albumin). The site of action is a component of one or more of these compartments. Drugs generally do not distribute evenly throughout these compartments. The specific compartments that a drug distributes into, and the extent to which it distributes, depend on the following:

- The chemical structure of the drug
- Blood flow to the tissue
- Structure of the capillaries feeding the tissue

Once a molecule is in the blood, regardless of its lipid or water solubility, it will eventually penetrate the endothelial cell of the capillaries because of their huge surface area and because, except for the CNS, the capillaries that feed tissues have some spaces between epithelial cells. Molecular size is a major hindrance for larger water-soluble molecules such as polypeptides, but they will eventually penetrate slowly, possibly between endothelial cells or by other mechanisms.

Blood flow to tissue will significantly affect drug distribution. Some tissues, such as the liver, kidney, and brain, have greater blood flow than fat or bone. Consequently, distribution will be faster to the sites with greater blood flow. Treating solid tumors or infections of the bone poses some therapeutic challenges because the blood flow to these sites is low. To obtain sufficient drug distribution at these sites of action, higher doses of drug, administration for longer periods, or injection directly into the tissue site is sometimes necessary.

Capillary structure varies among tissues and will affect drug distribution. For example, highly water-soluble drugs do not readily penetrate the CNS capillaries unless there is a specific transport process for them. The structural components around the CNS capillaries provide an additional barrier, and there are no spaces between the endothelial cells of the CNS capillaries. Therefore, in the CNS, passive diffusion is the major mechanism by which drugs cross the membrane; the more lipid-soluble drugs will cross the membrane more readily. In addition, there are transport mechanisms that remove some drugs that gain entry into the CNS. The *blood-brain barrier* is the term used to describe these attributes of the CNS. If the site of action is not the CNS, access to the CNS is a disadvantage because additional adverse effects are likely. Consider, for example, all the over-the-counter cold remedies that have drowsiness as an adverse effect. On the other hand, distribution into the CNS is desirable for sedatives and opiate analgesics because the site of action is within the CNS.

The placental barrier is somewhat similar to the blood-brain barrier in that there are mechanisms that restrict the entry of drugs from the mother to the developing baby. As with the blood-brain barrier, drugs that are more lipid soluble, such as alcohol, more readily diffuse into the baby's blood. However, the placental barrier is not as exclusionary as the blood-brain barrier, and thus most drugs will have at least some degree of entry into the unborn baby.

The chemical structure of the drug will determine the lipid solubility and chemical-binding characteristics. Lipid-soluble drugs will tend to distribute more readily into the CNS and into fat cells. The chemical-binding characteristics will determine to which receptors on which cells the drug will bind, and, as discussed earlier, the extent of plasma protein binding.

Section Summary

Drug distribution is the movement of drug into body fluids, tissues, and attachment to albumin; the greater the distribution into these sites, the lower the concentration available to reach the site of action. The degree of lipid solubility will determine the degree of distribution into the CNS and into fat tissue. The blood-brain barrier is a term used to describe the unique membrane structure of the capillaries of the CNS that primarily restricts entry to lipid-soluble drugs.

METABOLISM

Drug metabolism, also known as *biotransformation*, refers to the chemical alteration of the drug by one or more enzymes in the body (Figure 2-11). The liver is the primary site of this biotransformation, but the kidney and intestinal cells also have a significant level of drug metabolism, and to a lesser extent, so do the lungs and brain. The drug reacting with the metabolizing enzyme is called the parent drug or substrate; the products of the reactions are called metabolites.

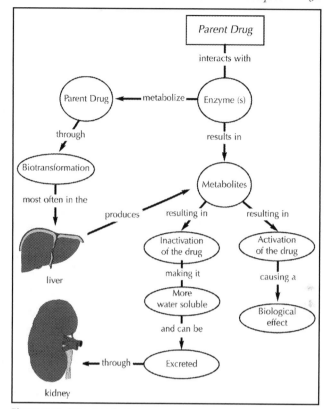

Figure 2-11. Drug metabolism.

$$\text{Parent Drug} \xrightarrow{\text{Enzyme}} \text{Metabolite(s)}$$
$$\text{(substrate)} \qquad\qquad \text{(product)}$$

It is common for a drug to be converted to more than one metabolite. Drug metabolism usually makes the drug inactive and more water soluble, which is important in preparation of the drug for excretion because the urine is aqueous and is the primary route for excretion. Drug metabolism and excretion provide the 2 mechanisms by which the actions of drugs are terminated.

A multitude of drug-metabolizing enzymes have been identified. Although most drug metabolism results in loss of biological activity, other scenarios also occur (Figure 2-12). Sometimes the biological activity of the metabolite is more, somewhat less than, or the same as the parent drug. For example, about 10% of codeine is metabolized to the more potent morphine, aspirin is quickly metabolized to the equipotent salicylic acid, and the major metabolite of diazepam (Valium) is less active than the parent compound. In some cases, such as diazepam, the active metabolite has a longer t½ than the parent drug and thus the observed duration of action is longer although potency is less. Sometimes the drug administered is in an inactive form, referred to as a *prodrug*, and the metabolizing enzymes convert the drug to the active drug. A prodrug is used when it provides an

advantage over the active drug, such as better oral absorption or diminished GI irritation.

Cytochrome P450 enzymes (CYP or P450) comprise a large group of enzymes that metabolize many drugs. The CYP group of enzymes is divided into families, subfamilies, and individual isoenzymes that are designated by a series of numbers and letters. Some drugs are metabolized by more than one CYP enzyme. Aside from being metabolized by P450 enzymes, some drugs either increase (induce) or decrease (inhibit) the activity of these enzymes. The concept of inhibiting and inducing enzymes is discussed further in the next chapter regarding drug interactions.

The effect of exercise on the rate of drug metabolism is complex, and research has not provided a set of useful general principles. During exercise, the blood flow to the liver is reduced, and therefore it would seem that the liver metabolism rate should also decrease. However, exercise increases the metabolism for some drugs that are highly protein bound, presumably because the liver becomes more efficient at extracting protein-bound drug as blood flow decreases. Sporadic vs routine exercise may also affect the metabolism rate differently; routine exercise seems to increase liver metabolism efficiency for some drugs. Some enzymes are induced whereas others are inhibited by exercise. The therapeutic significance of these effects on specific drugs has not been established.

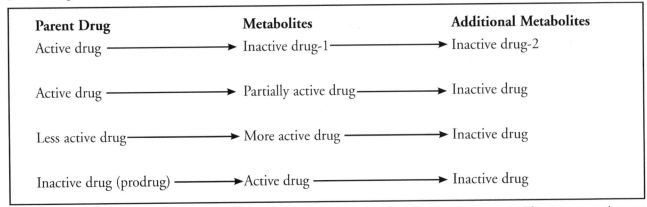

Parent Drug	**Metabolites**	**Additional Metabolites**
Active drug	⟶ Inactive drug-1	⟶ Inactive drug-2
Active drug	⟶ Partially active drug	⟶ Inactive drug
Less active drug	⟶ More active drug	⟶ Inactive drug
Inactive drug (prodrug)	⟶ Active drug	⟶ Inactive drug

Figure 2-12. Metabolism schemes. The parent drug can be converted to a metabolite by metabolizing enzymes. Oftentimes, more than one metabolizing enzyme will react with the drug to produce additional metabolites. The metabolites of some drugs may have therapeutic activity that is less than or more than the activity of the parent drug. Sometimes the form of the drug administered is inactive (also called a prodrug) to gain an advantage, such as enhanced absorption. An enzyme converts the prodrug to the active form, which is eventually inactivated.

Section Summary

The parent drug is the drug administered to the patient; the metabolite is the product after a metabolism reaction. Most drug metabolism occurs in the liver. Metabolism usually inactivates the drug and prepares it for excretion by the kidney by making the drug more water soluble. In some cases, however, drug metabolism produces a metabolite that also has biological activity. The CYP450 enzymes are a group of enzymes that metabolize many drugs. The activity of some of these enzymes is increased (induced) or decreased (inhibited) by other drugs and thus can be the cause of some drug interactions.

EXCRETION

Excretion of drugs is simply removal of the drug from the body. Water-soluble compounds are more readily excreted than lipid compounds; therefore, at least a portion of each dose of many drugs undergoes one or more metabolic reactions to make it more water soluble. The kidney is the most important organ for excretion of drugs, although the bile is also a significant route. Excretion of drugs by sweat, saliva, and lungs occurs for many drugs, but the quantity excreted through these routes is insignificant when exercise is not a factor. During exercise, there is an increased blood flow to the lungs and skin, but sufficient data are not available regarding the excretion of drugs to conclude any practical significance. Therefore, excretion of drugs by sweat, saliva, and lungs is not discussed further.

Renal Excretion

The kidneys contain more than 2 million nephrons, each containing various components, including a glomerulus and a renal tubule. The renal excretion rate of a drug depends on the net effect of glomerular filtration rate, tubular secretion, and tubular reabsorption. The rate of these mechanisms is dependent on rate of blood flow to the kidneys, concentration of drug in the blood, pH of the urine, and presence of other compounds that are actively transported by the same mechanism.

As shown in Figure 2-8, protein-bound substances remain in the blood and are not allowed to enter the renal tubule; free drug will enter as glomerular filtrate. The renal tubule provides additional mechanisms for compounds to enter from the blood (see Figure 2-8); these are active transport mechanisms, and the process is called *tubular secretion*. Because these mechanisms use protein carriers, the rate of tubular secretion depends on the blood concentration of the drug but the carriers can be saturated. Sometimes drugs that use the same transport mechanism will compete for the limited transport proteins, resulting in an altered rate of drug excretion. The classic illustration of this is penicillin G and probenecid. Penicillin G is rapidly secreted into the renal tubule by a secretion transporter. As a means to decrease the excretion rate of penicillin G, probenecid was developed, which competes for the same transporter and thus inhibits the renal tubular secretion of penicillin G so that it has a longer duration of action.

Although glomerular filtration excludes protein-bound drugs, the extent of protein binding does not significantly affect the rate of excretion of drugs. Because the drug is reversibly bound to plasma protein, as some of the free drug enters the renal tubule by filtration or by tubular secretion, some bound drug will release from the plasma protein to become free drug to quickly maintain the constant percentage of bound drug.

As the fluid passes through the various segments of the renal tubule, compounds can be reabsorbed back into the bloodstream. Active transport mechanisms exist for highly water-soluble endogenous compounds such as glucose and amino acids, although passive diffusion is the major mechanism for the reabsorption of drugs. The urinary pH can fluctuate from 5 to 8 as a result of diet, exercise, and presence of drugs and thus can affect the rate of excretion of some drugs. The excretion rate of salicylic acid, a metabolite of aspirin, is increased several-fold if the urine pH is 8 vs 6.

Exercise can decrease blood flow to the kidney and could decrease the renal clearance rate of all drugs excreted by this route. However, urinary pH can also decrease during exercise, which will alter the reabsorption of some drugs. Decreased urine output can increase the tubular concentration, leading to faster reabsorption by passive diffusion. Other factors that could affect excretion rate but have not been thoroughly studied are the intensity of exercise, hydration status of the patient, and extent of excretion from sweat. The impact of exercise also varies depending on the extent of drug metabolism vs kidney excretion as a means to terminate the drug activity. For example, if exercise increases liver metabolism for a drug but clearance of that drug is primarily by urinary excretion, then the net effect of exercise may be to decrease the clearance rate.

Biliary Excretion

Some drugs pass from the liver into the bile and are eventually secreted into the small intestine. These may be either lipid-soluble or water-soluble metabolites. If the drug enters the small intestine, it may be excreted in the feces or reabsorbed into the blood. Once the drug is reabsorbed, it may be excreted by the kidney or resecreted by the liver and reabsorbed from the intestine again. The reabsorption-secretion process is referred to as *enterohepatic recycling* and can extend the duration of the therapeutic effect of some drugs.

Section Summary

The kidney is the major site of drug excretion, although some drugs are also excreted in the bile. Drugs enter the renal tubule of the kidney through filtration at the glomerulus or through an active transport mechanism that secretes the drug into the renal tubule. The more lipid soluble the drug, the more likely it will be reabsorbed back into the blood from the renal tubule.

EFFECTS OF EXERCISE

The effect of exercise on absorption, distribution, metabolism, and excretion is quite complex. No doubt this is a prime reason that relatively little has been studied regarding this subject. Some studies present conflicting data or results that are of uncertain practical application. Because exercise affects so many functions, such as blood flow, respiration, fluid volume, and pH, more than one pharmacokinetic parameter may be altered at the same time.

During exercise, blood flow shifts to the muscles and skin and away from the visceral area, kidney, and liver. Blood flow can affect each of the pharmacokinetic parameters, but these have not been studied in a large number of drugs. Consequently, the effects of exercise could include more than one of the general actions listed in Box 2-5, depending on the drug, type of exercise, and intensity and duration of the exercise.

The bottom line for the athletic trainer is to be aware that, in some situations for some drugs in some patients, exercise could have a significant effect on the pharmacokinetic parameters. With currently available data, it is difficult to predict the occurrence of an exercise-induced problem (or advantage). However, the potential for a significant impact should not be discounted because the diminished clearance of a relatively toxic drug due to exercise could elicit some adverse or toxic effects.

CASE STUDY 1

After learning about pharmacokinetics, Rita realizes how complex the interactions between the body and medications are. Today, an athlete expressed concern to Rita about the frequency of one of his medications. He was recently prescribed the antibiotic amoxicillin for an upper respiratory tract infection. The antibiotic needs to be taken 3 times per day, and the athlete is having trouble remembering to take it. He asks Rita why the antibiotic has to be taken multiple times per day. Use a medication reference to review the pharmacokinetics of amoxicillin. Based on the pharmacokinetic parameters, what factor would be most involved in the frequency of dosing?

CASE STUDY 2

One of the athletes Rita works with has recently been diagnosed with diabetes mellitus. The athlete will be using insulin to control his blood sugar and will be injecting the insulin subcutaneously in the thigh. Rita is concerned about the effects that exercise will have on the activity of the insulin and the patient's blood sugar. Based on pharmacokinetic principles, what possible effect could exercise have on the insulin?

Box 2-5

POTENTIAL EFFECTS OF EXERCISE ON DRUG PHARMACOKINETICS

- Light exercise will decrease stomach emptying time, and strenuous exercise will increase stomach emptying time.

- Oral absorption of drugs is diminished by exercise due to decreased blood flow to the GI tract.

- Absorption from skin and skeletal muscle is increased by exercise due to increased blood flow to these areas.

- Exercise increases the duration of action by drugs cleared primarily by the kidney because of diminished clearance by this route. However, this may be modified for drugs that are acids and bases because renal tubular reabsorption of acids may increase and bases may decrease as urinary pH decreases during exercise. Duration and intensity of exercise may determine the extent to which kidney clearance of drugs is affected.

- Exercise results in diminished blood flow to the liver and thus increased duration of action by drugs that are inactivated by the liver. However, this is modified for drugs that are highly protein bound (eg, NSAIDs) because there is a longer time for the drug to separate from the protein-bound state and then be inactivated by the liver. Routine exercise may have the opposite effect by increasing the metabolic efficiency and activity of liver enzymes.

- Because fluid is lost during exercise, the volume of distribution should diminish, increasing the concentration of drug reaching the site of action. However, some drugs are excreted through sweat but the impact on overall excretion is relatively unknown.

- Drugs that have a significant first-pass effect may have enhanced blood concentrations when the exercise and oral administration are close together.

- A long-term exercise program may alter liver enzymes, hormone levels, and protein binding of some drugs, which can affect metabolism and excretion rates.

- The impact of exercise on pharmacokinetic parameters is more likely to be significant during intensive exercise of long duration, on therapeutic response occurring from drugs that have a shorter $t\frac{1}{2}$, from drugs that have an effective dose similar to the toxic dose, and with drugs for which a continuous therapeutic effect is most critical.

BIBLIOGRAPHY

Lenz TL. Pharmacokinetic drug interactions with physical activity. *Am J Lifestyle Med.* 2010;4:226-229.

Pandit NK. *Introduction to the Pharmaceutical Sciences.* 2nd ed. Philadelphia: Wolters Kluwer; 2012.

Ritschel WA, Kearns GL. *Handbook of Basic Pharmacokinetics Including Clinical Applications.* 7th ed. Washington, DC: American Pharmacists Association; 2009.

Shargel L, Wu-Pong S, Yu ABC. *Applied Biopharmaceutics and Pharmacokinetics.* 6th ed. New York, NY: McGraw-Hill; 2012.

CHAPTER 3: ADVANCE ORGANIZER

Foundational Concepts

- Additive Effect
- Synergistic Effect
- Antagonistic Effect
- Placebo Effect
- Tolerance
- Section Summary

Receptor Theory of Drug Action

- Section Summary

Dose-Response Relationships

- Single Dose
- Multiple Doses and Steady State
- Maintenance Dose and Loading Dose
- Section Summary

Therapeutic Considerations

- Patient Adherence
- Dose Calculations
- Therapeutic Drug Monitoring
- Age
- Liver and Kidney Function
- Section Summary

Drug Interactions

- Section Summary

Adverse Drug Reactions

- Section Summary

Pharmacogenetics

Medication Errors

Impact of Exercise

3

Pharmacodynamic Principles

Mechanism of Drug Action and Therapeutic Considerations

CHAPTER OBJECTIVES

At the end of this chapter, the reader will be able to:

- Explain the concept of pharmacodynamics and how it is applied to explaining the biological effects of drugs

- Differentiate between pharmacokinetics, pharmacodynamics, and therapeutics

- Explain the 2 major ways by which pharmacological tolerance occurs

- Summarize the receptor theory of drug action

- Explain the dose-response principle and how it is related to achieving a maximum dose response

- Explain the concept of potency and how it relates to producing a biological effect

- Explain how the relative safety of a drug is determined

- Explain how multiple doses of a drug reach a steady state of blood concentration to produce a biological effect

- Differentiate between a maintenance dose and a loading dose of a drug

- List variables that affect patient adherence with drug therapy and ways to improve adherence with the drug regimen

- Summarize the concept of therapeutic drug monitoring

- Explain why individuals respond differently to a drug regimen

- Describe how liver and kidney function can be used to determine appropriate drug dosage

- Define a drug interaction

- List and describe 7 mechanisms by which a drug interaction can occur

- Define an adverse drug reaction

- List and describe 8 categories of adverse drug reactions

- Identify several ways medication errors can occur and how they may be prevented

- Explain the potential impact that exercise has on pharmacodynamics

Houglum JE, Harrelson GL, Seefeldt TM.
Principles of Pharmacology for Athletic Trainers, Third Edition (pp 37-59).
© 2016 Taylor & Francis Group.

Box 3-1		
AREAS OF STUDY		
	DEFINITION	**FOCUS**
Pharmacokinetics	The study of the impact of the body on drugs	The rate and extent to which drugs are absorbed into the bloodstream, distributed throughout the body, metabolized, and finally excreted
Pharmacodynamics	The study of the impact of drugs on the body	The molecular mechanism by which drugs exert their therapeutic and adverse effects
Therapeutics	The study of the parameters that determine the most appropriate therapy for a patient	The parameters necessary to individualize treatment for the specific patient, including all of the patient's diseases, all of the drugs the patient may be using, the dosage regimen of each drug, and the impact of potential adverse effects

ABBREVIATIONS USED IN THIS CHAPTER

ADR. adverse drug reaction	**GI.** gastrointestinal
cAMP. cyclic adenosine monophosphate	**LD.** lethal dose
	NSAID. nonsteroidal anti-inflammatory drug
CNS. central nervous system	**OTC.** over-the-counter
DNA. deoxyribonucleic acid	**RNA.** ribonucleic acid
	TD. toxic dose
ED. effective dose	**TI.** therapeutic index

Pharmacodynamics is the study of the effect of drugs on the body. The primary focus of pharmacodynamics is on the molecular mechanism by which drugs exert their therapeutic and adverse effects. The molecular mechanism encompasses biochemical mechanisms and physiological responses. As the dose changes, the degree and type of response may also change as the drug occupies more receptors in a particular tissue and additional receptors in other tissues. Consequently, the dosage regimen required to optimize therapeutic effects and minimize adverse effects can be determined, at least in part, by the molecular mechanism of action. Stated another way, pharmacodynamics centers primarily on the mechanism of drug action.

Therapeutics is the study of the parameters that determine the most appropriate therapy for a patient. It considers the parameters necessary to individualize treatment for the specific patient, including all of the patient's diseases, all of the drugs the patient may be using, the dosage regimen of each drug, and the impact of potential adverse effects. Therefore, knowledge of the pharmacodynamic and pharmacokinetic principles is a necessary component of therapeutics (ie, to determine the most appropriate therapy

for the patient). The lines separating pharmacokinetics, pharmacodynamics, and therapeutics are not always clear (Box 3-1). For example, the dose-response effect of a drug occurs because of the absorption, distribution, metabolism, and excretion characteristics of the drug, but the specific dose-response effects are also a result of the mechanism of action, all of which will determine the therapeutic use of the drug.

In this chapter, we will discuss the theoretical basis for the mechanism of drug action, the dose-response relationship, the mechanisms for common adverse effects, and therapeutic considerations that may affect the treatment regimen for some patients.

FOUNDATIONAL CONCEPTS

Some of the foundational concepts discussed in the previous chapter will be used in this chapter; others are unique to pharmacodynamics and therapeutics. It is important to see the relationship among some of these principles to truly understand the significance of the concept. For example, it shows that protein binding discussed in Chapter 2 has an effect on the amount of drug reaching the receptor or that the response from a drug may be altered due to the effect of other drugs on liver-metabolizing enzymes.

Additive Effect

The term *additive effect* is self-explanatory: the response obtained from 2 or more drugs is equal to the sum of the responses obtained when the drugs are used individually. The therapeutic responses being measured are usually the same response (eg, pain relief or skeletal muscle relaxation). For example, the concurrent use of ibuprofen (Motrin) and naproxen (Naprosyn), 2 nonsteroidal anti-inflammatory drugs (NSAIDs), provides additive analgesic effect but no redeeming therapeutic benefit and thus is generally discouraged (see Chapter 6). As in this example, concurrent use of 2 or more drugs should be avoided if no therapeutic advantage is obtained. However, sometimes there is an advantage of using a combination of drugs that give additive effects, such as reducing the adverse effects of a drug by using a lower dose but yet obtaining the same net therapeutic effect with the addition of the second drug. For example, if a moderate dose of inhaled corticosteroid as long-term therapy does not adequately control asthma, the addition of another long-term drug (noncorticosteroid) is recommended as an alternative to increasing the corticosteroid dose, thereby decreasing the potential of adverse effects from a higher dose of corticosteroid yet controlling the asthma (see Chapter 9).

Synergistic Effect

When drugs exhibit a *synergistic effect,* it means that the use of 2 drugs together produces a response greater than what would be expected by adding the response observed from using each drug alone. To put it mathematically, if drugs A and B each produce X amount of response when used alone, but used together they produce $> 2\times$ response, they are synergistic. An example is the use of probenecid along with penicillin G, as discussed in Chapter 2. Probenecid alone does not have antibacterial activity, but it inhibits the renal tubular secretion of penicillin G and thus significantly increases the duration of action of penicillin G. Another example is the synergistic effect of any NSAID added to codeine for pain relief (see Chapter 7).

Antagonistic Effect

When the use of a second drug reduces the effect of another drug, the second drug has an *antagonistic effect* to the first. If one drug binds to a certain receptor as an agonist, it will initiate a certain response. If a second drug binds to the same receptor, thus preventing the agonist response, the second drug is an antagonist, also known as a *competitive antagonist, receptor antagonist,* or *blocker.* An antagonistic effect may be due to a receptor antagonist or to an unrelated mechanism (ie, the antagonist does not bind to the agonist's receptor). For example, the use of an antacid with a tetracycline antibiotic will have an antagonistic effect on the tetracycline by binding the tetracycline and preventing it from being absorbed. Drugs that have an antagonistic effect can sometimes be an advantage if it is desirable to reverse the effect of a drug. Naloxone (Narcan), for example, is an opioid receptor antagonist that is used to reverse the potentially fatal respiratory depression effects from an overdose of opioids such as heroin or morphine. Many over-the-counter (OTC) cold preparations combine a nasal decongestant with an antihistamine to gain an additive therapeutic effect (ie, improved air flow), but the decongestant also causes some central nervous system (CNS) stimulation, which has an antagonistic effect on the drowsiness side effect from the antihistamine.

Placebo Effect

It is important to differentiate between a placebo and a placebo effect. A *placebo effect* is either a therapeutic or adverse response that cannot be attributed to the pharmacological effect of the drug. A *placebo* is a dosage form that contains no active ingredient; capsules filled with lactose is an example. The most common, but not exclusive, source of the placebo effect occurs when treating symptoms associated with subjective responses. A variety of other symptoms have been shown to respond to placebo in as much as 35% of the population. These responses from placebo include relief of fever, headache, anxiety, nausea, and pain from many sources, including angina and ulcers. The placebo effect is not imaginary. It may be due in part to the release of hormones or neurotransmitters, not because of pharmacological activity of any drug, but due to the patient anticipating a response from what he or she believes is the drug. The use of a placebo is uncommon except in research and clinical drug studies, which use a placebo group of subjects to determine therapeutic efficacy of a drug.

Although the use of a placebo is rare for therapy, the placebo effect is a common phenomenon and can be used as a therapeutic advantage. Because the expectations of the patient can contribute to the placebo effect, this portion of the response can be fostered by the attending healthcare professional if he or she provides encouragement and an optimistic outlook regarding expected therapeutic outcomes. If a patient is convinced that pain relief is imminent upon administration of an analgesic, a placebo effect may bring greater or quicker relief than what would be expected from the drug alone.

Tolerance

Tolerance is the diminished response to a drug because of continued use. In other words, to get the same effect from the drug as previously obtained, the dose of the drug must be increased. Not all drugs produce tolerance. However, for those drugs known to produce tolerance, the effectiveness of the drug should be monitored so that the dose can be adjusted appropriately. Tolerance is especially prevalent among the opioid analgesics, CNS stimulants, benzodiazepines, barbiturates, and ethanol.

The benzodiazepines are a group of CNS-depressant drugs with muscle relaxant and anti-anxiety effects (see Chapter 13). Examples include diazepam (Valium) and clorazepate (Tranxene). Barbiturates are another group of CNS depressants with several uses including inducing sedation or sleep. Examples include phenobarbital (Luminal) and secobarbital (Seconal).

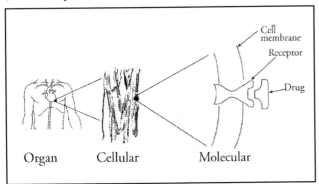

Organ   Cellular   Molecular

Figure 3-1. Site of action. The site of action is in specific tissues at the cellular and molecular levels, often at a receptor on the cell membrane to which the drug chemically fits.

When tolerance develops to one drug in a pharmacological category (eg, CNS depressants or CNS stimulants), there is usually cross-tolerance to other drugs within that category. If tolerance to morphine develops, there will be a degree of tolerance to the other morphine-like drugs such as codeine and meperidine (Demerol). Tolerance is a relatively slow process, taking at least days to weeks to develop depending on the drug. Rate of tolerance can also vary for different effects from the same drug. For example, tolerance to the appetite-suppressant effects of cocaine and amphetamines develops more quickly than tolerance to the euphoric effects.

There are 2 major mechanisms that cause pharmacological tolerance: liver enzyme induction and receptor effects. Using alcohol as an example, chronic alcohol use causes the liver to produce more molecules of drug-metabolizing enzymes (see Chapter 2). Because there are more molecules of enzymes, the rate of drug metabolism (alcohol in this case) by these enzymes will be increased. This results in a decreased level of drug in the blood. Consequently, the chronic alcohol user gradually requires more drinks to reach the same level of intoxication. As discussed later in this chapter, drugs that induce liver enzymes also have the potential to cause drug interactions by affecting the metabolism rate of other drugs.

Another mechanism for tolerance is a change in either the number of receptors or the affinity of the receptors for the drug. (As discussed later in this chapter, the *affinity* is the strength of the chemical bonding interaction between the drug and the receptor.) In this situation, the blood level of the drug is not being reduced, but rather the responsiveness at the receptor. Examples are opioid analgesics, CNS stimulants, and benzodiazepines. Because drugs of the same drug category typically bind to the same receptor, it is easy to see why a cross-tolerance is common within a category. In addition, if different effects from a drug are caused from the drug binding to different types of receptors, it is not surprising that the tolerance develops more rapidly to one effect than another. Tolerance to the pain relief from morphine is more rapid than to the constipation side effect. Barbiturates are a group of CNS depressants to which tolerance develops due to

both mechanisms: enzyme induction and changes in receptor activity. Regardless of mechanism, pharmacologic tolerance is reversible in that it eventually disappears after the drug is discontinued. In addition to the pharmacologically based tolerance discussed in this section, there is also learned tolerance, in which the person learns from experience to change his or her behavior while under the influence as a means to compensate for the CNS effects (eg, making a conscious effort to walk in such a way so as not to appear to be intoxicated).

Section Summary

Pharmacodynamics is a study of the impact that drugs have on the cells of the body, with a focus on the mechanism by which all the effects occur. Sometimes the magnitude of the observed effects is modified by the presence of other drugs. If the presence of more than one drug leads to a reduced total response, the drugs are antagonistic; if the total combined response is what would be expected by adding the individual responses, the drugs are additive; if the total is more than would be expected from adding the individual responses, the drugs are synergistic. If a drug is given that has no active ingredient, the drug is called a placebo, and any perceived response by the patient is called a placebo effect. If the response of a drug diminishes after continued use, the reduced response is a result of tolerance. Drugs that are CNS stimulants and depressants are particularly known for the tolerance they produce. Cross-tolerance occurs among drugs in the same drug category, so that if tolerance exists to morphine, it will also exist with codeine.

RECEPTOR THEORY OF DRUG ACTION

In a broad sense, any macromolecule to which a drug binds and initiates a biological response can be called a *receptor*. This would include enzymes, DNA, RNA, transport proteins, as well as receptors on membranes that bind endogenous hormones and neurotransmitters. Almost all drugs act by binding with these macromolecules. There are some exceptions, such as antacids, which directly neutralize stomach acid. In any case, the principle is that most drugs interact with some component of the cell, and this interaction causes a biochemical change. The point of interaction with the receptor is also called the *site of action* (see Chapter 2) for the drug (Figure 3-1).

When discussing receptors, it is most useful to focus on the receptors located on the surface of membranes because they are the most important type of receptor for a wide range of drugs. An understanding of the mechanism of drug action at these receptors also helps to understand other concepts. These cell surface receptors are the binding sites of many endogenous hormones and neurotransmitters. In fact, as shown in Figure 3-2, a drug that binds to a receptor is merely mimicking (agonist) or blocking (antagonist) the effect of endogenous compounds. The receptor only exists so that a biological response can be regulated through the binding of an endogenous compound.

Every cell has many different types of receptors embedded within the membrane, and there are multiple copies of each receptor that the cell produces. One means by which the cell self-regulates the amount of chemical signal that it receives through the receptors is to increase or decrease the number of receptors it makes. For example, a diminished concentration of cholesterol in the blood will cause an increased synthesis of low-density lipoprotein receptors on the surface of the cell so that more cholesterol will bind to the receptor and be taken into the cell. A constant exposure of cells to morphine-like drugs will cause cells to decrease the production of morphine receptors and, as previously discussed, will cause tolerance to the morphine. Therefore, the number of receptors on the cell's surface is in flux.

Cells contain the specific receptors that are responsible for regulating the metabolic functions of that cell. In other words, every cell does not contain every type of receptor. From a pharmacological standpoint, this cellular selectivity of receptors limits the adverse effects from drugs because the effects of each drug are limited to the cells that have the type of receptor for that particular drug (eg, if Drug A only binds to receptor type A, Drug A will only have an effect on cells that have receptor A). There are various classes of receptors, such as alpha (α)- and beta (β)-adrenergic, but there are also subtypes that are designated by subscripts, such as α_1, α_2, β_1, and β_2. Subtypes are also selective for tissues, and thus drugs that are selective for certain subtypes will be more selective for a particular tissue. Drugs that are β_1 adrenergic agonists will increase the heart rate but will not cause bronchial dilation because β_1 receptors are located on the surface of heart muscle cells, whereas β_2 receptors are located on bronchial muscle cells.

The interaction between a receptor and drug exists because the chemical structure of the drug corresponds (or matches), to some degree, with the chemical structure of the receptor (see Figure 3-2). This means that chemical bonds can form between the drug and the receptor. These bonds usually are reversible and thus the drug binds to the receptor and then releases, back and forth.

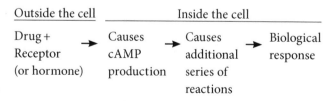

The strength of this bonding interaction is called the *affinity* of the drug for the receptor. The greater the affinity, the greater the chemical interaction, or chemical fit, of the drug for the receptor.

Affinity and efficacy are the two components of the drug's interaction with the receptor that determine the type and extent of biological response. The intrinsic efficacy is the

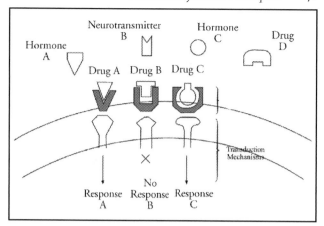

Figure 3-2. Drug-receptor activity. Drugs bind to the same receptors used by hormones and neurotransmitters. When agonists (Drugs A and C) bind to their respective receptor, they initiate a transduction mechanism, which causes a specific biological response. When an antagonist (Drug B) binds, it prevents initiation of the transduction mechanism. The ability of the drug to chemically bind (fit) with the receptor is its affinity. The ability of the drug to either initiate or prevent the transduction mechanism is its intrinsic efficacy. Only tissues that have a receptor for the drug will be affected by the drug. Drug A mimics hormone A; Drug B does not initiate transduction mechanisms and thus is a blocker of the response by neurotransmitter B; Drug C mimics hormone C; Drug D has no receptor on this cell, thus neither initiates nor inhibits any response from the cell.

ability of the drug to cause the receptor to initiate a domino effect of chemical reactions (*transduction mechanism*) that ultimately causes the biological response (see Figure 3-2), such as increased heart rate. There are several types of transduction mechanisms. One well-documented transduction mechanism involves the activation of the membrane protein called G-protein, which leads to the activation of the enzyme adenylyl cyclase inside the cell. This, in turn, produces cyclic adenosine monophosphate (cAMP), which continues the domino effect through several more steps. cAMP is one of many compounds called *second messengers* because they continue the signal (message) intracellularly from the first messenger (the hormone) located outside the cell. Regardless of whether the drug or the endogenous hormone combines with the receptor, the same chain of events is initiated, beginning with the transduction mechanism and ending with the biological response:

Outside the cell		Inside the cell	
Drug + Receptor (or hormone)	→ Causes cAMP production	→ Causes additional series of reactions	→ Biological response

The receptor theory of drug action explains how an agonist and antagonist can bind to the same receptor but have opposite effects (Figure 3-3). Drugs that bind to the same receptor as an endogenous compound and initiate the transduction mechanism will mimic the effects of the

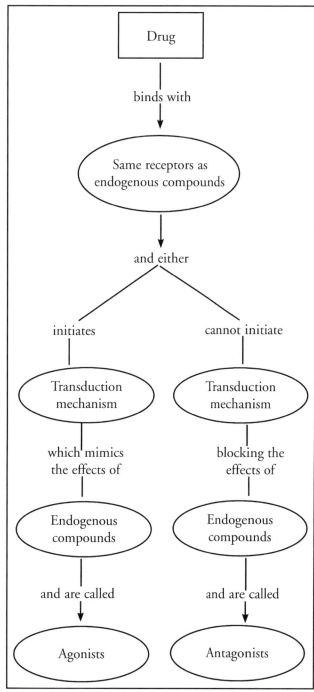

Figure 3-3. Receptor theory of drug action. When an agonist binds to the receptor, a transduction mechanism is initiated, and ultimately a response increases. The antagonist can also bind to the same receptor, which prevents the biological response. This theory explains how an agonist and antagonist can bind to the same receptor and have opposite effects.

endogenous compound and are agonists. Drugs that bind to the same receptor as the endogenous compound but are unable to initiate the transduction mechanism will block the effects of the endogenous compound and are antagonists.

To some extent, the receptor mechanism of drug action can be thought of as a lock (receptor) and key (drug) sys-

tem in which more than 1 key will fit into the lock but only the keys that are able to turn the tumblers in the lock will unlock the door (agonist); when the other keys (antagonist) are in the lock, they prevent the correct key from unlocking the door. To be able to unlock the door, the first criterion is that the key must fit into the keyhole (ie, the affinity). The second criterion is whether the key is able to turn the locking mechanism to unlock the door (ie, the efficacy). If both agonist and antagonist are present, the effect that will predominate is dependent on the relative agonist/antagonist concentration at the site of action, affinity for the receptor, and efficacy.

Section Summary

The mechanism of action of most drugs, for both therapeutic and adverse effects, is that the drug chemically combines with a component of the cell referred to as the receptor. A receptor is generally a large molecule, typically a protein, that has specific chemical characteristics that only allow it to bind to molecules (eg, hormones and drugs) with corresponding chemical characteristics (similar to a lock and key). When the drug binds to the receptor to initiate a sequence of events inside the cell, the drug is called an agonist; when the drug binds to the receptor to inhibit the sequence of events, the drug is an antagonist. The strength of the binding of the drug for the receptor is called the affinity of the drug for the receptor; like the fit of the key into the lock. The ability of the drug to produce the biological response is called the efficacy of the drug (like the ability of the key to turn the lock).

DOSE-RESPONSE RELATIONSHIPS

Aside from affinity and intrinsic efficacy contributing to the biological response, the receptor theory of drug action also assumes that the extent of drug response is directly and linearly dependent on the number of receptor sites occupied by the drug. As more drug is given, the concentration of drug at the site of action (ie, at the receptor) also increases. Once a drug molecule is in the vicinity of the receptor, the likelihood of the drug coming in contact with the receptor is a by-chance occurrence, and therefore the frequency that this event occurs is a matter of statistical probability based on the concentration of the drug and receptors; the more drug and/or receptor molecules, the greater the chances of the drug being in contact with the receptor. Drug-receptor interaction is generally a reversible process, with the drug response being initiated only when the drug and receptor are chemically interacting (drug-receptor).

Drug +   Drug -   Drug
Receptor   →   Receptor   →   Response

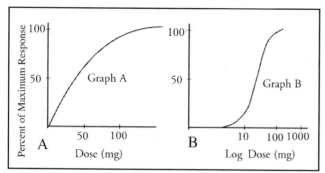

Figure 3-4. Dose-response principle. As the dose of the drug is increased, drug molecules will occupy a larger percentage of receptors and cause a larger biological response. If the observed response is plotted against the dose on a linear scale (Graph A), a hyperbolic curve results in which the response increases gradually until a maximum response is obtained when all of the receptors are occupied. If the same data are plotted using a logarithmic scale (Graph B) for the dose, a sigmoid curve results but the data show a linear relationship between dose and response for a significant portion of the dosage range.

Therefore, as the concentration of the drug increases, more drug molecules will occupy more receptors, which will then produce a greater response. This is the basis for the *dose-response principle* and is shown in Graph A of Figure 3-4. As more receptors are occupied by drug molecules, the chances of a drug finding a free receptor become less until the dose is high enough that all of the receptors are occupied by drug and therefore additional drug does not produce additional effect; maximal response is achieved. Once all of the receptors are occupied, there are no other variables to affect the magnitude of response by that drug. Therefore, increasing the dose further will not increase the response. If the same data are plotted using logarithmic scale for the dose (Graph B of Figure 3-4), a sigmoid curve results but provides a significant segment that is linear (between approximately 20% and 80% of maximal response). The logarithmic dose plot not only provides a more conveniently usable linear portion, but also allows a broader dose range to be represented on the same graph (Figure 3-5).

Single Dose

A typical dose-response curve for a single dose of 3 hypothetical drugs is shown in Figure 3-5. If pain relief is the response being measured, note that the maximal effect obtained by Drug C is lower than for Drugs A and B. In this example, Drugs A and B could represent the opioid analgesics morphine and codeine, and Drug C could represent aspirin, which relieves pain by a different mechanism compared with opioids.

The ED_{50} (effective dose) is the dose of drug that is effective in producing 50% of a specified response. The ED_{50} could represent the average dose needed to produce 50% of a maximal response in a group of people or the dose that will produce a specific effect in 50% of the patients.

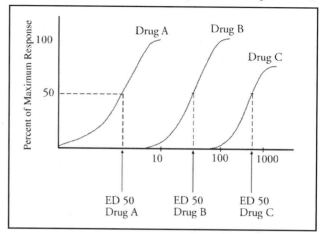

Figure 3-5. Dose response and potency. The dose-response curve is shown for 3 hypothetical pain relievers: Drugs A, B, and C. As the dose increases, more receptors are occupied by the drug and thus the percent of maximal pain relief increases until all the receptors are occupied and no additional relief is obtained. The dose that produces 50% of maximal response (ED_{50}) is shown for each. Drug A is the most potent because the dose to reach the same ED_{50} is lowest for Drug A. Drug C is the least potent but also does not have the intrinsic activity to produce the same maximal response as Drugs A and B.

For example, it could be the dose of codeine that reduced the frequency of coughing by 50%, or the dose of codeine that eliminated the cough in 50% of the patients. The ED_{50} allows a comparison of effective drug dosages among drugs being used for the same therapeutic effect. The ED_{50} can be used to calculate the *therapeutic index* (TI), which is an indicator of the relative safety of the drug.

Potency is a term used to compare the dose of a drug required to produce a particular effect relative to the dose of another drug that acts by a similar mechanism to produce that same effect. The position of the dose-response curve along the x-axis is indicative of potency. In Figure 3-5, Drug A is more potent than Drug B because it takes a considerably lower dose of Drug A to produce the same ED_{50} response compared to the dose for Drug B. Potency is determined by affinity, efficacy, and pharmacokinetic parameters but is of little therapeutic importance because drug dosages are adjusted to compensate for differences in potency. An *equipotent* dose is used when comparing the efficacy of similar drugs (ie, doses are adjusted to give the same response). Consequently, although ibuprofen is more potent than either aspirin or acetaminophen for minor pain relief, 200 mg of ibuprofen is considered equipotent as an analgesic to 650 mg of either aspirin or acetaminophen. However, potency does affect the feasibility of using a drug by some routes of administration, such as sublingual and transdermal, because it is physically very difficult to get large quantities of drug to quickly dissolve under the tongue or to diffuse through the skin. Therefore, potent drugs, such as nitroglycerin with an effective dose of less than 1 mg, are the most practical for these dosage forms.

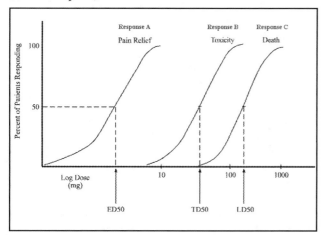

Figure 3-6. Dose response and TI. The dose-response curve is shown for 3 responses from a hypothetical pain reliever. Response A is pain relief, response B is a toxic symptom, and response C is death. The TI is an indication of relative safety of the drug as determined by the ratio of either LD_{50}/ED_{50} or TD_{50}/ED_{50}. The greater the ratio, the greater the safety because a larger dose can be given without occurrence of toxic effects. In this example, the dose required to achieve pain relief in 100% of the patients overlaps a portion of the toxicity curve. Therefore, for a small percentage of patients, a dose of drug necessary to relieve pain will also cause some of the toxic symptoms. However, there is no overlap between the curve representing pain relief and the curve representing death.

The dose-response curve is also useful for estimating the relative safety of a drug. The LD_{50} (lethal dose) is the dose that will cause death in 50% of the population as extrapolated from animal data (Figure 3-6). The ratio of the LD_{50}/ED_{50} is the TI. The larger the TI, the greater the margin of safety. Notice in Figure 3-6 that the dose required to produce pain relief in 100% of the population does not overlap the dose that will kill any of the population. However, from a practical standpoint, we may not want to use death as the determination point for relative safety. The TD_{50} (toxic dose) is the dose that will produce a specific toxic effect in 50% of the population. Generally, a specific toxic effect is used to determine the TI using the ratio TD_{50}/ED_{50}. In Figure 3-6, some patients receiving a dose at the higher end of the normal range will experience the toxic symptom and thus will require a change in therapy. Obviously, use of the normal dosage range of a drug with a TI of 10 will be less likely to cause death or toxicity than a drug with a TI < 5. Examples of drugs with a low TI are aminoglycoside antibiotics, warfarin (Coumadin), some cardiac drugs, and some anticonvulsants used to treat epileptic seizures; these drugs require closer therapeutic drug monitoring.

The significance of the TI is relative to the responses being used to calculate it. For example, if a drug has a TI of 3 when using ringing in the ears as the toxic effect, it would be considered safer than a drug with TI of 3 for which the lethal dose was used for the calculation. The TI provides an impression of the degree of safety associated with the drug but the specific value does not provide much clinically relevant information except as means of noting that additional

caution is necessary when using drugs that have a low TI. In fact, these drugs are likely to require additional clinical monitoring, such as a periodic check for changes in liver or kidney function as a result of drug toxicity.

> *An example of TI calculations is shown. If in a test group of animals, half go to sleep with 100 mg of the sedative phenobarbital and half die at a dose of 260 mg, then $TI = LD_{50}/ED_{50} = 260/100 = 2.6 = a$ low TI.*

Another type of monitoring for drugs with a low TI is therapeutic drug monitoring. This monitoring is used to check the blood (or serum) concentration of the drug and then alter the drug dosage based on that blood concentration. This type of dosage adjustment is used to keep the drug concentration within a certain range (or window). When the drug concentration is kept within this therapeutic window, the incidence of toxicity is minimized. The width of the therapeutic drug concentration is a more clinically useful indicator of safety than the TI; examples are given in Table 3-1. All of the drugs in Table 3-1 have a relatively narrow therapeutic window, which also means they are relatively more toxic (hence the need to monitor the blood concentration). The athletic trainer is not likely to encounter many patients taking drugs with a narrow therapeutic window, but understanding the concept is beneficial to the understanding of the relative safety of drugs. The blood concentrations of drugs that have a relatively wide therapeutic range are typically not monitored because they are safer.

Multiple Doses and Steady State

When multiple doses of a drug are administered (Figure 3-7), the blood concentration increases beyond the concentration obtained by a single dose and eventually levels off when the rate of drug becoming bioavailable equals the rate of drug being removed through metabolism and/or excretion (ie, clearance). This leveling effect is the *steady-state concentration*. Once steady state is reached, continued therapy at the same dose and dosing interval will not increase the peak blood concentration. If a drug is given at a regular dosing interval (eg, 4 times each day), at some point the rate of drug clearance will equal the rate of drug absorbed. The mathematics of this principle establish that if the same dose is administered at a regular dosing interval, the amount of drug in the body will be 87.5% of steady state after dosing has been continued beyond 3 half-lives (t½), approximately 94% after 4 t½, 97% after 5 t½, and 98.4% after 6 t½; this principle is shown in Figure 3-8. So, for therapeutically relevant purposes, steady state can be considered attained after dosing has continued for a time beyond 4 to 5 t½ of the drug. Using this principle, if 250 mg of naproxen (t½ 14 hours) is

			TABLE 3-1

THERAPEUTIC RANGE OF SERUM DRUG CONCENTRATION FOR SELECTED DRUGS

GENERIC NAME	TRADE NAME	DRUG CATEGORY	THERAPEUTIC CONCENTRATION[a]
amikacin	Amikin	aminoglycoside antibiotic	20 to 30 mg/L[b]
digoxin	Lanoxin	antiarrhythmic, congestive heart failure	0.8 to 2.5 µg/L
phenobarbital	Luminal	anticonvulsant	10 to 30 mg/L
phenytoin	Dilantin	anticonvulsant	10 to 20 mg/L
procainamide	Pronestyl	antiarrhythmic	4 to 8 mg/L
theophylline	Theo-Dur	antiasthmatic	10 to 20 mg/L
valproic acid	Depakene	anticonvulsant	50 to 100 mg/L

[a]Represents serum concentration appropriate for most patients.
[b]Represents peak concentration range for amikacin.

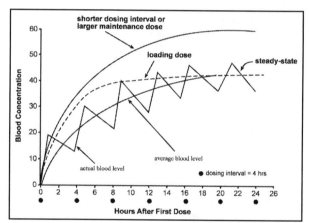

Figure 3-7. Multiple dose effect. A drug with a half-life (t½) of about 5 hours is given every 4 hours (•) beginning with time 0. After each dose, the blood concentration increases to a peak and then decreases to the lowest concentration just prior to the next dose. The blood concentration increases until steady state is reached beyond 4 t½ (>20 hours). A higher steady-state concentration is reached by either increasing the dose or decreasing the dosing interval. Giving a loading dose will increase the blood concentration quicker.

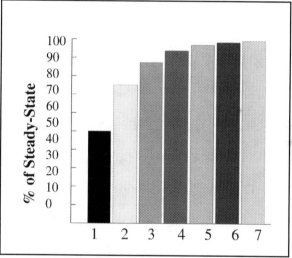

Figure 3-8. Achieving steady state. As a general principle, when dosing of a drug is at a regular interval (eg, every 12 hours), the blood level after each half-life reaches a concentration equal to ½ of the concentration remaining to reach steady state. Therefore, if t½ is 14 hours: (1) 14 hours (1 t½) after the first dose, the blood concentration is 50% of steady state; (2) 28 hours (2 t½) after the first dose, the blood concentration is 50%+½(50%)=75% of steady state; (3) 42 hours (3 t½) after the first dose, the blood concentration is 75%+½(25%)=87.5% of steady state; (4) 56 hours (4 t½) after the first dose, the blood concentration is 87.5%+½(12.5%)=93.8% of steady state; and (5) 70 hours (5 t½) after the first dose, the blood concentration is 93.8%+½(6.25%)=96.9% of steady state. When the sixth dose is given at 60 hours (the first dose being at 0 hours), steady state is reached (approximately), which is after 4 t½.

administered every 12 hours, the peak blood concentration will continue to increase after each 12-hour interval, reaching 94% of steady state after absorption of the sixth dose at 60 hours (first dose at time 0). Continued therapy at this dosage regimen for naproxen will not increase the peak blood concentration beyond another 6%.

The steady-state level obtained can be altered by one of 2 methods: changing the dosing interval or changing the dose. Figure 3-7 illustrates an increase in the blood concentration when the dosing interval is shortened (eg, from 4 hours to 3 hours), or if the maintenance dose is increased but the dosing interval is not changed. In either situation, the amount of drug that is bioavailable increases. If the dosing interval is made longer (eg, from 4 to 6 hours) or if the dose is reduced, the steady-state concentration will decrease.

Maintenance Dose and Loading Dose

A dose administered at a regular dosing interval on a repetitive basis is called a *maintenance dose*. This maintenance therapy could be a 10-day course of antibiotic therapy or 10 years (ie, long-term or chronic) of antihypertensive therapy. In Figure 3-7, the dosing interval is 4 hours and the $t\frac{1}{2}$ is about 5 hours. The blood concentration attained after the dose at 20 hours (after 4 $t\frac{1}{2}$) approximates the steady-state level. However, if it is important to more quickly reach a blood level approximating steady state, to treat an infection or a cardiac dysrhythmia, a loading dose can be given. The *loading dose* is one or more doses that are higher than the maintenance dose and administered at the beginning of therapy for the purpose of achieving the desirable therapeutic concentration quicker. The steady-state level obtained after the loading dose(s) is the same as it would be without the loading dose, assuming no change in the maintenance dose and dosing interval.

Section Summary

The larger the dose, the larger the number of receptors that will be occupied by the drug, and thus a larger response. When the dose reaches a certain concentration so that most of the receptors are occupied by drug, it is statistically less likely that the drug will find an available receptor, thus the response tapers off. These principles are the basis for the typical dose-response relationship in which the response increases with increasing dose, up to a point. The ED_{50} is the dose that produces the therapeutic effect in 50% of the population; the LD_{50} is the dose that is lethal to 50% of the population; and the TD_{50} is the dose that causes a specified toxic symptom in 50% of the population. One indicator of relative safety of a drug is the TI, which can be calculated based on the ratio of LD_{50}/ED_{50} or TD_{50}/ED_{50}; in either case, the larger the number, the greater the difference between the dose that is effective and the dose that causes significant problems. The therapeutic window is a target range of drug concentration in the blood that produces the best therapeutic effect while minimizing toxic effects.

When doses of a drug are given at a regular dosing interval, eventually the blood concentration will level off regardless of how much longer the dosing interval is maintained. This level of drug is called the steady-state blood concentration and occurs after the dosing has occurred for a time beyond approximately 4 to 5 $t\frac{1}{2}$ of the drug. For a drug with a $t\frac{1}{2}$ of 5 hours, steady state is approximately reached when dosing at regular intervals goes beyond 20 hours. The amount of drug given at regular intervals is called the maintenance dose. As a means of attaining steady state quicker than 4 $t\frac{1}{2}$, a loading dose can be given, which is an initial dose that is larger than the maintenance dose.

THERAPEUTIC CONSIDERATIONS

From the dose-response relationships, it is evident that a standard dose used in a population of patients will not produce the same response in each patient. Some patients will experience maximum therapeutic effect with minimal adverse or toxic effects, whereas the response of other patients will fall elsewhere on the dose-response curve. The latter group of patients may require an increase or decrease in dose to obtain the necessary balance between therapeutic effectiveness and adverse effects. Each patient's response to a particular therapy will be dictated by his or her specific pharmacokinetic and pharmacodynamic parameters, which are affected by genetics, age, sex, body size, and drug interactions from concurrent therapy.

Patient Adherence

Patient adherence refers to the extent to which the patient is taking the medication as prescribed. Obviously, medications will only produce the desired therapeutic outcome if the proper dosage regimen is maintained. Nonetheless, poor patient adherence is a major cause of poor therapeutic outcomes. Some of the reasons for patients not adhering to the prescribed dosage regimen are as follows:

- Cost of the medication is too high

- Forgetting to take the medication

- Inconvenient dosing regimen (eg, inhalation asthma medications or multiple-times-per-day dosing)

- Poor patient education regarding the necessity to take medications as prescribed

Patient adherence improves if the patient does not have to take the medication as frequently each day; thus, once-daily dosing significantly improves patient adherence compared with a 3-times-per-day dosing regimen.

The athletic trainer can have an impact on improving patient adherence by educating the patient as to the importance of adhering to the prescribed dosing regimen. An understanding of the mechanism of action of the drug, drug-dosing principles, and proper drug administration techniques can be useful. With this information, the athletic trainer can provide appropriate education to assist the patient in maintaining therapeutic outcomes from the use of chronic medications. For example, a patient taking half the prescribed dose to obtain half the benefit may in fact be obtaining no benefit because the minimum effective dose may not be reached. A patient using a corticosteroid inhaler prior to exercise rather than for daily, long-term therapy does not understand the proper dosing principle or mechanism of action of the drug and is obtaining little or no benefit from the inhaler. The patient should understand the purpose of each drug, the necessity of adhering to the prescribed dosage regimen, and the proper technique for drug administration.

Dose Calculations

The standard dose for drugs with a high TI is often set at 2 or 3 levels—children, adults, and elderly. The dose for children is sometimes refined according to age (eg, one dose for children aged 2 to 5 years and another dose for children aged 6 to 11 years). The basis for these divisions is to compensate for the increased volume of distribution that accompanies increased size. As the likelihood for toxicity or significant adverse effects increases (ie, lower TI), the calculation of the dose becomes more specific. The dose can be calculated based on weight (mg/kg) or body surface area (mg/m^2) of the patient. Body surface area correlates more closely with renal and metabolic capacity than does body weight, assuming normal kidney and liver function. Charts are available to determine the body surface area based on the patient's height and weight. As an example, a patient who is 6 feet tall and 170 pounds has a surface area of 2 m^2.

Therapeutic Drug Monitoring

Because there can be significant variability of response from one patient to another, drugs that have a low TI are sometimes monitored by measuring the blood (or plasma or serum) concentration of the drug. As mentioned previously, this is referred to as *therapeutic drug monitoring*. Measuring the blood concentration leaves no question regarding the extent to which age, genetics, disease, patient compliance, or other parameters have affected bioavailability. The blood level is determined after the patient is at steady state. For some drugs, a normal range of blood concentration has been established; above this level the incidence of toxic effects greatly increases, and below this level there is a greater likelihood the drug is subtherapeutic (ie, below the minimum effective concentration). The range between the low and high desired concentration is referred to as the *therapeutic range* or *therapeutic window*. As an example, theophylline (Theo-Dur) is used for the treatment of asthma (see Chapter 9) and has a therapeutic range of 10 to 20 mg/L. As the concentration of theophylline moves above 20 mg/L, the incidence of adverse effects increases, whereas concentrations below 10 mg/L are less likely to be therapeutically effective. Drugs with a small TI will have a narrow therapeutic window. Besides theophylline, other examples of drugs that are frequently monitored include some antidysrhythmic drugs, anticonvulsants, and aminoglycoside antibiotics, examples of which are shown in Table 3-1. Dosage adjustments are made based on the blood concentration after the drug has reached steady state. By keeping the concentration within the therapeutic window, toxic effects and ineffective dosage regimens can be avoided.

Age

Although the athletic trainer may not be working with infants, a discussion of some therapeutic problems from infants to the elderly illustrates the type of potential problems that may occur. Although dose adjustment based on size is an obvious necessity for therapy to newborns and infants, the capability for drug clearance by the liver and kidney is also reduced through the first year or so. Consequently, it is necessary to closely monitor the effects of drugs administered to newborns and infants, especially for drugs with a low TI. A reduced dosage range for children is established for drugs suitable for use in children. The adult oral dose for ampicillin to treat certain infections is 1 to 4 g/day, whereas for children it is 50 to 100 mg/kg/day. However, not all drugs have been approved for use in children, even at reduced doses. Other drugs, such as the asthma medication zafirlukast (Accolate), were first approved for use in adults and then approved later for use in young children.

There are other important issues related to drug administration in children. Some drugs should not be used in children due to adverse or toxic effects that are unique to children. Tetracycline antibiotics bind to developing teeth and will cause permanent staining. There is concern regarding the extent to which chronic use of corticosteroids for treatment of asthma in children may delay growth. Sometimes it is preferable to have special drug dosage forms and formulations for children. Liquids are easier for some children to swallow than solid dosage forms as long as the liquids are adequately sweetened and flavored. Because elixirs contain alcohol, they are usually avoided in children.

The elderly may also require adjustments in dosing for some drugs. The percentage of the population aged older than 60 years is increasing, and many elderly patients maintain an exercise routine as part of their lifestyle. As a person ages, several pharmacokinetic and pharmacodynamic parameters are altered, which may warrant an adjustment in drug dose, especially for drugs with a smaller TI (Box 3-2).

It is important to note that these changes occur gradually as a person ages, and thus the impact varies among patients. In addition, the picture is complicated by the fact that there are multiple changes occurring simultaneously in the same patient. Finally, it is not only the altered therapeutic effect that is of concern in the elderly, but also the adverse effects. Elderly patients tend to have an enhanced response to many adverse effects, such as the central and autonomic effects of drowsiness, confusion, urinary retention, constipation, and hypotension. It is very difficult to predict the extent of change on all of the pharmacokinetic parameters. Consequently, the best therapy is attained through therapeutic drug monitoring or by monitoring the outcomes of initial therapy, the occurrence of adverse effects, and the concurrent administration of other drugs to determine the need for therapy adjustments. If the therapeutic outcome or

---

Box 3-2

PHARMACOKINETIC AND PHARMACODYNAMIC PARAMETERS THAT ARE ALTERED IN THE ELDERLY

- Diminished function of liver-metabolizing enzymes and reduced blood flow decreases biotransformation rate of drugs and increases the duration of action.

- Reduced kidney function decreases the excretion rate of drugs and increases the duration of action.

- Reduced blood flow to the GI tract reduces the extent of oral absorption.

- Reduced gastric emptying and GI motility can alter drug absorption rates.

- There is an increased proportion of body fat as muscle mass decreases, which increases the volume of distribution of lipid-soluble drugs and thus decreases the concentration at the site of action.

- Diminished albumin concentration, primarily as a consequence of reduced liver function, can decrease the extent of protein binding and increase the response from drugs that are highly protein bound.

- An increased number of diseases in a given patient will increase the number of drugs being used and thus increase the likelihood of drug interactions.

- A change in level of exercise may alter pharmacokinetic parameters as discussed in Chapter 2.

---

adverse effects are not acceptable, age-related factors should be considered in the young and the elderly.

Liver and Kidney Function

Because the clearance of drugs occurs primarily by the liver and kidney, a reduction in the efficiency of these organs through disease, drug toxicity, or the aging process may necessitate a dosage adjustment to attain the proper therapeutic response but avoid adverse effects. The key question is how much dosage adjustment is needed. Sometimes the liver and kidney function must be monitored to determine the extent to which dosage adjustment is necessary. To detect the existence of liver damage, the blood level of aspartate aminotransferase, also known as serum glutamic oxaloacetic transaminase, and alanine aminotransferase, also known as serum glutamic pyruvate transaminase, must be evaluated. Although an elevated concentration of these enzymes in the blood is indicative of acute liver cell damage, they cannot be directly correlated with loss of drug-metabolizing activity. Other indicators of diminished liver function are elevated bilirubin concentration, decreased albumin, and prolonged blood clotting time; the liver is key in the metabolism of bilirubin, albumin, and blood-clotting factors. Again, although the levels of these compounds are indicators of diminished liver function, they do not provide a quantitative determination of the loss of drug-metabolizing capability.

In contrast to liver function, the extent of kidney function can be calculated. One measure of kidney function is creatinine clearance. Creatinine is a waste product of muscle metabolism that is produced at a relatively constant rate per day based on the amount of muscle mass. It is filtered at the glomerulus and is not reabsorbed; thus, creatinine excretion rate is a good measure of kidney function. *Creatinine clearance* refers to the rate (mL/min) at which the kidney clears the blood of creatinine; normal is 100 to 120 mL/min. If kidney function is diminished, less blood will be cleared of creatinine per minute. Dosage adjustment calculations of some drugs that are cleared primarily by the kidney have been established based on creatinine clearance. Aminoglycoside antibiotics and digoxin (Lanoxin) are among these drugs.

Section Summary

The optimal drug therapy is one that provides the right drug at a dose that produces the most effective therapeutic effect with the least adverse effects. Many factors affect the ability to reach optimal drug therapy. Lack of patient adherence (ie, the patient does not take the drug properly) is a major hindrance to optimal drug therapy. Poor adherence often occurs because the patient does not understand the proper use of the drug or the importance of adhering to the dosage regimen.

Proper dosage is obviously important if optimal effectiveness is to be attained. The dosage calculation may be based on the patient's age, weight, or body surface area, depending typically on the degree of toxicity associated with the drug. To fine-tune the dose, the response of the patient to the drug may be monitored so that the dosage regimen can be modified based on the patient's response. Alternatively, the blood concentration of the drug can be measured and used as the gauge for dosage adjustment. Infants, young children, and the elderly sometimes respond differently than the rest of the population, resulting in less-than-optimal response to therapy. Special monitoring and adjustments in therapy are often necessary for these populations.

Because the liver and kidneys are responsible for clearance of drugs, the level of efficiency of these organs affects the response to drug therapy. Sometimes these organs must be evaluated to determine the extent to which they are functioning. The measure of liver enzymes and creatinine clearance can be useful to assess whether the liver and kidneys, respectively, are functioning properly. Adjustment of drug dosage may be necessary if either organ is functionally deficient. There are a multitude of factors that can hinder the ability to achieve optimal drug therapy.

DRUG INTERACTIONS

A *drug interaction* occurs when the addition of another drug increases or decreases the effect obtained from the therapy. Some drug-drug interactions are beneficial and are incorporated into the therapeutic plan (eg, the use of multiple drugs to treat asthma and hypertension). In other situations, interactions between drugs are detrimental because they reduce therapeutic effectiveness, increase the incidence of adverse effects, or increase toxicity. For example, alcohol can increase the likelihood of toxicity of acetaminophen (see Chapter 7), and it increases the CNS depressant effects of all other CNS depressants (see Chapter 8). Some foods and herbs can cause drug-food and drug-herbal interactions (see Chapter 15), respectively. There are thousands of interactions of drugs with other drugs, food, and herbal remedies. Many drug handbooks (see Table 1-8) list some drug interactions for each drug, and some books focus exclusively on drug interactions (eg, *Drug Interactions Handbook*). Internet sites also provide drug interaction information; an example with search capability for prescription drugs, OTC products, and herbals is http://reference.medscape.com/drug-interactionchecker. It is beyond the scope and intent of this text to mention all of these interactions, but a few examples are provided in Table 3-2. As a general rule, drugs with a low TI and drugs for which a diminished response may have critical consequences must be particularly monitored for potential interactions. Obviously, the likelihood of drug interactions increases as the number of drugs being taken by the patient increases.

There are many mechanisms that cause drug interactions. Some are a result of changes in pharmacokinetic parameters, and others are due to pharmacodynamic changes. These mechanisms are described here and summarized in Table 3-3:

- *Receptor antagonist.* When 2 drugs have affinity for the same receptor, one drug will displace the other and thus diminish the response of the other, especially if one is an agonist and the other an antagonist. Propranolol (Inderal) is a β-adrenergic antagonist (ie, a β blocker); pirbuterol (Maxair) is a β-adrenergic agonist used for the treatment of asthma. If propranolol was being used to treat hypertension, it could diminish the effectiveness of pirbuterol at a time when the patient needs it to treat an acute asthma attack.

- *Enzyme induction.* This occurs when a drug (the inducer drug) increases the synthesis of one or more metabolizing enzymes. Often the inducer drug increases the amount of metabolizing enzyme that is responsible for metabolizing a second drug. Consequently, enzyme induction will diminish the response from the second drug. Occasionally, the metabolites are more active, in which case the inducer drug will increase the response from the second drug because the more active metabolite is produced faster. Enzyme induction is a relatively slow process requiring the inducer drug to be present for days to weeks to demonstrate a maximum effect. Cytochrome P450 enzymes (see Chapter 2) are particularly affected by inducers, although other enzymes can be too.

> Recall from Chapter 2 that liver enzymes metabolize drugs and typically inactivate the drug. The more enzyme molecules present, the faster the rate of metabolism and the faster the inactivation of the drug. A faster inactivation results in a diminished effect from the drug.

Drug A = Inducer of Enzyme B

$$\text{Drug B} \xrightarrow{\text{Enzyme B}} \text{Metabolite of Drug B}$$

Drug A increases the synthesis of Enzyme B. When Drug A and B are used concurrently, the induction of Enzyme B by Drug A increases the metabolism rate of Drug B.

Some anticonvulsants and alcohol are examples of liver enzyme inducers. Examples of drugs that are significantly affected by enzyme inducers are oral anticoagulants, estrogen contraceptives, antidepressants, and theophylline for asthma therapy; the therapy may need to be adjusted for these drugs to compensate for enzyme induction.

- *Enzyme inhibition.* This drug interaction occurs when 2 drugs bind to the same metabolizing enzyme, but one drug is the substrate for the enzyme whereas the other is an inhibitor. Because inhibition of a metabolizing enzyme will decrease the activity of that metabolizing enzyme, Drug B will be cleared from the body more slowly.

TABLE 3-2

EXAMPLES OF DRUG INTERACTIONS WITH OTHER DRUGS, FOOD, AND HERBS

DRUG	INTERACTING SUBSTANCE	POTENTIAL CONSEQUENCE (TABLES THAT PROVIDE EXAMPLES OF DRUGS)
ACE inhibitors	NSAIDs	Decreases antihypertensive effect (Tables 6-4, 12-8)
Acetaminophen	Alcohol	Increases toxicity
Ampicillin	Sulbactam	Increases effectiveness of ampicillin (Table 5-2)
Antianxiety drugs	Grapefruit juice	Increases absorption and potential toxicity
Antihistamines	Alcohol	Increases sedation, particularly with first-generation antihistamines (Table 10-3)
Antihypertensive drugs	Nasal decongestant	Decreases physiological effectiveness (Tables 10-2, 12-6, 12-7, 12-8, 12-9)
Antihypertensive drugs	Herbs	Some herbs (eg, black cohosh, California poppy, golden seal, coleus, quinine) may increase antihypertensive effect excessively
Antihypertensive drugs	Herbs	Some herbs (eg, ginger, ginseng, kola, bayberry, blue cohosh, cayenne, licorice) may decrease antihypertensive effect
Benzodiazepines	Alcohol, kava	Increases sedation (Table 8-2)
Caffeine	Grapefruit juice	Increases CNS stimulation of caffeine
Calcium channel blockers	Grapefruit juice	Increases occurrence of adverse effects (Table 12-9)
CNS depressants	Alcohol	Increases CNS depression effects (Table 8-2)
Corticosteroids, systemic	Antifungal drugs	Decreases metabolism and may increase toxic effects (Table 6-6)
Corticosteroids, systemic	NSAIDs	Increases incidence of ulceration and bleeding
Corticosteroids, oral	Antacids	Decreases oral absorption
Diazepam	Alcohol	Enhances CNS depression; potential toxicity
Fluoroquinolones	Dairy products and antacids	Diminishes absorption (Table 5-5)
Nasal decongestants	Caffeine	Increases cardiovascular adverse effects and CNS stimulation (Table 10-2)
Opioid analgesics	Acetaminophen, aspirin, ibuprofen	Synergistic analgesic effect (Table 7-2)
Oral contraceptives	Many drugs	Diminishes the effectiveness of oral contraceptives (Table 3-5)
Oral contraceptives	St. John's wort	Diminishes the effectiveness of progestin contraceptives
Tetracyclines	Dairy products and antacids	Diminishes absorption (Table 5-4)
Warfarin	Aspirin, other NSAIDs	Increases anticoagulant effect; potentially spontaneous bleeding
Warfarin	Broccoli, cabbage	Vitamin K–rich foods decrease anticoagulant effect
Warfarin	Antifungal agents	Enzyme inhibition; increases anticoagulant effect
Warfarin, aspirin, other NSAIDs	Herbs	Herbs that have anticoagulant or antiplatelet effects (eg, garlic, ginkgo biloba, ginseng, green tea, grape seed) may increase bleeding/bruising

(continued)

	TABLE 3-2 (CONTINUED)	

EXAMPLES OF DRUG INTERACTIONS WITH OTHER DRUGS, FOOD, AND HERBS

DRUG	INTERACTING SUBSTANCE	POTENTIAL CONSEQUENCE (TABLES THAT PROVIDE EXAMPLES OF DRUGS)
β agonist	β blocker	Physiologically oppose each other; diminishes asthma therapy effectiveness (Tables 9-5, 12-6)
β blockers	NSAIDs	Decreases antihypertensive effect
CNS = central nervous system; NSAIDs = nonsteroidal anti-inflammatory drugs.		

TABLE 3-3

TYPES OF DRUG INTERACTIONS SUMMARIZED

DRUG INTERACTION TYPE	DESCRIPTION
Receptor antagonist	When 2 drugs have an affinity for the same receptor, one drug will displace the other and thus diminish the response of the other; one is an agonist and the other an antagonist.
Enzyme induction	This occurs when a drug (the inducer drug) increases the synthesis of one or more metabolizing enzymes.
Enzyme inhibition	Occurs when 2 drugs bind to the same metabolizing enzyme, but one drug is the substrate for the enzyme whereas the other is an inhibitor.
Physiologic antagonism	The physiological effect of 2 drugs given concurrently oppose each other without either drug directly interfering with the mechanism of action or pharmacokinetic parameters of the other.
Physiologic agonists	Two or more drugs when used concurrently result in an increase in physiological effects, either additive or synergistic, but the drugs do not have the same mechanism of action or affect the pharmacokinetic parameters of the other.
Absorption effects	The use of one drug inhibits the absorption of another drug if given concurrently.
Excretion effects	One drug increases or decreases the excretion rate of another drug.

Drug A = Inhibitor of Enzyme B

Drug B ——✗——▶ Metabolite of Drug B
        Enzyme B

Drug A inhibits Enzyme B. Enzyme B metabolizes Drug B. When Drug A and B are used concurrently, the inhibition of Enzyme B by Drug A decreases the metabolism rate of Drug B.

When the substrate drug and inhibitor drug are used concurrently, the substrate drug will have a longer duration, increased blood concentration, and greater biological response than expected. This enhanced response may include adverse effects and toxicity. Examples of inhibitors of metabolizing enzymes that are known to affect the level of other drugs include erythromycin (Erythrocin), cimetidine (Tagamet), some antifungal agents such as fluconazole (Diflucan), antidepressants referred to as selective serotonin reuptake inhibitors such as fluoxetine (Prozac), and grapefruit juice.

As an example of enzyme inhibition, if cimetidine (Tagamet), a drug used to treat gastrointestinal (GI) problems (see Chapter 11) is added to therapy that includes a β blocker such as propranolol (Inderal) for treatment of hypertension (see Chapter 12), within a day the cimetidine will begin to inhibit the enzyme that had been metabolizing propranolol. Because less enzyme is available to metabolize propranolol, the blood level of propranolol will increase and may cause adverse effects. In this scenario, if the cimetidine is to remain as part of the therapy, the dose of propranolol should be reduced to decrease the incidence of adverse effects.

- *Physiologic antagonism.* In this situation, the physiological effect of the 2 drugs given concurrently oppose each other without either drug directly interfering with the mechanism of action or pharmacokinetic parameters of the other. For example, one drug decreases blood pressure, whereas the second drug increases blood pressure. This type of interaction is particularly important in treatment of diseases such as hypertension, diabetes mellitus, hypercholesterolemia, and asthma because there are many prescription and OTC products that have physiological effects that exacerbate these diseases. For example, nasal decongestants used to treat symptoms of the common cold can increase blood pressure and blood glucose and thus act as physiologic antagonists of therapy for hypertension and diabetes.

- *Physiological agonists.* Similar to physiological antagonism in that 2 or more drugs used concurrently do not have the same mechanism of action, but in this case the result is an increase in physiological effects, either additive or synergistic. An example is the use of the anticoagulant warfarin (Coumadin) with aspirin, which also prolongs blood clotting; the result may be excessive anticoagulation. Sometimes the physiological agonistic response is desirable and is the basis for using 2 or more drugs with different mechanisms of action to treat the same disease, such as for treatment of cancer or hypertension (see Chapter 12).

- *Absorption effects.* The use of one drug could inhibit the absorption of another drug if given concurrently. Laxatives, such as milk of magnesia, which contain divalent cations (ie, metal ions that have a charge of +2, such as Ca^{2+}, Mg^{2+}, Al^{2+}), will bind to tetracycline and fluoroquinolone antibiotics and inhibit their absorption (see Chapter 5). Typically, dosing of the interfering drug (eg, milk of magnesia) should be about 2 hours before or 1 hour after the other drug.

- *Excretion effects.* One drug could alter the excretion rate of another drug, for example by competing for the tubular secretion sites, as in the case for the concurrent use of probenecid with penicillin G (see Chapter 2).

It is impossible to remember all of the potential drug interactions associated with every drug. Even with the availability of drug handbooks and computer-based information, it is difficult to assess the practical significance of the interaction. Drugs with a wide therapeutic window are less likely to pose a noticeable difference in response due to a drug interaction. Nonetheless, it is important for the athletic trainer to understand the principles of drug interaction; if an unexpected drug effect is observed, a drug-drug, drug-herbal, or drug-food interaction should be considered and steps taken to refer the patient. The physician and pharmacist can determine whether a potential interaction exists so that appropriate modification of therapy can be made.

Section Summary

Drug interactions have a significant impact on the effectiveness of drug therapy in many patients. The more drugs that are used concurrently in a patient, the greater the probability for drug interactions. There are many mechanisms that can be responsible for these drug interactions. It is counterproductive to use 2 drugs that produce the opposite effects, such as an agonist and antagonist. Less obvious are the many instances in which groups of drugs share the same metabolizing enzymes. When one of these drugs increases the level of the metabolizing enzymes (ie, enzyme induction), it causes other drugs to be metabolized quicker by that same enzyme, thus reducing the duration of action of the other drugs. Inhibition of drug-metabolizing enzymes can also be the cause of drug interactions. When a new drug is added to existing therapy and the new drug inhibits the metabolizing enzyme that inactivates the initial drug, the initial drug will be metabolized slower and thus the duration of action will be extended. If adding a drug to therapy inhibits the absorption or increases the renal excretion of another drug, the effectiveness of drug therapy will be affected and an adjustment in dosage regimen may be necessary. In all cases of drug interactions, the need for dosage adjustment is dependent on whether the change in drug response is significant. The clinical significance of these interactions varies with the magnitude to which the drug response is altered and the degree of toxicity of the drugs affected.

ADVERSE DRUG REACTIONS

An *adverse drug reaction* (ADR) is any undesirable response from a drug. These reactions can range from dry mouth to life-threatening organ damage. The incidence of clinically significant ADRs is reflected in the fact that up to 7% of hospitalizations are a result of an ADR. In addition, more than 10% of hospitalized patients experience at least one ADR. Some ADRs may occur after just one dose of the drug, whereas others occur only after continued use of the drug. Sometimes a drug is removed from the market because a severe ADR is identified after the drug has been used in a large number of patients (ie, *postmarketing monitoring*). ADRs can be subdivided into the following categories, which are summarized in Table 3-4:

- *Side effects.* These are expected responses based on the pharmacologic action of the drug. They are also dose related so that larger doses will increase the frequency of side effects. Because of differences

TABLE 3-4
CATEGORIES OF ADVERSE DRUG REACTIONS

CATEGORY	DESCRIPTION
Side effects	Expected responses based on the pharmacologic action of the drug
Allergic reactions	Exaggerated immune response initiated by the exposure to certain drugs or other chemicals
Organ cytotoxic effects	Adverse effects on organs
Idiosyncratic reactions	Reaction that is peculiar to an individual or a defined group of people
Drug-drug interactions	Interaction of 2 or more drugs that results in a disadvantage to the patient
Drug-food interactions	Interaction of a drug with food that results in an adverse patient reaction
Drug-herb interactions	Interaction of a drug with herbal products that results in an adverse patient reaction
Drug use during pregnancy	It is assumed that most drugs cross the placenta barrier to some extent and thus pose the potential for adverse reactions in this selected population for whom the drug was not intended

among patients in the pharmacokinetic and pharmacodynamic parameters, not every patient will experience each side effect associated with a drug, but the percentage of the population that will experience any given side effect is predictable based on previous observations. Side effects are usually less severe compared with most other ADRs. Examples of side effects are dry mouth, constipation, increased heart rate, hypotension, gastrointestinal upset, and drowsiness. In some cases, the dose of the drug may have to be decreased to diminish the severity of the side effect. As discussed earlier, elderly patients are susceptible to diminished clearance of drugs and may require a lower dose to decrease the occurrence and intensity of side effects.

- *Allergic reactions.* Allergic reactions from drugs occur in approximately 5% of the population. Some patients have been misidentified as having a drug allergy due to the inaccurate identification of other ADRs as an allergy. The intensity of drug-induced allergic reactions is usually independent of dose. An initial sensitization exposure to the drug is required to initiate the allergic response. Allergic reactions are immune responses with symptoms that can vary considerably among patients, but the drug should be discontinued regardless of the severity of the allergic response. Symptoms can be as mild as urticaria or as severe as life-threatening bronchoconstriction and hypotension associated with an anaphylactic reaction. Dermatologic reactions are the most common type of allergic response, but these usually are mild and disappear after discontinuation of the drug. If a drug causes anaphylaxis, symptoms will usually occur within 30 minutes after exposure to

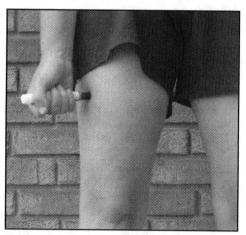

Figure 3-9. EpiPen administration.

the drug. The drug of choice for the initial treatment of anaphylaxis is epinephrine administered subcutaneously or intramuscularly. Generally, the most common device used to self-deliver the epinephrine intramuscularly is an autoinjector such as an EpiPen (Figure 3-9). Although the athletic trainer may help prepare the device for use, the patient must self-administer the medication. The procedure for self-administering an EpiPen is listed in Box 3-3. Because anaphylaxis is a medical emergency, the emergency medical plan should be activated upon its recognition. Even if an EpiPen is used, the patient needs to be seen by a physician immediately because additional medical treatment may be necessary.

The most common causes of allergic drug reactions are β-lactam antibiotics, NSAIDs, and sulfonamides (ie, certain sulfur-containing compounds).

Box 3-3

PROCEDURE FOR ADMINISTERING THE EpiPen AUTO-INJECTOR

TO ADMINISTER

STEP	ACTION
1	Grasp the unit, with the orange tip pointing downward
2	Form a fist around the unit (orange tip down)
3	With other hand, pull off the blue safety release
4	Hold orange tip near outer thigh
5	Swing and firmly push against outer thigh at a 90-degree angle to the thigh until you hear the EpiPen click; the EpiPen is designed to work through clothing
6	Hold firmly against the thigh for 10 seconds to deliver the medicine
7	Remove unit, massage injection area for 10 seconds

Note: Most of the liquid stays in the unit and cannot be reused.

AFTER USE

8	Get emergency help right away
9	Carefully put the EpiPen back into the carrying tube
10	Carrying tube cap will not close after EpiPen is used
11	Take unit to hospital so that the physician can inspect it and it can be disposed of properly

Adapted from https://www.epipen.com/en/about-epipen/how-to-use-epipen.

The β-lactam antibiotics consist of 2 groups of antibiotics with similar chemical structures: the penicillins and the cephalosporins (see Chapter 5). Allergic reactions occur more often with this group of drugs than with any others but the incidence is less than 10%. Although allergic reactions to the β-lactams are usually mild, anaphylaxis can occur. Aspirin and other NSAIDs can cause a variety of reactions, including urticaria and anaphylaxis. Aspirin and other NSAIDs can also induce asthma attacks or other respiratory symptoms in 4% to 20% of patients with chronic asthma, depending on the subpopulation of asthma patients. Sulfonamides include drugs in the categories of antibiotics, diuretics, and oral hypoglycemic agents used to treat type 2 diabetes mellitus. Allergic reactions to sulfonamide

antibiotics occur in approximately 5% of the general population and with a lower frequency in the other sulfonamide categories. The most common manifestations from sulfonamides are dermatologic and may include fever.

- *Organ cytotoxic effects.* Some drugs have adverse effects on organs, particularly the liver, kidney, and pancreas. Drugs such as acetaminophen and NSAIDs can cause hepatotoxicity, and susceptibility is increased if the liver function is already compromised by chronic alcohol use or disease. Most of the time hepatotoxicity is due to a metabolite, which either initiates an immune reaction or has direct toxicity on the liver cells. Nausea, anorexia, and jaundice are symptoms common to hepatotoxicity. Many drugs such as NSAIDs (ibuprofen, Chapter 6) and aminoglycoside antibiotics (amikacin, Chapter 5) have the potential to cause nephrotoxicity. Toxicity is usually dose related. Pancreatitis can also result from administration of some drugs such as estrogens, sulfonamides, and tetracyclines. Organ function tests are sometimes part of the standard protocol for use of some drugs to monitor for potential organ cytotoxicity. These ADRs typically require a reduction of drug dosage or discontinuation of the drug depending on the severity of the adverse response.

- *Idiosyncratic reactions.* An *idiosyncrasy* is a reaction that is peculiar to an individual or a defined group of people. Because of a genetic makeup that is different than the general population, a patient may be very sensitive to small doses of a drug or highly insensitive to high doses of a drug. For example, the gene that codes for a specific drug-metabolizing enzyme may code for an abnormal structure for the enzyme so that it metabolizes the drug much slower than the normal enzyme. Consequently, the drug may have an unusually long duration of action. Alterations of the receptor structure through a change in the structure of the gene that codes for the receptor could increase or decrease the affinity or efficacy related to that receptor. More information on the effects of genetics on the action of drugs can be found below in the section on pharmacogenetics.

- *Drug-drug interactions.* As discussed previously, as the number of drugs used concurrently in the same patient increases, there is an increased likelihood of drug interactions. When the drug interaction results in a disadvantage to the patient, the drug interaction is an ADR. These drug interactions may result from the use of prescription, OTC, or herbal medicines or alcohol. Oral contraceptives are examples of drugs that interact with several other drugs, resulting in either a decreased effectiveness of the oral contraceptive or an altered effect from the other

Pharmacodynamic Principles   55

| | | TABLE 3-5 | | |

EXAMPLES OF DRUG INTERACTIONS WITH ORAL CONTRACEPTIVES

GENERIC NAME	TRADE NAME	RESULT OF INTERACTION/COMMENTS
phenobarbital	Luminal	• Diminishes effectiveness of oral contraceptives • Other barbiturates may have same effect
carbamazepine	Tegretol	• Diminishes effectiveness of oral contraceptive • Other anticonvulsants such as phenytoin (Dilantin) and felbamate (Felbatol) have a similar effect
penicillins	see Table 5-2	• Anecdotal reports of diminished oral contraceptive effect, although pharmacokinetic data unsupportive
griseofulvin	Fulvicin	• Diminishes effectiveness of oral contraceptive • Other antifungal drugs may have a similar effect
rifampin	Rifadin	• Diminishes effectiveness of oral contraceptive by this antibiotic
St. John's wort		• May diminish effectiveness of oral contraceptive
tetracyclines	see Table 5-4	• Anecdotal reports of diminished oral contraceptive effect, although pharmacokinetic data unsupportive
warfarin	Coumadin.	• Decreases the anticoagulant effect of warfarin

drug. Table 3-5 lists some examples of drug interactions with oral contraceptives.

• *Drug-food interactions.* Because each patient's diet changes daily, it is difficult to incorporate the impact of drug-food interactions into the dosage regimen of the patient. Consequently, most significant drug-food interactions are considered ADRs. For example, warfarin (Coumadin) is an anticoagulant for which many drug-food interactions have been reported; all vitamin K–containing foods (eg, broccoli, cabbage, lettuce, green tea) are physiologic antagonists to warfarin activity. Dairy products are rich in calcium and can prevent the absorption of tetracycline antibiotics. Aged cheeses and meats should be avoided in patients being treated with monoamine oxidase inhibitors, a class of antidepressants, because they may enhance the effect of these drugs. Examples of monoamine oxidase inhibitors are tranylcypromine (Parnate) and phenelzine (Nardil). Grapefruit juice inhibits transport proteins in the intestinal cells and inhibits CYP enzymes to significantly increase the blood concentration of many drugs, including some antihypertensives, antianxiety drugs, and statins (used to reduce cholesterol blood levels).

• *Drug-herbal medicine interactions.* As with drug-food interactions, drug-herbal medicine interactions are generally considered ADRs because it is difficult to predict the extent of the interaction.

Contributing significantly in this regard is the lack of established standards of quality for these products. Nonetheless, many drug-herbal medicine interactions have been reported. For example, St. John's wort, which has been used to treat many conditions, including depression, may increase the activity of monoamine oxidase inhibitors used concurrently to treat depression. Ginkgo has been used to treat conditions such as peripheral vascular disease and dementia and may increase the effects of anticoagulant drugs being used concurrently. Athletic trainers should be aware that herbal medicines contain compounds that have the potential to cause interactions and thus should be considered along with prescription and OTC drugs when considering a patient's total drug usage. Herbal supplements are discussed in Chapter 15.

• *Use during pregnancy.* Because the placenta does not exclude molecules to the same extent as the blood-brain barrier, it is assumed that most drugs cross the placental barrier to some extent. This poses the potential for adverse reactions in a selected population for whom the drug is not intended. The US Food and Drug Administration (FDA) has a use-in-pregnancy rating system (Table 3-6) that considers the extent to which information about the drug has ruled out the drug as a risk factor for the developing baby against the potential benefit of the drug to the patient. The FDA has proposed a new system for describing risks of medication use during

TABLE 3-6	
US Food and Drug Administration Ratings for Drug Use-in-Pregnancy Safety	
Category A	Controlled studies show no risk. Controlled studies in pregnant women have failed to demonstrate a risk to the developing baby in any trimester of pregnancy.
Category B	No evidence of risk in humans. Controlled studies in pregnant women have not shown increased risk of abnormalities to the developing baby despite adverse findings in animals, or, in the absence of adequate human studies, animal studies show no risk. The chance of harm to the developing baby is remote but remains a possibility.
Category C	Risk cannot be ruled out. Controlled human studies are lacking, and animal studies have shown a risk or are lacking also. There is a chance of harm to the developing baby if the drug is administered during pregnancy; however, the potential benefits may outweigh the potential risk.
Category D	Positive evidence of risk. Studies in humans, or investigational or postmarketing data, have demonstrated risk to the developing baby. Nevertheless, potential benefits from the use of the drug may outweigh the potential risk (eg, in a life-threatening situation or serious disease).
Category X	Contraindicated in pregnancy. Studies in animals or humans, or investigational or post-marketing reports, have demonstrated positive evidence of abnormalities or risk in the developing baby, which clearly outweighs any benefit to the patient.

pregnancy and lactation; this proposed system will provide additional detail in the medication labeling information to guide decisions by prescribers and patients. No effort is made in this textbook to specify the pregnancy risk of the drugs discussed. However, such information is available in many drug information handbooks.

Section Summary

Adverse drug reactions is a broad term that refers to any undesirable response from a drug. Side effects are predictable, dose-related adverse effects. Allergic reactions range from relatively minor rash to life-threatening anaphylaxis. Most allergic drug reactions are caused by penicillins and cephalosporin antibiotics, NSAIDs, and sulfonamides (eg, certain diuretics, oral hypoglycemic drugs, and sulfa-containing antibiotics). Some drugs produce toxicity to selective organs, and thus therapy with these drugs requires periodic monitoring of organ function. Other drugs cause unusual and unpredictable adverse reactions to a small population of people due to some specific genetic makeup of that group of people. Interactions with food, herbal medicines, or other drugs also pose the potential for initiating ADRs. Use of drugs during pregnancy must be done with caution because of the potential harm to the developing baby. An FDA classification of use-in-pregnancy risk categories is a useful guide regarding the relative risk-to-benefit of using any drug during pregnancy.

PHARMACOGENETICS

A patient's genetic makeup can influence the therapeutic effects as well as the adverse effects of medications. The study of how these genetic changes affect drug action is referred to as *pharmacogenetics*. These genetic variations contribute to the different responses to medications among patients. Pharmacogenetics is an expanding area of medical research and practice. The goal of pharmacogenetics is to use a patient's genetic variations to design a drug regimen that is specific to that individual. This process is also referred to as personalized medicine. The choice of drug or the drug dose can be changed to fit the person's genetic makeup. For example, the FDA has included dosing instructions in the labeling for the anticoagulant warfarin based on genetic variations in the target for warfarin action or an enzyme that metabolizes warfarin. There is still a lot that is unknown about the effects of genetic variations on specific medications, and further research is needed in this area. A detailed description of what is known about pharmacogenetics is beyond the scope of this text. Instead, a brief description of the genetic variations observed in patients is provided.

Both pharmacokinetic and pharmacodynamic processes can be affected by genetic variations. Regarding pharmacokinetics, the most studied aspect of genetic variations and drug response has been on drug-metabolizing enzymes. Genetic variations have been observed in the cytochrome P450 enzymes as well as other drug-metabolizing enzymes. This leads to differences in the response to these drugs both in therapeutic effects and adverse effects. For example, the opioid analgesic codeine is normally metabolized by a cytochrome P450 enzyme to the more active analgesic morphine. Some patients have decreased activity of this enzyme, which causes less of the codeine to be converted to morphine. The pain relief from codeine in these patients is significantly lower compared with patients with normal enzyme activity. This example shows how genetic variations can lead to differences in therapeutic effect. As mentioned previously, warfarin's metabolism is affected by genetic variations. Patients who have lower activity of the enzyme that metabolizes warfarin experience more bleeding complications from the use of this drug. Decreasing the warfarin dose can reduce the risk of this adverse effect. The pharmacodynamics of a medication can be affected if there is a genetic variation in the target for the drug's action. An example of this phenomenon involves the β_1 receptor. Drugs that block this receptor are used in the management of cardiovascular disorders (see Chapter 12). Some patients have variations in the gene that codes for this receptor. Researchers are studying the changes in this gene to determine which patients would benefit the most from β_1 receptor antagonists and those who would be predicted not to benefit from this class of drugs.

MEDICATION ERRORS

Medication errors occur when some type of mistake occurs in the medication use process, such as the wrong dose or the wrong drug being administered to the patient. The consequences of these errors range from having relatively little effect to being fatal. These errors are often caused from miscommunication of oral or written instructions from one health care professional to another or to the patient (eg, a pharmacist who fails to repeat the verbal order back to the physician, or the notoriously poor handwriting of physicians that results in the misinterpretation of the prescription by the pharmacist). Contributing significantly to the problem is the fact that there is an increasing number of drugs that have similar spellings or pronunciations as another drug. For example, Levatol (penbutolol) and Lipitor (atorvastatin) are close in spelling but quite different in terms of their effects. Although this pair of drugs has only 3 letters in common, coupled with poor handwriting or misspelling, they can be confused. Table 3-7 lists some of the many examples of drug pairs that look or sound alike. The problem is compounded when the dosage unit is the same for the 2 drugs, such as Lanoxin (digoxin) 0.125-mg tablets and Levoxine (levothyroxine) 0.125-mg tablets. The Institute for Safe Medication Practices provides a website (www.ismp.org) that includes lists of medications that are more commonly associated with medication errors, educational resources for consumers and health care providers, and FDA safety alerts.

TABLE 3-7

PAIRS OF DRUGS WITH SIMILAR NAMES

acetazolamide	acetohexamide
alprazolam	lorazepam
aspirin	Asendin
aspirin	Afrin
albuterol	atenolol
Aldomet	Aldoril
Aldomet	Anzemet
Aleve	Alesse
Amicar	Amikin
Amicar	amikacin
ampicillin	aminophylline
atorvastatin	atomoxetine
Atrovent	Alupent
Avinza	Evista
bacitracin	Bactrim
bacitracin	Bactroban
baclofen	Bactroban
Benadryl	Bentyl
Benadryl	Benylin
Benadryl	benazepril
Bicillin	Wycillin
Brethine	Brethaire
bupropion	buspirone
cefazolin	cefprozil
Cefotan	Ceftin
cefoxitin	Cytoxan
cefoxitin	cefotaxime
cefoxitin	cefotetan
Celebrex	Cerebyx
clonidine	Klonopin
codeine	Cardene
codeine	Lodine
Cytoxan	Cytotec
Cytoxan	Cytosar U
Cytoxan	CytoGam
Cytoxan	cefoxitin
Cytoxan	Ciloxan

(continued)

TABLE 3-7 (CONTINUED)

PAIRS OF DRUGS WITH SIMILAR NAMES

dactinomycin	daptomycin
Demerol	Demulen
Demerol	Dymelor
Diabeta	Zebeta
digoxin	Desoxyn
digoxin	doxepin
dimenhydrinate	diphenhydramine
Ecotrin	Edecrin
Ecotrin	Akineton
ephedrine	epinephrine
ethanol	Ethyol
Femara	Femhrt
Flovent	Flonase
lamivudine	lamotrigine
Miralax	Mirapex
morphine	meperidine
morphine	hydromorphone
Neurontin	Noroxin
Nicoderm	Nitro-Derm
oxycodone	Oxycontin
penicillamine	penicillin
Percogesic	paregoric
PhosLo	PhosChol
prednisolone	prednisone
Prozac	Prilosec
Retrovir	ritonavir
rimantadine	ranitidine
Septra	Sectral
sulfasalazine	sulfisoxazole
sulfasalazine	Salsalate
sulfasalazine	sulfadiazine
Tylenol	Tylox
Tylenol	Tuinal
Valtrex	Valcyte
Verelan	Vivarin
Verelan	Voltaren
Viagra	Allegra
	(continued)

TABLE 3-7 (CONTINUED)

PAIRS OF DRUGS WITH SIMILAR NAMES

Vicodin	Hycodan
Volmax	Flomax
Zocor	Cozaar
Zyrtec	Zantac
Zyrtec	Zyprexa
Zyprexa	Celexa

Administering the wrong dose is another type of error. Misplaced decimal points have resulted in toxic symptoms or death. For doses that are less than 1 unit, use of a decimal without a 0 to the left of the decimal (ie, .5 rather than 0.5) has resulted in 10-fold error; a decimal point should never be used without a digit to the left (leading zero) when writing a dose. The lack of a leading zero can also cause a misinterpretation of the desired drug (eg, Flomax .4 mg mistaken for Volmax 4 mg).

Misinterpretation of oral instructions to the patient is also a significant contributor to medication errors. The health care professional cannot assume that the patient understands the directions exactly as they were intended. The best way to ensure that the patient understands when and how to take medications is to have him or her repeat back his or her interpretation of the instructions. In some cases, such as use of asthma inhalers, the patient should demonstrate the use of the medication so that there is no confusion as to proper technique. Because misinterpretation of instructions to the patient is a significant problem, the athletic trainer can play a role in reducing medication errors. As a checkpoint beyond the physician and pharmacist, the athletic trainer can ensure that the patient clearly understands medication-use instructions.

IMPACT OF EXERCISE

The effect of exercise on pharmacodynamics is primarily due to the pharmacokinetics discussed in Chapter 2. In other words, the dose-response effects, as a result of getting the drug to the site of action, depend on the absorption, metabolism, distribution, and excretion parameters. The effect of exercise directly on the pharmacodynamics (ie, the effect on the response from the drug once it is at the site of action) has not been extensively studied in humans. Exercise can affect the number and intrinsic efficacy of some receptors, such as β-adrenergic receptors, but the varied impact on the pharmacokinetic parameters deters any conclusive statement regarding therapeutically significant changes in the pharmacodynamics due to exercise.

Exercise is a component of nondrug therapy for treatment of some conditions such as diabetes mellitus, hypertension, cardiovascular disease, and arthritis. Theoretically, therefore, exercise should contribute to the effectiveness of the drugs used to treat these diseases. Yet, due to a change in multiple parameters, there is little evidence that exercise alone will improve the disease to the extent that a reduction in drug therapy is predictable. Complicating the picture of exercise effects on pharmacodynamics is that exercise alters the release of some endogenous hormone and neurotransmitters, which may alter the pharmacokinetics and pharmacodynamics of some drugs.

CASE STUDY

As the athletic trainer working at a Division III university, Susan is meeting with a women's golf team member. Patricia injured her back during a tournament last weekend and was instructed by the physician to take Nalfon, an anti-inflammatory drug, 4 times per day. Patricia reports that she doesn't feel the medication helps her much but she also admits that she usually remembers to take the drug only in the morning and has taken it 4 times a day only once over the past several days. What should Susan do in this situation?

BIBLIOGRAPHY

Brazeau DA, Brazeau GA. *Principles of the Human Genome and Pharmacogenomics*. Washington, DC: American Pharmacists Association; 2011.

Kuntz JL, Safford MM, Singh JA, et al. Patient-centered interventions to improve medication management and adherence: a qualitative review of research findings. *Patient Educ Couns*. 2014;97:310-326.

Seden K, Dickinson L, Khoo S, Back D. Grapefruit-drug interactions. *Drugs*. 2010;70:2373-2407.

CHAPTER 4: ADVANCE ORGANIZER

Use of Medications in the Athletic Training Room

- Over-the-Counter Medications
- Over-the-Counter Unit Dose
- Prescription Drugs
- Controlled Substances
- Compounded Pharmaceuticals
- Samples

Administering, Dispensing, and Treating

- Administering
- Dispensing
- Treating (Therapeutic Intervention)

Personnel, Authorizations, and Agents of Record

- Team Physicians
- Physician Licensing
- Athletic Training Staff
- Athletic Training Students
- Pharmacy Authorization
- Treatment Authorization
- Patient Authorization
- Unsecured Medication Authorization

Regulatory Agencies

- State Versus Federal Regulation
- General Interpretation of Regulatory Issues

Historical Perspective of Regulations

- Federal Agencies and Legislative Acts

Policies and Procedures

- Expired Medications
- Security
- Storage
- Refrigerated Medications
- Audit and Reconciliation
- Recordkeeping
- Signage
- Drug Enforcement Administration Requirements
- Practice Sites in Other Geographical Locations
- Traveling With Medications
  - International Travel

Chapter Summary

4

Medication Management in an Athletic Training Facility

Alan D. Freedman, MEd, ATC

Chapter Objectives

At the end of this chapter, the reader will be able to:

- Differentiate between an administered dose, dispensed dose, and treatment (or therapeutic intervention)

- Differentiate between over-the-counter (OTC) medications, prescription drugs, controlled substances, compounded pharmaceuticals, and drug samples; and explain pertinent regulations regarding each

- Write policies and procedures to meet state and federal laws regarding dispensing, administering, storing, packaging, labeling, and transporting of medications

- Explain the role of state and federal regulations regarding prescription medications

- Explain the role of various federal agencies in the regulation of medications

- Locate federal regulations that are pertinent to the dispensing, administering, storing, packaging, labeling, and transporting of medications

- Explain the relationship between team physician and athletic training staff regarding the use and storage of medications

- Differentiate between discretionary and nondiscretionary decisions

- Develop guidelines associated with domestic and international travel

ABBREVIATIONS USED IN THIS CHAPTER	
CAATE. Commission on Accreditation of Athletic Training Education	**OSHA.** Occupational Safety and Health Administration
DEA. Drug Enforcement Administration	**OTC.** over-the-counter
FDA. Food and Drug Administration	**Rx.** prescription

The roles and responsibilities of the certified athletic trainer have expanded and become more clearly defined over the past several years. It is the expectation of athletes, coaches, administrators, and the public that athletes return to competition as quickly as possible. To address the ongoing advancement in athletic training, many states have passed legislation to update state practice acts so that laws reflect the current practice of athletic training. The ultimate goal of the athletic trainer is to appropriately and

Houglum JE, Harrelson GL, Seefeldt TM.
Principles of Pharmacology for Athletic Trainers, Third Edition (pp 61-73).
© 2016 Taylor & Francis Group.

safely provide a standard of care, based in scientific principle, so that the athlete can return to practice and competition at the pre-injury/illness level. The standards of care are rapidly changing, expanding, and evolving. This has occurred because of the following:

- Changes to the educational proficiencies and competencies. Educational reform in athletic training has identified and addressed the need to better prepare athletic training students from a didactic and clinical application perspective as opposed to superficial information or personal experience. By having a working knowledge, sound and effective therapeutic interventions can be implemented. There is a need to progress from focusing on signs, symptoms, and diagnoses to more evidence-based principles and rationales as to how medication can operationally be used as an effective modality.

- Changes in, and the development of, official position statements, new technologies, and new scientific discoveries. The National Athletic Trainers' Association has developed a comprehensive consensus statement that serves as an excellent guideline in establishing and implementing policies and procedures with regard to the proper management of medication in the athletic training room.

Just as when performing a musculoskeletal evaluation, the same systematic approach needs to be used when considering the use of medications as a viable therapeutic intervention in providing care to an athlete.

USE OF MEDICATIONS IN THE ATHLETIC TRAINING ROOM

It is the expectation of all stakeholders of an athletic program that the care athletes receive will be expedited with efficiency and accuracy. Most athletic training facilities are multipurpose health care clinics that have designated areas for providing triage, rehabilitation, counseling, hydrotherapy, and general medical treatment. A common practice in athletic training is to facilitate an athlete's care with the use of medications. It is important for the athletic trainer to possess an understanding of the indications, contraindications, therapeutic effects, adverse effects, and dosages of these medications. Most importantly, the athletic trainer must possess the ability to exercise sound clinical judgment (within their scope of practice) in the use of any medication. Although athletic trainers need to have a working knowledge of the medications their athletes are taking, high quality care requires they have knowledge of how medications are used, stored, and labeled.

Over-the-Counter Medications

OTC medications can be purchased without a prescription and are not considered a food or dietary supplement. OTC medications are regulated by the US Food and Drug Administration (FDA). If the athletic trainer is asked by the athlete for a recommendation of an OTC medication, athletic trainers need to exercise caution in making a recommendation so that any discussion does not go beyond his or her scope of practice. Athletic training facilities should establish and maintain written protocols for the recommendations of OTC medications. These protocols should be written and approved by the team physician, athletic training staff, athletic administration, and the Office of Risk Management. A drug usage log should contain the athlete's name, date of service, name of medication, strength, dosage form, quantity, purpose, and initials of the athletic trainer and athlete. Athletic trainers must act within their scope of practice for athletic training at all times. The scope of practice is determined by the laws governing the practice of athletic training in a particular state as well as the Role Delineation Study published by the Board of Certification, Inc (www.bocatc.com).

Although athletic trainers are involved with medications on a routine basis, the following precautions must be considered in the event that the athlete has questions or a medical condition arises and information is requested by a hospital or other medical facility:

- Starting dose
- Frequency of the dosing
- Medication taken with or without food
- Photosensitivity
- Interactions with other medications

Over-the-Counter Unit Dose

OTC medications should not be left on the athletic training room counters in bulk containers for the athletes to help themselves whenever they think they need medication to cure their ills. In addition to creating recordkeeping and potential therapy problems, this can lead to cross-contamination from athletes pouring medications into their hands and then repouring them back into the container. Almost 90% of all OTCs are available as unit dose packs. A unit dose pack is designed as an administered dose and is prelabeled to meet the requirements of the FDA and the Occupational Safety and Health Administration (OSHA). Single-dose packs pose a budgeting issue because they are usually more expensive, yet the cost can be justified in that it is more hygienic and easier to regulate what is dispensed.

Prescription Drugs

Prescription medications must be prescribed by a physician, bought at a pharmacy, prescribed for and intended to be used by one person, and regulated by the FDA. The FDA stipulates that any container for prescription medications prior to dispensing must carry the designation "Rx only" on the label (see Figure 1-2). Even if it has been used in the athletic training room for years, if it bears the mark "Rx only," it must be considered a prescription drug and treated as such according to state and federal laws.

Controlled Substances

Controlled substances are prescription drugs the US Drug Enforcement Administration (DEA) has determined to be "drugs of abuse" or "drugs of potential abuse." The medications are placed into 5 separate schedules (see Table 1-7). As a general rule, controlled substances should not be stored in the athletic training room at any time. If the team physician deems it necessary to treat an athlete's condition with a controlled substance, a prescription must be written and filled at a pharmacy.

Compounded Pharmaceuticals

A *compounded pharmaceutical* is prepared from raw components in the pharmacy (Figure 4-1). Although all pharmacists are licensed to compound, it has become such a specialty that training and experience can make quite a difference in the effectiveness and quality of the compounded product. The athletic trainer should check the qualifications of the pharmacy if the team physician wishes to use compounded products. Never accept unsolicited compounded products that are mailed by a pharmacy directly to your athletic training facility. According to the FDA, any compounded product is a prescription drug and all regulations must be followed. There is no such thing as a "sample" compounded pharmaceutical. Compounded products may be extremely helpful in sports medicine and are used by many organizations.

Samples

Sample medications, which would require a prescription if filled by the athlete, are sometimes considered trivial or not as regulated. However, they are prescription medications (there can be OTC sample medications) and are governed by state and federal laws and enforced by the FDA. Sample medications are placed in small packages because they are designed to be administered doses. There are very specific guidelines that must be followed whenever sample medications are dispensed or administered by the physician (Box 4-1).

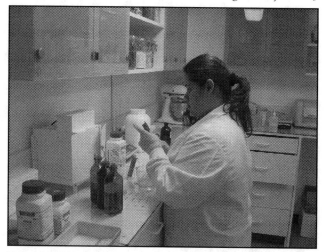

Figure 4-1. Compounded pharmaceuticals. All pharmacists are licensed to compound; however, it has become such a specialty that training and experience can make quite a difference in the effectiveness and quality of the compounded product.

ADMINISTERING, DISPENSING, AND TREATING

There are 3 ways in which medications can be delivered by the physician. Each way has a clear regulatory definition (Box 4-2). Medications can be administered, dispensed, or used as a treatment option when providing a therapeutic intervention within athletic training facilities. Because the athletic trainer may deal with athletes of varying heights and weights, and prescribed medications may have recommended dosages that are based on age or body weight, it may be useful to have a standard dosing chart available as a reference guide that is kept in the physician's examination room.

Administering

An *administered dose* is defined by law as a medication given to the athlete that is consumed within 24 hours. Essentially, this is a dose that is intended as a one-time treatment. The labeling requirements for an administered dose are quite different from those of a dispensed dose. According to the FDA, a dose administered by the licensed entity has minimal labeling requirements, such as directions for use and athlete's name, yet still must adhere to the same recordkeeping requirements such as inventory, reconciliation, and drug usage logs. There are tangible reasons why manufacturer samples come in such small quantities. Although it seems wasteful to have excessive packaging for 2 small tablets/capsules in one small container, it stands to reason that a sample is designed by law to serve as an administered dose. However, if the physician grabs a handful of sample containers, the medication now becomes a

---

Box 4-1

GUIDELINES FOR DISPENSING OR ADMINISTERING SAMPLE MEDICATIONS BY A PHYSICIAN

1. A pedigree or chain of custody must exist. A pedigree is a receipt that must be supplied by the licensed entity or person delivering the sample medications to the receiving entity or person. The receipt must include the name of physician or manufacturer representative delivering and receiving, the name of the medication, the strength, the dosage form, the quantity, the lot number, the expiration date, the date of transfer, and the signatures of the physicians. The concept behind a pedigree is that the FDA inspector should be able to follow the trail of the sample medication from the manufacturer to the end user.

2. A separate audit and reconciliation must be maintained. The FDA requires a separate audit and reconciliation for all sample medications, which shall account for each and every dose and dosage form being received and administered or dispensed by the physician's office or athletic training facility.

3. Samples must be stored separately from other prescription drugs. Samples must be stored in a locked and secured cabinet separate from all other prescription drugs and controlled substances because they are not labeled in advance and can only be administered directly by the physician.

Box 4-2

DIFFERENCE AMONG ADMINISTERED DOSE, DISPENSED DOSE, AND TREATMENT

DELIVERY MECHANISM	DEFINITION
Administered dose	A medication given to a patient as a one-time dose that is consumed within 24 hours
Dispensed dose	An amount of medication to be consumed by the patient over > 24 hours
Treatment (therapeutic intervention)	Medications applied or injected within the athletic training facility

---

Box 4-3

INFORMATION REQUIRED ON LABEL AND IN DISPENSING LOG

- Patient name
- Date of service
- Physician name
- Medication name
- Strength
- Dosage form
- Quantity
- Expiration date
- Lot number
- Initials of medical assistant recording data and initials of the dispensing physician
- Address of the athletic training facility where the medications were dispensed

---

dispensed dose and must be labeled and recorded according to state and federal dispensing laws.

Dispensing

A *dispensed dose* is an amount of medication to be consumed by the athlete over more than 24 hours and includes the interpretation of the prescription order. This is usually the case with prescription medications such as antibiotics and anti-inflammatory drugs. The best method of delivery for a dispensed dose in athletic training facilities is a therapeutic dose pack, which is packaged by a licensed FDA repackager to be used in an appropriate course of therapy. The FDA requires that any entity that packages medications in advance for anyone other than the patient must obtain licensure to do so. An athletic training facility, student health center, local pharmacy, or hospital should not package their therapeutic dose packs for physician dispensing unless they are licensed by the FDA to repackage. All dispensed doses are subject to state and federal laws for packaging, labeling, and recordkeeping requirements. The label and dispensing log must contain the information contained in Box 4-3.

Treating (Therapeutic Intervention)

Finally, a medication can be administered as a treatment (therapeutic intervention). Because the treatment is applied or injected within the athletic training facility, there are

Date	Name of Athlete	Sport	Medication and Strength	Amount Dispensed	ATC	Prescribing Physician	Time Medication Administered
10/26	Sara Smith	Women's Basketball	Amoxicillin 500 mg	20	AF	Dr. Jones	4:30 pm

Figure 4-2. An example of a form with necessary information that must be completed when any medication is given.

Date	
Diagnosis	
Medication	
Strength and dosage	
Duration	
Prescribing physician	

Figure 4-3. An example of a form with necessary information that should be kept in an athlete's medical record.

no labeling requirements; however, all records must still be maintained. *Treatments* are either injections used during a surgical or medical procedure or medications applied according to the physician's prescription for iontophoresis or phonophoresis as part of an ongoing treatment plan. When any medication is provided for an athlete, the appropriate documentation needs to occur (Figure 4-2) and the documentation log kept in a secure location.

In addition to having a general medication log, a record should be kept of medications that have been prescribed to each athlete and placed in a designated section of his or her medical record (Figure 4-3). This fundamental step in the documentation process ensures the accuracy of the care being provided to the athletes. This can be useful in the event that athletes are competing in organizations that have strict guidelines about what medications are allowed to be taken while competing. Additionally, this documentation can be a valuable reference in the event of a positive drug test to show what medications athletes have been taking.

PERSONNEL, AUTHORIZATIONS, AND AGENTS OF RECORD

Team Physicians

Anytime there are medications stored in an athletic training facility, there must be a licensed physician who accepts responsibility for the medications. This is required if there is only one medication, such as an inhaler or EpiPen for emergencies, or an entire dispensary that contains medications that are dispensed by the physician in the athletic training room. All medications ordered, received, stored, dispensed, and/or administered to the athlete are the legal responsibility of the licensed physician providing care.

Physician Licensing

Most physicians maintain a DEA registration to prescribe controlled substances. However, the DEA requires an additional and separate registration for all locations where controlled substances are ordered, received, stored, administered, and dispensed. In some cases, a team physician will maintain up to 5 or 6 separate DEA registrations, depending on the number of teams and organizations he or she is representing. In some states, a state-controlled substance license is required in addition to the DEA registration. To ensure that a facility is in full compliance with state and federal law, it is recommended that appropriate regulatory agencies are consulted on an ongoing basis.

Athletic Training Staff

The athletic training staff needs to have a working knowledge of the various medications that athletes may take so that sound clinical decisions can be made. This includes an understanding of indications, contraindications, effects, and

---

BOX 4-4

INFORMATION THAT MUST BE DOCUMENTED WHEN ANY IONTOPHOREIS OR PHONOPHORESIS TREATMENT IS GIVEN

- Name and strength of medication
- Amount of medication used
- Type of modality
- Date of treatment
- Name of the athletic trainer
- Name of the authorizing physician
- Amount of time for the treatment

---

dosing parameters. In some instances, the team physician, who is responsible for supervising the athletic training staff, is not employed by the university, professional team, or institution. Likewise, the athletic training staff is not usually employed by the team physician. In most cases, the institution pays for the medications and medical supplies that are used by the physician within the athletic training facility. Therefore, the physician must implement a strict agency of authorization for all individuals working within the facility. The agency statements should reflect the nondiscretionary decisions and actions to be performed by the athletic training staff and should include the following:

- Authorization to forward prescription orders on behalf of the physician
- Authorization to access the medication cabinet for purposes of inventory control and recordkeeping
- Authorization to assist the physician with nondiscretionary decisions
- A statement to the fact that this agency is created in the best medical interest of the athletes according to the physician

The agency statement should be signed annually and updated as necessary by all practicing team physicians and all athletic trainers acting as agents for the physicians.

Athletic Training Students

Commission on Accreditation of Athletic Training Education–accredited athletic training education programs require athletic training students to gain real-life experience under the direct supervision of certified athletic trainers who are appropriately credentialed within their respective states or under the supervision of other state-licensed allied health professionals. At no time should it be left to the discretion of the athletic training student to administer or dispense

any medication to athletes. It is important to note that athletic training students do not have a legally defined scope of practice, and therefore these types of responsibilities should not be delegated by the athletic trainer.

Pharmacy Authorization

The team physician must sign a separate annual acknowledgment directed to the pharmacy designating which members of the medical staff are authorized to forward prescription orders on the physician's behalf. The document must also contain the exact physical address of the athletic training facility where the medications will be sent.

Treatment Authorization

In most athletic training facilities, the athletic trainer decides when to use iontophoresis or phonophoresis according to the standing orders and protocols of the athletic health care team. Because these treatments involve the use of prescription medications, state and federal regulations must be followed and written authorization must be obtained from the physician according to established protocol. The parameters of the treatment need to be documented and are included in Box 4-4.

In some states, these treatments have been recognized specifically in law, and every individual treatment prescription must be in the patient's name. Because iontophoresis and phonophoresis involve the use of prescription medications, these forms of treatment should be implemented by the athletic trainer and not delegated to a student.

Patient Authorization

It is prohibited by law for anyone to pick up a prescription for someone other than immediate family unless he or she has been granted permission in writing. The pharmacy is responsible for ensuring this procedure. In many cases, the athletic training staff will act on behalf of the athlete by either picking up medications at the local pharmacy or signing for deliveries of medications. Each year, athletes should sign an authorization granting permission to specific members of the athletic training staff to forward prescription orders, receive, pick up, secure, store, travel with, and/or administer medications that have been prescribed and dispensed for them by a licensed physician.

Unsecured Medication Authorization

Under certain circumstances, there may be a need for prescription medication to be left in an unsecured location of the athletic training facility. Federal law specifically states that all medications are to be locked and secured. However, in the practice of medicine, the physician may want certain medications available for emergency reasons or treatments and may therefore choose to store them in an unsecured area. If this situation arises in the athletic training facility, it is a discretionary decision of the physician that is documented in writing. This documentation must list the medication to be left unsecured and the reason for the request; it should be signed by the physician, maintained on file, and renewed annually. Some of the medications most commonly stored in this way are ethyl chloride, silver sulfadiazine, albuterol (inhaler), sodium chloride (for irrigation), Bactroban, EpiPen, and dexamethasone.

REGULATORY AGENCIES

The purpose of regulatory agencies is to protect the consumer and the public from the unlawful production, use, and distribution of certain medications. The concerns of these regulatory entities include issues relating to drug diversion, negligence, licensure, and wrongful medical practice. Through the enforcement of regulations written by legislatures and consumer boards, regulatory agencies ensure the provision of health care by qualified practitioners. There are instances where there is no specific language addressing regulatory issues either at the state or federal level with regard to athletic training, although states are engaging in legislation to address this concern. It is vital for the athletic trainer to understand the laws that govern each allied health profession and conform to each state's respective practice act. The laws provide the guidelines needed to establish standards of practice with respect to administering and dispensing medications, as well as the required documentation associated with this practice. To prevent and eliminate any discrepancy as to working within one's scope of practice, national and state bodies governing athletic training are often proactive in establishing policies and standards of practice.

State Versus Federal Regulation

State and federal regulations for prescription medications are closely aligned. If state and federal laws are in conflict, the licensed professional should follow the more restrictive regulation. Most state laws are directed toward physicians who are dispensing for profit to the general population, which may create a conflict of interest or competition with local pharmacies. Only a few states, including Ohio, South Carolina, Virginia, California, and Florida, have acknowledged that medical practice exists in athletic training facilities. Federal and state laws are consistent when the physician is dispensing or administering directly to his or her patients in a closed environment. It is illegal for an athletic trainer to dispense medication, although there is some variability in state laws

regarding the administration of nonprescription medication in a single-dose pack by licensed health providers.

General Interpretation of Regulatory Issues

When a regulatory agency is investigating an alleged drug-related mismanagement complaint, it will need to determine who has made discretionary vs nondiscretionary decisions. The persons making discretionary decisions must be licensed to do so. Within the athletic training facility, discretionary decisions such as diagnosing, prescribing, dispensing, treating, and administering can only be made by the physician and may not be delegated to unlicensed personnel. An illustration of the discretionary decision process is as follows:

1. The diagnosis of the patient is considered a discretionary decision. In some cases, the team physician may contact the athletic trainer and discuss the condition of the athlete. The physician may want to review previous medications the athlete has used and may rely on the athletic trainer for evaluation. However, the physician must make the final assessment for the medical diagnosis.

2. After making the medical diagnosis, the physician may make the discretionary decision of prescribing a medication or treatment. The physician may ask the athletic trainer which medications the athlete has taken in the past (OTC/prescription). The athletic trainer may help identify possible allergies, yet the choice of which medication to be administered or dispensed must be made by the physician. When physicians are dispensing or administering medications from their own office or practice location, they are not required to write a prescription, although they must keep an accurate record of the transaction. A written prescription is required when a licensed entity other than the physician is dispensing the medication. Part of the definition of dispensing is the interpretation of a prescription order.

3. The dispensing or administering of medications is considered a discretionary decision. Only a physician or other duly licensed authorized person, such as a pharmacist, nurse practitioner, or physician assistant, is allowed to dispense or administer medications. The athletic trainer may assist in nondiscretionary roles such as recordkeeping and the labeling process.

A physician may use assistants or medical staff to assist in the process of dispensing under supervision. Recordkeeping, delivery, and minor labeling are among several nondiscretionary decisions appropriate for the athletic trainer to perform. Only the physician can make the final decision and authorize the medication to the patient.

BOX 4-5	
FUNCTION OF FEDERAL AGENCIES IN REGULATING MEDICATIONS	
AGENCY	FUNCTION
Food and Drug Administration (FDA)	Responsible for overseeing and regulating the manufacturing, repackaging, and relabeling of prescription drugs. The FDA also regulates sample medication and is responsible for the enforcement of regulation resulting from food, dietary supplements, injuries, and complaints
Drug Enforcement Administration (DEA)	Oversee licensure and certification of all locations where controlled substances are ordered, received, stored, administered, or dispensed
Occupational Safety and Health Administration (OSHA)	Responsible for public safety regarding contamination, storage, disposal, and public exposure to medication risks
Federal Trade Commission (FTC)	Responsible for regulating medications transported over state lines that have not yet been prescribed and/or dispensed to the patient

HISTORICAL PERSPECTIVE OF REGULATIONS

Federal Agencies and Legislative Acts

Several federal agencies are responsible for different functions related to the regulation of medications (see Chapter 1). These include the FDA, DEA, OSHA, and the Federal Trade Commission. The function of each of these organizations is outlined in Box 4-5.

There are also numerous federal legislative acts designed to regulate medication control and distribution. Table 4-1 shows a chronological time line of creation and implementation based on changes in society and in the practice of medicine. Box 4-6 highlights specific federal regulations pertinent to athletic training facilities.

POLICIES AND PROCEDURES

A policies and procedures manual should be kept current and on file. This manual should be reviewed and revised annually by a committee consisting of the team physician(s), the athletic training staff, representatives from the athletic administration, and the institution's Office of Risk Management. The purpose of this manual is to clearly define all aspects of the practice and operations of the athletic training facility. Every athletic training facility will have its own separate and unique policies and procedures. However, the general concepts mentioned in this chapter should be consideration for inclusion in the manual.

Expired Medications

There is no justification for expired medications being stored in a facility or being administered or dispensed to an athlete. Expired medications must be removed from the active supplies and disposed properly. The medication name, strength, dosage form, quantity, lot number, and expiration date and the initials of the staffperson doing the recording should be noted. A copy of the log should accompany the prescription medications to the outside agency contracted to handle their destruction. OTC medications that are expired should be disposed in a biohazard waste container. Expired prescription and OTC medications should not be flushed down a toilet.

Security

According to state and federal laws, all medications must be stored in a locked and secured cabinet or container. There are no specific laws to define secure; it is left up to the licensed professional to determine what is considered reasonable. Accordingly, "Rx Only" medications should not be unsecured on an athletic training room counter. If the athletic training facility maintains medications that must be refrigerated, the refrigerator must have a lock and should be in a secure area with limited access. All access to keys or combination locks to the medical cabinet or locations where medications are stored and secured must be included in the policies and procedures manual. The team physician(s) must specifically identify and authorize by signature which staff members are granted access. This authorization should be kept on file and maintained in a readily retrievable format for at least 3 years. All necessary precautions need to be taken to ensure that only authorized personnel have keys to these storage areas.

	TABLE 4-1	
FEDERAL ACTS RELATED TO MEDICATION CONTROL AND DISTRIBUTION		
DATE	**ACT**	**PURPOSE**
1938	Federal Food, Drug and Cosmetic Act (FDCA) (52 Stat, 1040; 21USC 301 et al)	Established to regulate the safety, quality, purity, strength, and labeling of drugs
1951	Humphrey Amendment	Enacted in 1951 and took effect in 1952. This amendment established 2 classes of drugs by differentiating between prescription and non-prescription or OTC medications
1962	Good Manufacturing Practice (GMP) Regulations	Established by the Kefauver-Harris Amendment, which required all repackaging operations to meet minimum standards for the repack-aging of medications
1970	Federal Comprehensive Drug Abuse Prevention and Control Act	Regulated the manufacture, distribution, and dispensing of drugs that have a potential of abuse. Registration with the DEA is required to legally assume any of these responsibilities
1970	Poison Prevention Act	Passed to regulate the packaging of prescription and nonprescription drugs in child-resistant safety containers
1983	Federal Anti-Tampering Act	Established to mandate tamper-resistant packaging on all nonprescription drugs
1983	Fair Packaging and Labeling Act	Mandated labeling of contents of nonprescription drugs to assist con-sumers in identifying similar products
1987	Prescription Drug Marketing Act	Mandated the accountability of sample drugs from the manufacturer to the physician to the end user
1988	Anti-Drug Abuse Act	Reclassified anabolic steroids as controlled substances
1990	Omnibus Reconciliation Act (OBRA 90)	Mandated drug review, patient medication records, and verbal patient education as part of the dispensing of prescription medications
2003	Health Insurance Portability and Accountability Act (HIPAA)	Mandated the protection of patient information and confidentiality by all health practitioners involved with protected health information

Storage

Most medications must be stored at room temperature and in a dry environment. They should be stored in containers that allow for easy identification of the labeling. Controlled substances must be stored separately from all other prescription drugs. Each facility must decide if controlled substances will be kept on site; it is advisable to avoid this practice. Medications should be stored in a secured and locked location within the athletic training facility with access being granted to a small number of people.

Refrigerated Medications

All medications, including those that require refrigeration, must be locked and secured. If there are vaccines or injections that require refrigeration, the refrigerator must be located in the licensed area at all times. Refrigerator temperatures should be checked and documented on a regular basis to ensure that the medication(s)

are stored at the correct temperature. The temperature of the refrigerator should be calibrated and certified with the other therapeutic modalities on a yearly basis. It is a violation of federal and state law to store food or other nonpharmaceutical items in the same refrigerator as medications.

Audit and Reconciliation

All medications should be completely audited and reconciled at least once a year. This includes every dose and dosage form dispensed or administered. The audit should balance and the data maintained on file in a readily retrievable format for a period of 3 years.

Recordkeeping

It is imperative that all administered and dispensed medications be documented (see Figure 4-2). It is the responsibility of the licensed professional to maintain

---

Box 4-6

FEDERAL REGULATIONS SPECIFIC TO THE MANAGEMENT OF PRESCRIPTION MEDICATIONS IN THE ATHLETIC TRAINING FACILITY

PRESCRIPTION DRUG MARKETING ACT

- 21 CFR 5.115—Sample medication control
- 21 CFR 1301.23(1)—DEA certificate required for separate locations
- 21 C.F.R. 1301.75—Storage of controlled substances
- 21 C.F.R. 1301.44—DEA certificate readily retrievable
- 21 C.F.R. 1301.90—Security of personnel for handling of controlled substances
- 21 C.F.R. 1304.4—Recordkeeping requirements for controlled substances
- 21 C.F.R. 1304.02(d)—Defines a physician who prescribes, administers, and dispenses controlled substances
- 21 C.F.R. 1304.11-12(b)—Inventory requirements for controlled substances
- 21 C.F.R. 1304.13—Reconciliation requirements for controlled substances
- 21 C.F.R. 1305.12—Reporting a theft of a controlled substance
- 21 C.F.R. 1301.92—Responsibility to report drug diversion

FOOD, DRUG, AND COSMETIC ACT

- 21 U.S.C. 360(g)—Requirement to utilize a FDA-licensed pharmacy repackager
- 21 U.S.C. 353(b)(2)—Labeling of prescription medications

POISON PREVENTION PACKAGING ACT

- 15 U.S.C. 1471—Packaging of controlled substances and prescription medications
- 15 U.S.C. 1473 (b)—Exception to PPPA for prescriber dispensing of non-child safety container

FEDERAL CONTROLLED SUBSTANCE ACT

- 21 U.S.C., 824(a)(f)—DEA certificate required
- 21 U.S.C. 802(10)—Prescriber dispensing
- 21 U.S.C. 823 (f)—DEA certificate required for separate locations
- 21 U.S.C. 802(10)—Defines a dispensing physician versus an individual practitioner
- 21 U.S.C. 827(c) (1) (A) (B)—Acquisition and disposition recordkeeping requirements for individual practitioners dispensing controlled substances

---

accurate and up-to-date records. The team physician is required by law to maintain all prescription data in a readily retrievable location for 3 years. These data should include the athlete's name; date of service; Rx number; physician name; medication name, strength, dosage form, quantity, expiration date, and lot number; initials of the staff member; and initials of the physician. The records must also show a complete audit and reconciliation of all medications used within the athletic training facility. Auditing and reconciling should be done on no less than an annual basis.

Basic records should include copies of all licenses for physicians, pharmacies, and waste disposal companies. Inventory records should include invoices, drug use logs, reconciliation reports, separate controlled substance inventories, return drug reports, sample receipt logs and use, and copies of any agency statements made by the physician. Records must be kept in storage for a minimum of 3 years and must be readily retrievable at all times.

Signage

Each athletic training facility should have an area or room specifically designated for the team physicians for examination of athletes and the practice of medicine. That room should have proper signage signifying the space as a licensed medical office or clinic. This designated room should also be the site for medication storage.

Drug Enforcement Administration Requirements

The DEA has a few specific regulations for controlled substances that are different from those for prescription drugs. The DEA requires:

- That controlled substances be stored securely and separately from all other prescription drugs

- A biannual inventory of all controlled substances; the inventory must be kept on file in a readily retrievable format

- Any nonlicensed personnel who have been previously convicted of a crime relating to controlled substances to notify the licensed professional who is responsible for the controlled substances of this conviction in writing

- A separate registration for every physical location where controlled substances are received, stored, administered, or dispensed

- Separate records for acquisition and disposition of controlled substances

Practice Sites in Other Geographical Locations

It is not unusual for an organization to operate a summer or spring practice camp in another state. Even if this camp is used for only one month, the licensure laws must be followed. According to most state and federal agencies, if a physician sets up practice for more than 5 days (this is an average; the amount of time can vary from 2 days to 1 week depending on the agency and the inspector answering the question) at a location and stores, dispenses, administers, or receives medications of any kind, he or she is required to license the additional athletic training facility and to maintain a personal license to practice medicine in that state. For example, if an organization is located in New York and has a summer practice camp in Philadelphia, the physician(s) must obtain a license to practice in Pennsylvania, or the organization must affiliate with a local physician licensed to practice medicine in that state. Additionally, a large university may have more than one athletic training facility on campus. Several states have amended practice acts to allow physicians to perform their functions when traveling with teams in another state. Athletic trainers should refer to state practice acts and regulatory bodies to determine how they may affect the way services may be provided if traveling to another state.

Traveling With Medications

Traveling with athletic teams is commonplace in athletic training. As a means of preparation, athletic trainers routinely carry all of the necessary equipment and supplies that may be needed on a trip, including medications. It is good practice to do as much advanced planning as possible regarding the local medical contact information when traveling domestically and internationally. Most host athletic trainers or venue organizers have information for visiting teams that include emergency phone numbers and the name and address of local hospitals and pharmacies. Athletic trainers should take the time to review this information in advance. It is also helpful to check with the front desk staff at the hotels in which they are staying because they can provide additional information.

It is generally not a good idea to travel with medications that have not been prescribed for a specific individual. Medications that have not been dispensed and labeled for a specific user must be transported by a licensed individual or become the responsibility of the licensed individual upon reaching the intended destination. Some states have allowed the athletic trainer to transport medications under the condition that he or she has access to a local physician or the team physician who is traveling separately. In other states, such as Ohio, it is prohibited by law for anyone other than the physician to transport medications that are not designated for the end user. In all cases, the medications must be locked and secured at all times. These drugs are the responsibility of the team physician and must be tracked according to established policies and procedures of the athletic training facility.

International Travel

Anytime an athletic team is traveling outside of the United States, several precautions need to be taken to mitigate any potential problems. The organizations listed in Box 4-7 provide relevant, up-to-date information that will help guide travel preparation. State and federal laws do not specifically address international travel; therefore, every effort must be made to follow the policies and procedures of the athletic training facility. When traveling internationally:

- Keep an inventory of all medications that an athlete has been prescribed

  - Maintain multiple copies of this inventory in addition to all travel documents and keep the copies in different locations

  - Record generic and trade names of the medications; generic names are more commonly known internationally than trade names

  - Record the strength and dosage of the tablet being taken because it may not be universal outside of the United States even if it is the same product made by the same company

BOX 4-7	
WEBSITES TO CHECK BEFORE INTERNATIONAL TRAVEL	
AGENCY	WEBSITE
US Department of State	www.travel.state.gov/content/passports/english/go/checklist.html
Transportation Security Administration	www.tsa.gov/traveler-information
Centers for Disease Control and Prevention	www.nc.cdc.gov/travel/page/pack-smart#travelhealthkit
World Health Organization	www.who.int/precautions/medical_conditions/en

- Take digital photographs of the medication labels and the medications themselves
- Separate the medication into 2 containers
  - Pack in separate pieces of luggage in the event that luggage gets lost or delayed, so the athletes are not without their medication; one of the bottles should be kept in the athlete's carry-on baggage
- Carry a letter from the prescribing physician or team physician outlining the athlete's diagnosis, the medication being taken, and any other pertinent information to help expedite the Customs process in the event the medical status of an athlete is questioned

CHAPTER SUMMARY

The use of medications is a common practice in athletics. It is important for athletic trainers to know the federal and state laws that regulate their scope of practice. Federal agencies responsible for different functions related to medications are the FDA, DEA, and OSHA. If there is a conflict in federal and state laws, the more restrictive of the 2 should be followed. The team physician has the legal responsibility of all medications and all discretionary decisions related to diagnosing, prescribing, dispensing, and administering drugs. The physician must have proper licensure in the state in which the team practices.

Additionally, it is illegal for athletic trainers to dispense medication or to use prescription drugs for iontophoresis or phonophoresis without written authorization from a licensed physician. Responsibilities of the athletic training staff relative to medications include assisting the physician, conducting inventory control, participating in the development of policy and procedures manual, and maintaining appropriate records. Basic records should include a copy of the licenses for the physicians, pharmacies, and waste disposal companies; drug use logs; annual medication audit reports; policies and procedures manual; record of athletes receiving or being administered medications; controlled substance inventories; and documentation to authorize drugs to be in an unsecured area.

All drugs must be stored in a locked and secured cabinet or container, whether they are prescription, controlled substances, compounded pharmaceuticals, or samples. Refrigerated medications must be stored in a locked refrigerator with the temperature monitored and no food in the refrigerator. Controlled substances must be stored separately from other prescription drugs. Repackaging of medication must also be according to FDA regulations. Storage, security, and repackaging regulations also apply to drugs in the athletic trainer's kit. Adhering to state and federal regulations is important for the safety, health, and well-being of the athletes.

CASE STUDY

Miranda is a Division I field hockey player who underwent a partial medial meniscectomy on her left knee during the winter break. When she enters the athletic training facility approximately 3 weeks post-op, she is nonweight bearing, has a 20-degree extension lag, is unable to voluntarily contract her quadriceps, has moderate effusion, and reports 7/10 pain at rest. During the initial evaluation, she communicates that she has been unable to do any of the prescribed exercises because of the intense pain. When asked what she has done for the pain, Miranda says that the only thing that relieves her pain is Vicodin taken in conjunction with vodka. She explains that she has been taking the narcotic since she was released from the hospital. When asked how she was able to refill her prescription, Miranda states that she has been sneaking Vicodin from her parents' medicine cabinet and obtaining some more from an athlete in another sport who had some left over from a previous injury. How would you handle this situation?

ACKNOWLEDGMENTS

The chapter author and editors would like to thank Robert Nickell, RPh, FACA, FAPO, for his previous contribution to this chapter in the first and second editions.

BIBLIOGRAPHY

Balka E, Kahnamoui N, Nutland K. Who is in charge of patient safety? Work practice, work processes and utopian views of automatic drug dispensing systems. *Int J Med Inform.* 2007;76(suppl 1):S48-S57.

Beran RG, Docking J. Travelling with medications. *Aust Fam Physician.* 2007;36(5):349-350.

Boggess BR, Bytomski JR. Medicolegal aspects of sports medicine. *Prim Care.* 2013;40(2):525-535.

Boss M, Campbell D, Carey L, Ragland D. Efficient dispensing of medications by a traveling health care team. *Am J Health Syst Pharm.* 2010;67:1992-1994.

Centers for Disease Control and Prevention. Pack smart. January 13, 2011. http://www.cdc.gov/travel/page/pack-smart#travelhealthkit. Accessed January 30, 2015.

Ciocca M, Stafford H, Laney R. The athlete's pharmacy. *Clin Sports Med.* 2011;30:629-639.

Diehl J, Kinart C, Cohen R, et al. *BOC facility principles.* http://www.bocatc.org/images/stories/resources/facility_safety%202015.pdf. Omaha, NE: Board of Certification, Inc.

Ferguson A, Delaney B, Hardy G. Teaching medication administration through innovative simulation. *Teaching and Learning in Nursing,* 2014;9(2):64-68.

Kahanov L, Abdenour T, Falustick J, Pavlovich M, Swann EH, Walters DR. Consensus statement: Managing prescriptions and non-prescription medication in the athletic training facility. http://www.nata.org/sites/default/files/ManagingMedication.pdf. Accessed January 30, 2015.

Kahanov L, Furst D, Roberts J. Adherence to drug-dispensation and drug-administration laws and guidelines in collegiate athletic training rooms. *J Athl Train.* 2003;38:252.

Kary JM, Lavallee M. Travel medicine and the international athlete. *Clin Sports Med.* 2007;26:489-503.

Lundén J, Vanhanen V, Myllymäki T, Laamanen E, Kotilainen K, Hemminki K. Temperature control efficacy of retail refrigeration equipment. *Food Control.* 2014;45:109-114.

Minguet F, Van Den Boogerd L, Salgado TM, Correr, CJ, Fernandez-Llimos F. Characterization of the medical subject headings thesaurus for pharmacy. *Am J Health Syst Pharm.* 2014;71(22):1965-1972.

Mutie M, Cooper G, Kyle G, Naunton M, Zwar N. Travelling with medications and medical equipment across international borders. *Travel Med Infect Dis.* 2014;12(5):505-510.

Posner J. Clinical pharmacology: the basics. *Surgery (Oxford).* 2002;30(4):174-180.

Ragland D, Campbell D, Boss M, Carey L. Efficient dispensing of medications by a traveling health care team. *Am J Health Syst Pharm.* 2007;67:1992-1996.

Richir MC, Tichelaar J, Geijteman E, de Vries T. Teaching clinical pharmacology and therapeutics with an emphasis on the therapeutic reasoning of undergraduate medical students. *Eur J Clin Pharmacol.* 2008;64(2):217-224.

Transportation Security Administration. Traveler information. www.tsa.gov/traveler-information. Accessed July 19, 2015.

United States Department of State. Traveler's checklist. www.travel.state.gov/content/passports/english/go/checklist.html. Accessed January 30, 2015.

World Health Organization. International travel and health. http://www.who.int/ith/precautions/medical_conditions/en/. Accessed January 30, 2015.

CHAPTER 5: ADVANCE ORGANIZER

Foundational Concepts

- Microorganisms and Terminology
- Categories of Antibiotics
- Antimicrobial Resistance
- Superinfections
- Selection of Antimicrobial and Dosage Regimen
- Respiratory Infections
- Section Summary

Antibacterial Drugs

- Penicillins
- Cephalosporins
- Carbapenems
- Tetracyclines
- Macrolides
- Sulfonamides
- Aminoglycosides
- Fluoroquinolones
- Topical Antibacterial Drugs
- Section Summary

Antifungal Agents

- Antifungal Agents for Systemic Infections
- Antifungal Agents for Superficial Infections
- Section Summary

Antiviral Agents

Antiseptics and Disinfectants

Treatment of Sexually Transmitted Diseases

Role of the Athletic Trainer

5

Drugs for Treating Infections

CHAPTER OBJECTIVES

At the end of this chapter, the reader will be able to:

- Explain the differences among infections caused by bacteria, fungi, or viruses
- Explain the mechanism(s) of action for antimicrobial, antifungal, and antiviral medications
- List and describe the categories of antibiotics
- Describe the process that results in a microorganism becoming resistant to an antibiotic drug
- Explain how superinfections result from antibiotic therapy
- List 3 considerations in prescribing an antibiotic medication
- Discuss the role that antibiotics have in treating upper and lower respiratory infections
- Differentiate between 9 categories of antibiotic drugs
- Explain the differences between superficial and systemic fungal infections
- Summarize the causes, characteristics, and drug regimens for various types of fungal infections
- Indicate the use of antiseptics and disinfectants
- Summarize the role of the athletic trainer for patients who are taking antibiotic medication(s)

ABBREVIATIONS USED IN THIS CHAPTER	
AIDS. acquired immunodeficiency syndrome	**OTC.** over-the-counter
	PABA. para-aminobenzoic acid
CSF. cerebrospinal fluid	
DNA. deoxyribonucleic acid	**RNA.** ribonucleic acid
	Rx. prescription
FDA. Food and Drug Administration	**STD.** sexually transmitted disease
GI. gastrointestinal	**THFA.** tetrahydrofolic acid
HIV. human immunodeficiency virus	
	TI. therapeutic index

This chapter discusses basic information regarding infections and their treatment. Although the focus is on bacterial infections, fungal and viral infections are also discussed. Antimicrobial agents are among the most frequently prescribed drugs, and thus it is important for the athletic trainer to have a clear understanding of the appropriate use of these drugs. Infections such as bacterial respiratory infections or systemic fungal infections have the potential to affect physical performance. Use of the most effective antimicrobial agent at the most effective dosage will allow the athlete to return to optimal performance more quickly.

Houglum JE, Harrelson GL, Seefeldt TM.
Principles of Pharmacology for Athletic Trainers, Third Edition (pp 75-94).
© 2016 Taylor & Francis Group.

FOUNDATIONAL CONCEPTS

Antimicrobial refers to any drug used to treat any microorganism (eg, bacteria, fungi, or viruses). Some principles will be referred to throughout the discussion of antimicrobial agents, including terminology related to the infecting microorganism, microbial resistance, superinfections, selection of antimicrobial drugs, and categorization of antimicrobial drugs.

Microorganisms and Terminology

Bacteria are single-cell organisms that, unlike human cells, contain a rigid outer cell wall in addition to a cell membrane. Although much of the cellular metabolism is similar to human cells, there are significant differences, which are the target of drug therapy. For example, in bacteria, the enzymes and ribosomes required for replication, transcription, and protein synthesis are somewhat different from in human cells. The term *antibiotic* usually refers to a drug used to treat bacterial infections, although the origin of the term is broader and sometimes refers to any antimicrobial agent. *Antibacterial* specifically applies to treatment of bacterial infections. Fungi also contain metabolic processes that are unique from human cells, but some of the differences that exist with bacteria do not exist with fungi. Consequently, it is often more difficult to treat fungal infections without also affecting similar processes in human cells. Viruses can only propagate by using the enzymes and genetic replicating system of the host cell, and thus drugs that target these processes affect human cells. Because there are fewer biochemical processes that are unique to viruses, there are fewer antiviral drugs to treat these infections.

Categories of Antibiotics

As will be discussed later, the most frequently used method of grouping antibiotics is by the chemical structure. Penicillins, tetracyclines, and sulfonamides ("sulfa drugs") are examples of three classes of antibacterial agents that are based on chemical structure. Another classification is by mechanism of action, such as drugs that inhibit the synthesis of the bacterial cell wall, alter the integrity of the cell membrane, inhibit protein synthesis, inhibit nucleic acid synthesis, and inhibit utilization of nutritional compounds.

A broader categorization classifies the drug as bactericidal or bacteriostatic. *Bactericidal* refers to a drug that kills bacteria, whereas *bacteriostatic* drugs will slow the normal growth rate of the bacteria so that the patient's immune system has a better opportunity to eliminate the infecting organisms. If the patient's immune system is not functioning optimally due to a disease (eg, acquired immunodeficiency syndrome [AIDS]) or use of another drug (eg, an anticancer drug that suppresses the immune system), a bacteriostatic drug may not be effective in treating the

infection. Although occasionally the concentration of drug at the site of action will determine whether an antibiotic is bactericidal or bacteriostatic, usually the mechanism of action is the determining factor. For example, antibiotics that inhibit cell wall synthesis are bactericidal, whereas those that act solely by inhibiting protein synthesis are typically bacteriostatic.

Another means of grouping antibiotics is according to their spectrum of activity: narrow vs broad spectrum. *Narrow-spectrum* drugs are effective against a smaller number of similar organisms; *broad-spectrum* drugs are effective against a larger number of organisms of a more varied grouping. For example, narrow-spectrum antibacterial drugs may be effective against a few gram-positive organisms, whereas a broad-spectrum antibacterial drug may be effective against several gram-negative and gram-positive bacteria.

> *A Gram stain (named after Christian Gram) is a relatively simple laboratory test to determine whether the bacteria being tested will retain a certain dye. Whether the bacteria retains the dye (gram-positive) or not (gram-negative) is dependent upon the chemical structure of the bacterial cell wall. The Gram stain test quickly eliminates many bacteria as the cause of the infection and narrows the choices of potentially effective antibiotics. For example, a test result confirming the presence of gram-negative bacteria eliminates all antibiotics that are not effective against gram-negative bacteria.*

Table 5-1 illustrates various means of categorizing antimicrobial drugs. It should be noted that not even broad-spectrum antibacterial drugs are effective against fungi or viruses; antifungal agents are generally only effective against fungi, and antiviral agents are only effective against viruses. Consequently, it is ineffective to use antibacterial drugs such as penicillin to treat viral infections such as the common cold or flu.

Antimicrobial Resistance

If a microorganism is sensitive (ie, susceptible) to an antimicrobial drug, the drug is effective in treating infections caused by that microorganism. If a microorganism that was sensitive to an antimicrobial agent becomes less sensitive or loses its sensitivity, the organism has become resistant to the drug. The terms *sensitive*, *resistant*, and *susceptible* are referring to the response of the microorganism to the drug; these terms are not referring to the patient and should not be confused, for example, with reference to a patient being sensitive (ie, allergic) to a drug.

Drug resistance develops because of a change in the genetic makeup of microorganisms (Figure 5-1). This

TABLE 5-1				
CLASSIFICATION OF ANTIBIOTICS				
EXAMPLE (GENERIC NAME)	CHEMICAL STRUCTURE	MECHANISM OF ACTION	BACTERICIDAL OR BACTERIOSTATIC	SPECTRUM
amikacin	aminoglycoside	Inhibit protein synthesis and other mechanisms	Bactericidal	Narrow
cephalexin	cephalosporin	Inhibit cell wall synthesis	Bactericidal	Narrow
ciprofloxacin	fluoroquinolone	Inhibit DNA synthesis	Bactericidal	Broad
doxycycline	tetracycline	Inhibit protein synthesis	Bacteriostatic	Broad
erythromycin	macrolide	Inhibit protein synthesis	Bacteriostatic	Narrow
imipenem	carbapenems	Inhibit cell wall synthesis	Bactericidal	Broad
penicillin G	penicillin	Inhibit cell wall synthesis	Bactericidal	Narrow
sulfamethoxazole	sulfonamide	Metabolic inhibitor	Bacteriostatic	Broad

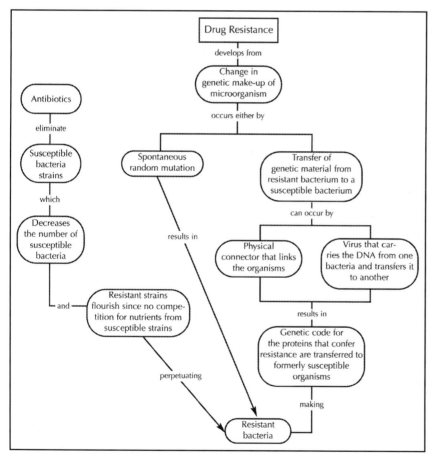

Figure 5-1. Process of developing resistance to antibiotic drug therapy.

change can occur by spontaneous, random mutation, which results in an advantage for the organism. The altered genetics are then passed on to successive generations of the organism. Although mutations are an important cause of resistance in bacteria, it is less common than the transfer of genetic material from a resistant bacterium to a susceptible bacterium. This transfer of genetic material can occur by any one of several mechanisms, including through a physical connector that links the organisms or through a virus that copies the DNA from one bacteria and transfers it to another. Regardless of the mechanism, the genetic material that is transferred contains the genetic code for the protein(s) that confer resistance, thus making a formerly susceptible organism resistant. Because resistance by this mechanism results in the transfer of multiple genes, susceptible bacteria can become resistant to several classes of drugs at the same time.

Overuse of antibiotics promotes the development of resistant strains of microorganisms. As susceptible strains are eliminated by exposure to antibiotics, the resistant strains flourish without the competition for nutrients from the susceptible strains. The existence of more resistant strains increases the likelihood of these strains passing their drug resistance genetic characteristics to other susceptible strains. Overuse of broad-spectrum antibiotics is particularly problematic because they diminish the population of several strains of competing organisms at the same time.

The change in genetic makeup results in resistance by any one of several mechanisms. More than one mechanism may be the cause of resistance to a particular antibiotic.

- Production of an enzyme that inactivates the drug. The β-lactamases comprise a group of enzymes that inactivate some penicillins and cephalosporins by breaking apart a key chemical structure of these antibiotics. These enzymes are also referred to as penicillinases and cephalosporinases. Other antibiotics, such as the aminoglycosides, are also inactivated by bacterial enzymatic action on the antibiotic.

- Altered structure of the target-binding site of the antibiotic. If the DNA of the bacteria codes for an altered structure for the target-binding site, the drug will no longer bind as effectively and thus the activity of the drug will be diminished. Antibiotics such as the macrolides, penicillins, cephalosporins, and fluoroquinolones can be inactivated by this mechanism.

- Altered mechanism for entry of the drug into the microorganism. Some antibiotics enter the microorganism through transport mechanisms such as membrane channels and protein carriers. If the microorganism obtains DNA that codes for altered proteins responsible for the transport process, the rate of entry of the antibiotic into the microorganism will be diminished. Aminoglycosides and tetracyclines are examples of antibiotics to which resistance can develop by this method.

A topic related to antimicrobial resistance is *nosocomial infections*, also called *hospital-acquired infections*. These are infections that a patient contracts while in the hospital or other institution such as a nursing home. Often these infections are acquired from equipment or supplies associated with intravenous infusions, dialysis, catheters, and mechanical ventilators. Because hospitals frequently use antibacterial drugs, the bacteria that survive in the hospital environment are often resistant organisms. Additionally, patients in the hospital setting are typically more severely ill and may have compromised immune responses. Nosocomial infections sometimes pose a serious treatment challenge and may markedly hinder, or even prevent, the patient's recovery.

Superinfections

Superinfections are sometimes also referred to as *supra-infections*. These are infections that develop during the treatment of an initial infection. If the antibiotic used to treat a specific infection also kills a sufficient number of normal flora in the gastrointestinal (GI), respiratory, or urinary tract, for example, the growth of resistant microorganisms will increase. The growth of the resistant strains is normally held in check by the large number of normal flora. The resistant microorganisms may be fungi or bacteria, which are not susceptible to commonly used antimicrobial agents. Broad-spectrum antimicrobials and longer duration of therapy are more likely to cause superinfections because these factors will have a larger impact on the normal flora. For the purpose of minimizing the development of drug resistance and occurrence of superinfections, it is best that the antibiotic selected has the narrowest spectrum possible while simultaneously being effective against the invading microorganism and that the drug therapy not be continued beyond the time necessary to eradicate the microorganism.

Aside from superinfections, another adverse effect that can develop due to disruption of the normal GI flora is diarrhea. Antibiotics with a broad spectrum of activity have a greater propensity for affecting GI flora and thus causing diarrhea, but also antibiotics that are absorbed poorly from the GI tract will have a greater impact on the normal flora. An example is a comparison of the incidence of diarrhea between amoxicillin (Amoxil) and ampicillin (Omnipen). These are 2 penicillins with almost identical antimicrobial activity, but amoxicillin is absorbed more completely after oral administration and also has a lower incidence of diarrhea. It should be noted that there are other causes of antibiotic-induced diarrhea other than disruption of normal flora (eg, direct irritation of the intestine by the tetracyclines).

Selection of Antimicrobial and Dosage Regimen

Selection of an antibiotic should take into consideration the microorganism, the site of the infection, and the patient. Although all of these factors are important, effectiveness of the antibiotic against the infecting organism is the first consideration; if the drug cannot kill or inhibit the growth of the infecting microorganism, it is futile to give the drug to treat that infection.

Ideally, the appropriate antibiotic is determined by identifying the infecting organism and determining which antibiotic the organism is most susceptible to. However, it may be necessary to begin therapy prior to the availability of the identification and susceptibility laboratory results, especially in cases of severe infection. The patient's symptoms will often provide sufficient information for the physician to select an antibiotic that is likely to be effective. For example, most acute ear infections are caused by *Streptococcus pneumoniae*, *Haemophilus influenzae*, or *Moraxella catarrhalis*, and amoxicillin is effective against many strains of all 3 of these organisms. In other situations, the antibiotic can be changed, if necessary, to optimize therapy based on the susceptibility lab results.

The site of the infection may limit the selection of antibiotics available because some of the drugs that are effective against the microorganism may not be able to penetrate to the site of the infection. If the cerebrospinal fluid (CSF) is infected, the antibiotic must cross the blood-brain barrier, and thus antibiotics that have a greater degree of lipid solubility (see Chapter 2) will penetrate more effectively than highly water-soluble antibiotics. However, note that inflammation from bacterial infections increases the penetration of some drugs into the CSF. Similarly, some drugs penetrate lower respiratory tract infections better than others do. Again, drugs that are more lipid soluble penetrate these infected sites more effectively, and thus more readily reach the effective concentration for treating lower respiratory tract infections. Penetration of the antibiotic into the tissue can also be an issue for treating infections of various other tissues such as the heart, urinary tract, or prostate.

Factors regarding the patient must also be considered (eg, drug allergies, pregnancy, age, and existence of other diseases). Although amoxicillin is effective in the treatment of most acute ear infections, an alternative antibiotic must be selected for the penicillin-allergic patient. Some antimicrobial agents cause an increased risk for significant adverse effects to the mother or the unborn child and should be avoided. Tetracyclines can affect developing bones and teeth in young children and should be avoided. Neurological disorders can occur in newborns from the use of sulfonamides, which release bilirubin from protein-binding sites on albumin, thus increasing the concentration of free bilirubin to toxic levels. Antibiotics that are excreted by the kidney or metabolized by the liver must be used with greater caution in patients who also have kidney or liver disease, respectively. Patients being treated for an infection but who also have a compromised immune system, such as patients undergoing cancer chemotherapy or patients with HIV/AIDS, may require bactericidal rather than bacteriostatic antimicrobial agents to eliminate the infecting organism.

The proper dosage regimen is also important for successful eradication of the infecting organism. The dosage and duration of therapy depends on several factors. Higher doses are required if the infected site is difficult for the antibacterial drug to penetrate. Dosage can also vary because all bacteria do not have the same degree of susceptibility to a particular antibacterial drug. The immune defense of some patients is not as effective against some bacteria, and thus a longer duration of therapy may be necessary for

them. As with the treatment of other diseases, poor adherence with the appropriate duration of therapy is a common cause of treatment failure. The patient should clearly understand that all of the doses of the antimicrobial drug should be taken as prescribed. Too often patients discontinue using the drug when they begin to feel better, but unfortunately, the infection may still exist although the symptoms are gone. Discontinuation of the antimicrobial is a common cause of a recurrent infection.

Respiratory Infections

Respiratory tract infections are among the most common reasons patients seek medical attention and are one of the most common groups of illnesses associated with inappropriate drug therapy. Consequently, it is worthwhile to tie together some previously mentioned foundational principles with respect to these infections. Pharyngitis is the most common upper respiratory tract infection. Most cases of pharyngitis are viral infections, and it is often associated with the common cold. Treatment of these viral infections with an antibiotic is a scenario that contributes to the overprescribing of antibiotics. A significant percentage of the antibiotic prescriptions written for patients outside the hospital are unnecessary. Such use of antibiotics is a potential cause of resistant strains and unnecessary adverse drug reactions. Laboratory tests of throat cultures can identify whether the infection is bacterial.

The other 2 most common upper respiratory tract infections, otitis media and sinusitis, are typically bacterial infections, but inappropriate use of antibiotics also occurs when infections at these sites are viral. However, sometimes sinusitis may be difficult to differentiate from allergies or symptoms of the common cold. Sinusitis infections are sometimes caused by bacterial strains that have developed resistance to the first-line antibiotics (from the penicillin category). This necessitates the use of an alternative therapy specific for the resistant organism. Some sinusitis infections become difficult to eradicate and require treatment beyond the usual 10 to 14 days.

The 2 most frequent lower respiratory tract infections are acute bronchitis and pneumonia. Acute bronchitis is usually viral, but bacterial infections also occur. Bacteria are typically the infecting causative organism of pneumonia in adults, whereas viruses are the predominant cause in children. Pneumonia can be life threatening; therefore, appropriate treatment is critical. Because numerous pathogens can be the cause, a broad-spectrum antibiotic is typically used initially until the results of cultures can identify the most effective therapy. As described above, regardless of whether the infection is in the lower or upper respiratory tract, the specific site of the infection, the ability of the drug to penetrate to the site of action, and the patient's medical history must be considered in addition to the susceptibility of the organism to the drug.

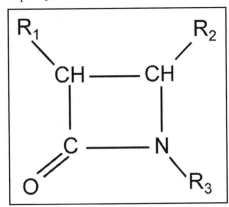

Figure 5-2. The β-lactam ring is a structure common to the penicillins, cephalosporins, and carbapenems. Specific drugs in each of these categories differ from one another by the various chemical groups, designated by R₁, R₂, and R₃, that are attached around the β-lactam ring.

Section Summary

There are several means of categorizing antibacterial drugs, but grouping them by chemical structure is common. Drug resistance refers to a change in the susceptibility of the organism to a particular drug or group of drugs; therefore, drugs that were once effective against the microorganism are no longer effective. This resistance can occur by several mechanisms but always results from a change in the genetic makeup of the microorganism. The development of resistance is a significant problem that hinders effective antimicrobial therapy.

Another problem related to antimicrobial therapy is the development of superinfections, which are secondary infections that occur because of the treatment of the primary infection. Often superinfections result from bacteria or fungi that exist in the body at low levels because of the much larger number of nonpathogenic microorganisms (normal flora) that prevent their growth. As antibiotic therapy reduces the normal flora along with the primary infection, it provides an opportunity for other pathogenic microorganisms to flourish as a superinfection. The potential for superinfections and development of resistant organisms adds to the importance of selecting the appropriate antimicrobial agent for the infection; use of broader spectrum drugs for longer periods enhances the potential for these problems. Therefore, the goal of therapy is to select an antibiotic that most selectively targets the infecting bacteria and minimizes adverse effects at the same time.

ANTIBACTERIAL DRUGS

As would be expected, antibiotics with similar chemical structures are placed in the same category, and the drugs in that category will have some pharmacological and therapeutic similarities. Discussion in this section focuses on these similarities, although some important differences are also mentioned. Discussion is also limited to drugs that are members of antibiotic categories because they encompass the majority of available antibacterial drugs. However, it is noteworthy that there are several other antibiotics that do not fall into these categories and are not discussed.

Penicillins

A drug is categorized as a *penicillin* if it has certain chemical structural components, including a component referred to as a β-lactam ring (Figure 5-2). It is the β-lactam ring that is key to the binding of the penicillin molecule to the active site of the bacteria. However, it is also this ring that makes these antibiotics potentially vulnerable to β-lactamases (penicillinases), enzymes produced by some bacteria that break apart the β-lactam ring, thus imparting resistance to the bacteria. Penicillin G was the first of this group to be discovered when in 1928 it was observed that a mold produced a substance that killed bacteria. After clinical trials, penicillin G became available to the US military in the early 1940s. Although penicillin G was a tremendous discovery, it has some limitations. For example, most of an oral dose is inactivated by stomach acid, it has a narrow spectrum of activity, and it is inactivated by penicillinase. Consequently, chemically modified penicillins have been produced to alleviate these limitations. There are now several penicillins available, and their properties are typically compared with the characteristics of penicillin G (Table 5-2). Some penicillins are more stable to stomach acid (eg, acid-stable), are resistant to penicillinase, or have a broader spectrum of activity. Note the terms *resistant* and *sensitive* are also used to describe the susceptibility of the drug to penicillinase just as they are used to describe the susceptibility of the microorganism to the drug. Thus, a bacteria that is penicillinase producing will be resistant to a penicillinase-sensitive drug (eg, penicillin G), whereas a penicillinase-producing bacteria will be sensitive to a penicillinase-resistant drug (eg, nafcillin).

A few penicillins are available in combination with drugs that have little antibacterial activity but are inhibitors of β-lactamases. Sulbactam, clavulanic acid, and tazobactam are β-lactamase inhibitors that are available together in the same dosage form with some penicillins, such as ampicillin and amoxicillin, which are not β-lactamase resistant. The combination of one of these agents with a penicillin gives the penicillin greater effectiveness against otherwise resistant bacteria.

Penicillin G is the only natural penicillin used therapeutically. It was an impure product when it was first used, and therefore the dose was based on units (U) of biological activity rather than a weight basis. Although penicillin G is now available in pure form, units are often used to designate

TABLE 5-2

SELECTED CHARACTERISTICS OF PENICILLINS

GENERIC NAME	TRADE NAME	ORAL	PENICILLINASE	SPECTRUM
amoxicillin	Amoxil	Yes	Sensitive	Broad
amoxicillin plus clavulanate	Augmentin	Yes	Resistant	Broad
ampicillin	Principen	Yes	Sensitive	Broad
ampicillin plus sulbactam	Unasyn	No	Resistant	Broad
dicloxacillin	Dynapen	Yes	Resistant	Narrow
nafcillin	Unipen	No	Resistant	Narrow
oxacillin	Bactocill	No	Resistant	Narrow
penicillin G	generic	No	Sensitive	Narrow
penicillin V	Pen-Vee K	Yes	Sensitive	Narrow
piperacillin	Pipracil	No	Sensitive	Extended
piperacillin plus tazobactam	Zosyn	No	Resistant	Extended
ticarcillin plus clavulanate	Timentin	No	Resistant	Extended

dose. The approximate conversion is 400,000 U = 250 mg of penicillin G.

The penicillins that are acid stable are more effectively absorbed by the oral route than penicillin G. For example, amoxicillin is more acid stable than either penicillin G or ampicillin, and therefore a larger percentage of an oral dose of amoxicillin is absorbed. The penicillins are excreted rapidly by the kidney through glomerular filtration and tubular secretion. Consequently, concentrations of penicillin are high in the urine.

Penicillins have a high therapeutic index. The most notable adverse effect is the potential for allergic reactions, which occurs in up to 10% of patients, depending on the specific study. Symptoms range from skin rash to life-threatening anaphylaxis. Any of the penicillins can elicit a response in susceptible patients, and thus if a patient is allergic to one penicillin, all of them should be avoided. Previous exposure to a penicillin is necessary for an allergic reaction to occur.

Penicillins are bactericidal drugs. Unlike mammalian cells, bacteria have a high osmotic pressure within the cell and thus have a rigid cell wall that prevents the cell from bursting. Penicillins inhibit the activity of various enzymes that are responsible for the synthesis of the cell wall, thus causing gaps in the cell wall and lysis of the bacteria. These antibiotics are more effective when the bacteria are actively growing and undergoing cell division.

The specific susceptible bacteria vary with each penicillin, and therefore it is advantageous to identify the infecting organism and conduct susceptibility testing. In general, however, penicillins are effective against more gram-positive than gram-negative bacteria. Penicillins generally distribute into most tissue and thus are used to treat

Box 5-1

FACTS ABOUT PENICILLINS

- Contain a β-lactam structure
- Mechanism of action: inhibit cell wall synthesis
- Bactericidal
- Spectrum of activity: narrow to broad; contain subcategories based on increasing spectrum of activity; in general, effective against gram-positive and gram-negative bacteria
- Adverse effects: cause allergic reactions in up to 10% of patients
- Primary uses: infections of urinary tract, respiratory tract, and heart, as well as treating syphilis
- Excretion: primarily urine
- Other notes: most are inactivated by β-lactamases (penicillinases)

susceptible microorganisms that cause infections of various tissues, including the urinary tract, respiratory tract, heart (endocarditis), and middle ear (otitis media), as well as syphilis. Penicillin is also used to prevent recurrences of rheumatic fever and to prevent bacterial endocarditis prior to certain dental and surgical procedures in patients with prosthetic cardiac valves, mitral valve prolapse, history of previous bacterial endocarditis, or rheumatic heart disease (Box 5-1).

TABLE 5-3

SELECTED CEPHALOSPORINS

GENERIC NAME	TRADE NAME	GROUPING	ADMINISTRATION
cefaclor	Ceclor	Second generation	PO
cefadroxil	Duricef	First generation	PO
cefazolin	Ancef	First generation	IM, IV
cefdinir	Omnicef	Third generation	PO
cefditoren	Spectracef	Third generation	PO
cefepime	Maxipime	Fourth generation	IM, IV
cefixime	Suprax	Third generation	PO
cefotaxime	Claforan	Third generation	IM, IV
cefotetan	Cefotan	Second generation	IM, IV
cefoxitin	Mefoxin	Second generation	IM, IV
cefprozil	Cefzil	Second generation	PO
ceftaroline	Teflaro	Fifth generation	IM, IV
ceftazidime	Fortaz	Third generation	IM, IV
ceftibuten	Cedax	Third generation	PO
ceftriaxone	Rocephin	Third generation	IM, IV
cefuroxime	Ceftin, Zinacef	Second generation	IM, IV, PO
cephalexin	Keflex	First generation	PO

IM=intramuscular; IV=intravenous; PO=oral.

Cephalosporins

There are over a dozen cephalosporins available, about twice the number of penicillins. About half are effective by the oral route. Cephalosporins are similar to penicillins in many ways:

- They contain a β-lactam structure
- They inhibit cell wall synthesis
- They are bactericidal
- They have a high therapeutic index
- They are inactivated by β-lactamases (cephalosporinases)
- They cause allergic reactions
- They are excreted primarily by glomerular filtration and tubular secretion
- They contain subcategories based on increasing spectrum of activity

Allergic reactions to cephalosporins occur less frequently than with penicillins, and anaphylaxis is rare. Some cross-reactivity exists between these 2 categories of antibiotics; if a patient is allergic to either the penicillins or cephalosporins, there is an increased likelihood that the patient will also be allergic to the other category. Cross-reactivity is estimated to occur in approximately 3% to 5% of patients allergic to penicillins. Mild allergic reaction to penicillin should not hinder the use of cephalosporins in that patient, but patients who have a severe allergic reaction to penicillins should not be given cephalosporins.

Cephalosporins are grouped as first-generation through fifth-generation drugs. First-generation drugs are effective primarily against gram-positive bacteria. Second-generation drugs are more effective against some gram-negative bacteria and are more likely to be resistant to cephalosporinases. Third-generation cephalosporins are broader spectrum and have increased resistance to cephalosporinases. The fourth-generation continues this trend with broader spectrum of activity and/or better resistance to cephalosporinases. Recently, a fifth-generation agent, ceftaroline, was approved by the US Food and Drug Administration; this agent has activity against a drug-resistant bacteria called methicillin-resistant *Staphylococcus aureus*. Examples of these drugs are included in Table 5-3 (see also Box 5-2).

Carbapenems

Like the penicillins and cephalosporins, the carbapenems are β-lactam antibiotics that also inhibit cell wall

+---

BOX 5-2

FACTS ABOUT CEPHALOSPORINS

- Contain a β-lactam structure

- Mechanism of action: inhibit cell wall synthesis

- Bactericidal

- Spectrum of activity: narrow to broad; contain subcategories based on increasing spectrum of activity

- Adverse effects: cause allergic reactions; may have cross-reactivity with penicillins (approximately 3% to 5%)

- Primary uses: respiratory tract, urinary tract, bacteremia, skin, and soft tissue infections

- Excretion: primarily urine

- Other notes: inactivated by β-lactamases (cephalosporinases)

BOX 5-3

FACTS ABOUT CARBAPENEMS

- Contain a β-lactam structure

- Mechanism of action: inhibit cell wall synthesis

- Bactericidal

- Spectrum of activity: broad

- Adverse effects: cross-reactivity may exist in patients allergic to other β-lactams

- Primary uses: infections of the skin and urinary tract, pneumonia, and intra-abdominal and pelvic infections

- Excretion: primarily urine

---

synthesis and are bactericidal. These newest β-lactams have traditionally been resistant to β-lactamases and therefore are broad spectrum, parenteral β-lactam antibiotics used to treat infections with gram-negative bacteria that are resistant to other antibiotics. However, in recent years, resistance to the carbapenems has been an increasing problem. Certain bacteria, particularly a group of gram-negative bacteria termed the Enterobacteriaceae, produce β-lactamases called carbapenemases that degrade the β-lactam structure in the carbapenem. The carbapenemases can also break down other β-lactam antibiotics, leading to resistance to multiple antibiotics. These drugs—imipenem (Primaxin), meropenem (Merrem), doripenem (Doribax), and ertapenem (Invanz)—can be used to treat infections of the skin, urinary tract, lower respiratory tract, intra-abdominal area, and pelvis. The carbapenems are usually well tolerated, but adverse effects include diarrhea, nausea, and vomiting. Cross-reactivity may exist in patients allergic to the other β-lactam antibiotics (Box 5-3).

Tetracyclines

The tetracyclines have been on the market for more than 50 years, but their use as a first-line drug has decreased because of increased incidence of bacterial resistance and the availability of other more effective and less toxic antibiotics. However, they remain highly effective to treat some infections such as Rocky Mountain spotted fever, cholera, Lyme disease, and pneumonia from *Mycoplasma pneumoniae*. Doxycycline (Vibramycin) is effective for postexposure prophylaxis to anthrax (see also ciprofloxacin). Tetracyclines are an alternative therapy to treat many infections when the drug of choice is not suitable for the patient (eg, due to allergy or resistance).

The mechanism of action of the tetracyclines is to inhibit protein synthesis. An active transport mechanism is necessary for sufficient drug to reach the site of action inside the bacteria. Tetracyclines bind to specific active sites on the ribosomal RNA to inhibit protein synthesis. Mammalian cells do not have the active transport system necessary to attain sufficient concentrations of tetracyclines at the site of action, and the structure of mammalian ribosomal RNA is different from that of bacteria. Inhibition of protein synthesis with tetracyclines will diminish the growth of the bacteria (bacteriostatic) but will not kill the microorganism. All of the tetracyclines are broad-spectrum antibiotics, effective for many gram-positive and gram-negative bacteria.

A major difference among the tetracyclines is the duration of action (Table 5-4), with the 2 most lipid-soluble tetracyclines, doxycycline and minocycline, having the longest duration of action. These 2 tetracyclines also have the greatest ability to penetrate into the brain and CSF compared with the other tetracyclines. Although all of the tetracyclines are effective orally, they are not completely absorbed, and the presence of food will further diminish their absorption. However, the greater lipid solubility of doxycycline and minocycline contributes to their more complete absorption from the GI tract and the diminished impact from food on the absorption. The extent of absorption is an important factor because unabsorbed tetracycline can alter the intestinal flora and result in the development of resistant organisms and bacterial and fungal superinfections.

All tetracyclines bind to certain minerals, primarily calcium, magnesium, aluminum, zinc, and iron, although doxycycline and minocycline are affected to a lesser extent. When tetracycline molecules bind to these minerals that

TABLE 5-4				
SELECTED CHARACTERISTICS OF TETRACYCLINES				
GENERIC NAME	TRADE NAME	LIPID SOLUBILITY	APPROXIMATE HALF-LIFE (HR)	EXTENT OF ORAL ABSORPTION
demeclocycline	Declomycin	Intermediate	14	Intermediate
doxycycline	Vibramycin	High	20	High[a]
minocycline	Minocin	High	15	High[a]
tetracycline	Sumycin	Intermediate	9	Intermediate
[a]Oral absorption not significantly affected by food.				

Box 5-4
FACTS ABOUT TETRACYCLINES

- Mechanism of action: inhibit protein synthesis

- Bacteriostatic

- Spectrum of activity: broad

- Adverse effects: epigastric burning, nausea, vomiting, diarrhea, and photosensitivity (up to 2% of patients); may affect bones and teeth in patients younger than 8 years

- Primary uses: infections such as Rocky Mountain spotted fever, cholera, Lyme disease, and pneumonia form *Mycoplasma pneumoniae*; alternative therapy to treat many infections when the drug of choice is not suitable for the patient

- Other uses: additive to animal feed to increase the growth rate of livestock, treat peptic ulcers caused by *H pylori*, and treat acne

- Excretion: primarily urine but some excreted in bile

- Other notes: absorption is affected by the presence of food; unabsorbed tetracycline can alter the intestinal flora and result in the development of resistant organisms and bacterial and fungal superinfections

children younger than 8 years or to pregnant or nursing mothers because these drugs cross the placenta and are found in breast milk.

In addition to the potential to affect teeth and bones in children, the tetracyclines may also cause other adverse effects. GI symptoms such as epigastric burning, nausea, vomiting, and diarrhea can occur, especially when the tetracycline is administered on an empty stomach. These antibiotics can also produce photosensitivity in some patients, which may cause the patient to become sunburned more readily when exposed to direct sunlight or sunlamps. Protective clothing is advised to avoid direct sunlight, and sunscreens are of little benefit. Some patients may need to discontinue therapy, and photosensitivity may persist for weeks after the drug is discontinued.

Besides treatment of some systemic and respiratory infections, tetracyclines have 3 other specific uses. Oxytetracycline and chlortetracycline, in particular, are used in agriculture as an additive to animal feed to increase the growth rate of livestock. This use continues to be controversial due to its possible impact on contributing to the development of resistant strains of bacteria. Another use particularly of tetracycline, in combination with other drugs, is to treat peptic ulcers caused by *Helicobacter pylori* (*H pylori*), a bacterium that is a major cause of peptic ulcer disease (see Chapter 11). A third use is to treat acne. The mechanism involved in acne therapy is through inhibition of *Propionibacterium acnes*, which produce fatty acids that initiate an inflammatory response. Daily oral use of tetracycline as low-dose therapy is effective to treat acne with minimal adverse effects (Box 5-4).

Macrolides

This group of antibiotics includes the original macrolide, erythromycin (Eryped), and the newer macrolides, clarithromycin (Biaxin) and azithromycin (Zithromax). These drugs can be administered orally and are generally bacteriostatic, although at higher concentrations they become bactericidal to some bacteria. The macrolides

are contained in foods, laxatives, and mineral supplements, the drug is not absorbed from the GI tract. Consequently, oral doses of these drugs should only be taken 1 hour before or 2 hours after the consumption of food, particularly dairy products. The binding of tetracyclines to the calcium in bones and teeth causes these drugs to affect bone development and causes permanent discoloration of tooth enamel. Therefore, the tetracyclines should not be administered to inhibit protein synthesis of sensitive bacteria. The spectrum of activity of these antibiotics is somewhat similar to the penicillins, and the macrolides are often the alternate drug recommended in penicillin-allergic patients. They are used as an alternative to penicillins and other antibacterial therapy to treat infections of the GI, genital, and respiratory tracts, as well as skin and soft tissue infections. Resistance can occur by several mechanisms: an altered transport mechanism that decreases the amount of macrolide inside the bacterial cell, a change in the structure of the binding site, or an increased production of an enzyme that inactivates the macrolide. Erythromycin is also used topically to treat acne by inhibiting *P acnes*, which contribute to the inflammation.

The most common adverse effects from macrolides are GI and include epigastric irritation, diarrhea, nausea, and vomiting. Among the macrolides, erythromycin has the highest incidence of these effects, but they can be minimized by administration of the drug with food. However, erythromycin is not stable to stomach acid, and food diminishes absorption. Consequently, various dosage formulations, such as acid-resistant coatings (also known as *enteric coatings*), have been developed to facilitate adequate absorption even when given with food. Clarithromycin is not affected by stomach acid or presence of food as much as erythromycin, but it does undergo first-pass metabolism, which diminishes its bioavailability. This macrolide is also manufactured in an extended-release dosage form, which should be administered with food. The food slows the rate at which the drug passes through the small intestine and thus increases the bioavailability of the extended-release clarithromycin. Azithromycin is affected by food and thus should be given either 1 hour before or 2 hours after meals.

The macrolides provide an example of some of the pharmacokinetic principles discussed in Chapter 2. Erythromycin is inactivated by stomach acid and thus is incompletely absorbed. Administration with food decreases the absorption of the acid-sensitive erythromycin; to com-

pensate for this, erythromycin is manufactured with acid-resistant coatings, which allow adequate absorption even when given with food. Both erythromycin and clarithromycin inhibit cytochrome P450 enzymes and are therefore involved in several drug interactions (Box 5-5).

Sulfonamides

Sulfonamides were the first systemic antibacterial agents used therapeutically. They have been referred to as *sulfa drugs* because of the sulfur atom in the chemical structure. The use of these drugs has diminished as additional antibiotics have become available and strains of sulfonamide-resistant bacteria have developed. Sulfonamides are broad-spectrum bacteriostatic antibiotics. Their mechanism of action (Figure 5-3) is to inhibit an enzyme needed for synthesis of tetrahydrofolic acid (THFA) from para-aminobenzoic acid (PABA). THFA is necessary for the synthesis of DNA, RNA, and proteins, and therefore sulfonamides are referred to as *metabolic inhibitors*. A deficiency of THFA will prevent cell growth and division. THFA must be synthesized inside certain bacteria because they cannot transport extracellular folic acid into the cell as an alternative means to make THFA. Mammalian cells cannot synthesize THFA from PABA but must obtain folic acid from the diet; it is a vitamin. Consequently, sulfonamides do not affect folic acid use in mammals.

Bacterial resistance to sulfonamides can be due to several mechanisms. Sometimes bacteria acquire a different enzyme that uses PABA but to which sulfonamides bind less effectively. Some bacteria develop characteristics that diminish the rate of entry of sulfonamides into the cell. Alternatively, other bacteria develop resistance by synthesizing much more PABA to compete for the active site on the enzyme that uses PABA as substrate.

Oral sulfonamides, such as sulfamethoxazole, are excreted by the kidney and thus reach a relatively high concentration in urine and are useful in treating urinary tract infections. Other uses for these sulfonamides include

Figure 5-3. Mechanism of action of sulfonamides and trimethoprim. Sulfonamide antibiotics inhibit (X) the enzyme that uses para-aminobenzoic acid (PABA) as the substrate in the synthesis of tetrahydrofolic acid (THFA) in some bacteria. Humans cannot use PABA in this manner but rather ingest the vitamin folic acid, which is more directly converted to THFA. Consequently, the sulfonamide antibiotics do not inhibit folic acid metabolism in humans. Trimethoprim is not a sulfonamide, but it also inhibits the synthesis of THFA at another step along the same pathway. Trimethoprim is often used concurrently with a sulfonamide because both drugs together produce a synergistic antibacterial effect.

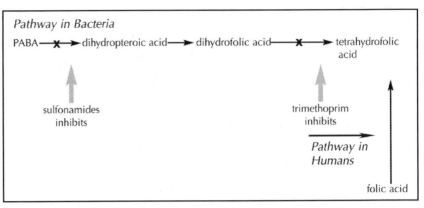

Box 5-6

FACTS ABOUT SULFONAMIDES (SULFA DRUGS)

- Mechanism of action: inhibit an enzyme needed for synthesis of THFA from PABA

- Bacteriostatic

- Spectrum of activity: broad

- Adverse effects: crystallization of sulfonamides in the urine if not enough water is consumed, resulting in renal damage; skin rashes, photosensitivity; hypersensitivity to topical sulfonamides

- Primary uses: urinary tract infections, pneumonia, and upper respiratory infections; topical sulfonamides used to treat eye infections and second- and third-degree burns

- Excretion: urine

---

treatment of pneumonia and upper respiratory tract infections caused by susceptible bacteria. Topical use of sulfonamides results in a high incidence of hypersensitivity reactions and therefore is confined to treatment of eye infections with sulfacetamide (Sulamyd) and to prevent infections following second- and third-degree burns, silver sulfadiazine (Silvadene) being the preferred sulfonamide. Mafenide (Sulfamylon) can also be used to prevent topical infections, although unlike silver sulfadiazine, mafenide causes pain on application to wounds and can cause blood acid-base imbalance.

It is common to use another antibiotic, trimethoprim, together in the same dosage form as the sulfonamides to obtain a synergistic effect. As shown in Figure 5-3, trimethoprim also inhibits the synthesis of folic acid but in an enzymatic step in the pathway following the site of action of sulfonamides. Use of trimethoprim with sulfamethoxazole together (Bactrim) has extended the usefulness of the sulfonamides. This combination is used in the treatment of urinary tract infections and respiratory infections.

Several adverse effects are of significant concern when sulfonamides are being used. If sulfonamides crystallize in the urine, they can cause renal damage. This is less of a problem with the currently used sulfonamides, but nonetheless patients should be cautioned to drink enough liquid to produce 1200 to 1500 mL of urine per day. Mild hypersensitivity reactions are relatively common and are usually manifested by skin rash or photosensitivity. Infants should not be given sulfonamides because they can displace bilirubin from the albumin-bound sites to increase the concentration of free bilirubin in the blood, which can reach toxic levels. Near-term pregnant women and nursing mothers should also not be treated with sulfonamides (Box 5-6).

Aminoglycosides

The aminoglycosides are bactericidal antibiotics that are used primarily to treat infections from gram-negative bacteria. These antibiotics inhibit protein synthesis, which typically results in bacteriostatic activity. However, aminoglycosides also disrupt other aspects of the bacterial cell, such as cell membrane integrity, which contribute to the bactericidal activity. As with the other antibiotics, resistance can develop to these antibiotics by several mechanisms, including a change in the cell permeability to the drug and inactivation of the drug by the resistant bacteria.

Streptomycin was the first antibiotic developed among this group but is used less frequently since the advent of more active aminoglycosides such as gentamicin (Garamycin), tobramycin (Nebcin), and amikacin (Amikin). None of the aminoglycosides are absorbed orally due to their water-soluble nature. Thus, they are used only parenterally for a systemic effect, and some are used topically to treat eye infections. Neomycin, another aminoglycoside, is too toxic for systemic use but is used orally to suppress intestinal bacteria prior to surgery and is used in several topical antibiotic preparations, both alone and in combination with other drugs. For example, Neosporin ointment and triple

Table 5-5

FLUOROQUINOLONE ANTIBIOTICS

GENERIC NAME	TRADE NAME	ADMINISTRATION
ciprofloxacin	Cipro	PO, IV
gemifloxacin	Factive	PO
levofloxacin	Levaquin	PO, IV
moxifloxacin	Avelox	PO, IV
norfloxacin	Noroxin	PO
ofloxacin	Floxin	PO
IV = intravenous; PO = oral.		

antibiotic ointment contain a combination of neomycin with 2 other topical antibiotics, polymyxin B and bacitracin. A unique characteristic of aminoglycosides is their synergistic activity when used in combination with cell wall synthesis inhibitors (penicillins).

The aminoglycosides have a relatively low therapeutic index. A significant adverse effect of the aminoglycosides is their potential to cause ototoxicity and nephrotoxicity. Ototoxicity results in impaired balance and hearing, which may be irreversible. Nephrotoxicity may result in diminished renal function but this is usually reversible upon discontinuation of the drug. Patients on aminoglycoside therapy must be monitored for early signs of ototoxicity (eg, tinnitus, dizziness) and nephrotoxicity (eg, elevated blood creatinine) (Box 5-7).

Fluoroquinolones

The fluoroquinolones (Table 5-5) is a group of antibiotics with several favorable characteristics:

- They are bactericidal and broad spectrum; thus, one or more of these drugs can be used to treat infections caused by many gram-negative and gram-positive bacteria.
- They penetrate into many tissues and thus are effective in treating infections of the urinary tract, respiratory tract, prostate, GI tract, bones, joints, and soft tissues.
- They are effective orally (however, the absorption of fluoroquinolones is reduced by certain minerals; therefore, these antibacterial drugs should not be given with food, drugs, or mineral supplements that contain calcium, magnesium, aluminum, zinc, and iron).
- They have relatively mild adverse effects; the most frequently reported include nausea, vomiting, headache, and dizziness.

In addition, ciprofloxacin (Cipro) and levofloxacin (Levaquin) are approved for postexposure prophylaxis to anthrax (see also doxycycline). The favorable characteristics of the fluoroquinolones have made them very popular antibiotics. However, the extensive use of these agents has led to a significant increase in resistance over the years.

Some adverse effects are of particular note to the athletic trainer. The fluoroquinolones have demonstrated some potential to cause tendonitis and rupture of tendons; this risk is greater for patients older than 60 years and for those taking corticosteroids. Fluoroquinolones should be discontinued if symptoms of tendonitis occur and should be avoided in patients with any existing symptoms of tendonitis (eg, pain, swelling, inflammation in tendon area). These drugs may also cause lesions on the cartilage of weight-bearing joints. Consequently, fluoroquinolones are not currently recommended for use in patients aged younger than 18 years or in pregnant women. Additionally, some fluoroquinolones cause phototoxicity to direct or indirect sunlight or to artificial ultraviolet light (eg, sunlamps). Symptoms such as skin burning, redness, rash, and itching are indications the drug should be discontinued.

The mechanism of action for fluoroquinolones is to inhibit DNA synthesis. The corresponding process in mammalian cells is not affected by the fluoroquinolones. As with other antibiotics, resistance can develop to the fluoroquinolones by more than one mechanism (Box 5-8).

Topical Antibacterial Drugs

Several antibacterial drugs are available for topical use as creams, ointments, lotions, and ophthalmic solutions. Some

---

Box 5-8

FACTS ABOUT FLUOROQUINOLONES

- Mechanism of action: inhibit DNA synthesis
- Bactericidal
- Spectrum of activity: broad
- Adverse effects: nausea, vomiting, headache, and dizziness and have demonstrated some potential to cause rupture of tendons and articular cartilage lesions; phototoxicity
- Primary uses: infections of the urinary tract, respiratory tract, prostrate, GI tract, bones, joints, and soft tissues
- Excretion: varies within the group, some primarily in urine but other through GI tract
- Other notes: should not be given with foods, drugs, or mineral supplements that contain calcium, magnesium, aluminum, zinc, or iron, as they can affect absorption

---

antibiotics are available as prescription products to treat or prevent infections on the skin from wounds or burns and to treat ophthalmic infections. Many of these antibiotics have already been discussed and include sulfonamides, fluoroquinolones, erythromycin, and tobramycin. Some topical antibiotics are available without a prescription and are used primarily to prevent infection from minor wounds and burns. To treat infections from a wider array of bacteria, several products contain more than one antibiotic. They typically include the following antibiotics:

- *Bacitracin.* This is a bactericidal antibiotic that inhibits cell wall synthesis. It is primarily effective against gram-positive bacteria.

- *Neomycin.* As previously discussed, neomycin is a bactericidal aminoglycoside antibiotic. It is effective against gram-negative bacteria. Potentially any topical antibiotic could cause an allergic skin reaction, although neomycin has the highest incidence (approximately 5%) among these over-the-counter (OTC) antibiotics.

- *Polymyxin B.* This is bactericidal primarily against gram-negative bacteria and is available OTC to treat skin infections and by prescription as an ophthalmic solution. It alters cell membrane structure and thus changes the permeability characteristics of the membrane.

Section Summary

There are many chemical categories of antibacterial drugs, but they can also be grouped by mechanism of action. Antibiotics that inhibit the synthesis of bacterial cell walls are bactericidal and include the penicillins, cephalosporins, and carbapenems. These are also called β-lactam antibiotics because they contain a chemical structural entity called a β-lactam ring. Protein synthesis inhibitors are bacteriostatic and include the tetracyclines and macrolides. Aminoglycosides inhibit protein synthesis but also disrupt other cellular activity and thus are bactericidal. The sulfonamides inhibit the production of THFA, a compound synthesized by some bacteria and necessary for their cell growth; inhibition of THFA synthesis does not kill the cell. Fluoroquinolones inhibit DNA synthesis and are bactericidal.

Resistance can develop to the β-lactam antibiotics as a result of some bacteria being able to produce enzymes called β-lactamases that break apart the β-lactam ring. Antibiotics that are inactivated by these enzymes are β-lactamase sensitive; those that are not inactivated are β-lactamase resistant. Penicillinases and cephalosporinases are subgroups of these enzymes. Numerous penicillins and cephalosporins are effective in treating infections of many tissues. The primary differences among these drugs are their effectiveness against specific bacteria, their effectiveness when administered orally, and their sensitivity to β-lactamases. The most significant adverse effect is the potential for allergic reactions; cross-reactivity among the β-lactam antibiotics exists in some patients.

The tetracyclines are broad-spectrum agents; doxycycline and minocycline are the tetracyclines most commonly used to treat systemic infections. Tetracyclines bind to calcium, magnesium, aluminum, zinc, and iron although doxycycline and minocycline are affected the least. Therefore, these drugs should not be administered within about 1 to 2 hours of using nutritional supplements or foods that are rich in these minerals. The tetracyclines should also be avoided in children and during pregnancy because they bind to the calcium in teeth and bone. These antibiotics are especially useful as an alternative therapy for many infections. Macrolides are useful to treat many of the same infections as the tetracyclines.

The aminoglycosides are only used parenterally to treat systemic infections. They have the potential to cause ototoxicity and nephrotoxicity, and thus blood concentrations and adverse effects are monitored closely.

The fluoroquinolones are broad spectrum, bactericidal, and effective when administered orally. Because they have the potential to cause tendons to rupture and lesions on cartilage, fluoroquinolones are not recommended in patients aged younger than 18 years, for use during pregnancy, or in patients with tendonitis.

ANTIFUNGAL AGENTS

The key biochemical processes that are targets of antibacterial drugs are different for fungi, and thus drugs used to treat bacterial infections are not effective against fungi. The biochemical processes of fungi more closely resemble human cells than bacteria cells, which makes it more difficult to treat fungal infections (called *mycoses*) without also affecting human cells. Treatment of fungal infections is a serious concern because of the increase in incidence of these infections and the development of resistance to antifungal therapy. Contributing to the increased incidence of fungal infections is the use of broad-spectrum antibiotics that may result in fungal superinfections, more medical procedures that have the potential to introduce fungal infections, and an increased number of immunocompromised patients (eg, patients with cancer, transplant, or AIDS).

Compared with superficial fungal infections, systemic fungal infections have a greater potential for morbidity. However, to the athletic trainer, superficial fungal infections are important because they occur much more frequently and they can hinder athletic performance. Yeasts and molds are fungi; molds are multicellular and thread-like in appearance, whereas yeasts are oval-shaped single-cell organisms. Yeasts are typically in a parasitic form that infects tissue. Fungi can cause systemic infections through the respiratory, GI, or urinary tracts, as well as through compromised skin. Fungal infections increase in patients whose immune defenses are diminished through disease or drugs (eg, corticosteroids) or as superinfections through the disruption of normal flora due to use of broad-spectrum antibiotics. For example, *Candida* is a part of the normal flora of skin and mucous membranes. The number of *Candida* organisms at these sites is usually relatively low because the predominance of the normal flora competes for nutrients with *Candida* and prevents them from proliferating. However, the use of a broad-spectrum antibiotic can cause the number of normal bacterial flora to be diminished sufficiently to allow the *Candida* to proliferate, thus becoming an infection of the skin, GI tract, mouth, or vagina.

Antifungal Agents for Systemic Infections

Except for fungal infections that may be obtained due to invasive medical procedures or use of broad-spectrum antimicrobial agents, most systemic fungal infections are contracted by inhalation of the fungus. Once the lungs are infected, the fungus can spread to other organs and become life threatening. Patients who are immunocompromised, such as those receiving certain cancer therapies or immunosuppressive drugs (eg, corticosteroids) or those with HIV/AIDS are more susceptible.

The mechanism of action of many antifungal agents is to disrupt the normal functioning of the cell membrane causing leakage of cellular contents. For some of these drugs, whether they have fungistatic or fungicidal activity depends on the concentration of the drug at the site of action, with higher concentrations being fungicidal. Amphotericin B (Fungizone) is a very effective antifungal agent and remains the treatment of choice for some fungal infections, but it has the significant disadvantages of not being absorbed orally and causing a relatively high incidence of nephrotoxicity. It is also associated with other adverse effects such as fever, chills, nausea, and headache. For many years, amphotericin B was the primary antifungal agent, but other drugs have been developed that are less toxic and are effective orally, particularly the azole group. This is a group of broad-spectrum antifungal agents that includes fluconazole (Diflucan), itraconazole (Sporanox), voriconazole (VFEND), and posaconazole (Noxafil). Nausea and vomiting are the most common adverse effects but can be reduced by administration of the drug with food. Other adverse effects vary among the antifungal agents but include headache and abdominal pain. Systemic use of some antifungal agents (eg, itraconazole, terbinafine) has the potential to cause hepatotoxicity, and thus monitoring liver function is recommended. There is also a significant drug interaction potential with the azole antifungals due to cytochrome P450 enzyme inhibition.

Antifungal Agents for Superficial Infections

Superficial fungal infections affect mucous membranes (eg, vaginal, oral, GI), skin, scalp, and nails. Examples of topical antifungal drugs are listed in Table 5-6, and additional antiseptic agents used for ringworm of the scalp are listed in Table 5-7. Some antifungal therapy for superficial infections requires oral administration because of the site or severity of the infection. For example, nystatin (Mycostatin) can be used orally to treat GI fungal infections because the drug is not absorbed from the GI tract. When topical therapy alone is ineffective, oral dosage forms of griseofulvin (Fulvicin), itraconazole (Sporanox), fluconazole (Diflucan), and terbinafine (Lamisil) are used to treat fungal infections of the skin, scalp, and/or nails because these drugs penetrate into these sites. Although improvement in symptoms is typically observed after 1 week of treating some fungal infections, weeks to months of treatment are usually necessary to eliminate the infection, depending on the drug used and the site of the infection. Consequently, adherence throughout the duration of therapy is sometimes a challenge to achieve but necessary to attain success.

Fungal infections of skin, scalp, and nails are most often caused by several species of fungi referred to as *dermatophytes*. These fungal infections are collectively termed *tinea*, *dermatomycoses*, or *ringworm* (which are not worms or rings but produce an itching and painful red-ringed

TABLE 5-6

EXAMPLES OF TOPICAL ANTIFUNGAL AGENTS

GENERIC NAME	TRADE NAME	OTC/RX	DOSAGE FORM
amphotericin B[a]	Fungizone	Rx	Cream, lotion
butenafine	Mentax	Rx	Cream
	Lotrimin Ultra	OTC	Cream
ciclopirox	Loprox	Rx	Cream, gel, lotion, shampoo
	Penlac	Rx	Nail lacquer
clotrimazole	Lotrimin	OTC, Rx	Cream, lotion, solution
	Gyne-Lotrimin	OTC	Vaginal suppositories, cream
econazole	Spectazole	Rx	Cream
ketoconazole	Nizoral	Rx	Cream
miconazole	Micatin	OTC	Cream, powder, spray
	Monistat	OTC	Vaginal suppositories, cream
naftifine	Naftin	Rx	Cream, gel
nystatin[a]	Mycostatin	Rx	Cream, ointment, powder
	Nystatin	Rx	Vaginal tablets
oxiconazole	Oxistat	Rx	Cream, lotion
sulconazole	Exelderm	Rx	Cream
terbinafine	Lamisil AT	OTC	Cream, spray
tolnaftate[b]	Tinactin	OTC	Cream, powder, spray

OTC = over the counter; Rx = prescription.
Except where indicated, these products are effective against infections of tinea pedis, tinea cruris, and tinea corporis.
[a]Not for tinea infections.
[b]Also used for onychomycosis although tolnaftate only as adjunct to systemic therapy.

patch). These and other superficial infections include several characteristics:

- *Tinea pedis (ringworm of the foot; athlete's foot).* This is the most common of the dermatomycoses. Infection is facilitated through the moist environment of sweating feet and poorly ventilated shoes. Symptoms vary from cracking and itching between the toes to swelling, severe inflammation, and occurrence of secondary bacterial infection. Treatment with appropriate OTC products is typically sufficient unless there is serious inflammation, the toenails are affected, or the infection prevents normal activity. Treatment may be necessary for 2 to 4 weeks to resolve the infection.

- *Tinea capitis (ringworm of the scalp).* Occurs more frequently in children and is spread by direct contact with animals, humans, or inanimate objects (eg, combs) that are contaminated with the fungus. Symptoms include painful inflammation, which may result in temporary or permanent hair loss. Treatment requires systemic antifungal therapy (eg, griseofulvin, itraconazole) for 1 to 3 months. Topical agents can also be used but cannot cure the infection and are generally antiseptic.

- *Tinea corporis (ringworm of the body).* Occurs on the skin of the trunk and limbs. The infection is spread by direct contact with animals, humans, or inanimate objects infected with this microorganism. Topical agents are usually sufficiently effective (see Table 5-6), although systemic agents such as griseofulvin and terbinafine are also available.

- *Tinea cruris (ringworm of the groin; jock itch).* Tight-fitting clothes and moisture facilitate the infection and recurrence is common. Symptoms are typically redness and itching in the groin area and the inside of the thigh. Recurrence of the infection is common. Topical OTC antifungal therapy is usually sufficient,

		TABLE 5-7	
		EXAMPLE ANTISEPTICS	
GENERIC NAME	**TRADE NAME**	**DOSAGE FORMS**	**USED AGAINST**
benzalkonium chloride	Zephiran	Solution, tincture	Bacteria, fungi, viruses
benzalkonium chloride/ salicylic acid	Ionil	Shampoo	Tinea capitis
camphor/phenol	Campho-Phenique	Gel, liquid	Bacteria, fungi, viruses
chlorhexidine	Hibiclens	Solution, towelettes	Antibacterial
hydrogen peroxide	hydrogen peroxide	Liquid	Bacteria, viruses
iodine	Iodine Tincture	Tincture	Bacteria, fungi, viruses
isopropyl alcohol	isopropyl alcohol	Liquid	Bacteria
phenol	Unguentine	Cream, ointment	Bacteria, fungi, viruses
povidone-iodine	Betadine	Aerosol, cream, gel, ointment, shampoo	Bacteria, tinea capitis and other fungi, viruses
selenium sulfide	Selsum Blue	Shampoo	Tinea capitis
thimerosal	Mersol	Solution, tincture	Bacteria, fungi
triclosan	Septisol	Soap, solution	Bacteria

although a systemic antifungal drug may be necessary if severe inflammation exists. Treatment should continue for 1 to 2 weeks, although symptoms may disappear after a few days. Topical hydrocortisone (see Chapter 6) for 2 to 3 days may also be used to relieve itching.

- *Tinea unguium (ringworm of the nails; onychomycosis).* Infected nails become discolored with debris accumulating underneath and may eventually be destroyed. Topical antifungal agents are usually not as effective as systemic therapy. Oral itraconazole and terbinafine are effective. Because nails are slow growing, treatment with systemic antifungal agents is necessary for 6 weeks to 12 months, depending on the severity and the drug used.

- *Tinea versicolor (pityriasis versicolor).* This is not actually a ringworm but is similar in appearance. It is a mild, chronic skin infection, usually of the upper trunk, caused by a fungus that is part of the normal skin flora (*Malassezia furfur*). Some patients experience mild pruritus (itching); otherwise it is usually asymptomatic. Because the fungus is part of the normal flora, the disease is recurrent, occurring more frequently in hot, humid weather; during excessive sweating; or because of corticosteroid therapy (see Chapter 6). Typical lesions are scaly and have discoloration as patches of white, tan, or pink. Almost all topical or oral antifungal drugs are effective treatment.

- *Vaginal candidiasis. Candida albicans* is a part of the normal vaginal flora and causes most vaginal yeast infections. Use of topical therapy such as intravaginal tablets or creams for a few days to 2 weeks is necessary, depending on the antifungal agent. Oral therapy with a single dose of fluconazole is also used for treatment of vaginal candidiasis. *Candida* infections are also referred to as *monilial infections.*

- *Oral candidiasis (thrush). Candida* infection of the mucous membranes of the mouth. Topical therapy is usually effective, with treatment continuing for 1 to 2 weeks after symptoms relieved. Asthma patients using corticosteroids by inhalation have a higher incidence of thrush, especially if they do not rinse their mouth with water after using the inhaler or do not use a spacer with it (see Chapter 9).

Section Summary

Fungal infections can occur from inhalation of airborne fungus, from contamination of a wound, as a superinfection during treatment with broad-spectrum antibiotics, or in immunocompromised patients. There are several antifungal agents available to treat systemic fungal infections, and although resistance to these drugs can occur, it is less frequent than bacterial resistance to antibiotics. Examples of superficial fungal infections are athlete's foot, jock itch, and ringworm of the scalp and nails. Both topical and systemic antifungal agents are used to treat certain superficial fungal infections. Unlike most bacterial infections,

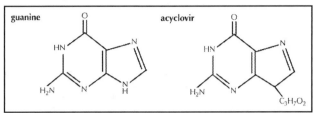

Figure 5-4. Chemical comparison of antiviral drug, acyclovir, with DNA component, guanine. Some antiviral drugs have a chemical structure very similar to components of RNA and DNA. Acyclovir is an antiviral drug that has a structure similar to guanine, a building block for DNA. Thus, acyclovir interferes with DNA synthesis in cells infected with certain viruses.

which require days to weeks of treatment, fungal infections typically require weeks to months of antifungal therapy.

ANTIVIRAL AGENTS

As previously mentioned, the development of drug therapy to treat viral infections poses unique challenges because viruses use the enzymes and genetic processes of the host cell to propagate. Consequently, drugs used to treat bacterial and fungal infections are not effective for treatment of viral infections. Nonetheless, millions of prescriptions are written each year for antibiotics to treat infections that are not bacterial. This inappropriate use of antibiotics costs hundreds of millions of dollars, unnecessarily exposes the patient to potential adverse effects, and contributes to the occurrence of antimicrobial resistance.

Viruses contain DNA or RNA enveloped within a protein coat. Examples of diseases caused by DNA viruses include smallpox, chickenpox, shingles, herpes simplex infections, hepatitis B, and warts. German measles, rabies, common cold, influenza, and mumps are caused by RNA viruses. Medications for herpes virus infections and influenza are discussed in this section. Drugs used to treat the RNA virus that causes AIDS (HIV) and viruses that cause hepatitis will not be discussed because of the complexity of the medications and therapy of these infections.

Many of the antiviral drugs have chemical structures similar to the building blocks of RNA and DNA (Figure 5-4). Therefore, these drugs interfere with the synthesis of viral RNA and DNA. As with antibacterial and antifungal agents, resistance can also develop to the antiviral agents. Adverse effects range from neurotoxicity and nephrotoxicity to nausea and vomiting, depending on the drug. Each drug is effective against only a narrow spectrum of viruses, and most are effective orally but some are also available for parenteral or topical use.

Acyclovir (Zovirax) is the drug of choice to treat the herpes simplex virus (eg, genital herpes and encephalitis) or varicella-zoster virus (eg, chickenpox and shingles). GI upset and headache are common adverse effects from oral use.

Valacyclovir (Valtrex) is a prodrug, metabolized to acyclovir after oral administration and provides better bioavailability than acyclovir. Famciclovir (Famvir) is also a prodrug but converted to a different metabolite that is not orally absorbed. Penciclovir (Denavir) is a topical antifungal used to treat cold sores, a herpes simplex virus. Docosanol (Abreva) is an OTC product that is also used to treat cold sores.

Oseltamivir (Tamiflu) and zanamivir (Relenza) are used in the prophylaxis and treatment of influenza A and B. Adverse effects include anorexia, nausea, nervousness, anxiety, lightheadedness, and insomnia.

ANTISEPTICS AND DISINFECTANTS

Antiseptics and disinfectants are used only externally to kill (*germicide*) or inhibit the growth (*germistatic*) of microorganisms. *Antiseptics* are preparations applied to tissue such as hands or a site of injection or incision. *Disinfectants* are products applied to inanimate objects such as surgical areas or instruments. The mechanism of action of these compounds is generally nonspecific compared with the site-specific action of the antimicrobials previously discussed, and consequently they are too toxic for internal use. Some antiseptics and disinfectants are toxic to bacteria, fungi, and viruses. They may facilitate the physical removal of cells from surfaces, denature protein, or physically disrupt membranes due to the harsh chemical nature of the compound. See Table 5-7 for some examples of antiseptics used primarily as skin and wound cleansers. Continuous exposure of wounds to some antiseptic products may delay wound healing through a cytotoxic effect on some cells necessary for the healing processes.

TREATMENT OF SEXUALLY TRANSMITTED DISEASES

Sexually transmitted diseases (STDs) are a significant health problem in the United States. The number of sexual partners is the biggest risk factor for contracting an STD: the more partners, the higher the risk. The incidence is also greater for homosexual men than for heterosexuals. For some infections, the treatment regimen differs depending on the age of the patient (child vs adult), location of the infection, and whether the patient is pregnant. Treatment of some STDs has changed over the years because of the development of resistant strains of some organisms. Table 5-8 lists the causative organism for common STDs and a drug of choice for treating the disease in adults. Most of the drugs in Table 5-8 have been previously mentioned in this chapter; however, there are others:

- *Metronidazole* (Flagyl). This drug is effective against certain bacteria and protozoa. Bacterial infections include *H pylori* in some people with ulcers

TABLE 5-8				
EXAMPLES OF SEXUALLY TRANSMITTED DISEASES AND TREATMENTS[a]				
DISEASE	INFECTING ORGANISM	GENERIC NAME	TRADE NAME	ADMINISTRATION
Chlamydia	*Chlamydia trachomatis*	azithromycin	Zithromax	Oral
		doxycycline	Vibramycin	Oral
Gonorrhea	*Neisseria gonorrhoeae*	ceftriaxone	Rocephin	IM
		azithromycin	Zithromax	Oral
Syphilis	*Treponema pallidum*	penicillin G	Bicillin LA	IM
		doxycycline	Vibramycin	Oral
Trichomoniasis	*Trichomonas vaginalis*	metronidazole	Flagyl	Oral
Bacterial vaginosis	*Gardnerella vaginalis, Mycoplasma hominis*	metronidazole	Flagyl	Oral
Genital herpes	Herpes simplex virus	acyclovir	Zovirax	Oral
		valacyclovir	Valtrex	Oral
		famciclovir	Famvir	Oral
Genital warts	Human papillomavirus	podofilox	Condylox	Topical
		imiquimod	Aldara	Topical
Pubic lice (crabs)	*Phthirus pubis*	permethrin	Nix[b]	Topical
Pubic mites (scabies)	*Sarcoptes scabiei*	permethrin	Elimite	Topical

[a]In adults. Selection of drug may vary depending on the site of the infection.
[b]Available OTC. All others by prescription.

(see Chapter 11) and bacterial vaginosis; protozoal infections include amebiasis and trichomoniasis. Metronidazole interferes with DNA function in these organisms. It is absorbed orally, metabolized by the liver, and excreted primarily by the kidney. The most common adverse effects include dizziness, headache, nausea, vomiting, diarrhea, metallic taste in the mouth, and loss of appetite. Metronidazole may be taken with food if GI upset occurs. The drug discolors the urine dark or reddish-brown. An unpleasant disulfiram-like reaction occurs if the patient ingests alcohol or is exposed to topically applied products with alcohol within 72 hours of taking metronidazole.

Disulfiram (Antabuse) is a drug that is used in the management of chronic alcoholism. It produces an unpleasant response if alcohol is consumed while taking it. Some other drugs, such as metronidazole, also produce a similar unpleasant disulfiram-like reaction when combined with alcohol. The unpleasant reaction is characterized by headache, nausea, vomiting, flushing, sweating, and tachycardia.

- *Podofilox* (Condylox). Podofilox is used topically as a solution or gel to treat genital warts. It is applied twice daily in a cycle of 3 days with application, followed by 4 days without applying the drug. It causes erosion of the wart tissue. Adverse effects are pain, inflammation, burning, and itching.

- *Imiquimod* (Aldara). Imiquimod is a topical cream used to treat genital warts. It induces cytokines and other factors that enhance the immune response at the local site. Imiquimod is applied at bedtime 3 times per week and then removed by washing in the morning. Adverse effects are local itching, burning, erosion, flaking, and edema.

- *Permethrin* (Elimite, Nix). Permethrin is used topically as a liquid (Nix) to treat lice infestation (also called *pediculosis*) and as a cream (Nix) to treat mite infestation (also called *scabies*). It is effective against not only pubic lice (crabs) but also head and body lice. It causes paralysis and death of the parasite. For treatment of scabies or lice, a single application is usually sufficient. Adverse effects are mild and include temporary burning or stinging.

ROLE OF THE ATHLETIC TRAINER

- *Educate regarding infections.* Many patients do not understand that the occurrence of an infection does not mean automatic treatment with an antibiotic. Antibiotics are not effective in the treatment of viral infections, the most common cause of most upper respiratory infections. Unnecessary use of antibiotics can lead to unnecessary adverse effects, including the occurrence of superinfections.

- *Educate regarding adherence.* As with therapy for many diseases, nonadherence with appropriate antimicrobial therapy is a significant cause of treatment failures. Typical antibiotic therapy requires 7 to 14 days of the prescribed dosage regimen for a cure, although the recommended length of therapy varies with the type of infection, site of infection, and treatment regimen. Sometimes patients discontinue use of the drug after a few days because the symptoms disappear; treatment for the entire prescribed time is necessary to most efficiently eradicate the infection. It is particularly difficult to continue with treatment of fungal infections that require weeks to months of therapy. The athletic trainer can encourage the patient to continue treatment for successful recovery.

- *Monitor for allergies.* Patients who develop a rash during systemic or topical treatment with any antimicrobial drug may not realize that the rash could be the result of an allergic response to the drug. The athletic trainer can be observant concerning these connections so that a change in antimicrobial therapy can be initiated if necessary.

- *Monitor for common adverse effects.* The athletic trainer can help avoid adverse effects other than allergic reactions. Tetracyclines, for example, should not be used by children younger than 8 years. Also, potential problems associated with photosensitivity with these drugs and the fluoroquinolones should be monitored so that the adverse effects can be minimized through use of protective clothing or the therapy can be changed. Also, fluoroquinolones should be avoided in patients younger than 18 years and in patients with tendonitis. The occurrence of any symptom that did not exist before therapy was initiated should be suspected as a potential adverse effect.

- *Monitor for effectiveness.* Because infections are caused by so many microorganisms, and because resistance to antimicrobial agents is a significant problem, some patients on antimicrobial therapy may not have improved symptoms as therapy progresses. The athletic trainer can check with the patient to be sure the infection is being responsive to the drug therapy. For example, are the symptoms ameliorating? If they are not, reevaluation of the therapy may be necessary.

CASE STUDY

Although Violet, the athletic trainer working with the university's intercollegiate wrestling team, has made sure the wrestling mats are cleaned on a regular basis, she also realizes that infections, especially skin infections, are expected during the wrestling season. Will, a 20-year-old, 149-pound wrestler on the team, comes to Violet in a panic. Will has noticed a large round area of redness on his leg and is afraid that he has Lyme disease. Violet inspects the lesion and notices that it has a very distinct circular pattern similar to a donut with a healed center. It is red, raised, and scaly. She suspects that Will's lesion is not Lyme disease but tinea corporis. Violet knows that Will must be seen by the physician to determine his contagion status for competition, but she also knows what can be done to resolve the problem. What kind of infection is this? What agents are used in the treatment of tinea corporis? What education should the athletic trainer provide regarding this infection?

BIBLIOGRAPHY

Gallagher JC, MacDougall C. *Antibiotics simplified.* 3rd ed. Burlington, MA: Jones and Bartlett Learning; 2013.
Hendricks KA, Wright ME, Shadomy SV, et al. Centers for Disease Control and Prevention expert panel meetings on prevention and treatment of anthrax in adults. *Emerg Infect Dis.* 2014;20(2).
Katzung BG. *Basic and clinical pharmacology.* 12th ed. New York, NY: McGraw-Hill Companies; 2011.
Rabenberg VS, Ingersoll CS, Sandrey MA, Johnson MT. The bacterial and cytotoxic effects of antimicrobial wound cleansers. *J Athl Training.* 2002;37:51-54.
Rodvold KA, File TM, Nicolau DP, Drew RH. START (stewardship tactics for antimicrobial resistance trends). *J Manag Care Pharm.* 2009;15(supplement):S3-S26.

CHAPTER 6: ADVANCE ORGANIZER

Foundational Concepts

- Inflammatory Process
- Arachidonic Acid Metabolites
- Rheumatoid Arthritis and Gout
- Section Summary

Nonsteroidal Anti-Inflammatory Drugs

- Therapeutic Uses of Nonsteroidal Anti-Inflammatory Drugs
- Pharmacokinetics and Dosage
- Adverse Effects
- Drug Interactions
- Therapy Guidelines
- Section Summary

Corticosteroids

- Therapeutic Uses of Corticosteroids
- Pharmacokinetics and Dosage
- Adverse Effects
- Drug Interactions
- Therapy Guidelines
- Section Summary

Glucosamine

- Use and Effects
- Pharmacokinetics and Dosage
- Adverse Effects
- Section Summary

Treatment for Rheumatoid Arthritis and Gout

- Drug Therapy for Rheumatoid Arthritis
- Drug Therapy for Gout
- Section Summary

Topical Anti-Inflammatory Products

- Section Summary

Role of the Athletic Trainer

6

Drugs for Treating Inflammation

CHAPTER OBJECTIVES

At the end of this chapter, the reader will be able to:

- Describe and explain the inflammatory process

- List the common chemical mediators, explain how they affect physiological functions, and summarize their role in the inflammatory process

- Differentiate how the pathophysiology of rheumatoid arthritis and gout differ from other inflammatory reactions

- Explain the difference between COX-1 and COX-2 enzymes

- Explain how nonsteroidal anti-inflammatory drugs (NSAIDs) affect blood clotting and how aspirin differs from other NSAIDs in this mechanism

- Describe the pharmacokinetics of NSAIDs and corticosteroids

- Recall the general dosing regimen for NSAIDs and corticosteroids

- List the signs and symptoms and explain the pathophysiology of specific adverse effects and drug interactions with NSAID and corticosteroid therapy

- Explain the physiological effects of increased dosage and treatment duration for corticosteroids

- Describe how corticosteroids exert their therapeutic effect on the inflammatory process

- Recall the most appropriate drug therapy for the treatment of rheumatoid arthritis and gout

- Describe the potential value of glucosamine to treat osteoarthritis

- Recall the 3 types of drugs that can be components in a topical over-the-counter (OTC) anti-inflammatory medication

- Explain how topical anti-inflammatory medications exert their therapeutic effects

- Summarize the role of the athletic trainer for patients who are on NSAID or corticosteroid drug therapy

Inflammation can be caused by a variety of stimuli, including physical injury, infections, heat, and antigen-antibody interactions. The inflammatory response is generally a beneficial mechanism that allows the body to combat the injury or infection more effectively. However, sometimes the inflammatory response is excessive in duration or intensity, and the use of drug therapy to reduce the response is beneficial. This chapter discusses the key cellular components of the inflammatory response as a basis for an understanding of the mechanism of action of anti-inflammatory drugs, the pharmacological characteristics that are common among the agents within the nonsteroidal and steroidal categories

Houglum JE, Harrelson GL, Seefeldt TM.
Principles of Pharmacology for Athletic Trainers, Third Edition (pp 97-122).
© 2016 Taylor & Francis Group.

TABLE 6-1

DRUGS ONLY USED TO TREAT INFLAMMATION CAUSED BY A SPECIFIC DISEASE PROCESS

GENERIC NAME	TRADE NAME	USE	MECHANISM
cromolyn	Intal	Asthma	Mast cell stabilizer
montelukast	Singulair	Asthma	Diminishes effect of LTs
nedocromil	Tilade	Asthma	Mast cell stabilizer
zafirlukast	Accolate	Asthma	Diminishes effect of LTs
zileuton	Zyflo	Asthma	Diminishes effect of LTs
allopurinol	Zyloprim	Gout	Inhibits uric acid formation
colchicine	Colcrys	Gout	Inhibits leukocyte infiltration
probenecid	Benemid	Gout	Increases urinary excretion of uric acid
sulfinpyrazone	Anturane	Gout	Increases urinary excretion of uric acid
adalimumab	Humira	Rheumatoid arthritis	Prevent inflammatory activity of TNF
azathioprine	Imuran	Rheumatoid arthritis	Immunosuppression, inhibits DNA synthesis
etanercept	Enbrel	Rheumatoid arthritis	Prevents inflammatory activity of TNF
hydroxychloroquine	Plaquenil	Rheumatoid arthritis	Immunosuppression, but unknown mechanism
leflunomide	Arava	Rheumatoid arthritis	Inhibits T-cell and antibody production
methotrexate	Rheumatrex	Rheumatoid arthritis	Several, including immunosuppression
penicillamine	Cuprimine	Rheumatoid arthritis	Immunosuppression, but mechanism unknown

LTs = leukotrienes.

ABBREVIATIONS USED IN THIS CHAPTER

ACTH. adrenocortico-tropic hormone

CNS. central nervous system

COX. cyclooxygenase

CRH. corticotropin-releasing hormone

CYP. cytochrome P450

DNA. deoxyribonucleic acid

DMARD. disease-modifying antirheumatic drug

FDA. Food and Drug Administration

GI. gastrointestinal

HPA. hypothalamic-pituitary-adrenal

IL. interleukin

LT. leukotriene

MI. myocardial infarction

NSAID. nonsteroidal anti-inflammatory drug

OTC. over-the-counter

PG. prostaglandin

PGI$_2$. prostacyclin

RNA. ribonucleic acid

SLE. systemic lupus erythematosus

TI. therapeutic index

TIA. transient ischemic attack

TNF. tumor necrosis factor

TX. thromboxane

TXA$_2$. thromboxane A$_2$

of anti-inflammatory drugs, and some specific examples of drugs in each of these 2 categories.

The NSAIDs and corticosteroids discussed in this chapter have a direct effect on the inflammatory response mechanism. There are other drugs that also diminish inflammation indirectly by improving the inflammatory-causing disease and thus are used to relieve the inflammation associated with that specific disease. For example, antimicrobial drugs (see Chapter 5) reduce the inflammation associated with an infection by affecting the infecting organism, but these drugs do not have direct anti-inflammatory activity. In a similar fashion, inflammation is abated by some drugs that are unique to the treatment of rheumatoid arthritis, gout, or asthma (Table 6-1) because of the impact of these drugs on the disease process. Drugs used to treat asthma will be discussed in Chapter 9; drugs used selectively for rheumatoid arthritis and gout are discussed later in this chapter.

FOUNDATIONAL CONCEPTS

The major purpose for using anti-inflammatory drugs is to reduce inflammation. Consequently, a brief discussion of the inflammatory process is provided. The mechanism

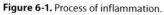

Figure 6-1. Process of inflammation.

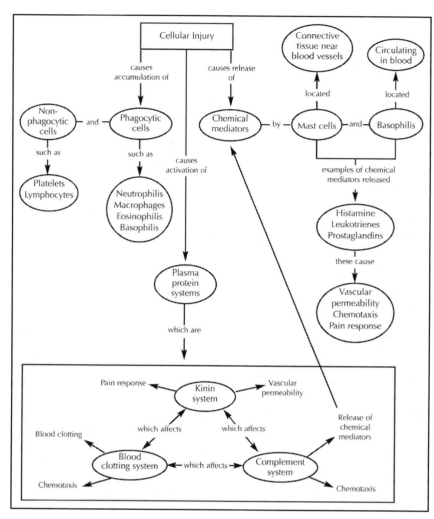

of action of steroidal and nonsteroidal anti-inflammatory agents centers on the biochemical production of arachidonic acid metabolites; therefore, those pathways will also be a focus.

Inflammatory Process

The inflammatory process is normally a beneficial process, initiated immediately after injury and intended to facilitate repair and expedite a return of the tissue to normal function. Often times the inflammatory process is either bothersome or excessive in intensity or duration so that it must be treated to reduce the negative impact of the process, which may merely be acute discomfort or pain or may be chronic and debilitating. Regardless of the cause of the inflammation, there are many chemical mediators, numerous types of activated cells, and a few plasma protein systems that become a part of the inflammatory response (Figure 6-1). *Chemical mediators* are compounds that are released by one cell type, attach to the receptor of a second cell type, and affect the response of that second cell. There is considerable interaction among these mediators, various cell types, and plasma protein systems, which are

intended to regulate the rate and extent of the inflammatory response. In other words, some of these interactions stimulate the progress of the inflammatory response, whereas other interactions prevent the process from spreading beyond certain limits.

The inflammatory response is initiated within seconds after cellular injury caused by a wide range of stimuli, including physical trauma, radiation (eg, ultraviolet light, x-rays), chemicals (toxins, caustic substances), heat, infectious microorganisms, or hypersensitivity reactions. These stimuli cause the release of several chemical mediators by *mast cells* and *basophils*, which are key cells in initiating the inflammatory response. Mast cells are located in connective tissue near blood vessels, whereas basophils are circulating in the blood. Both of these cell types have storage pockets (granules) for specific chemical mediators. For example, histamine dilates local capillaries, which increases blood flow to the site of inflammation. Histamine also increases vascular permeability; when vascular permeability increases, the vessels are more leaky, which facilitates access to the site by other components of the inflammatory response from the blood. Chemotactic factors are also

TABLE 6-2

MAJOR COMPONENTS OF THE INFLAMMATORY PROCESS

	COMPONENTS	FUNCTION
Chemical mediators	Bradykinin	Causes vasodilation and pain response
	Cytokines	Cause wide range of effects in inflammation and immune response; subgroups include interleukins (IL) and interferons (INF) of which there are several of each, such as IL-1, IL-2, INF-a, INF-b, etc
	Eosinophil chemotactic factor	Attracts eosinophils to inflammatory site
	Histamine	Increases capillary blood flow and vascular permeability
	LTs	Increases vascular permeability and chemotaxis
	Neutrophil chemotactic factor	Attracts neutrophils to inflammatory site
	Platelet-activating factor	Stimulates activity of platelets
	PGs	Increases vascular permeability and chemotaxis; induces pain; suppresses some aspects of inflammation
	Serotonin	Increases capillary blood flow and vascular permeability
Cell types	Basophils	Storage/release of several chemical mediators
	Eosinophils	Phagocytic; inactivates some chemical mediators (eg, histamine, LTs)
	Lymphocytes	Key cells of immune reactions; production/release of antibodies, including during inflammation
	Macrophages	Key phagocytes; primarily after 24 hours from initial inflammatory response
	Mast cells	Storage/release of chemical mediators.
	Neutrophils	Key phagocytes; within 6 to 12 hours of initial inflammatory response
	Platelets	Interact with clotting system for clot formation; releases chemical mediators
Plasma protein systems	Clotting system	Prevents bleeding and traps debris; affects chemotaxis; increases kinin response
	Complement system	Initiates inflammation; chemotaxis; destroys microorganisms; increases vascular permeability
	Kinin system	Increases vascular permeability and vasodilation; affects clotting system; causes pain response with PGs

LTs = leukotrienes; PGs = prostaglandins.

released; these are compounds that cause *chemotaxis*, the attraction of specific types of cells to the area. *Leukotrienes* (LTs) and *prostaglandins* (PGs) are also chemical mediators that are released by mast cells and play a role in vascular permeability, chemotaxis, and pain response; these mediators are discussed in more detail next. See Table 6-2 for a list of other chemical mediators.

Besides mast cells and basophils, many other cell types accumulate at the site of inflammation, either through chemotaxis or adhesion mechanisms, which hold the cells in the area of inflammation. Some cells are phagocytic, removing dead cells, debris, and bacteria from the site by engulfing them (*phagocytosis*). *Neutrophils* are at the scene early to carry out this task, whereas *macrophages* arrive later and persist longer. The regulatory processes that control the activity of these and other phagocytic cells (eg, eosinophils and basophils) are complex but are important to prevent an excessive inflammatory response. Platelets and lymphocytes are examples of nonphagocytic cells that also have specific roles during inflammation (see Table 6-2).

The *plasma protein systems* are composed of proteins with specific important functions in the inflammatory response. A unique feature of these systems is that they are composed of multiple proteins that are activated in a specific sequence in order to produce their biological effects. For example, the clotting system is a sequence of proteins that activates other proteins, leading to the formation of a clot. Some of the proteins generated through the clotting process also have other functions, such as chemotaxis and enhancing the kinin system. The *kinin system* is another plasma protein system; the most notable protein is *bradykinin*, which increases vascular permeability and produces pain. The *complement system* is also a plasma protein system that affects inflammation. This biochemical sequence of activated proteins can be initiated by the presence of bacterial or fungal cells. Among the many functions of the complement system are to kill microorganisms, cause chemotaxis, and initiate the release of chemical mediators from mast cells.

The inflammatory response is a complex process, and therefore it is difficult to completely control. Drug therapy can have an impact on the process; however, the prime focus of their mechanism of action is to alter the effect that chemical mediators have on the inflammatory response.

Arachidonic Acid Metabolites

The metabolism of arachidonic acid plays an important role in the inflammatory process and is worthy of separate consideration because much of anti-inflammatory drug therapy affects these pathways. *Arachidonic acid* is an unsaturated fatty acid that is the starting point (substrate) for the biosynthesis of several groups of compounds. In other words, these compounds are metabolites of arachidonic acid that contribute to the inflammatory response. These metabolites of arachidonic acid are also called *eicosanoids*. The eicosanoids are a part of a larger group of compounds referred to as chemical mediators. As discussed previously, the extent of inflammation is largely controlled by the extent of release of *chemical mediators* from various cell types. Aside from eicosanoids, other chemical mediators that are noneicosanoids include histamine, cytokines, and platelet-activating factor (see Table 6-2).

As shown in Figure 6-2, arachidonic acid is attached to phospholipids that are components of the membrane structure. An enzyme, phospholipase A_2, catalyzes the intracellular release of arachidonic acid from the membrane-bound phospholipid. Arachidonic acid then follows 1 of 2 pathways depending on which enzymes are active within that cell type. The 2 pathways are the cyclooxygenase (COX) pathway and the lipoxygenase pathway. These pathways lead to 4 groups of eicosanoid mediators: PGs, prostacyclin (PGI_2), thromboxanes (TXs), and LTs. The specific eicosanoids

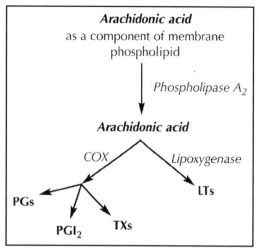

Figure 6-2. Pathways for the synthesis of arachidonic acid metabolites. Phospholipase A_2 releases arachidonic acid from the stored site as a component of membrane phospholipid. The released arachidonic acid is converted to various metabolites by either lipoxygenase or COX. COX = cyclooxygenase, PGs = prostaglandins, PGI_2 = prostacyclin, TXs = thromboxanes, LTs = leukotrienes.

produced in these pathways were given letter designations as they were discovered, such as PGs A through I (ie, PGA, PGB, PGC, etc) and LTs A through E. The names for the eicosanoids also have a subscript that designates the number of carbon-carbon double bonds in the molecule. For example, PGE_2 and LTC_4 have 2 and 4 such double bonds, respectively. Table 6-3 identifies some physiological functions that have been attributed to individual eicosanoids.

One or more of the eicosanoids are produced by virtually all cells, and they play an important role of regulating many physiological functions in addition to inflammation. In some cases, one eicosanoid modulates the response from another eicosanoid to maintain homeostasis. Trauma, disease, or drugs can offset the balance between these and other eicosanoids. One example is regarding the physiological effects of prostaglandin I_2 (PGI_2, also called *prostacyclin*) and thromboxane A_2 (TXA_2). Prostacyclin is produced in blood vessel walls and inhibits platelet aggregation, whereas TXA_2 is produced by platelets and enhances platelet aggregation (Figure 6-3). The normal balance between the effects of PGI_2 and TXA_2 is disrupted when the blood vessel wall is damaged by a laceration or by atherosclerosis. In this situation, the production of PGI_2 is reduced and the effects of TXA_2 predominate; hence, platelets aggregate and contribute to blood clot formation. A disruption of this normal balance also occurs due to some cardiovascular diseases, resulting in unwanted platelet aggregation and eventual thrombosis.

Related to inflammation, the arachidonic acid metabolites contribute to the symptoms of inflammation, including redness, swelling, and pain. During an allergic reaction or

TABLE 6-3	
PHYSIOLOGICAL EFFECTS OF SELECTED ARACHIDONIC ACID METABOLITES (EICOSANOIDS)	
EICOSANOID	**PHYSIOLOGICAL EFFECT**
LTB_4	Chemotactic for polymorphonuclear neutrophils (PMNs)
LTC_4 LTD_4 LTE_4	Bronchoconstriction, increases mucus secretion, increases microvascular permeability
PGD_4	Bronchoconstriction
PGE_4	Protects gastric mucosa by increasing mucus and decreasing acid secretion, increases edema during inflammation, potentiates bradykinin-induced pain, increases renal blood flow by renal vasodilation, bronchodilation, causes fever and increased perception of pain in the brain
PGF_{2a}	Bronchoconstriction
PGI_2	Inhibits platelet aggregation, increases local vasodilatation, increases edema during inflammation, potentiates bradykinin-induced pain, protects gastric mucosa by increasing mucus production and decreasing acid secretion, increases renal blood flow by renal vasodilation
TXA_2	Bronchoconstriction, increases platelet aggregation, increases local vasoconstriction, decreases renal blood flow
LT = leukotriene; PG = prostaglandin; TX = thromboxane.	

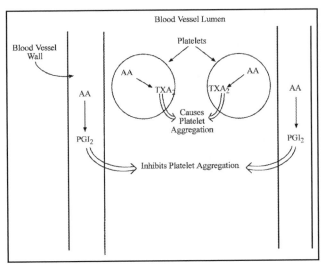

Figure 6-3. Platelet aggregation effects of PGI_2 and TXA_2. As platelets flow through blood vessels, they produce and release thromboxane A_2 (TXA_2), which causes platelets to aggregate. The cells that compose the blood vessel wall produce and release PGI_2, which inhibits platelet aggregation, thus off-setting the potentially deleterious effects of TXA_2. Under normal conditions, there is no need for platelet aggregation, and the proper balance between the effects of PGI_2 and TXA_2 is important to prevent an unwanted blood clot. If there is trauma to the blood vessel wall (eg, laceration or atherosclerosis), some of the cells are damaged and production of PGI_2 is diminished. Because PGI_2 is not produced to off-set the effect of TXA_2, platelets aggregate at the site of the laceration and facilitate blood clot formation. PGI_2 and TXA_2 are made from arachidonic acid (AA), as shown in Figure 6-2.

eicosanoid necessary to regulate certain normal ("housekeeping") functions. Similarly, COX-2 is produced in the brain, female reproductive tract, blood vessel walls, and kidneys to maintain normal function in these tissues. However, the production of COX-2 is also induced in response to inflammation and tissue injury, resulting in an increase in the synthesis of mediators that contribute to inflammation. PGs increase blood flow and erythema in the local area of the inflammatory response, initiate chemotaxis, sensitize pain receptors at the local site of inflammation, and cause a central nervous system (CNS) pain response.

Recall from Chapter 3 that when an enzyme is induced, the number of molecules of enzyme synthesized by the cell is increased due to an effect on the regulatory mechanism at the gene level. The result is an increased level of enzyme activity.

the bronchial hyper-responsiveness of an asthma attack, these same mediators are released as an exaggerated response to stimuli (see Chapter 9).

Because the COX pathway leads to the production of TX, PG, and PGI_2, drugs that block this pathway (COX inhibitors) will affect the processes controlled by these eicosanoids (Figure 6-4). There are 2 forms of the COX enzyme, COX-1 and COX-2, referred to as *isoforms*. Although these 2 enzymes catalyze the same reaction, they are produced under different conditions and by different tissues. COX-1 is produced in virtually all tissues at a relatively stable rate so that there is a sufficient amount of the appropriate

Various hormones and physical stimuli activate phospholipase A_2, which increases the release of stored arachidonic acid from the phospholipid structure. After the eicosanoids are produced from arachidonic acid, they are released by the cell. These mediators have a relatively short half-life, and thus their primary site of action is at or near the tissue that produces them; they are *local hormones*. For

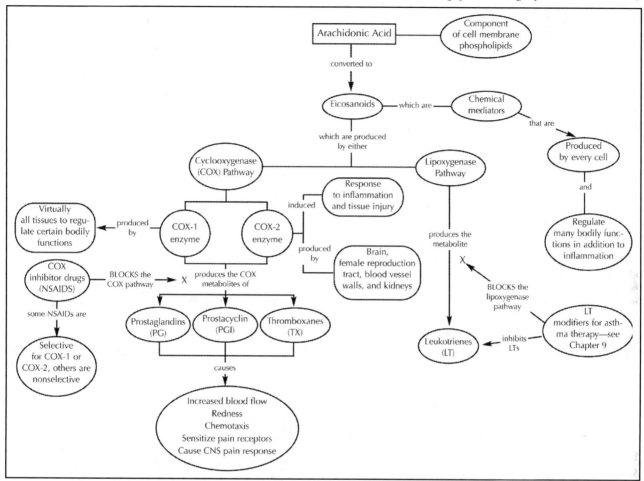

Figure 6-4. Effects of arachidonic acid metabolites and sites of drug action.

example, PGE_2 affects gastric acid secretion and is produced by gastric cells (see Chapter 11), the LTs that constrict bronchial smooth muscle are produced in the respiratory tract (see Chapter 9), and kidney function is altered by eicosanoids produced by renal cells. Once in the extracellular space, the eicosanoids can attach to their corresponding receptors to initiate an intracellular sequence through a second messenger system similar to the process described in Chapter 3. These intracellular reactions lead to the physiological responses shown in Table 6-3, including swelling, redness, and pain at the site of inflammation.

Rheumatoid Arthritis and Gout

Although the etiologies for rheumatoid arthritis and gout are different, inflammation is the principal characteristic of both. In addition to the inflammatory mechanism already discussed, other mechanisms also contribute to these diseases, and thus a discussion of additional drugs is necessary.

Rheumatoid arthritis is a common systemic inflammatory disease caused by an autoimmune response, possibly initiated as a result of a bacterial or viral infection.

Chemical mediators are released and contribute to the inflammatory response. Among these is *tumor necrosis factor* (TNF), a cytokine that has been identified as one of the chemical mediators that contributes to the autoimmune process in rheumatoid arthritis. Symptoms of rheumatoid arthritis often begin with joint stiffness and progress at varying rates among patients but can lead to total destruction of the cartilage, erosion of the bone, and destruction of the joint. Stiffness and swelling in the small joints of the hands, wrists, and feet are the most common, although other joints can also be involved. Chronic inflammation leads to deformity. Other tissues, such as lungs, heart, and eyes, may also be affected and pose serious complications. Some patients experience periods of spontaneous remission. The disease can occur at any age and is more common in women than in men.

Gout is inflammation and joint pain due to elevated uric acid blood concentration. Uric acid is a waste product of purine metabolism. The *purines* are a group of compounds produced in the body for use as part of the building blocks of DNA and RNA synthesis and they are one of the breakdown products of DNA and RNA. Patients with gout have an increased production or reduced excretion of uric acid and therefore have an elevated blood level of uric acid (ie, *hyperuricemia*). When the blood concentration of uric acid becomes too high, some crystallization of sodium urate (the sodium salt of uric acid) occurs in the synovium of joints and surrounding tissue. The deposit of these crystals initiates the inflammatory response at these sites, resulting in pain and swelling. Although symptoms can eventually occur at any joint, the most distal joints are most frequently affected, the first metatarsophalangeal joint often being the first. A possible explanation for the distal sites being favored is that the solubility of sodium urate is temperature dependent and the more distal joints are cooler. Although deposit of sodium urate in other tissues (eg, hips, shoulders, Achilles tendon, hands) is an eventual occurrence if untreated, drug therapy has immensely reduced this effect. However, crystallization of uric acid and sodium urate in the kidney remains a concern. Problems range from the more common formation of uric acid stones in urine to the less common acute renal failure.

Patients with gout experience acute, extremely painful attacks at varying intervals (initially months), which become shorter as the disease progresses. Initially, the time between acute attacks is pain free, but as chronic gout develops, the periods between acute attacks are not completely pain free. Duration of acute attacks also varies from hours to weeks if untreated. The incidence of gout peaks at age 30 to 50 years and is higher in men than women in this age group but becomes more evenly distributed in the elderly. Genetic factors related to the synthesis and excretion of uric acid can predispose a patient to develop gout, but other factors that cause increased uric acid blood levels are obesity, alcoholic beverages, hyperlipidemia, renal disease, hypertension, diuretic therapy (see Chapter 12), and low-dose aspirin therapy (aspirin at low doses blocks normal renal excretion mechanism of uric acid, whereas doses > 5 g/day increase uric acid excretion).

Section Summary

The inflammatory response involves numerous types of cells, chemical mediators, and plasma protein systems, which, when functioning properly, produce an inflammatory response that aids in the repair of damaged tissue. There are regulatory mechanisms as a part of the inflammatory response that affect the rate and extent of the response. The chemical mediators play a significant role in these regulatory mechanisms. These are compounds that are released by certain cells or, in some cases, produced by a plasma protein system and affect the response from other cells. The major mechanism of most anti-inflammatory drugs is to alter the response from chemical mediators.

Among the chemical mediators is a group called eicosanoids. These are compounds produced from the metabolism of arachidonic acid. There are 2 pathways that produce the eicosanoids: the COX enzyme initiates the COX path-

way, which produces the PG, TX, and PGI eicosanoids, whereas the lipoxygenase enzyme initiates the pathway that produces the LT eicosanoids. There are 2 forms of the COX enzyme, referred to as COX-1 and COX-2. Although most cells contain COX-1 activity, some cells contain a significant amount of COX-2 (see Figure 6-4). These include cells at the site of an inflammatory response and cells of the kidney and blood vessels.

Rheumatoid arthritis and gout are inflammatory diseases but with unique pathophysiology. The basis of rheumatoid arthritis is an autoimmune reaction that may be initiated by an infection, whereas gout results from crystallization of sodium urate. In both diseases, the joints are the primary site of pain and inflammation.

NONSTEROIDAL ANTI-INFLAMMATORY DRUGS

NSAIDs are among the most frequently prescribed drugs and frequently used OTC drugs; one estimate places the use of aspirin in the United States at more than 10,000 tons per year. Aspirin, also abbreviated ASA for the chemical name acetylsalicylic acid, has been used since the late 1800s. There are other compounds that also have salicylic acid as part of the chemical structure and thus are referred to as salicylates, but aspirin is the most frequently used.

Aspirin is the prototype NSAID to which the effects of other NSAIDs are often compared. There are now more than 20 NSAIDs on the market. Table 6-4 lists selected NSAIDs with the typical anti-inflammatory adult daily dosage. The major mechanism of action of these drugs is to decrease PG production (see Figure 6-2) by inhibiting either one or both of the COX isoforms (COX-1, COX-2). The NSAIDs have little or no clinically significant effect on the lipoxygenase pathway, which produces LT. Because LTs and several noneicosanoid mediators contribute to the inflammatory response, the extent to which noneicosanoids are involved may affect the effectiveness of NSAIDs in relieving the symptoms of inflammation.

As previously discussed, COX-2 activity is enhanced in response to pain and inflammation, and thus for anti-inflammatory effectiveness it would seem advantageous for NSAIDs to primarily inhibit this isoform rather than inhibiting both COX-1 and COX-2 (see Table 6-4). Additionally, inhibition of COX-1 would cause some of the adverse effects, especially in the gastrointestinal (GI) tract. Selective COX-2 NSAIDs have been developed in response to these anticipated advantages. The selective COX-2 NSAIDs (also called *coxibs*) have a greater specificity for inhibiting COX-2 as relative to COX-1 at therapeutic doses and may have a lower incidence of some adverse effects but have not achieved a therapeutic advantage to the extent originally anticipated. In fact, of the first 3 selective COX-2 NSAIDs approved by the

TABLE 6-4

SELECTED NONSTEROIDAL ANTI-INFLAMMATORY DRUGS

GENERIC NAME	TRADE NAME	ANTI-INFLAMMATORY TYPICAL DOSE (MG)	DOSES/DAY
aspirin	Many	650 to 975	4
celecoxib[a]	Celebrex	200	1 to 2
diclofenac	Voltaren	50	3 to 4
etodolac	Lodine	300	2 to 3
fenoprofen	Nalfon	300 to 600	3 to 4
flurbiprofen	Ansaid	50 to 75	2 to 4
ibuprofen	Advil	400 to 800	3 to 4
indomethacin	Indocin	50	2 to 4
ketoprofen	Orudis	50 to 75	3 to 4
meloxicam	Mobic	7.5	1
nabumetone	Relafen	1000	1
naproxen	Naprosyn	250 to 500	2
oxaprozin	Daypro	600 to 1200	1
piroxicam	Feldene	20	1
sulindac	Clinoril	150	2
tolmetin	Tolectin	200 to 600	3
[a]Indicates selective COX-2 inhibitor.			

US Food and Drug Administration (FDA), 2 (Bextra, Vioxx) have been withdrawn from the market because of increased incidence of heart attack and stroke. The other NSAIDs are nonselective inhibitors because they significantly affect both COX isoforms, although the relative selectivity for COX-1 and COX-2 varies among this group. For example, aspirin has a greater selectivity for COX-1, whereas etodolac (Lodine) and meloxicam (Mobic) have greater selectivity for COX-2 than for COX-1 and are considered nearly selective, or preferential, COX-2 inhibitors.

Therapeutic Uses of Nonsteroidal Anti-Inflammatory Drugs

NSAIDs are used to treat both acute and chronic inflammation. All of the NSAIDs are equally effective, although response varies from one patient to another; one particular NSAID may not be effective in a patient, whereas another may be. A week or 2 of therapy is typically long enough to determine whether the anti-inflammatory effect of the drug is sufficiently effective. There are no clinical guidelines to determine which NSAID will be most effective in a particular patient. Selection of an NSAID should be made based on experiences of the physician, preference of the patient, cost,

and adverse effects. The principal use of NSAIDs is to treat the pain and inflammation associated with musculoskeletal disorders such as osteoarthritis, rheumatoid arthritis, gout, tendonitis, sprains, and strains. Treatment with an NSAID reduces pain, swelling, and stiffness and increases mobility. Because eicosanoid-induced inflammatory responses are a COX-2 response, either selective or nonselective COX inhibitors are effective treatment.

Although it is clear that NSAIDs (selective or nonselective) reduce pain and inflammation, it is not clear whether they decrease the healing time to allow a person to return more quickly to activity following musculoskeletal injury. Results of research studies are conflicting; some demonstrate increased and others decreased healing rate. Pain and inflammation are beneficial components to the healing process, but when excessive they are detrimental not only to the healing process but also to the patient's ability to return to activity. Several factors may affect whether healing is expedited. As mentioned previously, mediators other than eicosanoids are involved to various extents during the inflammatory response, and therefore the type and extent of injury may influence the effectiveness of the NSAID. Timing between injury and drug therapy may also be important because the NSAIDs inhibit the synthesis of eicosanoids but do not affect the response of the eicosanoids once they are produced. Obviously, there are pharmacokinetic and/or pharmacodynamic factors that are significantly different from patient to patient because there is a wide range of intrapatient responses with any particular NSAID. Consequently, selection of the NSAID, dosing, and duration of therapy can also affect the potential for improved healing rate. Use of other treatment modalities (eg, ice, compression, ultrasound, etc) along with NSAID therapy may be of particular benefit when excessive inflammation is involved. Use of acetaminophen offers an alternative to NSAIDs for pain relief if a negative impact on healing rate is a concern with the use of NSAIDs.

All of the NSAIDs also have analgesic and antipyretic (fever-reducing) activity; however, not all of them are approved for these uses. Use of NSAIDs as analgesics is covered in the next chapter. Fever production is a COX-2 response that occurs in the brain. Aspirin and ibuprofen are the 2 NSAIDs most frequently used to reduce fever. Acetaminophen (Tylenol), which is not an NSAID, is also frequently used to reduce fever and is discussed in the next chapter with the other analgesics. NSAIDs and acetaminophen do not lower body temperature below normal or lower body temperature when it has been elevated by exercise.

NSAIDs are effective in inhibiting uterine synthesis of eicosanoids that contribute to cramps and excessive bleeding during menstruation. Therefore, these drugs are effective for treatment of dysmenorrhea.

NSAIDs that inhibit COX-1 have antiplatelet activity and thus have an anticoagulant effect. The importance of the balance between TXA_2 and PGI_2 regarding platelet aggregation has been discussed (see Figure 6-3). COX-1 produces TXA_2, which stimulates platelet aggregation; COX-2 produces PGI_2, which inhibits platelet aggregation. Platelet aggregation stimulates activation of blood coagulation factors that can lead to a thromboembolism and subsequent myocardial infarction, transient ischemic attack, or stroke. Therefore, inhibition of TXA_2 production in platelets is useful therapy to prevent the development of thromboembolisms in susceptible patients. Aspirin differs from other NSAIDs in this respect because it is an irreversible inhibitor of the COX enzymes (ie, when aspirin binds to a molecule of COX, the enzyme remains inactive). All other NSAIDs are reversible inhibitors (they bind and release, back and forth) and thus are less effective for antiplatelet therapy. Unlike most other cells, platelets do not have significant protein synthesis capacity so platelets cannot regenerate more molecules of COX. Because aspirin binds irreversibly to COX, it prevents the production of TXA_2 for the lifespan of the platelet (approximately 8 days). Once TXA_2 production is inhibited, the PGI_2 effect of inhibiting platelet aggregation will predominate. Low-dose aspirin (40 to 325 mg/day, but most commonly 81 mg) is effective for antiplatelet therapy and is used to reduce the risk for transient ischemic attacks and stroke, to decrease the risk for myocardial infarction in patients with previous myocardial infarction or unstable angina, and to decrease the incidence of emboli formation in patients with various cardiovascular diseases. The other nonselective NSAIDs are less effective because they are not irreversible inhibitors of COX. There is an increased risk for heart attack or stroke with the use of selective COX-2 inhibitors compared with nonselective NSAIDs, possibly because the selective COX-2 inhibitors affect the production of PGI_2 but not TXA_2. Another use for aspirin is to prevent the intense upper body flushing associated with high-dose niacin, which is used for treatment of elevated blood cholesterol. This flushing is caused by release of PGD_2, which can be inhibited by low-dose aspirin.

Pharmacokinetics and Dosage

All NSAIDs are absorbed rapidly from the GI tract, and thus almost all NSAIDs are available only as oral preparations. Administration with food or milk is generally advised to reduce gastric upset. Use of enteric-coated aspirin will also reduce gastric upset but will delay absorption. This delay is not of clinical significance for chronic anti-inflammatory use but may be important if quick pain relief is desired.

NSAIDs distribute into the CNS. They also distribute into breast milk and cross the placenta; thus, they are generally not recommended for use by pregnant or lactating women. NSAIDs, including selective COX-2 inhibitors, are extensively bound to plasma protein. Ibuprofen, fenoprofen, naproxen, and tolmetin are 99% bound to plasma protein.

Clearance of NSAIDs generally involves liver metabolism to form various metabolites, followed by excretion in the urine. For example, aspirin is rapidly converted by the liver to several metabolites, which are excreted in the urine, including the active metabolite salicylic acid. Both glomerular filtration and/or renal tubular excretion are used in the kidney to get NSAIDs and their metabolites into the renal tubule.

> *Recall from Chapter 2 that there are 2 active transport mechanisms in the kidney that actively transport many drugs from the blood into the renal tubule for urinary excretion.*

The antipyretic dose for aspirin and ibuprofen is similar to the dose for relief of mild to moderate pain. However, there is a risk for potentially fatal Reye's syndrome associated with the use of aspirin in children with fever, and therefore aspirin should be avoided as antipyretic therapy in children younger than 19 years; acetaminophen (Tylenol) or ibuprofen (Motrin, Advil) is preferred. Symptoms of Reye's syndrome occur following a viral infection (eg, flu, chickenpox) and include persistent vomiting, lethargy, and confusion.

Reye's syndrome is a potentially fatal condition that causes liver and brain damage. It occurs in some children who have chickenpox or influenza and are treated with aspirin. Because these 2 diseases are viral infections, and because it is often difficult to distinguish between influenza symptoms and other viral upper respiratory infections, use of aspirin and aspirin-containing products should be avoided in children and teenagers with any cold or flu-type symptoms.

The anti-inflammatory and analgesic dosage for NSAIDs will vary among patients depending on the extent of inflammation and pain, but generally the maximum anti-inflammatory dosage is greater than the maximum analgesic dosage. A typical analgesic dose for ibuprofen (Advil) in treating mild to moderate pain is 400 mg 4 times a day, whereas a typical anti-inflammatory dose is 600 mg 4 times a day. Similarly, for aspirin, the maximum daily analgesic and anti-inflammatory doses are 4 g and 6 g per day, respectively.

A typical adult aspirin tablet is 325 mg, whereas an adult low-dose aspirin is 81 mg. These amounts of aspirin per tablet seem to be an odd strength considering that all dosage forms for virtually all other NSAIDs are round numbers such as 10 mg, 100 mg, or 150 mg per tablet. The reason for the difference is that aspirin and some other drugs that have been available for more than 100 years (eg, morphine and codeine) were originally marketed in tablet strengths based on the system of weight called grains. Adult-strength aspirin tablets have historically been marketed as 5-grain tablets, which is approximately 325 mg, and low-dose aspirin as 1.25 grain, which is 81 mg. Consequently, these strengths are still used today. The extra-strength or maximum-strength products were marketed later and contain 500 mg per tablet, although some extended-release products continue to use multiples of 325 mg (ie, 650, 975). Some naproxen products are also marketed in an unusual strength because they exist in the product as the sodium salt of naproxen. Consequently, as stated on the OTC packaging, 220 mg naproxen sodium (Aleve) contains 200 mg of naproxen. Similarly, one drug company markets 500 mg/tablet of naproxen under one trade name and 550 mg/tablet of naproxen sodium under another trade name; both products contain the same amount of active drug (500 mg naproxen/tablet).

Aspirin overdose is a significant concern, especially regarding accidental poisoning in children. The initial symptom of toxicity often is tinnitus, but other symptoms may include nausea, vomiting, hyperthermia, sweating, disorientation, lethargy, and hyperventilation, followed by respiratory depression, coma, and death. Toxicity from other NSAIDs rarely causes death. Outdated bottles of aspirin will have an odor of vinegar (acetic acid) because the acetylsalicylic acid has decomposed to acetic acid and salicylic acid. These should be discarded because the salicylic acid will have greater gastric irritation effects.

Adverse Effects

The morbidity and mortality of the adverse effects associated with NSAID use are significant, especially with daily use and in certain at-risk patients. Over 16,000 patients die each year and more than 100,000 are hospitalized because of NSAID-related adverse effects. The toxicity from NSAIDs may be underestimated by patients because of the ready accessibility of NSAIDs as OTC products.

The most common adverse effects of NSAIDs are GI irritation, heartburn, nausea, upper GI bleeding, and gastric and duodenal ulcers or related complications, including perforation, bleeding, obstruction, and death. Patients may experience gastric upset without ulceration, and patients with a developing ulcer may be asymptomatic until ulceration has occurred. Two mechanisms are involved in the development of these GI adverse effects. A direct local irritation effect occurs when the drug is in direct contact with gastric mucosa. The other mechanism is through the systemic inhibition of COX. Gastric upset and some blood loss are a result of local irritation and can occur with the first dose, whereas the incidence of serious GI bleeding (potentially to the point of anemia) or ulceration increases significantly with higher doses of NSAID and with longer duration of therapy. Risk of these serious adverse effects is also greater in patients older than 60 years; patients who have a history of peptic ulcer disease; and patients who are also using oral corticosteroids, anticoagulants, alcoholic beverages, or cigarettes. Among the OTC NSAIDs, GI adverse effects occur most frequently with aspirin and least frequently with ibuprofen. COX-2 selective inhibitors have demonstrated a lower incidence of GI damage and symptoms of ulcers compared with nonselective NSAIDs. However, it should be noted that adverse effects related to the GI tract occur with the COX-2 selective inhibitors as well, and celecoxib has the same warning about GI complications in its labeling as the nonselective NSAIDs. In addition, because the incidence of GI effects is most significant with long-term use, there may be no advantage of COX-2 inhibitors for short-term use (less than 2 weeks) in patients with no other risk factors for GI ulceration. Symptoms of GI toxicity include dark/tarry stools, indigestion, nausea, vomiting, and abdominal pain.

Gastric irritation can be minimized by administration of NSAIDs with milk, food, or antacids (except for enteric-coated products because milk and antacids may cause the coating to dissolve prematurely). A disadvantage of antacid use with chronic aspirin therapy is that antacids can alkalinize the urine, which increases the excretion rate of aspirin. Enteric-coated aspirin also reduces gastric mucosal damage by preventing dissolution of the aspirin until it

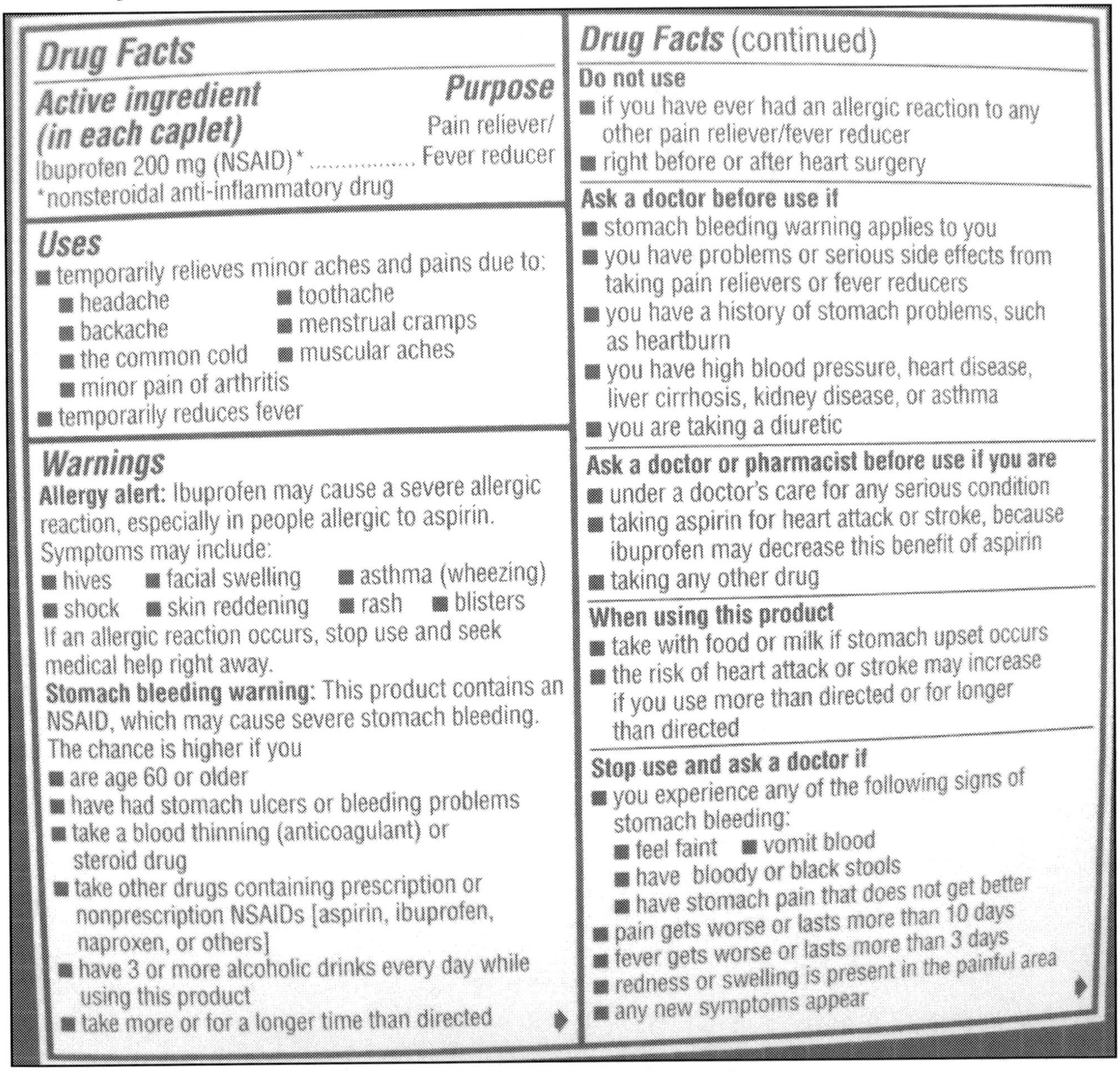

Drug Facts

Active ingredient (in each caplet)   Purpose

Ibuprofen 200 mg (NSAID)* .... Pain reliever/ Fever reducer

*nonsteroidal anti-inflammatory drug

Uses
- temporarily relieves minor aches and pains due to:
  - headache
  - backache
  - the common cold
  - minor pain of arthritis
  - toothache
  - menstrual cramps
  - muscular aches
- temporarily reduces fever

Warnings

Allergy alert: Ibuprofen may cause a severe allergic reaction, especially in people allergic to aspirin. Symptoms may include:
- hives
- shock
- facial swelling
- skin reddening
- asthma (wheezing)
- rash
- blisters

If an allergic reaction occurs, stop use and seek medical help right away.

Stomach bleeding warning: This product contains an NSAID, which may cause severe stomach bleeding. The chance is higher if you
- are age 60 or older
- have had stomach ulcers or bleeding problems
- take a blood thinning (anticoagulant) or steroid drug
- take other drugs containing prescription or nonprescription NSAIDs [aspirin, ibuprofen, naproxen, or others]
- have 3 or more alcoholic drinks every day while using this product
- take more or for a longer time than directed

Drug Facts (continued)

Do not use
- if you have ever had an allergic reaction to any other pain reliever/fever reducer
- right before or after heart surgery

Ask a doctor before use if
- stomach bleeding warning applies to you
- you have problems or serious side effects from taking pain relievers or fever reducers
- you have a history of stomach problems, such as heartburn
- you have high blood pressure, heart disease, liver cirrhosis, kidney disease, or asthma
- you are taking a diuretic

Ask a doctor or pharmacist before use if you are
- under a doctor's care for any serious condition
- taking aspirin for heart attack or stroke, because ibuprofen may decrease this benefit of aspirin
- taking any other drug

When using this product
- take with food or milk if stomach upset occurs
- the risk of heart attack or stroke may increase if you use more than directed or for longer than directed

Stop use and ask a doctor if
- you experience any of the following signs of stomach bleeding:
  - feel faint
  - vomit blood
  - have bloody or black stools
  - have stomach pain that does not get better
- pain gets worse or lasts more than 10 days
- fever gets worse or lasts more than 3 days
- redness or swelling is present in the painful area
- any new symptoms appear

Figure 6-5. Warnings on labels for OTC NSAIDs include risk for GI and cardiovascular adverse effects.

reaches the small intestine and may be particularly useful, compared with buffered or plain aspirin, for patients on chronic aspirin therapy. Another means of protecting the gastric mucosa during NSAID therapy is the administration of the PG substitute, misoprostol (Cytotec), or a proton-pump inhibitor. Misoprostol is a chemical modification of PGE_1 and acts by the same mechanism as PGE_2 and thus is a PGE_2-substitute during NSAID therapy but is contraindicated in women of child-bearing age because it has abortifacient properties. Proton-pump inhibitors such as omeprazole (Prilosec) reduce the amount of acid pumped into the stomach lumen by the stomach cells (see Chapter 11). The incidence of peptic ulcers associated with long-term NSAID therapy can be reduced when misopros-

tol or proton-pump inhibitors are used in conjunction with NSAID therapy.

All NSAIDs, except aspirin, have been associated with an increased incidence of heart attack and stroke. Because of this, warnings have been added to the labeling of these medications regarding cardiovascular and GI risks on OTC and prescription drugs of selective and nonselective NSAIDs (Figure 6-5). As mentioned earlier, inhibition of PGI_2 (and not TXA_2) by COX-2 selective inhibitors may be the cause of the enhanced risk of heart attack and stroke associated with selective COX-2 inhibitors.

Hypersensitivity to NSAIDs is another adverse effect of significant concern. Symptoms typically occur within 3 hours of ingestion of the drug and range from rhinitis, urticaria, and flushing to bronchospasm and asthmatic attack. Hypersensitivity reactions to NSAIDs are more frequent in patients with chronic urticaria, asthma, or nasal polyps. Fatal reactions of anaphylaxis or asthma are rare but have occurred. There is a cross-sensitivity among the NSAIDs, and therefore these drugs should be avoided in patients who have experienced any allergic symptoms from use of any of the NSAIDs. Currently, this recommendation also applies to the COX-2 inhibitors, although there is some evidence that COX-2 inhibitors (celecoxib in particular) may not cause the pulmonary effects in patients with aspirin-induced asthma.

One theory for the hypersensitivity mechanism is that as the NSAIDs inhibit COX-1, additional arachidonic acid is available as a substrate for the lipoxygenase pathway (see Figure 6-2), resulting in increased levels of LTs, which are the cause of asthmatic bronchospasms and anaphylaxis in susceptible patients. Patients with known intolerance to NSAIDs must be careful when selecting OTC medication because NSAIDs are components of many analgesic and anti-inflammatory products, as well as combination products such as for cold and sinus relief. Examples of OTC products containing NSAIDs are shown in Table 6-5. Patients who are allergic to aspirin also have a greater likelihood of being allergic to tartrazine (FDA yellow #5), which is a coloring agent added to some foods and drugs. Finally, patients who are allergic to sulfonamides (sulfur-containing drugs), such as sulfa antibiotics, certain diuretics, and oral antidiabetic drugs, have a possibility of a cross-allergy to celecoxib (Celebrex), which also contains a sulfur. Therefore, this selective COX-2 inhibitor should not be used in these patients.

All NSAIDs have the potential to cause renal toxicity. PGs play a role in maintaining appropriate salt and water balance and cause renal vasodilation as a countermeasure to maintain renal blood flow when it is diminished by other factors such as age, heart failure, hypertension, or kidney disease. Consequently, all NSAIDs should be used with caution in patients with these or any other conditions associated with fluid retention and edema because the NSAID may reduce kidney function and thus accentuate the problem. These patients should also be aware that reduced urine output and edema are symptoms of diminished kidney function.

The incidence of liver toxicity is less than the risk of renal toxicity. Nonetheless, caution is necessary when using NSAIDs in patients with reduced liver function or history of liver disease. If NSAIDs are used in these patients, reduced dosage may be necessary because most NSAIDs have a significant liver metabolism component to the clearance. If symptoms of nausea, fatigue, jaundice, pruritus, right-upper-quadrant abdominal pain, and flu-like symptoms occur, hepatotoxicity should be considered.

Because of the antiplatelet action of aspirin, it should be avoided in patients with blood-clotting disorders. Similarly,

TABLE 6-5

EXAMPLES OF OVER-THE-COUNTER PRODUCTS CONTAINING ASPIRIN OR OTHER NONSTEROIDAL ANTI-INFLAMMATORY DRUGS

TRADE NAME PRODUCT	NSAID COMPONENT[a]
Advil Cold & Sinus	ibuprofen
Aleve	naproxen
Anacin	aspirin
Ascriptin Regular Strength	aspirin
Bayer Low Dose	aspirin
Dristan Sinus Pain	ibuprofen
Ecotrin Adult Low Strength	aspirin
Empirin	aspirin
Excedrin Migraine	aspirin
Excedrin Extra Strength	aspirin
Midol Extended Relief	naproxen
Motrin IB	ibuprofen
Vanquish	aspirin

[a]The product may contain other active components in addition to the NSAID.

other nonselective NSAIDs should be used with caution in these patients. Selective COX-2 inhibitors do not diminish platelet aggregation.

Of additional interest for the athletic trainer are animal studies that have shown delayed new bone growth with use of NSAIDs, including selective COX-2 inhibitors, which may have a larger impact than nonselective COX inhibitors on delaying bone healing. Only a few human studies have examined this issue, and results have been inconclusive. Use of non-NSAID analgesics (see Chapter 7) rather than NSAIDs for pain relief is advisable for patients with fractures. In addition, the effect of NSAIDs on the healing rate of musculoskeletal injuries is unclear.

Drug Interactions

NSAIDs can increase the response from several drugs. Because aspirin prolongs clotting time through its antiplatelet activity, it will enhance the effect of other anticoagulants such as warfarin (Coumadin), a frequently used oral anticoagulant. Aspirin must be used with caution with warfarin, especially considering that aspirin can cause gastric bleeding, which may be enhanced significantly in conjunction with the anticoagulant effects of warfarin. Although the antiplatelet activity is less pronounced with the other NSAIDs, caution is also warranted when these drugs are used with warfarin. Even selective COX-2 inhibitors may affect warfarin response, possibly by inhibiting CYP450 enzyme metabolism (see Chapter 2) of warfarin. For mild-to-moderate analgesia, acetaminophen is preferred for patients on warfarin therapy because acetaminophen does not have anticoagulant effects. NSAIDs can also increase the hypoglycemic effect in patients taking oral antidiabetic drugs and can cause potentially toxic effects from methotrexate when it is used at anticancer dosages.

> *Recall from Chapter 2 that cytochrome P450 (CYP450) enzymes are a large group of enzymes that metabolize drugs. Some drugs are metabolized by more than one CYP enzyme. Additionally, recall from Chapter 3 that some drugs increase or decrease the activity of CYP enzymes, which results in drug interactions.*

NSAIDs can diminish the effects of some drugs. The effectiveness of antihypertensive drugs (see Chapter 12) such as diuretics, angiotensin-converting enzyme inhibitors, and β-blockers are diminished by the concurrent use of NSAIDs. The antiplatelet cardioprotective effect of low-dose aspirin can be diminished by the concomitant use of ibuprofen (see Figure 6-5); although not studied to the same extent as ibuprofen, presumably other NSAIDs have a similar interaction with the antiplatelet effect from aspirin. Because aspirin is an irreversible inhibitor of COX enzymes but ibuprofen is not irreversible, ibuprofen is less effective than aspirin. When ibuprofen is used with aspirin, some of the ibuprofen binds to COX-1 in platelets in place of aspirin (ie, inhibiting aspirin from binding). Although the risk of altering the clinical response from aspirin is minimal with an occasional dose of ibuprofen, it is recommended that the ibuprofen be used either 8 hours or more prior to the aspirin dose or at least 30 minutes after to minimize the effect on aspirin (assuming immediate-release aspirin).

Use of a systemic corticosteroid or alcoholic beverages has the potential to cause peptic ulcers. Consequently, patients on NSAID therapy, particularly aspirin, should be warned about the additional risk of using alcoholic beverages concurrently with NSAIDs (see Figure 6-5). The enhanced risk of ulcer formation from the concurrent use of corticosteroids and long-term NSAID therapy warrants that consideration be given to using misoprostol (Cytotec) or a proton-pump inhibitor as a preventative measure.

There are other such potential interactions, but the point is that because NSAIDs affect pathways that have an impact on so many physiological functions, NSAIDs have the potential for several adverse effects as well as a significant potential for drug interactions. Therefore, the patient's response to multiple drug therapy should be monitored by a physician and/or pharmacist. As a general rule, if a patient experiences a change in symptoms or response after the addition of another drug, it is reasonable to suspect a drug interaction; an adjustment in therapy may be necessary.

Therapy Guidelines

Because NSAIDs have the potential for several significant adverse effects and because the goal of therapy with these drugs is generally to attain specific symptomatic relief, the lowest dose for the shortest duration of therapy that accomplishes the therapeutic goal should be used. Because response varies significantly among patients, it may be necessary to switch from one NSAID to another before an acceptably effective one is identified for a specific patient. A suitable therapeutic response is generally evident within 2 weeks after beginning therapy.

There is no clinically effective means of determining which NSAID may be effective for a patient. However, the patient's medical history, anticipated duration of therapy, cost, and experiences can be a guide to the selection. For example, an OTC NSAID of the patient's choice may be suitable for short-term therapy to treat pain and inflammation of an acute sprain in a young and otherwise healthy person. On the other hand, long-term therapy to treat arthritis in an active older adult may require consideration of once-per-day dosing, history of GI ulcers, cost, and other medications the patient is taking.

Treatment with NSAIDs should be limited to one of these drugs at a time. There is no significant therapeutic advantage to combining NSAIDs. In fact, because some NSAIDs have a greater tendency for one adverse effect or drug interaction, using a combination of 2 NSAIDs at the same time adds the potential for adverse effects from both drugs.

Studies regarding the use of NSAIDs in children are limited; therefore, dosing recommendations for use in children and children's dosage forms are not available for most NSAIDs. The exception is for ibuprofen. Studies have demonstrated that ibuprofen is safe and effective for use in children, and appropriate pediatric dosage forms are available. Approved dosages for children older than 2 years are also reported for naproxen, meloxicam, tolmetin, and celecoxib.

Section Summary

Arachidonic acid is a fatty acid that is a component of membrane phospholipids in virtually all cells. Arachidonic acid is converted to a series of metabolites, also known as eicosanoids, by either the COX or lipoxygenase pathways. The metabolites of the COX pathway include PGs, prostacyclin, and TXs. These metabolites affect many physiological functions, including decreasing the production of stomach acid, increasing the production of protective mucus in the stomach, producing renal vasodilation, contracting uterine smooth muscle, promoting and inhibiting platelet aggregation, sensitizing pain receptors at peripheral and CNS sites, causing an increased body temperature, and contributing significantly to the inflammatory response by increasing blood flow, edema, and release of other inflammatory mediators. There are 2 isoforms of COX, and each tissue produces a predominance of one or the other. COX-1 is produced by gastric mucosal and renal cells, and inhibition of COX-1 by NSAIDs is the cause of the most frequent significant adverse effects. Production of COX-2 occurs at sites that cause pain, inflammation, menstrual cramps, and fever. Inhibition of COX-2 is usually the intent of therapy (the exception is to prevent platelet aggregation). Therefore, NSAIDs that selectively inhibit COX-2 theoretically should have a therapeutic advantage when treating pain and inflammation, but other disadvantages have hindered their use.

Aspirin is a nonselective NSAID and is the prototype with which both selective and nonselective NSAIDs are often compared. Therapy with NSAIDs should be tailored to the needs of each patient and involve the lowest dose used for the shortest time necessary to achieve the desired therapeutic outcome. The patient should be aware of potential adverse effects, particularly gastric upset and ulceration. Use of NSAIDs with food or milk helps diminish gastric adverse effects. NSAIDs should be used with caution in patients with kidney or liver disease. NSAIDs may also be deleterious to patients with risk factors associated with cardiovascular disease. NSAIDs may also inhibit healing of bone fractures. The primary potential for drug interactions exists with patients who are also using corticosteroids, alcoholic beverages, or warfarin.

CORTICOSTEROIDS

The adrenal cortex produces 2 types of corticosteroids: the glucocorticoids and the mineralocorticoids. The primary endogenous glucocorticoid is cortisol (hydrocortisone) and the primary mineralocorticoid is aldosterone. As the name suggests, the mineralocorticoid response has a significant impact on mineral balance; aldosterone increases urinary reabsorption of sodium and excretion of potassium. The glucocorticoid response has a significant impact on glucose metabolism but also affects several other physiological processes. The extent to which corticosteroids exhibit these glucocorticoid physiological effects generally increases as dose and duration of therapy increase. Box 6-1 lists the most significant physiological effects.

Because there is some chemical structure similarity between cortisol and aldosterone, it is not surprising that cortisol has some degree of mineralocorticoid effect (eg, sodium retention). Development of corticosteroids for therapeutic use has focused on increasing the relative potency of the anti-inflammatory, compared with mineralocorticoid, effect. For example, hydrocortisone has equal potency of

---

Box 6-1

PHYSIOLOGICAL EFFECTS OF INCREASED DOSAGE AND TREATMENT DURATION OF CORTICOSTEROIDS

- Glucose production by the liver is increased using glycerol and amino acids (gluconeogenesis), and the glucose is released into the blood (hyperglycemia).

- The rate of protein breakdown is increased to supply amino acids to the liver for glucose synthesis.

- Skeletal muscle wasting occurs with high-dose, long-term use.

- Triglyceride hydrolysis (lipolysis) is increased to supply glycerol for glucose synthesis. Fatty acids become more available as the other product of lipolysis, and thus there is an increased use of fatty acids as an energy source in peripheral tissues.

- Fat is redistributed away from extremities with high-dose, long-term use.

- Calcium absorption from the GI tract is diminished and excretion of calcium by the kidney is increased.

- The aldosterone-like effects (eg, sodium and water retention, potassium excretion) from corticosteroids are generally low but vary depending on which corticosteroid is used.

- Several components of the immune and inflammatory responses are diminished.

---

anti-inflammatory and sodium retention activity. On the other hand, dexamethasone is 25 times more potent than hydrocortisone regarding anti-inflammatory activity and has no sodium retention effects. Prednisone is 4 times more potent than hydrocortisone but has almost the same degree of mineralocorticoid effect as hydrocortisone. Table 6-6 lists some corticosteroids and their anti-inflammatory dosages.

Therapeutic Uses of Corticosteroids

The major use of corticosteroids is to suppress immune and inflammatory responses. These 2 processes are interconnected such that immune responses often have an inflammatory component. The anti-inflammatory mechanism of action for the corticosteroids encompasses a broader effect than that of the NSAIDs. The corticosteroids inhibit the activity of phospholipase A_2 (see Figure 6-2) to

TABLE 6-6		
DOSAGE RANGE OF SELECTED CORTICOSTEROIDS		
GENERIC NAME	**TRADE NAME**	**DOSAGE RANGE[a] (MG/DAY)**
betamethasone	Celestone	0.25 to 9
cortisone	Cortone	25 to 300
dexamethasone	Decadron	0.75 to 9
hydrocortisone	Cortef	15 to 240
methylprednisolone	Medrol	4 to 60
prednisolone	Delta-Cortef	5 to 60
prednisone	Deltasone	5 to 60
triamcinolone	Aristocort	2.5 to 60
[a]Represents adult dosage range, but dosage must be individualized based on patient's response and the specific disease being treated.		

decrease both PG and LT production. Inhibition of these eicosanoid chemical mediators reduces the swelling and pain associated with inflammation. However, they also inhibit the infiltration of phagocytes and lymphocytes at the site of inflammation and inhibit the release of additional chemical mediators that affect the inflammatory and immune responses, such as histamine and some cytokines.

Corticosteroids are used to treat rheumatoid and gouty arthritis, systemic lupus erythematosus, bronchial asthma (see Chapter 9), inflammatory bowel disease (see Chapter 11), tendonitis, bursitis, inflammatory ocular disorders, allergic reactions, and dermatologic diseases. Table 6-6 lists examples of corticosteroids used to treat these conditions. Aside from these conditions, which have an inflammatory component, corticosteroids are also used to treat certain cancers, to suppress organ transplant rejection, and as replacement therapy for adrenocortical insufficiency.

Pharmacokinetics and Dosage

Doses and duration of therapy with corticosteroids vary considerably depending on the specific inflammatory or immune disorder being treated. For example, long-term, low-dose therapy with prednisone for a patient with systemic lupus erythematosus may be 15 mg/day given as a single dose in the morning. On the other hand, short-term therapy at 60 mg/day in divided doses may be used to treat ulcerative colitis until remission occurs. Except for life-threatening situations, such as immunosuppressive therapy in organ transplantation or as cancer chemotherapy, corticosteroid

therapy should be initiated at the lowest dose and for the shortest time possible to achieve the therapeutic outcomes. Determining the dosage regimen for each patient for systemic treatment is somewhat trial and error and necessitates monitoring the extent of therapeutic, as well as adverse, effects. As therapy extends beyond 1 week, the incidence of adverse effects generally increases in a dose-related fashion.

Corticosteroids are available for use by several routes of administration. Inhalation products used to treat asthma are discussed in Chapter 9. Topical application of corticosteroids is used only for local, not systemic, effects and should be used whenever possible in place of systemic therapy to treat dermatological inflammatory conditions. Local injections are also useful to minimize systemic adverse effects in situations where inflammation is limited (eg, in a specific joint or soft tissue, such as tendons). For a systemic effect, the oral route is preferred because corticosteroids are almost completely absorbed from the GI tract. Intramuscular injections are available in which the corticosteroid exists as an ester form, which has lower aqueous solubility and thus slowly dissipates from the site of injection. These forms of the corticosteroid have a longer duration of action of several days to weeks depending on the specific product. Examples are betamethasone acetate (Celestone Soluspan), dexamethasone acetate (Decadron-LA), methylprednisolone acetate (Depo-Medrol), and triamcinolone diacetate (Aristocort Forte).

The primary mechanism of clearance for corticosteroids is liver metabolism to form inactive metabolites that are excreted in the urine.

> *An ester form means that another molecule (eg, acetate) is chemically bonded to the corticosteroid. The addition of the acetate makes the corticosteroid less water soluble, and thus it will not be dissolved in the extracellular fluid as rapidly. These are sometimes referred to as* depot *injections.*

Adverse Effects

An alteration of the normal physiological regulation of corticosteroid production is the cause of significant adverse effects associated with corticosteroid therapy. The amount of corticosteroid produced by the adrenal gland is regulated through a feedback regulation process by the amount of corticosteroid in the blood. The corticosteroid level in the blood fluctuates; when it starts decreasing, the hypothalamus releases corticotropin-releasing hormone (CRH), which signals the anterior pituitary to release adrenocorticotropic hormone (ACTH), which signals the adrenal gland to produce more corticosteroid (ie, cortisol). When the cortisol level in the blood is sufficient, it signals the hypothalamus and pituitary to stop releasing hormone.

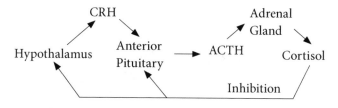

This control system is referred to as the *hypothalamic-pituitary-adrenal (HPA) axis*. If a corticosteroid is given as drug therapy, it mimics the action of cortisol on the HPA axis and thus suppresses the synthesis of cortisol by the adrenal gland. The amount of HPA suppression, and subsequent adrenal suppression, is dependent on the dose and duration of corticosteroid therapy. There is also variation among patients as to the time it takes to recover from adrenal suppression. It could take weeks to months for normal HPA axis function to return. If adrenal suppression occurs and the dose of corticosteroid is removed too quickly, the patient can experience various symptoms, including nausea, vomiting, anorexia, headache, lethargy, fever, and pain in the muscles and joints. Abrupt discontinuation after long-term therapy can be fatal.

Treatment with corticosteroids for only a few days usually does not elicit the significant adrenal suppression or the other adverse effects listed in Box 6-2. However, even when short-term treatment is warranted for acute inflammation, it may be worth considering whether the metabolic effects on glucose, protein, and lipid metabolism may have an impact on the patient's athletic performance. The incidence and extent of adverse effects increases with duration of therapy and increased dose. The impact on athletic performance will depend on the extent of the adverse effect, level of athletic participation, and specific athletic event of concern. Muscle weakness from long-term corticosteroid therapy would likely affect the athletic performance of all individuals on this therapy, whereas a fungal infection, with treatment, would not.

Drug Interactions

The major drug interactions are related to the adverse effects discussed previously. Patients on NSAIDs have an increased risk of peptic ulcers when corticosteroids are added to therapy. In addition, because corticosteroids can cause hyperglycemia, they are working against the desired effect of insulin or oral hypoglycemic drugs used to treat diabetic patients; adjustment of diabetic therapy may be necessary. The effect on potassium excretion can accentuate the potassium loss associated with certain diuretics that can cause hypokalemia.

Therapy Guidelines

Although dosages of corticosteroids vary considerably depending on the disease and the individual responses,

there are some general therapy guidelines. Among the major concerns with corticosteroid therapy is the existence of adrenal suppression. It is difficult to determine exactly what dose, duration of therapy, and dosing schedule will result in adrenal suppression. However, in general, short-term therapy is considered to be less than 1 week. In general, as doses of prednisone increase above 5 mg/day, the dose is considered supraphysiologic and therefore capable of causing adrenal suppression. When corticosteroid therapy is to be discontinued in patients who are likely to have adrenal suppression, the dose of corticosteroid is tapered to provide time for HPA axis to recover. Many protocols have been reported for tapering corticosteroid dosages, but the process can take weeks to months depending on the duration and dosage of corticosteroid that the patient received. Alternate-day dosing is sometimes used in patients receiving long-term therapy after initial management of the disease has been accomplished. This dosing schedule provides a means of diminishing some of the adverse effects associated with corticosteroid therapy as well as reducing the effect on the HPA axis.

Section Summary

Use of corticosteroids is an effective means of treating inflammation associated with rheumatoid arthritis, bronchial asthma, tendonitis, bursitis, osteoarthritis, allergic reactions, systemic lupus erythematosus, and dermatologic diseases. However, systemic use poses the potential for several significant adverse effects. Consequently, except for life-threatening conditions, use of systemic corticosteroids should be at the lowest dose for the shortest time necessary. The mechanism of action of corticosteroids is multifaceted and includes inhibition of the synthesis of arachidonic acid metabolites, diminished action of phagocytic cells, and reduced release of other mediators. Besides adrenal suppression, examples of other adverse effects are hypertension, osteoporosis, cataracts, behavioral disturbances, infection, peptic ulcer, glucose intolerance, increased appetite, and muscle weakness. Adverse effects are minimized when corticosteroids are used topically, by inhalation, or by local injection at the site of inflammation. Alternate-day dosing is another means of decreasing adverse effects and HPA axis effects in patients who require long-term therapy. Drug interactions are primarily associated with concurrent use of NSAIDs and drugs used to treat diabetes mellitus.

GLUCOSAMINE

Glucosamine is classified as a dietary supplement and thus does not fall under the same FDA scrutiny as drugs. Although the product labeling includes a statement that the product is not intended to treat or prevent disease,

---

Box 6-2

Potential Adverse Effects of Corticosteroid Therapy

- Adrenal suppression is a significant concern, especially as dose and duration of therapy increase. Consequently, withdrawal of long-term corticosteroid therapy must be tapered over a time determined by the extent of adrenal suppression. Using alternate-day dosing of systemic corticosteroids, rather than dosing every day, helps minimize the adrenal suppression.

- Flare-up of the disease being treated is a problem associated with the withdrawal of corticosteroid therapy because the symptoms of the disease are no longer being suppressed.

- Hypertension and hypokalemia can occur in part as a result of sodium and water retention (edema) and potassium depletion. This is minimized by use of corticosteroids with predominantly glucocorticoid rather than mineralocorticoid activity (see Table 6-6). Consequently, corticosteroids should be used with caution in patients on diuretics that deplete potassium (see Chapter 12) or patients with reduced kidney function.

- Osteoporosis is a frequent result of long-term corticosteroid therapy. Steps to minimize this effect include use of calcium supplements, vitamin D supplements, and any one of a group of drugs called bisphosphonates (brand names Fosamax, Actonel, Boniva), which inhibit bone resorption. However, caution is needed with the use of corticosteroids in patients with existing osteoporosis.

- Increased susceptibility to infection because of suppression of the immune response, or activation of an infection that had been held under control by the immune system. Because inflammation often contributes to the infection symptoms, corticosteroids may also mask the existence of an infection. It is reasonable advice for patients on oral corticosteroid therapy to take extra precautions to avoid contact with people who have a communicable disease. Also, because of the immune suppression effects of corticosteroids and because fungal infections are often difficult to treat, patients with fungal infections should avoid corticosteroid therapy if possible.

- There is an increased risk for peptic ulcers, especially when combined with other ulcer-causing agents such as NSAIDs.

- Suppression of growth in children can occur with relatively small doses of systemic corticosteroids. This effect can be reduced by alternate-day dosing.

- Myopathy can occur but is more frequently associated with prolonged, high-dose use of corticosteroids. The muscle weakness is primarily of the arms and legs but may include generalized weakness. Discontinuation of therapy is warranted, and reversal of the effect occurs after several months.

- Cataracts are a relatively common adverse effect from long-term corticosteroid use. Consequently, periodic eye exams are recommended for early detection. Glaucoma can also occur, especially in patients with diabetes mellitus or a family history of glaucoma.

- A variety of effects on the CNS results in an array of possible responses, including elevated mood, euphoria, insomnia, irritability, nervousness, and depression. These effects occur within days of initiating therapy and are more likely to occur with higher daily doses.

- In addition to the CNS effects, there are various other adverse effects that can occur with short-term therapy (eg, appetite stimulation, GI irritation, headache, and exacerbation of acne).

- Many of the corticosteroids cross the placenta and also enter breast milk and can affect the infant.

- Increased blood glucose may diminish control of hyperglycemia in diabetic patients and therefore should be used with caution in these patients.

- Fat redistribution can occur with long-term, high-dose therapy. The fat moves from the extremities to the face and trunk, causing a moon face, buffalo hump, and enlarged abdomen.

glucosamine has been widely used for reducing osteoarthritis symptoms and thus is included in this chapter.

Use and Effects

Glucosamine is not an analgesic and is not considered an anti-inflammatory agent; it does not affect the COX pathway. Glucosamine is an aminomonosaccharide that is used to make glycosaminoglycans, which are components of proteoglycans used to make cartilage. Use of glucosamine is based on the belief that it stimulates the production of cartilage to replace damaged cartilage. Unlike the anti-inflammatory drugs, glucosamine reportedly may stop or reverse the progression of osteoarthritis, a disease characterized by continued breakdown of articular cartilage. Effects of glucosamine therapy have included reduced restriction of active and passive movement, articular pain, and joint tenderness and swelling. Glucosamine is sometimes marketed in the same dosage form with chondroitin sulfate, which is a glycosaminoglycan. The proposed action of this compound is similar to glucosamine.

Several clinical studies have been conducted to examine the effectiveness of glucosamine in reducing the symptoms of osteoarthritis. The results of these studies have yielded conflicting results, with some showing benefit and others showing no difference from placebo. Many of these studies have been interpreted with caution due to poor study design and/or small sample size. However, results from a large randomized placebo-controlled trial (the GAIT trial) failed to show a statistically significant benefit from glucosamine, chondroitin, or a combination of glucosamine and chondroitin.[1,2] The American College of Rheumatology released osteoarthritis treatment guidelines in 2012 that included a conditional recommendation against the use of glucosamine and chondroitin in arthritis patients.

Pharmacokinetics and Dosage

Glucosamine is absorbed by the oral route, although the first-pass effect (see Chapter 2) reduces bioavailability to about one-fourth the oral dose. The majority of the unaltered glucosamine is excreted by the kidney. The most common oral dosage used in clinical trials is 500 mg 3 times per day given as glucosamine sulfate. Glucosamine is available in most pharmacies and food supplement stores. Because dietary supplements are not subject to the same standards of potency and purity (nor efficacy and safety) as drug products, the characteristics of each glucosamine product are unknown.

Adverse Effects

The adverse effects reported for glucosamine have been minimal. When adverse effects have been reported, the major complaint has been GI discomfort, but other complaints include headache, skin rash, and itching. Although no systematic study has been conducted regarding drug interactions with glucosamine, some of the clinical trials of therapeutic effectiveness of glucosamine included patients taking medications for various diseases; no significant drug interactions were reported.

Section Summary

Glucosamine has been used in the treatment of osteoarthritis. However, recent data from a well-designed clinical trial did not show a significant benefit from glucosamine. Adverse effects are minimal, the most predominant being GI discomfort.

TREATMENT OF RHEUMATOID ARTHRITIS AND GOUT

NSAIDs and corticosteroids are used to treat rheumatoid arthritis and gout, but unique features of these diseases also necessitate the use of other drugs.

Drug Therapy for Rheumatoid Arthritis

For treatment of rheumatoid arthritis, NSAIDs are usually part of initial therapy and are useful to provide anti-inflammatory activity and as an analgesic to quickly reduce the pain. All of the NSAIDs are effective in reducing these symptoms, although some patients respond better to one drug vs another. The likelihood of toxicity from the long-term use of anti-inflammatory doses of NSAIDs limits their use. Additionally, NSAIDs only reduce the symptoms; they do not affect the progression of the disease. More aggressive therapy is recommended as a part of initial therapy and includes disease-modifying antirheumatic drugs (DMARDs) along with NSAIDs. Long-term use of DMARDs may be able to delay or stop the progression of the disease. In the meantime, NSAIDs are useful to alleviate the symptoms but then can be discontinued when the effect of the DMARD is sufficient. Table 6-7 lists DMARDs and summarizes their characteristics. Among the DMARDs, methotrexate (Rheumatrex) is often the first choice. Hydroxychloroquine (Plaquenil), leflunomide (Arava), and sulfasalazine (Azulfidine) are also used to treat mild to moderate rheumatoid arthritis. These drugs are also used in combination with methotrexate or with other DMARDs to treat patients who do not respond sufficiently to a single agent. The mechanism of action of some DMARDs is unknown, whereas some specific immunosuppressive and/or anti-inflammatory activity has been identified for others. One of the major disadvantages of traditional DMARDs is that they have a slow onset of action; it takes weeks to months to see benefit from these agents.

TABLE 6-7

DRUGS FOR TREATING RHEUMATOID ARTHRITIS

GENERIC NAME	TRADE NAME	SELECTED CHARACTERISTICS
adalimumab	Humira	Monoclonal antibody against TNF. Given by subcutaneous injection every other week. May cause flu-like symptoms and increase risk of infections, including serious respiratory infections.
abatacept	Orencia	Inhibits the activation of T-cells. Given by subcutaneous injection once weekly. Can also be given IV. May increase risk of infections.
anakinra	Kineret	Blocks the action of IL-1. Given by subcutaneous injection once daily. May increase risk of infections.
azathioprine	Imuran	Monitor liver function and signs of bone marrow suppression. Contraindicated during pregnancy.
certolizumab	Cimzia	Monoclonal antibody against TNF. Given by subcutaneous injection every other week. May increase risk of infections, including serious respiratory infections.
cyclosporine	Neoral	Monitor kidney function. May cause hypertension, hyperglycemia, increased incidence of infection, and GI effects. Use if other DMARDs not effective.
etanercept	Enbrel	Decreases activity of TNF. Given by subcutaneous injection once per week. May cause headache and increase risk of infections, including serious respiratory infections.
golimumab	Simponi	Monoclonal antibody against TNF. Given by subcutaneous injection once a month. Also can be given IV. Given in combination with methotrexate. May increase risk of infections, including serious respiratory infections.
hydroxychloroquine	Plaquenil	Relatively safe but monitor for retinal toxicity. Give with food to minimize GI effects.
infliximab	Remicade	Must be given with methotrexate to prevent antibody production against infliximab. May increase the risk of infections, including serious respiratory infections. Dose given by IV infusion at certain week intervals.
leflunomide	Arava	Monitor liver function. Contraindicated during pregnancy. May cause reversible hair loss, respiratory infections, GI effects. Long half-life so loading dose given.
methotrexate	Rheumatrex	Monitor liver and kidney function and blood cell counts. GI effects. Contraindicated during pregnancy. Dosage is once/week.
penicillamine	Cuprimine	May cause autoimmune diseases, GI effects, metallic taste, skin rash, oral mucosal lesions. Use when other DMARDs not effective. Caution if penicillin allergy.
rituximab	Rituxan	Monoclonal antibody to a receptor on B-cells. Given by IV infusion. May cause serious infusion reactions and increase risk of infections.
sulfasalazine	Azulfidine	Prodrug converted to active sulfapyridine by GI bacteria and then absorbed. GI effects common but decreased by using enteric-coated dosage forms, take with food, or using divided daily dosage. May cause rash and harmlessly turn skin and urine yellow-orange.

(continued)

TABLE 6-7 (CONTINUED)		
DRUGS FOR TREATING RHEUMATOID ARTHRITIS		
GENERIC NAME	**TRADE NAME**	**SELECTED CHARACTERISTICS**
tocilizumab	Actemra	Monoclonal antibody that blocks action of IL-6. Given by subcutaneous injection weekly or every other week. May increase risk of infections, including serious respiratory infections.
tofacitinib	Xeljanz	May increase risk of infections, including serious respiratory infections.
DMARDs = disease-modifying antirheumatic drugs; GI = gastrointestinal; IV = intravenous.		

Several biologic DMARDs are available to treat rheumatoid arthritis. An advantage of this class compared with traditional DMARDs is that the onset of action is faster (usually 1 to 3 weeks). Examples of these drugs include etanercept (Enbrel), adalimumab (Humira), and infliximab (Remicade). All of the biologic DMARDs are proteins and thus must be administered by injection. The mechanism of action involves blocking components of the immune system that contribute to the progression of rheumatoid arthritis. These agents block the effects of chemical mediators of inflammation such as TNF, interleukin-1 (IL-1), and IL-6 or block receptors on immune system cells. The biologic DMARDs are used alone or in combination with other DMARDs to treat moderate to severe rheumatoid arthritis that is not responding to traditional DMARDs. A significant concern is the occurrence of serious infections, including tuberculosis and fungal infections. Patients should be screened with a tuberculin skin test.

Similar to NSAIDs, corticosteroids alleviate symptoms of rheumatoid arthritis but do not delay the progression of the disease. Several days of high-dose corticosteroid therapy are useful in controlling flare-ups of rheumatoid arthritis. Corticosteroid therapy is also used to control symptoms while DMARD therapy is being initiated if NSAIDs are not effective. Intra-articular and intramuscular injections are an alternative to oral therapy, and slow-release forms of the corticosteroid provide weeks to months of relief. Long-term therapy, even at low doses, is not preferred but is useful in patients who do not respond sufficiently to any other therapy. As always, long-term use poses the problems of potentially serious adverse effects such as osteoporosis, glaucoma, cataracts, hyperglycemia, hypertension, and increased susceptibility to infections. Consequently, some precautions that should be taken are monitoring blood pressure and blood glucose, watching for symptoms of osteoporosis (eg, bone pain), and using calcium and vitamin D supplements to prevent osteoporosis.

Drug Therapy for Gout

Drug therapy for gout centers on 2 approaches: alleviate the pain associated with acute attacks and prevent recurrent attacks by decreasing the blood uric acid level. The most frequently used drugs to treat acute gout (Table 6-8) are colchicine and indomethacin (Indocin). The exact mechanism for colchicine is not clear, but it does not have generalized anti-inflammatory or analgesic activity; its effectiveness is relatively specific for gout. Colchicine is most effective if given within 48 hours after onset of symptoms. Pain is diminished within hours of the first dose, and inflammation is usually gone within 3 days. This drug has a low therapeutic index and therefore the dosage regimen is quite specific (1.2 mg orally as the initial dose, followed in 1 hour by 0.6 mg). GI adverse symptoms are an indication of toxicity. Although colchicine is very effective, patients must be well advised regarding the use of this drug.

Indomethacin is considered the drug of choice to treat acute gout attacks. It has a quick onset of action, is comparable with colchicine in effectiveness, and is much less toxic than colchicine. After an initial higher oral dose, the dose of indomethacin is reduced until symptoms are gone, and then the dose is tapered off over several days. Many other NSAIDs are also effective (eg, naproxen, fenoprofen, ibuprofen) and can be used to treat acute attacks. However, aspirin should not be used because it can block the excretion of uric acid, depending on the dose. Although there are some advantages of indomethacin and NSAIDs compared with colchicine, patients with a history of GI bleeding or renal disease should avoid indomethacin and other NSAIDs.

If colchicine or an NSAID is not effective or is inappropriate for a patient, corticosteroid therapy can be used to treat acute attacks. Oral, parenteral, or intra-articular administration is effective. The oral dose must be tapered gradually after the acute attack subsides.

There are 4 drugs used to lower uric acid blood levels (antihyperuricemic therapy). Two of them, probenecid (Benemid) and sulfinpyrazone (Anturane), increase the excretion rate of uric acid by blocking the reabsorption of uric acid from the renal tubule. The other antihyperuricemic drugs, allopurinol (Zyloprim) and febuxostat (Uloric), inhibit the synthesis of uric acid from purines (xanthine oxidase inhibitors). The xanthine oxidase inhibitors are the preferred agents for lowering uric acid levels. The antihyperuricemic drugs are of no benefit to treat acute

		TABLE 6-8	
		DRUGS FOR TREATING GOUT	
GENERIC NAME	**TRADE NAME**	**SELECTED CHARACTERISTICS**	**USE**
colchicine	Colcrys	Low TI. GI effects are sign of toxicity. Avoid in pregnancy. Must be taken within 48 hours of onset of symptoms. Pain subsides within hours; swelling subsides within few days. Not effective for other inflammatory conditions.	Treat acute episodes
indomethacin	Indocin	Pain subsides within hours; swelling subsides within few days. May cause severe frontal headache, GI effects, and gastric ulcers. Avoid use if history of ulcers or kidney disease.	Treat acute episodes
allopurinol	Zyloprim	May cause hypersensitivity reaction; discontinue if skin rash. May increase likelihood of acute attack within first several months but use with colchicine or NSAID decreases incidence. Use with large volume of fluid/day to prevent uric acid damage to kidney. No anti-inflammatory/analgesic effect.	Long-term preventative; blocks uric acid synthesis
febuxostat	Uloric	May increase likelihood of acute attack within first several months but use with colchicine or NSAID decreases incidence. Use with large volume of fluid/day to prevent uric acid damage to kidney. No anti-inflammatory/analgesic effect.	Long-term preventative; blocks uric acid synthesis
probenecid	Benemid	GI effects; use with food. May increase likelihood of acute attack within first several months but use with colchicine or NSAID decreases incidence. Use with large volume of fluid/day to prevent uric acid damage to kidney. No anti-inflammatory or analgesic effect. Avoid in patients with impaired kidney function.	Long-term preventative; increases uric acid excretion
sulfinpyrazone	Anturane	GI effects; use with food. May increase likelihood of acute attack within first several months but use with colchicine or NSAID decreases incidence. Use with large volume of fluid/day to prevent uric acid damage to kidney. No anti-inflammatory or analgesic effect. Avoid in patients with impaired kidney function.	Long-term preventative; increases uric acid excretion
GI=gastrointestinal; TI=therapeutic index.			

gout attacks, but long-term therapy reduces the incidence of acute attacks. However, the incidence of an acute attack is increased during the initial several months of therapy with antihyperuricemic drugs; therefore, colchicine or an NSAID can be added during these months to decrease the incidence of acute attacks. A large daily intake of water is recommended during therapy to avoid the development of uric acid stones. In addition, antihyperuricemic therapy should not be started during an acute attack because these drugs may exacerbate the symptoms. Finally, for patients who have gout that fails to respond to traditional therapies, a medication called pegloticase (Krystexxa) can be used. Pegloticase breaks down uric acid; therefore, blood levels of uric acid drop. A major disadvantage of this agent is that it has to be given by intravenous infusion and causes infusion reactions.

Recall from Chapter 2 that there is an active transport mechanism that transports endogenous compounds (eg, amino acids, glucose) back into the blood from the renal tubule. Uric acid is reabsorbed by this active transport mechanism.

Section Summary

Drug therapy for rheumatoid arthritis and gout has 2 major aspects: treat acute pain and inflammation and use long-term therapy to decrease the incidence of acute episodes. NSAIDs play a role to treat acute pain and inflammation for both diseases and corticosteroid therapy can

TABLE 6-9

SELECTED TOPICAL NONPRESCRIPTION ANTI-INFLAMMATORY/ANALGESIC PRODUCTS

TRADE NAME	DOSAGE FORM	PRIMARY INGREDIENTS
Absorbine Jr Plus	Liquid	4% menthol
Aspercreme	Cream	10% trolamine salicylate
Ben-Gay Cold Therapy	Gel	5% menthol
Ben-Gay Greaseless Pain Relieving Cream	Cream	15% methyl salicylate, 10% menthol
Ben-Gay Ultra Strength	Cream	30% methyl salicylate, 10% menthol, 4% camphor
Eucalyptamint	Gel	16% menthol, eucalyptus oil
Heet	Liniment	18% methyl salicylate, 3.6% camphor, 0.25% capsaicin
Cortizone-10	Ointment	1% hydrocortisone
Icy Hot Balm	Ointment	29% methyl salicylate, 7.6% menthol
Icy Hot Cream	Cream	30% methyl salicylate, 10% menthol
Icy Hot Stick	Gel	30% methyl salicylate, 10% menthol
Sportscreme	Cream	10% trolamine salicylate
Vicks VapoRub	Ointment	4.8% camphor, 2.6% menthol, 1.2% eucalyptus oil

be used if NSAIDs are not effective. Colchicine and indomethacin are particularly useful to treat acute gout. The use of DMARDs is part of the more aggressive therapy to reduce the progression of rheumatoid arthritis. Drugs such as methotrexate and hydroxychloroquine are DMARDs, but the response from therapy must be monitored because they can cause serious adverse effects. Sulfinpyrazone, probenecid, febuxostat, and allopurinol are antihyperuricemic drugs that may be life-long therapy to reduce the incidence of acute gout attacks.

TOPICAL ANTI-INFLAMMATORY PRODUCTS

Topical anti-inflammatory products are available by prescription to treat various topical inflammatory conditions, but there are numerous gels, creams, and ointments available OTC that contain a salicylate, a counterirritant, and/or a corticosteroid (eg, hydrocortisone). There may also be an analgesic component added to some of these compounds. Table 6-9 lists examples of these OTC anti-inflammatory/analgesic products.

Salicylate is the only NSAID used topically in the United States. The form of salicylate is usually methyl salicylate (see Table 6-9). Topically applied salicylate may be effective when applied at the site of strains, sprains, and muscle soreness from strenuous exercise, although most of the reports

are regarding analgesic rather than anti-inflammatory effectiveness for the treatment of these conditions. Topical application has not been shown to be more effective than oral use of NSAIDs.

Salicylates act primarily by penetrating directly to the tissue rather than by absorption into the systemic circulation and distribution to the tissue site. The rate and extent of absorption into the systemic circulation varies depending on the site of application (eg, greater on the abdomen or forearm and less on the foot) and increases with multiple applications at the same site. Regardless of the site of application, the amount absorbed is too low for systemic therapeutic purposes (ie, it is not a transdermal route) and is used for a local response only. Nonetheless, topically applied salicylates must be used with the same caution as oral NSAIDs in patients with known risk factors such as NSAID hypersensitivity, renal disease, liver disease, alcohol use, and history of GI bleeding.

Counterirritants are oftentimes a component of OTC anti-inflammatory/analgesic products. These are compounds that are applied topically to relieve pain; they act by producing less severe pain (via skin irritation) to essentially distract the patient from a more severe pain. Although the exact mechanism is unclear, counterirritants appear to indirectly stimulate sensations such as cold, hot, or itching, which directs the attention away from the more severe pain in the muscles, joints, or tendons. This mechanism contributes to the analgesic action of methyl salicylate, allyl isothiocyanate (mustard oil), turpentine oil, camphor,

```
╔══════════════════════════════════════╗
║              BOX 6-3                  ║
╠══════════════════════════════════════╣
║        CONSIDERATIONS FOR THE         ║
║   TOPICAL USE OF CORTICOSTEROIDS      ║
╠══════════════════════════════════════╣
```

- Because corticosteroids inhibit the immune response, do not use topical corticosteroids to treat inflammation associated with skin infection.

- Prescription topical corticosteroids can cause local skin reactions such as skin atrophy, acneiform eruptions, and perioral dermatitis.

- Topical use of corticosteroids for long periods, particularly the more potent prescription products, can cause systemic adverse effects.

- Systemic absorption of topically applied corticosteroids will increase if applied to inflamed skin.

- In addition to the anti-inflammatory effect, topical corticosteroids also relieve the itching associated with insect bites and contact dermatitis from poison ivy, harsh chemicals, cosmetics, and other minor irritants.

menthol, and capsicum (from hot chili peppers). In addition to the counterirritant effect, methyl salicylate, allyl isothiocyanate, and turpentine oil are also *rubefacients* (ie, they cause redness due to cutaneous vasodilation). On the other hand, menthol and camphor cause a cooling effect, whereas capsicum causes a feeling of warmth without vasodilation. Although these compounds are considered safe and effective counterirritants, they may also have a placebo component. The feeling of warmth or coolness and the sensations of irritation, as well as some odors associated with topical application, may give the patient the confidence that the drug is working, thus producing a beneficial psychological effect. Methyl salicylate and menthol are also used in smaller amounts as components of wintergreen oil and peppermint oil, respectively, as flavoring agents.

Increased irritation and possible tissue damage (eg, blistering) can occur if methyl salicylate is applied to tissue and then occlusive bandaging or heating pads are used. Use of counterirritants during hot and humid weather or application after strenuous exercise can pose similar problems. Counterirritants should only be applied to intact skin, not to wounds or damaged skin.

Capsicum has been used 2 to 4 times daily to reduce the pain associated with osteoarthritis and rheumatoid arthritis by rubbing the product around the affected joints. Capsicum appears to inhibit substance P, a neurotransmitter that is thought to be involved in pain sensation at peripheral sites. It may also have some anti-inflammatory properties. For treatment of arthritis, pain relief may not occur until after 1 to 2 weeks of treatment, with maximum

relief after several weeks. A local burning sensation occurs with initial therapy but subsides with continued use.

Camphor and menthol are also used topically to relieve itching (antipruritic) caused from contact with numerous irritants such as poison ivy, chemicals, and cosmetics. These local analgesics are typically used in combination with other compounds, such as topical anesthetics, which also contribute to the antipruritic response.

Hydrocortisone is the only topical corticosteroid available without a prescription, but several more potent corticosteroids are available in topical dosage forms by prescription. The mechanism and therapeutic use of these products have already been discussed, but some additional noteworthy points are listed in Box 6-3.

There are other substances that reportedly have anti-inflammatory and/or counterirritant properties and are added to some OTC products, although evidence is less convincing regarding their effectiveness. These substances include eucalyptus oil, wormwood, and echinacea.

Section Summary

The advantage of topical application of anti-inflammatory agents is the reduced incidence of systemic effects and the potential of some placebo effect. Methyl salicylate is the most frequently used NSAID for topical application, although methyl salicylate exerts its action primarily as a counterirritant. Other counterirritants include camphor, menthol, and capsicum. Pain and itching may be associated with inflammation, and counterirritants are used for their topical analgesic and antipruritic activity rather than for any specific anti-inflammatory action. Hydrocortisone is the only topical corticosteroid available OTC, although other topical corticosteroids are available by prescription for their anti-inflammatory effectiveness.

ROLE OF THE ATHLETIC TRAINER

A comparison of the characteristics of NSAIDs and corticosteroids is presented in Table 6-10. Regarding the use of NSAIDs, the athletic trainer can have a positive impact on ensuring therapeutic outcomes and reducing adverse effects. The dose and duration of therapy will depend on the therapeutic goal; low-dose, long-term therapy with aspirin is typical to prevent heart attack or stroke in certain predisposed patients, whereas short-term, higher-dose therapy with any one of many NSAIDs is expected for treatment of an acute inflammatory condition. The athletic trainer should understand these differences and encourage the patient to adhere to the prescribed therapeutic regimen. Regardless of dose and therapeutic intent for use of NSAIDs, the following are important to consider:

- The benefits and risks must be weighed to determine whether anti-inflammatory drugs should be

TABLE 6-10

CHARACTERISTICS OF NONSTEROIDAL ANTI-INFLAMMATORY DRUGS AND CORTICOSTEROIDS

CHARACTERISTIC	NSAIDS	CORTICOSTEROIDS
Availability	OTC and Rx	OTC topical and Rx
Primary route	Oral	Oral, injection, topical
Therapeutic uses	Anti-inflammatory	Anti-inflammatory
	Analgesic	Immunosuppressant
	Antipyretic	Adrenal replacement therapy
	Anticoagulant	Anticancer
Primary clearance route	Liver metabolism	Liver metabolism
	Urinary excretion	Urinary excretion
Primary adverse effects	Gastric irritation	Adrenal suppression
	Peptic ulcers	Increased blood glucose
	Diminished kidney function	Peptic ulcers
	Allergic reaction	Osteoporosis
	Increased clotting time	Susceptibility to infection
		Muscle weakness
Primary drug interactions	Increased warfarin response	Decreased effect of insulin and oral antidiabetic drugs
	Increased oral antidiabetic drug effect	Increased ulcer risk with NSAIDs
	Decreased effect of some antihypertensives	
	Increased ulcer risk with corticosteroids	
Examples	Aspirin, ibuprofen, naproxen	Cortisone, dexamethasone, prednisone
Mechanism	Inhibits COX	Inhibits phospholipase

OTC = over-the-counter; Rx = prescription.

used for any specific patient. There is significant potential for adverse effects with the use of NSAIDs and corticosteroids, and the benefits of faster healing and shorter time before a return to full activity are not assured.

- NSAIDs should be taken with food or milk, or at least with a full glass of water, to reduce gastric discomfort.

- Only one NSAID should be used at a time.

- The use of NSAIDs should be avoided in patients who have had a hypersensitivity response to any NSAID.

- The likelihood of gastric ulceration increases with longer-term, higher-dose use of NSAIDs and in patients who are elderly, have a history of peptic ulcer disease, are concurrently taking corticosteroids, or are consuming alcoholic beverages. Patients with severe or persistent gastric pain should be referred to their physician.

- NSAIDs should be avoided in patients who are pregnant or breastfeeding. Aspirin should be avoided in children and teens with viral infections.

- NSAIDs can cause diminished renal function, although athletes at risk for this are primarily those with existing heart, liver, or kidney impairment. NSAIDs should be discontinued and the athlete referred to his or her physician when signs of edema or reduced urine output are present.

Corticosteroids are often used in bursts of short-term therapy to treat acute inflammation; the frequency of adverse effects is greatly reduced when these drugs are used for only a few days. Nonetheless, the athletic trainer should be aware of the potential for adverse effects and drug interactions, particularly in athletes who are being treated with corticosteroids for longer periods. Use of corticosteroids is associated with these key points:

- Diabetic athletes should be keenly aware that they may require an adjustment in anti-diabetic drug therapy.

- Athletes who are also on NSAIDs should know that black, tarry stools may indicate GI bleeding.

- Athletes should be alerted that fever and sore throat are often signs of infection.

- Signs of swelling and weight gain may indicate sodium and water retention and may warrant a change in therapy.

CASE STUDY

Two days ago, Tyler suffered a moderate ankle sprain during basketball when his ankle rolled into severe inversion as he landed after going up for a rebound. The team physician was in attendance at practice; after examining Tyler, Dr. Becki gave him Voltaren with instructions for use and dosage. Tyler reports to you that he doesn't feel the medication is doing anything because he still has all the symptoms he had when the injury occurred. You explain to him that because he has been taking it long enough to achieve a steady-state of the drug in his system, you will contact Dr. Becki to see if she has suggestions for another NSAID that may work better for him. How would you explain to Tyler what NSAIDs do therapeutically and why the Voltaren might not have been working?

REFERENCES

1. Clegg DO, Reda DJ, Harris CL, et al. Glucosamine, chondroitin sulfate, and the two in combination for painful knee osteoarthritis. *N Engl J Med.* 2006;354(8):795-808.

2. Sawitzke AD, Shi H, Finco MF, et al. Clinical efficacy and safety over two years use of glucosamine, chondroitin sulfate, their combination, celecoxib or placebo taken to treat osteoarthritis of the knee: a GAIT report. *Ann Rheum Dis.* 2010;69(8):1459-1464.

BIBLIOGRAPHY

Chen MR, Dragoo JL. The effect of nonsteroidal anti-inflammatory drugs on tissue healing. *Knee Surg Sports Traumatol Arthrosc.* 2013;21(3):540-549.

Curtiss FR. Relative value of the NSAIDs, including COX-2 inhibitors and meloxicam. *J Manag Care Pharm.* 2006;12(3):265-268.

Elnachef N, Scheiman JM, Fendrick AM, Howden CW, Chey WD. Changing perceptions and practices regarding aspirin, nonsteroidal anti-inflammatory drugs, and cyclooxygenase-2 selective nonsteroidal anti-inflammatory drugs among US primary care providers. *Aliment Pharmacol Ther.* 2008;28(10):1249-1258.

Geusens P, Emans PJ, de Jong JJ, van den Bergh J. NSAIDs and fracture healing. *Curr Opin Rheumatol.* 2013;25(4):524-531.

Harirforoosh S, Asghar W, Jamali F. Adverse effects of nonsteroidal anti-inflammatory drugs: an update of gastrointestinal, cardiovascular and renal complications. *J Pharm Pharm Sci.* 2013;16(5):821-847.

Hochberg MC, Altman RD, April KT, et al. American College of Rheumatology 2012 recommendations for the use of nonpharmacologic and pharmacologic therapies in osteoarthritis of the hand, hip, and knee. *Arthritis Care Res.* 2012;64(4):455-474.

Khanna D, Fitzgerald JD, Khanna PP, et al. 2012 American College of Rheumatology guidelines for the management of gout. Part 1: systemic nonpharmacologic and pharmacologic therapeutic approaches to hyperuricemia. *Arthritis Care Res.* 2012;64(10):1431-1446.

Singh JA, Furst DE, Bharat A, et al. 2012 update of the 2008 American College of Rheumatology Recommendations for the use of disease-modifying antirheumatic drugs and biologic agents in the treatment of rheumatoid arthritis. *Arthritis Care Res.* 2012;64(5):625-639.

Stockl K, Cyprien L, Chang EY. Gastrointestinal bleeding rates among managed care patients newly started on COX-2 inhibitors or nonselective NSAIDs. *J Manag Care Pharm.* 2005;11(7):550-558.

Warden SJ. Cyclooxygenase-2 inhibitors, beneficial or detrimental for athletes with acute injuries. *Sports Med.* 2005;35(4):271-283.

Chapter 7: Advance Organizer

Foundational Concepts

- Perception of Pain
- Terminology

Nonsteroidal Anti-Inflammatory Drugs

Acetaminophen

- Effects and Uses
- Pharmacokinetics and Dosage
- Adverse Effects, Toxicity, and Drug Interactions
- Section Summary

Opioid Analgesics

- Mechanism of Action
- Effects and Uses
- Pharmacokinetics and Dosage
- Drug Interactions
- Specific Opioids
- Section Summary

Caffeine

Topical Analgesics

Local Anesthetics

- Mechanism and Effects
- Parenteral Use
- Topical Anesthetics

Role of the Athletic Trainer

7

Drugs for Treating Pain

Chapter Objectives

At the end of this chapter, the reader will be able to:

- Explain how nonsteroidal anti-inflammatory drugs (NSAIDs) also have an analgesic effect

- Explain the pharmacokinetics, effects, uses, and dosage regimen for acetaminophen and opioid drugs

- Recall and recognize the signs and symptoms of possible adverse effects and toxicity for acetaminophen and opioid drugs

- Identify common drug interactions for acetaminophen and opioid drugs

- Compare and contrast the therapeutic advantages and disadvantages of aspirin and acetaminophen

- Describe the mechanism of action for opioid drugs

- Explain the difference between drug addiction and physical dependence

- Explain the concept of agonist-antagonist opioids

- Differentiate between several types of opioid drugs

- Identify specific drugs that belong to the opioid drug category

- Explain how caffeine can affect analgesia of other drugs

- Recall the physiological effects that caffeine has on the body

- Recall the 2 main compounds that are used as topical analgesics and how they achieve their topical analgesic effects

- Explain the mechanism of action, uses, and therapeutic effects of local anesthetics

- Recall the therapeutic uses of topical anesthetics

- Summarize the role of the athletic trainer for patients who are taking analgesic medications

Abbreviations Used in This Chapter

CNS. central nervous system	**MI.** myocardial infarction
COX. cyclooxygenase	**NSAID.** nonsteroidal anti-inflammatory drug
FDA. Food and Drug Administration	**OTC.** over-the-counter
GI. gastrointestinal	**PG.** prostaglandin
LT. leukotriene	**VAS.** visual analog scale
	t½. half-life

Houglum JE, Harrelson GL, Seefeldt TM.
Principles of Pharmacology for Athletic Trainers, Third Edition (pp 125-137).
© 2016 Taylor & Francis Group.

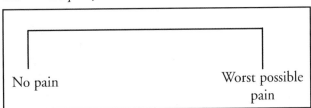

Figure 7-1. Visual analog pain scale (VAS).

Pain can be a symptom of underlying disease or chronic injury, or it may result from obvious acute trauma to musculoskeletal tissue from an athletic injury. The need for pain relief may require a single dose of pain reliever or long-term use of daily medication. Pain is the most common complaint among patients. Not surprising, therefore, is the abundance of analgesic products available by prescription and over the counter (OTC) to treat pain. The availability of OTC name-brand and generic analgesics as single-drug entities and combination products facilitates, even encourages, self-medication by patients. In addition, athletic injuries often necessitate the use of prescription pain relievers as part of short-term or long-term rehabilitation therapy. Obtaining optimal therapeutic outcomes of analgesic drug therapy requires not only use of the appropriate drug and dosage for the patient but also appropriate adjustments of therapy if adverse effects or drug interactions occur. Because of the ready availability of OTC analgesic products, achieving optimal outcomes can be a bigger challenge for the athletic trainer than it may seem.

This chapter discusses OTC and prescription analgesics, which include NSAIDs, acetaminophen, opioid analgesics, and caffeine. The uses, adverse effects, and potential drug interactions are discussed. Some of the information regarding the NSAIDs is repeated from the previous chapter regarding anti-inflammatory drugs, whereas other information regarding these drugs will focus on their specific use for analgesia.

FOUNDATIONAL CONCEPTS

Except for a few items of terminology discussed below, the major fundamental principle required to understand this chapter is the mechanism for pain perception as analgesics function by affecting this mechanism.

Perception of Pain

Pain is not a disease but rather a symptom of disease or a result of actual or potential damage to tissue. Alleviating the pain does not cure the underlying disease or repair the damaged tissue but is an important part of the treatment regimen. Relief from pain may also allow other treatment modalities, such as electrotherapy and heat and cold, to be performed more effectively. There is both a physical and an emotional component to pain, and thus it continually interferes with the patient's ability to focus on other tasks (eg, athletic performance). For example, even the anticipation of pain because of a previous injury can affect the patient's concentration and performance during athletic competition.

Pain is often described as an unpleasant sensory or emotional experience. It involves both the peripheral system and central nervous system (CNS) and it may be acute (eg, sprained ankle) or chronic (eg, arthritis). Sometimes pain is described as peripheral or visceral; *peripheral pain* is located in muscles, bones, and joints, whereas *visceral pain* originates from internal organs. Stimuli that damage tissue through chemical, mechanical, or thermal means will cause the activation of pain receptors called *nociceptors*, which exist on nerve endings in nearly all tissue. These stimuli may directly activate or sensitize nociceptors, or may do so indirectly by causing the release of various chemical mediators that subsequently activate or sensitize the nociceptors. Examples of these mediators are prostaglandins (PGs), leukotrienes (LTs), substance P, bradykinin, histamine, and cytokines. These and other chemical mediators may also be involved in the transmission of the nerve impulse (then called neurotransmitters) to the spinal cord and to the brain, which results in pain perception. Other neurotransmitters called *endorphins* (from "endogenous morphine") are released in the CNS as a means to control the pain. These endogenous opioid analgesics combine with specific receptors to inhibit the pain impulse. Other neurotransmitters in the CNS, such as serotonin and gamma-aminobutyric acid, may also be involved in inhibiting pain impulses.

There is no accurate means of quantifying pain because pain is a patient-specific perception of discomfort; pain exists if the patient says it exists. However, use of various pain scales is a common means of estimating the extent of pain as perceived by the patient and to determine the relative change in the pain for a given patient. For example, ask the patient to identify the level of pain on a scale of 0 to 10, where 0 is no pain and 10 is the worst pain possible. The visual analog scale (VAS) is another means of obtaining the patient's perception of pain level (Figure 7-1). The VAS uses a 10-cm line that represents a continuum of no pain at one end and the worst possible pain at the other end. The patient assesses the pain level and marks the place on the line to represent the level of pain. The distance is measured in millimeters from the "no pain" end and can be used to quantify the level of pain. Not only do pain scales give the athletic trainer an idea of the patient's pain level, but they also provide a baseline to determine whether the pain is lesser or greater at another time. Some patients may not give an accurate report of the pain. For example, athletes may underreport pain because of a desire to return to activity. Additionally, it is possible to decrease pain perception through relaxation, distraction, or elevated mood. On the other hand, pain perception may be increased by fatigue, anxiety, and depression.

Terminology

An understanding of the following terms will be useful with this chapter:

- An *analgesic* is a drug that is used to alleviate pain without causing the loss of consciousness. Drugs that induce sleep will alleviate the perception of pain while the patient is asleep but they do not selectively inhibit the transmission of pain impulses. Some drugs will alleviate the pain associated with a disease by treating the disease, but these drugs are not effective in treating pain associated with other causes. For example, pain from a urinary tract infection is alleviated because of treatment with an antibiotic; pain from gout is alleviated by the treatment with a drug that increases uric acid excretion.

- *Opiates* are drugs that are obtained from the opium poppy, opium being the extract from the plant. Morphine and codeine are 2 of the components of opium and thus are opiates.

- *Opioids* is a term broader than *opiates* and refers to drugs that have effects similar to the opiates. Oxycodone (OxyContin) and meperidine (Demerol) are 2 examples.

- *Narcotic analgesic* is another term used to refer to opioids. They can produce a state of narcosis (drowsiness or sleep) and relieve pain.

- *Narcotic* is also used in a legal context to refer to any controlled substance. Therefore, morphine is classified pharmacologically as a narcotic analgesic but also as a narcotic in the legal sense because it is a controlled substance. On the other hand, cocaine and amphetamine are classified pharmacologically as CNS stimulants, but because they have an abuse potential, they are also classified from a legal perspective as controlled substances and thus also referred to as narcotics. For clarification and differentiation, *narcotic analgesic* is the term used to refer to pain relievers that have an abuse potential, whereas the term *narcotic* can be used to refer to any controlled substance (including the narcotic analgesics).

NONSTEROIDAL ANTI-INFLAMMATORY DRUGS

The previous chapter discussed the mechanism of action of NSAIDs along with their therapeutic uses, pharmacokinetics, dosages, adverse effects, potential drug interactions, and therapy guidelines. As a review, the following points should be kept in mind:

- NSAIDs inhibit cyclooxygenase (COX), an enzyme that catalyzes the production of PGs.

- There are 2 isoforms: COX-1 and COX-2. Production of PGs has different function in various tissues. In general, COX-1 is the predominant isoform that produces PGs in most tissues but is particularly significant in the stomach, kidneys, and platelets. COX-2 is the predominant isoform that produces PGs because of tissue injury and contributes to pain, inflammation, and fever but also plays a role in renal function and inhibition of platelet aggregation.

- The most common adverse effects of NSAIDs are gastric irritation and ulceration, reduced renal function, and allergy.

- COX-2 selective NSAIDs may have a diminished incidence of some gastrointestinal (GI) adverse effects but not necessarily regarding some clinically significant effects such as the risk for GI bleeding.

- Whether selective or nonselective NSAIDs affect tissue healing (either beneficial or detrimental) is unclear.

- Caution is warranted regarding the use of all NSAIDs, including selective NSAIDs, in patients with reduced renal function or a history of kidney disease.

- Use of NSAIDs has been associated with an increased incidence of heart attack and stroke. All selective and nonselective NSAIDs, except aspirin, have warnings regarding this risk in their labeling.

- Concomitant use of NSAIDs with low-dose aspirin may reduce the antiplatelet response from aspirin.

- NSAIDs should be given with food or milk to reduce gastric irritation.

- PGs contribute to pain by sensitizing peripheral nerves and relaying the pain impulse in the CNS.

- All NSAIDs have equally effective analgesic and anti-inflammatory activity, but the effectiveness of NSAIDs varies among patients, and there is no way to predict which NSAID will be more effective than another in any given patient.

NSAIDs are effective for relief of mild-to-moderate pain. Generally, the maximum analgesic dose is less than the maximum anti-inflammatory dose, although there is overlap for the dosage range for the analgesic and anti-inflammatory effects. NSAIDs are used to treat pain associated with osteoarthritis, rheumatoid arthritis, dental pain, postsurgical pain, menstrual pain, headache, and trauma to tissue such as with musculoskeletal injury. Table 7-1 lists selected NSAIDs with their usual adult analgesic dosage.

TABLE 7-1			
SELECTED NONSTEROIDAL ANTI-INFLAMMATORY DRUG ANALGESICS			
GENERIC NAME	**TRADE NAME**	**TYPICAL ADULT ANALGESIC DOSE**	**OTC**
aspirin	many	500 to 1000 mg every 4 to 6 hours	Yes
celecoxib[a]	Celebrex	100 to 200 mg every 12 hours	No
diclofenac	Voltaren	50 mg every 8 hours	No
etodolac	Lodine	200 to 400 mg every 6 to 8 hours	No
fenoprofen	Nalfon	200 mg every 4 to 6 hours	No
ibuprofen	Advil	200 to 400 mg every 4 to 6 hours	Yes
ketoprofen	Orudis	12.5 to 25 mg every 6 to 8 hours	Yes
naproxen sodium	Aleve	220 mg every 8 to 12 hours	Yes
[a]Indicates selective COX-2 inhibitor.			

ACETAMINOPHEN

The chemical name for acetaminophen is N-acetyl-p-aminophenol, and thus it is referred to as *APAP*. Another, less common name for acetaminophen is *paracetamol*. Tylenol is the most common of many brand-name OTC analgesics. In addition, there are many generic label combination analgesic products and cold/allergy/sinus products that contain acetaminophen (see Chapter 10).

Effects and Uses

Use of acetaminophen is widespread because it has analgesic and antipyretic efficacy comparable with aspirin but does not have some of the adverse effects associated with aspirin and other NSAIDs. In fact, some names of acetaminophen products incorporate the terms *nonaspirin* or *aspirin free* to emphasize that it is an aspirin-like product but is without aspirin. The following are points of comparison of acetaminophen with aspirin:

- Acetaminophen inhibits COX in the brain but not in the peripheral sites. Consequently, acetaminophen is an effective antipyretic but does not have significant anti-inflammatory activity and hence it is not an NSAID.

- Acetaminophen does not have the risk of causing Reye's syndrome as aspirin does (see Chapter 6). Therefore, acetaminophen is safe to use in children and teenagers to treat muscle aches and fever associated with viral infections.

- Except for inhibition of COX in the brain, the mechanism of action of the analgesic activity for acetaminophen is unclear.

- Acetaminophen does not cause gastric irritation or ulceration.

- Platelet aggregation is not affected by acetaminophen and thus it does not affect blood clotting time and can be used in patients with clotting disorders. Occasional use of acetaminophen does not interfere with the effectiveness of warfarin (Coumadin) therapy (see Chapter 6), but daily use can inhibit warfarin metabolism and increase bleeding time.

- Acetaminophen does not have adverse effects on the kidney.

As discussed later in this chapter, aspirin and acetaminophen are used in combination with opioid analgesics (Table 7-2).

Pharmacokinetics and Dosage

Acetaminophen is readily and completely absorbed from the gastrointestinal tract, reaching peak blood concentration within 1 hour after oral administration. The half-life is approximately 2 hours. Most of the drug is metabolized by the liver to form metabolites that are more water soluble than the parent drug and thus increase the rate of urinary excretion.

Acetaminophen has similar potency as aspirin. The most effective adult dose is 325 to 1000 mg for acute pain every 4 to 6 hours, but daily dosage should not exceed 4000 mg. Like the NSAIDs, but in contrast to the opioids, acetaminophen has a ceiling effect for the analgesic activity such that increasing the dose beyond this ceiling will not achieve additional analgesia. For aspirin and acetaminophen, the ceiling effect for a single dose is usually between 650 and 1300 mg. Acetaminophen is available in many

TABLE 7-2

SELECTED OPIOIDS AND ANALGESIC COMBINATIONS

OPIOID (GENERIC)	TRADE NAME	DEA SCHEDULE	TYPICAL ORAL DOSE[a]	OTHER ANALGESICS (MG PER TABLET OR CAPSULE)
codeine	(generic)	II	15 to 60 mg	
codeine	Fiorinal w/Codeine	III	30 mg	325 mg aspirin 40 mg caffeine
codeine	Tylenol w/Codeine No. 3	III	30 mg	300 mg acetaminophen
hydrocodone	Vicodin	II	5 to 10 mg	300 mg acetaminophen
hydrocodone	Norco	II	7.5 to 10 mg	325 mg acetaminophen
hydrocodone	Vicoprofen	II	7.5 mg	200 mg ibuprofen
hydromorphone	Dilaudid	II	2 to 4 mg	
levorphanol	Levo-Dromoran	II	2 to 4 mg	
meperidine	Demerol	II	50 to 150 mg	
methadone	Dolophine	II	2.5 to 10 mg	
morphine	(generic)	II	5 to 30 mg	
oxycodone	OxyContin	II	10 to 20 mg[b]	
oxycodone	Percocet	II	5 mg	325 mg acetaminophen

[a]Represents adult dose of the opioid.
[b]Represents 12-hour, controlled-release dose.

dosage forms, including tablets, capsules, suppositories, chewable tablets, drops for infants, elixirs, and suspensions.

Adverse Effects, Toxicity, and Drug Interactions

There are fewer frequent adverse effects for acetaminophen compared with aspirin. Various allergic reactions, including skin rashes, occur occasionally. Rarely is there cross-hypersensitivity with aspirin or the other NSAIDs. Acetaminophen doses of <650 mg also pose little risk of bronchospasm in patients with aspirin-induced asthma.

The most serious adverse effect is due to overdose of acetaminophen. More calls are made to poison control centers for acetaminophen overdose than for overdose with any other drug. Contributing to the incidence of acetaminophen toxicity is the fact that there are so many OTC and prescription products that contain this drug. Because of the many combination products, patients often do not know that acetaminophen is one of the components of one or more products they are taking. Toxicity occurs when the amount of acetaminophen exceeds the capacity of the liver to metabolize it (Figure 7-2). Over 90% of an acetaminophen dose is metabolized by the liver by conversion to several products. With therapeutic doses of acetaminophen, a small portion of these products is toxic to the liver cell but is quickly detoxified within the liver cell. When an overdose occurs, the amount of toxic product produced exceeds the liver's ability to detoxify it, and consequently some of the toxic product reacts with other components of the liver cell, which can cause fatal hepatic necrosis. Any dose of acetaminophen >7.5 g in adults or 150 mg/kg in children is considered potentially toxic.

To decrease the occurrence of acetaminophen toxicity, some recent changes to dosing recommendations have been made. The manufacturer of Tylenol has reduced the maximum daily dose recommendations for its products. The maximum daily dose for Regular Strength Tylenol is now 3250 mg (2 tablets every 4 to 6 hours), and Extra Strength Tylenol's maximum daily dose has been lowered to 3000 mg (2 caplets every 6 hours). Note that the US Food and Drug Administration (FDA)–approved maximum daily dose of acetaminophen is still 4000 mg, although an FDA advisory panel has recommended lowering this dosing maximum. Acetaminophen is found in many combination products, which contributes to the risk of unintentional overdose. Many of these combination products contained 500 mg of acetaminophen per dosage form. The FDA has now limited the amount of acetaminophen in prescription combination products to a maximum of 325 mg per dosage form with

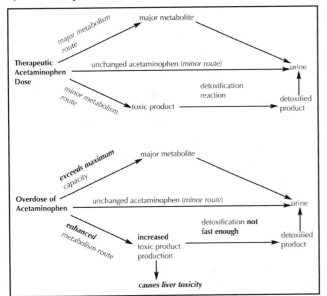

Figure 7-2. Mechanism of acetaminophen toxicity. Two pathways in the liver metabolize most of the acetaminophen. At therapeutic doses, the major pathway metabolizes most of the acetaminophen to form the major metabolite that is excreted in the urine. Because most of the therapeutic dose of acetaminophen is metabolized by this pathway, only a small amount is normally metabolized by another, typically minor pathway. The product of the minor pathway is a toxic product, which is quickly converted to a detoxified product and is then excreted in the urine. When too much acetaminophen is ingested, the capacity of the major pathway is exceeded and more acetaminophen is shunted to the minor pathway. The increased production of the toxic product in the minor pathway exceeds the amount that can be handled by the detoxification reaction. Consequently, some toxic product remains in the liver cell, reacts with other components of the cell, and becomes lethal to the cell.

the goal of reducing risk of unintentional overdose from these products.

Initial symptoms of acetaminophen toxicity may not occur for hours after overdose but include nausea, vomiting, drowsiness, and abdominal pain. Clinical evidence of hepatotoxicity becomes evident 2 to 4 days after overdose as determined by elevated liver enzymes and bilirubin in the blood.

> *Recall from Chapter 3 that the blood level of the liver enzymes aspartate and alanine aminotransferase (also called transaminase and abbreviated AST and ALT, respectively) increase in the blood as a result of liver toxicity.*

Treatment of overdose varies depending on the dose of acetaminophen and time since ingestion, but mainstays of treatment are activated charcoal and acetylcysteine (Mucomyst). These are most effective if administered within 1 hour and 10 hours of the acetaminophen, respectively. Acetylcysteine provides a substitute for the natural substance used in the detoxification reaction, thereby increasing the rate of detoxification. Activated charcoal is a nonspecific

absorbent that can decrease the absorption of some of the acetaminophen from the GI tract. Because of the potential for liver toxicity, patients with existing liver disease should be cautious regarding the use of acetaminophen.

Alcohol consumption provides the most significant potential for drug interaction with acetaminophen. Alcohol increases the amount of toxic product produced from acetaminophen metabolism. In addition, liver function may be compromised because of chronic alcohol consumption. The FDA recommendation is that patients who consume more than 3 alcoholic drinks per day should consult their physician before using acetaminophen. Another potential drug interaction is with warfarin (Coumadin). Although occasional use of acetaminophen is generally considered acceptable for patients on warfarin therapy, daily use may inhibit warfarin metabolism and increase bleeding time.

Section Summary

Acetaminophen is a drug that is equipotent with aspirin in relieving mild to moderate pain and reducing fever. Like aspirin, acetaminophen is used in combination with opioid analgesics for relief of moderate to severe pain. However, in contrast to aspirin, acetaminophen does not have an effect on blood clotting; does not cause GI adverse reactions; does not elicit the same hypersensitivity reactions; and when used as an antipyretic in children, it is not associated with Reye's syndrome. The major concern regarding the use of acetaminophen is the potential for high doses to cause liver toxicity. Concurrent use of alcohol can cause toxicity at lower doses of acetaminophen. In addition, the use of multiple products that each contain acetaminophen can inadvertently cause a toxic dose of acetaminophen.

OPIOID ANALGESICS

Opioid analgesics are drugs that have pharmacological activity similar to morphine, which is the prototype for this drug category. The major characteristics of these drugs are that they relieve moderate to severe pain, produce drowsiness, and have an abuse potential (Box 7-1).

Mechanism of Action

The effects of opioids are the result of them combining with the opioid receptors located primarily in the CNS but also in the peripheral nervous system. There are 3 main opioid receptor classes, designated *mu* (μ, MOP), *kappa* (κ, KOP), and *delta* (δ, DOP). Evidence indicates that subtypes of these receptors also exist. The brain produces natural analgesics that combine with these receptors to provide natural pain relief. The 3 main families of endogenous opioids are peptides called β-*endorphins*, *enkephalins*, and *dynorphins*; collectively these are referred to as

Box 7-1
FACTS ABOUT OPIOID ANALGESICS

- Used to relieve moderate to severe pain
- Reduce anxiety and distress
- Cause drowsiness
- Have an abuse potential for addiction and physical dependence
- All opioids are controlled substances except for nalbuphine
- Cause constipation
- Suppress coughing
- Adverse effects: respiratory depression, miosis, urinary retention, orthostatic hypotension, nausea, and vomiting
- Tolerance occurs to most of the opioid effects
- Drug interactions: significant CNS depressant effects if combined with other CNS depressants, including alcohol

endorphins. These compounds have various functions as neurotransmitters and neurohormones, but a primary role is to act as natural opioid analgesics to alter the perception of pain and stress. Not surprisingly, the endogenous opioids act through a second messenger after combining with the receptor.

Recall that second messengers are compounds that are produced within the cell in response to the initial signal received by a receptor outside the cell. The second messenger carries the signal within the cell by initiating a cascade of reactions, a transduction *mechanism, that ultimately result in the biochemical response (see Chapter 3).*

Effects and Uses

The effects of most clinically effective opioids, including analgesic and euphoric effects, are a result of their interaction with the mu receptor. Some opioids also combine with the kappa receptor, which contributes to analgesia but has the potential to cause dysphoria. Because morphine is the prototype opioid, a look at the effects of this drug is a good picture of the effects of the other opioids. However, there is some variation in the degree to which each of these effects occurs with each opioid; particularly significant variations will be specified.

The major therapeutic use of morphine is to relieve moderate to severe pain, such as pain associated with surgery, cancer, and myocardial infarction. Constant, dull pain is more effectively relieved at lower doses than sharp, intermittent pain. Besides analgesia, morphine also causes diminished anxiety and distress, which may contribute to pain relief by affecting the emotional aspect of pain perception. Drowsiness is also common, although sleep is not necessary for pain relief. The other senses, such as smell and touch, are not affected.

A specific aspect of opioid analgesics that separates them from acetaminophen and NSAIDs is their abuse potential (ie, their ability to cause addiction/psychological dependence). *Addiction* is a behavioral disorder that is characterized by obsessive drug use typically accompanied by extreme measures to obtain the drug. The driving force that causes addiction is the desire for the euphoria from the drug. However, addiction rarely occurs when opioids are used to treat pain except in patients who have a prior predisposition to drug addiction. Moderate to severe pain seems to antagonize the euphoric effects such that most patients do not experience euphoric effects. Because of the abuse potential, all of the opioid analgesics except nalbuphine are controlled substances. They are schedule II drugs with the exception of certain opioid products that are marketed in combination with aspirin or acetaminophen (codeine with acetaminophen [Schedule III]) and the partial agonist opioids buprenorphine (Schedule III), pentazocine (Schedule IV), and butorphanol (Schedule IV).

Physical dependence also exists among all opioid analgesics but is a characteristic separate from addiction. *Dependence* occurs because of cellular changes within the body in response to continual exposure to the drug. The nature of these changes is not known, but in essence the many functions of the body that are affected reach a new state of balance. When the drug is removed, the body must readjust to a different state of balance and this abrupt adjustment causes a withdrawal syndrome. The existence of a withdrawal syndrome when the use of a drug is terminated is the only criterion to define the existence of physical dependence.

Opioid withdrawal syndrome is unpleasant, but rarely fatal. The duration and severity of the withdrawal symptoms depend on the duration of action of the specific drug that was used and degree of physical dependence. Drugs with a longer duration of action produce a longer but milder syndrome. Those with a shorter duration of action produce a shorter but more intense syndrome. The longer the dependence period and the higher the dose that was used, the longer and more intense the syndrome. Symptoms begin several hours after the last dose and are alleviated if any opioid analgesic is used; otherwise, the duration of the symptoms is about 7 to 10 days (Box 7-2). Patients on chronic opioid therapy for more than 1 week are likely to have a degree of physical dependence. For these patients, a gradual

Box 7-2
Opioid Withdrawal Symptoms

- Sweating
- Runny nose
- Irritability
- Tremor
- Anorexia

- Nausea
- Vomiting
- Diarrhea
- Cramps
- Muscle spasms

reduction of the dosage for a few days will minimize withdrawal symptoms. Consequently, neither addiction nor physical dependence should be a clinical concern when opioids are necessary for pain management.

Morphine combines with opioid receptors in the GI tract to reduce intestinal motility and secretion of fluids into the intestine. Consequently, constipation is of significant concern and is one of the most common adverse effects. Constipation develops within days of initiating treatment, although it can be minimized by appropriate treatment with laxatives such as stool softeners or milk of magnesia, increased fiber, and adequate hydration. Because of the constipating effect, some opioids are used therapeutically to treat diarrhea. Paregoric (Schedule III) and opium tincture (Schedule II), which contain opium and thus contain morphine, are commercially available but are not used very frequently because of the availability of other opioids with less abuse potential. For example, diphenoxylate (Lomotil, Class V) and difenoxin (Motofen, Class IV) are effective antidiarrheal agents. Loperamide (Imodium) is also an opioid but has a very low abuse potential and consequently is not a controlled substance. It is available OTC to treat diarrhea.

Morphine also has sedative properties. There are more effective sedatives available than opioids, and thus these drugs are not used therapeutically for their sedative properties. However, sedation is sometimes advantageous when treating a patient for pain and may contribute to the reduced perception of acute pain. For other patients, drowsiness is an adverse effect as it is not conducive to some activities such as driving a car. Tolerance quickly develops to the sedative properties.

Opioid analgesics affect the cough center in the medulla to cause cough suppression. Two opioids, codeine and hydrocodone, are each available in combination with various compounds to treat upper respiratory conditions. The antitussive dose is lower than the analgesic dose; codeine dosage is every 4 to 6 hours at 10 to 20 mg for cough compared with 15 to 60 mg for pain.

Other effects of opioid analgesics include respiratory depression, miosis (pupil constriction), urinary retention, orthostatic hypotension (feeling faint when standing up),

nausea, and vomiting. These effects do not offer any therapeutic advantage and hence are adverse. At therapeutic doses, respiratory depression is not of significant concern unless the patient already has compromised respiration such as with chronic obstructive pulmonary disease. However, respiratory depression is the cause of death in most overdose cases. A competitive opioid antagonist can be administered to reverse respiratory depression; an example is naloxone (Narcan). An antagonist combines with the same opioid receptor as the opioid agonists without initiating the effects of the agonist. Consequently, the antagonists reverse the respiratory depression, analgesia, sedation, and euphoria and will initiate withdrawal syndrome in a physically dependent patient.

Orthostatic hypotension *is also called* postural hypotension. *The patient feels faint or dizzy when standing too quickly from a sitting or lying position. Normally, autonomic reflexes such as increased heart rate and constriction of blood vessels increase blood pressure and prevent orthostatic hypotension. However, drugs like opioid analgesics that cause dilation of peripheral blood vessels, or antihypertensive drugs (see Chapter 12), which inhibit the autonomic reflexes, will cause orthostatic hypotension.*

Miosis is of relatively little concern, although additional lighting may be necessary in some settings. Urinary retention is also a relatively minor problem, although the physician should be contacted if the patient is unable to urinate adequately. Because opioids cause some hypotensive effects, patients should be cautioned about the potential for orthostatic hypotension. They should be instructed regarding the potential for experiencing dizziness when standing up, and thus patients may need to stand slowly, especially from a supine position. Nausea and vomiting are CNS responses, occur more frequently in ambulatory patients, and are most pronounced as a result of the first dose.

Tolerance occurs to most of the effects of the opioids. Most importantly, tolerance occurs to the respiratory depression, sedative, and euphoric effects. Tolerance also develops to the analgesic effect but the rate of tolerance varies among patients. Fortunately, there is no ceiling effect for the analgesia so the dose of the opioid can be increased as tolerance develops. This is helpful for patients with terminal diseases (eg, some cancer patients) who need long-term pain relief with opioids. Tolerance does not develop significantly to the constipating and pupil-constricting effects. Because the opioid analgesics all combine with the mu receptor, it is not surprising that *cross-tolerance* exists among the opioid analgesics (ie, tolerance to one results in tolerance to the others). When tolerance occurs, the duration of the pain relief becomes shorter followed by reduced analgesic effectiveness of each dose.

> *Recall from Chapter 2 that* tolerance *is a diminished response to a drug because of continued use. In other words, the dose of the drug must be increased to achieve the same response that was previously obtained.*

Pharmacokinetics and Dosage

Morphine, as well as most other opioids, is available in dosage forms for use by oral, rectal, and parenteral routes. Morphine undergoes first-pass effect in the liver to a larger extent than other opioids; only about 25% of morphine is bioavailable after oral administration. Consequently, the oral dose is considerably higher than parenteral doses. Peak effectiveness occurs about 1.5 hours after oral administration. Most of the morphine is metabolized by the liver and excreted by the kidney. Patients with compromised liver or kidney function will have a higher blood concentration of morphine after repeated doses because of delayed drug clearance; these patients may require a reduced dosage. The typical adult parenteral dose of morphine is 10 mg, and the duration of action is about 4 hours. A typical oral starting dosage is 5 to 30 mg every 4 hours, although sustained-release tablets and capsules are available that have a duration of action of 8 to 24 hours. Table 7-2 provides a selected list of opioid analgesics and the typical adult oral dosage regimen for comparison, although the dosage regimen for each patient should be individualized to attain adequate pain relief.

> *Recall that* synergism *refers to an effect that occurs when 2 drugs used in the same therapy provide an effect greater than would be expected from the addition of their individual effects.*

Opioid analgesics are often combined with acetaminophen, or sometimes with aspirin or ibuprofen, because the combination of an opioid and nonopioid analgesic provides a *synergistic effect*, which enhances the analgesia without adding to the adverse effects of either drug. There are many of these brand name and generic name combination products; some examples are included in Table 7-2.

Drug Interactions

The most notable drug interaction of potentially significant consequence is the combination of opioids with other CNS depressants, including alcohol. The cause of death from an overdose of CNS depressant drugs is respiratory depression. The same result can occur when an opioid is combined with another CNS depressant drug. Examples of CNS depressants (see also Table 8-2) are the barbiturates that are used as sedatives and anticonvulsants (eg, phenobarbital) and the benzodiazepines that are used as sedatives, hypnotics, skeletal muscle relaxants, and antianxiety agents (eg, Valium, Restoril, Xanax, Ativan).

Specific Opioids

Table 7-2 lists examples of opioid analgesics and typical oral doses. Although the pharmacological effects of these drugs are much like morphine, there are some differences in effects and uses among the group. Hydromorphone and levorphanol are more potent than morphine, but this is of little clinical significance because the therapeutic dose is adjusted accordingly. Levorphanol has a longer half-life and can be given fewer times per day.

Codeine is less potent than morphine and is used to treat mild to moderate pain. It is often used in combination with either aspirin or acetaminophen; caffeine is also incorporated in some products. To designate an amount of codeine per dosage unit (ie, per tablet or capsule), the numbers 2, 3, or 4 are sometimes included in the product name to indicate the content of codeine equal to 15, 30, or 60 mg, respectively. For example, acetaminophen w/codeine no. 3 contains 30 mg of codeine. Much of the analgesic effect is attained because a portion of codeine is being metabolized to morphine. Hydrocodone is a chemical derivative of codeine with an analgesic effectiveness between codeine and morphine. It is available in combination with aspirin, acetaminophen, or ibuprofen; a hydrocodone-only product was recently approved by the FDA. Codeine and hydrocodone are also effective antitussive agents and are available in combination with antihistamines or decongestants for the treatment of colds.

Meperidine (Demerol) has a pharmacological profile similar to morphine but has a shorter duration and can cause additional adverse effects such as tremor, muscle twitching, and seizures. Meperidine should not be used with monoamine oxidase inhibitors because this combination can cause significant adverse effects (eg, severe respiratory depression, convulsions, and death).

> *Monoamine oxidase inhibitors comprise a group of drugs that are categorized therapeutically as antidepressants. They are notorious for adverse effects and drug interaction (see Chapter 13).*

Oxycodone has similar pharmacological effects, potency, and duration as morphine; is available in a controlled-release form; and is frequently combined with aspirin or acetaminophen. Of special note for oxycodone is the abuse associated with the controlled-release product (OxyContin). This product contains a larger quantity of oxycodone because the drug is meant to be taken every 12 hours rather than every 4 to 6 hours. If the controlled-release tablets are chewed, crushed, or dissolved in water, the controlled-release aspect is eliminated and the entire dose is available quickly by ingesting, snorting, or injecting the drug. Consequently, abuse of the controlled-release product (also known as *oxy*) has become a major problem. Recently, the FDA approved a new OxyContin formulation designed to reduce its abuse potential. The new formulation is more difficult to break and make into a form for injection or snorting.

Methadone has a longer duration than morphine and has good oral absorption. These are beneficial characteristics for treatment of chronic pain such as is needed for patients with cancer. Oral methadone is also used to treat heroin addicts as a means of preventing withdrawal syndrome while gradually diminishing the dependence.

Tramadol (Ultram) binds to the mu receptor with less effectiveness than codeine but also decreases pain perception through other mechanisms. As a result, tramadol has a significantly reduced risk for respiratory depression in overdose. Like several other opioids, tramadol is available in combination with acetaminophen (Ultracet), which enhances the overall analgesic effectiveness. Tramadol alone or in combination with acetaminophen is indicated for treatment of moderate to moderately severe pain with efficacy similar to codeine and codeine with acetaminophen. It was originally believed that tramadol had a lower potential for physical dependence and addiction than other opioids. This perceived low abuse potential resulted in the drug not being scheduled as a controlled substance. However, more recent data have indicated that tramadol has a higher potential for physical dependence and addiction than previously thought. In 2014, the US Drug Enforcement Administration (DEA) announced that tramadol has been added to the federal controlled substances list as a Schedule IV controlled substance.

Additional mu-agonist opioids that are not used orally are fentanyl (Sublimaze), alfentanil (Alfenta), sufentanil (Sufenta), and remifentanil (Ultiva). These are analgesic adjuncts to general anesthesia. They are much more potent than morphine (100-fold for fentanyl); thus, the dose is much smaller. Fentanyl is also available as a transdermal patch (Duragesic) for treatment of chronic severe pain. Onset is slow and thus is not for acute pain, but the duration is about 72 hours.

Heroin is not used therapeutically (Schedule I) but is available through illicit markets. Heroin is more lipid soluble than morphine and therefore has better access to the brain than morphine, resulting in a high abuse potential but with no advantage as an analgesic. In the heroin-dependent person, withdrawal begins about 6 to 12 hours after the last dose.

Section Summary

The opioid analgesics mimic the naturally occurring analgesics, endorphins, enkephalins, and dynorphins, by combining primarily with the mu, and to some extent the kappa, opioid receptors in the CNS. Morphine is the prototype opioid analgesic with which the effectiveness of others is compared. Besides effectively relieving moderate to severe pain, initial doses of morphine also cause drowsiness, diminished anxiety, orthostatic hypotension, and constipation. Tolerance develops quickly to these effects; however, constipation remains. Although euphoria is also a potential effect from opioids, it usually does not occur in patients being treated for moderate to severe pain. Because euphoria is the driving force for addiction, rarely does addiction occur in these patients. Physical dependence occurs with chronic use of opioids, and thus, when the drug is to be discontinued, the dosage of the opioid should be gradually decreased in patients who have been receiving therapy for 5 to 7 days. Several opioids are used in combination with an NSAID or acetaminophen to enhance the analgesic effectiveness. Besides analgesia, other common uses for selected opioids are to treat diarrhea and cough.

CAFFEINE

Caffeine is not often thought of as an analgesic, but it does enhance the analgesic properties of acetaminophen, aspirin, and ibuprofen when used in combination with them. Used alone, caffeine has little value as an analgesic. Table 7-3 provides examples of some aspirin and acetaminophen-containing OTC products that also contain caffeine. The mechanism by which caffeine enhances the effectiveness of analgesic products is unclear, but studies have demonstrated a shorter onset of action and a longer duration of action for relief of mild to moderate pain with use of OTC analgesics that also contain caffeine.

Although caffeine is frequently used in analgesic products, by far the most common use by the general public is as a CNS stimulant. Approximately 80% of adults in the United States consume caffeine daily, most commonly in the form of coffee, tea, soft drinks, and chocolate-containing foods (see Table 16-3). As a stimulant, caffeine will decrease drowsiness and fatigue and increase alertness at doses of 50 to 200 mg. At higher doses, caffeine causes restlessness, insomnia, nervousness, headache, diarrhea, and irritability. Caffeine-containing stimulant products such as NoDoz (available in 200-mg tablets) and Vivarin (available in 200-mg tablets) are marketed to help people stay awake.

Daily use of caffeine can result in physical dependence. Therefore, as with opioid dependency, abrupt discontinuation of caffeine use will cause withdrawal symptoms, which begin within the first day after discontinuing the drug. Peak withdrawal symptoms occur within 48 hours and then taper off but may last for a week with the primary symptoms being fatigue and headache (Box 7-3). To again highlight the difference between physical dependence and addiction, note that although caffeine can cause physical dependence, caffeine is not listed as an addictive substance because very few people lose control over the amount of caffeine they ingest or are unable to decrease or eliminate

TABLE 7-3			
EXAMPLES OF OVER-THE-COUNTER ANALGESICS THAT CONTAIN CAFFEINE			
TRADE NAME	ANALGESIC (MG)		CAFFEINE (MG)
	Aspirin	*Acetaminophen*	
Anacin Maximum Strength	500		32
Excedrin Tension Headache		500	65
Excedrin Extra Strength	250	250	65
Vanquish	227	194	33

intake if they so choose. Nonetheless, caffeine is a restricted substance in athletic competition (see Chapters 16 and 17).

TOPICAL ANALGESICS

Topical analgesics were discussed in the previous chapter with the topical anti-inflammatory products because some of them are specifically used to relieve the pain associated with inflammation. There are 2 main groups of compounds used as analgesics, the salicylates and the counterirritants. These compounds are used to relieve pain in muscles, joints, and tendons but, like topical anesthetics, are also indicated for the relief of cutaneous pain such as from insect bites, minor burns, and sunburn. Methylsalicylate and trolamine salicylate are components of many products; methyl salicylate is also a counterirritant. Other counter-irritants include menthol, camphor, allyl isothiocyanate, and capsicum. The counterirritants stimulate sensations of cold, warmth, or itching to distract the patient from the greater pain being experienced. These products also have a *rubefacient effect*, in that they cause localized vasodilation, which results in redness and a feeling of warmth. Menthol initially causes a cooling sensation followed by warmth. See Table 6-9 for examples of topical OTC analgesic products.

LOCAL ANESTHETICS

Local anesthetics are used as topical preparations to alleviate pain but are covered separately from the other topically applied analgesics because the mechanism is distinctly different and because some are also injected for a local or regional anesthetic effect. Examples of local anesthetics are shown in Table 7-4.

Mechanism and Effects

Local anesthetics act by inhibiting the nerve impulse transmission in the area where they are applied. Although sensation to pain is readily blocked, transmission of all

BOX 7-3
CAFFEINE WITHDRAWAL SYMPTOMS

- Fatigue
- Headache
- Irritability
- Restlessness
- Anxiety
- Yawning
- Runny nose

nerve impulses is also blocked, resulting in diminished perception of hot, cold, and touch. The advantage of these agents is that they act quickly, affect only the localized area, and, even with parenteral administration, do not cause loss of consciousness.

Some absorption occurs into the bloodstream from topical application, especially from mucous membranes. Adverse effects from therapeutic doses of local anesthetics are few, even following parenteral administration. Allergic reactions occur only rarely. At higher concentrations in the blood, local anesthetics can affect cardiac conduction, leading to heart block and cardiac arrest. Elevated blood levels can also stimulate the CNS, resulting in restlessness, tremor, and convulsions, followed by CNS depression. This can progress to coma and respiratory depression.

Parenteral Use

Local anesthetics are often used parenterally by infiltration or nerve block anesthesia in preparation for dental procedures, minor surgery, and diagnostic procedures. Infiltration anesthesia involves the injection of the local anesthetics at or near areas where anesthesia is desired. Nerve block anesthesia involves injection into or near nerves that supply a specific area. The area is usually larger than that which would be covered by infiltration and is more distant from the injection site. Epidural anesthesia specifically involves the injection of anesthetic and/or opioid in the epidural space of the spine to obtain effective relief of pain in a region, such as to the lower

TABLE 7-4				
SELECTED LOCAL ANESTHETICS				
GENERIC NAME	**TRADE NAME**	**TOPICAL**	**PARENTERAL**	**AVAILABLE OTC[a]**
articaine	Septocaine		X	
benzocaine	Lanacane	X		X
bupivacaine	Marcaine		X	
chloroprocaine	Nesacaine		X	
cocaine[a]	(generic)	X		
dibucaine	Nupercainal	X		X
lidocaine	Xylocaine	X	X	X
mepivacaine	Polocaine		X	
pramoxine	Tronolane	X		X
procaine	Novocain		X	
tetracaine	Pontocaine	X	X	
[a]Only topical dosage forms available.				

back. With these methods, the duration of anesthesia is dependent on the lipid solubility of the anesthetic and the amount of blood flow at the site of injection; more blood flow carries the drug away from the site more quickly. Sometimes a low concentration of a vasoconstrictor (eg, epinephrine) is added to the local anesthetic to diminish the local blood flow and thus extend the duration of action. For example, lidocaine (Xylocaine) has a duration of 10 to 20 minutes without epinephrine and 2 hours with epinephrine.

Topical Anesthetics

Local anesthetics are applied topically to obtain pain relief at that site on the surface of the skin or mucous membranes. Products are available as solutions, sprays, gels, ointments, creams, lozenges, and suppositories. Topically applied local anesthetics are used to treat pain and/or itching due to many causes, including sunburn, minor burns, insect bites, poison ivy, hemorrhoids, sore throat, and minor sports injuries, and to prevent pain at the site of parenteral injections.

Ethyl chloride is a topical anesthetic but differs from those listed in Table 7-4 in that its effectiveness is a result of a cooling effect (skin refrigerant). The usefulness of ethyl chloride is similar to the use of ice, but the effectiveness is much quicker. Ethyl chloride is applied as a spray, and it cools the skin as it rapidly evaporates. For the temporary relief of sports injuries, ethyl chloride is sprayed on the injured area until the skin just turns white (about 5 seconds). Duration of response is a few seconds to a minute but provides some relief from the initial trauma of the injury. Some

caution is necessary in handling and storing ethyl chloride because it is flammable and the spray containers are pressurized. Inhalation of ethyl chloride should be avoided as general anesthetic and cardiac effects may occur.

Cocaine is a topical anesthetic worthy of specific note. It causes CNS stimulation and euphoria by a mechanism unrelated to the local anesthetic action. Consequently, cocaine has a high abuse potential and is the only local anesthetic that is a controlled substance (Schedule II). However, it is an effective local anesthetic that is used topically for anesthesia of the ear, nose, and throat. Cocaine is also unique from the other local anesthetics in that it causes constriction of the local vasculature and thus eliminates the need for adding epinephrine. Absorption occurs from the mucous membranes and, as indicated, the effects on the CNS are more pronounced than with the other local anesthetics. Stimulatory effects occur first and are followed by depressant effects. Small doses of cocaine cause bradycardia, but moderate doses cause more significant cardiovascular effects such as tachycardia and hypertension.

ROLE OF THE ATHLETIC TRAINER

Use of analgesics by patients is a frequent occurrence and thus offers many opportunities for the athletic trainer to help ensure proper use of these medications. Unlike the use of antibiotics or long-term asthma medications in which poor adherence does not always initiate symptoms, poor adherence to analgesic therapy initiates a definite undesirable symptom—pain. The desire to relieve pain, coupled with the ready accessibility of OTC pain relievers, contributes to the overuse of analgesic drugs and the potential for significant adverse or toxic effects. Therefore, the athletic trainer can assist the patient in preventing these effects by being aware of the content of OTC and prescription analgesics and by being alert to the conditions that would cause a patient to be more susceptible to adverse effects. In this regard, the following are some key points and general statements that should be useful to the athletic trainer:

- Do not doubt the existence of pain reported by a patient. Everyone's pain threshold is different.

- Realize that to treat systemic pain there are 2 main groups of analgesics: NSAIDs/acetaminophen and opioids. NSAIDs and acetaminophen are effective for mild to moderate pain; opioids are effective for moderate to severe pain.

- Encourage patients who are using NSAIDs to take them with food or milk to reduce gastric irritation.

- Realize that acetaminophen is often used as an alternative to aspirin and other NSAIDs for relief of mild to moderate pain for patients who have a history of ulcers, are also taking warfarin, have diminished kidney function, have aspirin-induced asthma, or are allergic to any NSAID.

- Recognize that acetaminophen may be a better choice than NSAIDs as an analgesic for relief of mild to moderate pain while participating in strenuous exercise of long duration because acetaminophen does not affect kidney function as significantly and the termination of its activity does not depend on kidney function.

- Understand that although certain patients should not be taking either NSAIDs or acetaminophen, patients may not realize that they are ingesting an NSAID or acetaminophen as a component of an OTC product(s).

- Advise patients to be cautious regarding the use of multiple prescription and/or OTC products as they may each contain acetaminophen or aspirin, which can result in toxicity. Initial signs of toxicity for aspirin include tinnitus, dizziness, and headache; for acetaminophen, they include nausea, vomiting, and anorexia.

- Alert patients who require opioid analgesics to the likelihood of constipation as an adverse effect. Recommend use of laxatives (see Chapter 11) for relief of constipation.

- Ensure that all use of opioid analgesics is under the direction of a physician.

- Do not use counterirritants on open wounds or abraded skin. Do not wrap the treated area with occlusive bandages or expose the area to heat because excessive irritation or skin damage can occur (see Chapter 6).

CASE STUDY

Ella, a 21-year-old senior and your intercollegiate women's team's star soccer goalie, suffers from chronic tension headaches. Midterm exams are being held, so her headaches have increased to what she says give her pain of 7 on a 10-point scale. Her physician told her that he thought an OTC medication would be sufficient to take care of her headache complaints. However, he did not give Ella any additional information on what she should take. She comes to you asking about the kinds of OTC medications that are available for her pain and what are the pros and cons of each. How would you respond?

BIBLIOGRAPHY

Chou R, Fanciullo GJ, Fine PG, et al. Clinical guidelines for the use of chronic opioid therapy in chronic noncancer pain. *J Pain.* 2009;10(2):113-130.

Hodgman MJ, Garrard AR. A review of acetaminophen poisoning. *Crit Care Clin.* 2012;28:499-516.

Houglum JE. Pharmacologic considerations in the treatment of injured athletes with nonsteroidal anti-inflammatory drugs. *J Athl Training.* 1998;33:259-263.

National Drug Intelligence Center. OxyContin diversion, availability, and abuse. Intelligence Bulletin. US Department of Justice; August 2004. Product no. 2004-L0424-017.

Nicholson B. Acute pain management: overcoming barriers and enhancing treatment. MedscapeCME. http://www.medscape.com/viewprogram/14826_pnt. Accessed July 21, 2015.

Chapter 8: Advance Organizer

Foundational Concepts

- Central Nervous System Depression
- Anticholinergic Adverse Effects

Mechanism of Action

Effects and Dosage

Chapter Summary

Role of the Athletic Trainer

8

Drugs for Relaxing Skeletal Muscle

CHAPTER OBJECTIVES

At the end of this chapter, the reader will be able to:

- Explain the uses of skeletal muscle relaxant drugs

- Explain the adverse effects of drugs used to relax skeletal muscle

- Recognize the signs and symptoms of an anticholinergic adverse effect

- Identify drug categories that have anticholinergic adverse effects

- Explain the mechanism of action, therapeutic effects, and dosage regimen for drugs used to relax skeletal muscle

- Summarize the role of the athletic trainer for patients who are taking skeletal muscle relaxants

ABBREVIATIONS USED IN THIS CHAPTER

CNS. central nervous system	**GABA.** gamma aminobutyric acid
FDA. Food and Drug Administration	**OTC.** over-the-counter

This chapter discusses the use and effects of skeletal muscle relaxants that function through the central nervous system (CNS; ie, centrally acting) to alleviate muscle spasms. Peripherally acting skeletal muscle relaxants are generally used to block neuromuscular function during surgery or other medical procedures. Examples are succinylcholine (Anectine), atracurium (Tracrium), and vecuronium (Norcuron). Another group of muscle relaxants, which include baclofen (Lioresal) and dantrolene (Dantrium), are used to treat spasticity caused by diseases such as multiple sclerosis and cerebral palsy. Neither the peripherally acting muscle relaxants nor those used specifically for treatment of spasticity will be discussed.

Centrally acting skeletal muscle relaxants are a relatively small group of drugs used to prevent or relieve muscle spasms (Table 8-1). Muscle spasms are involuntary localized muscle contractions that are caused by pain, trauma, or muscle inflammation. Pain is often associated with muscle spasms, and, consequently, analgesics may be a part of drug therapy. Some muscle relaxants are available in combination with codeine, acetaminophen, aspirin, or aspirin with caffeine (see Table 8-1). Some physical agents, such as cryotherapy, moist heat, massage, and stretching, are also effective for relieving muscle spasms and associated pain. Muscle relaxants alone, and in combination with analgesics, are also used to treat back and neck pain, although the extent to which they are effective for this use is somewhat unclear.

Houglum JE, Harrelson GL, Seefeldt TM.
Principles of Pharmacology for Athletic Trainers, Third Edition (pp 139-144).
© 2016 Taylor & Francis Group.

TABLE 8-1			
SKELETAL MUSCLE RELAXANTS			
GENERIC NAME	ANALGESIC ADDED (MG)	TRADE NAME	TYPICAL ADULT ORAL MAINTENANCE DOSE
carisoprodol		Soma	350 mg 3 to 4 times/day
carisoprodol	aspirin (325)	Soma Compound	1 to 2 tablets 4 times/day
carisoprodol	aspirin (325) + codeine (16)	Soma Compound w/codeine	1 to 2 tablets 4 times/day
chlorzoxazone		Parafon Forte DSC, Lorzone	250 to 750 mg 3 to 4 times/day
cyclobenzaprine		Flexeril	5 mg 3 times/day
diazepam		Valium	2 to 10 mg 3 to 4 times/day
metaxalone		Skelaxin	800 mg 3 to 4 times/day
methocarbamol		Robaxin	1 g 4 times/day
orphenadrine		Norflex	100 mg 2 times/day
orphenadrine	aspirin (385) + caffeine (30)	Norgesic	1 to 2 tablets 3 to 4 times/day

FOUNDATIONAL CONCEPTS

There are some adverse effects that are predominant among the skeletal muscle relaxants and are also prevalent among other categories of drugs. Therefore, an understanding of the concepts related to these adverse effects is important.

Central Nervous System Depression

Depression of the CNS can result in drowsiness and dizziness; higher doses result in more significant sedation and respiratory depression. Overdose of CNS depressants results in coma and death from respiratory depression. As shown in Table 8-2, several categories of drugs cause CNS depression. When 2 or more of these drugs are used concurrently or used in combination with alcohol, the sedative effects are enhanced. For example, coma and death have resulted from the combination of alcohol and benzodiazepines. Even when therapeutic doses of these drugs are combined, a significantly enhanced drowsiness response can adversely affect the patient's activity, including athletic performance. Drowsiness is a safety concern if the patient is operating a motor vehicle, but this concern is even greater when CNS depressant drugs are combined.

Anticholinergic Adverse Effects

Several of the skeletal muscle relaxants are particularly noted for causing anticholinergic adverse effects. *Anticholinergic effects* is a term that refers to a group of adverse effects that are similar to the effects from drugs in the pharmacological category called anticholinergic drugs, such as atropine and scopolamine. Anticholinergic drugs, and other drugs with anticholinergic effects, block the cholinergic receptors at the site where the parasympathetic nervous system innervates smooth muscle and organ tissue. This receptor is also called the muscarinic receptor, and thus these drugs are also called *antimuscarinic drugs* or *muscarinic blockers*. Inhibition of the parasympathetic system by drugs with anticholinergic effects has the potential to cause responses that are opposite of stimulating the parasympathetic system (ie, cause anticholinergic effects, as listed in Table 8-3). There are several categories of drugs that cause anticholinergic adverse effects (Box 8-1). However, at therapeutic doses, not all of the drugs in these categories cause all of the responses listed in Table 8-3; the type of response and extent of response varies among these drugs and depends on the dosage being used.

MECHANISM OF ACTION

The skeletal muscle relaxants exert their activity on skeletal muscle through the CNS, although the exact mechanism is unknown. All of these drugs have some CNS sedative properties, and it is possible that these properties contribute to muscle relaxation. Diazepam (Valium) is a drug from the chemical category of drugs called benzodiazepines. Besides having sedative properties, diazepam combines with the GABA receptor. Stimulation of this receptor causes an inhibitory effect on nerve impulse transmission in the CNS, which may also contribute to muscle relaxation.

TABLE 8-2

SELECTED DRUGS THAT HAVE CENTRAL NERVOUS SYSTEM DEPRESSANT EFFECTS

DRUG CATEGORY	GENERIC NAME	TRADE NAME
Antianxiety	Benzodiazepines	
	alprazolam	Xanax
	clorazepate	Tranxene
	chlordiazepoxide	Librium
	diazepam	Valium
	lorazepam	Ativan
	oxazepam	Serax
Anticonvulsants	Benzodiazepines	
	clonazepam	Klonopin
	clorazepate	Tranxene
	diazepam	Valium
	Others	
	carbamazepine	Tegretol
	ethosuximide	Zarontin
	phenobarbital	Luminal
	primidone	Mysoline
Antidepressants	amitriptyline	Elavil
	doxepin	Sinequan
Antihistamines	diphenhydramine	Benadryl
	diphenhydramine and acetaminophen	Tylenol PM
	promethazine	Phenergan
	hydroxyzine	Vistaril
Antipsychotics	chlorpromazine	Thorazine
	clozapine	Clozaril
Opioid analgesics	codeine	(generic)
	hydromorphone	Dilaudid
	meperidine	Demerol
	morphine	(generic)
Sedative-hypnotics	Benzodiazepines	
	estazolam	ProSom
	flurazepam	Dalmane
	temazepam	Restoril
	triazolam	Halcion
	Barbiturates	
	amobarbital	Amytal
	pentobarbital	Nembutal
	phenobarbital	Luminal

(continued)

TABLE 8-2 (CONTINUED)		
SELECTED DRUGS THAT HAVE CENTRAL NERVOUS SYSTEM DEPRESSANT EFFECTS		
DRUG CATEGORY	GENERIC NAME	TRADE NAME
Sedative-hypnotics	Others	
	chloral hydrate	(generic)
	eszopiclone	Lunesta
	zaleplon	Sonata
	zolpidem	Ambien
CNS depressant effects may be enhanced when any of these drugs are used concurrently or with skeletal muscle relaxants in Table 8-1. Alcohol is also a CNS depressant but is not shown.		

TABLE 8-3	
ANTICHOLINERGIC ADVERSE EFFECTS	
RESPONSE	COMMENTS
Blurred vision	Affects near vision
Constipation	Increase fluid/fiber; may require stool softener or laxative
Decreased sweating	Potential for hyperthermia, especially on hot day
Dry mouth	Increase fluids; stimulate saliva with hard candy or gum
Increased heart rate	Potential problem for patients with cardiac problems
Pupil dilation	May cause sensitivity to light; prefer dim light/sunglasses
Increased intraocular pressure	Avoid anticholinergic drugs in patients with glaucoma
Urinary hesitancy	If significant, should consider change in therapy
Urinary retention	If significant, should consider change in therapy

BOX 8-1
EXAMPLES OF DRUG CATEGORIES THAT HAVE ANTICHOLINERGIC ADVERSE EFFECTS

- Antihistamines such as diphenhydramine (Benadryl) are used to treat colds and allergies (see Chapter 10) but are also used to treat motion sickness and are contained in OTC sleep-aid products to treat insomnia. These antihistamines are not the H_2 antihistamines (H_2-receptor antagonists) that are used to treat peptic ulcers (see Chapter 11).
- Opioid analgesics (see Chapter 7)
- Tricyclic antidepressants such as amitriptyline (Elavil) and imipramine (Tofranil). The term *tricyclic* identifies a specific chemically related group of drugs that share a common therapeutic role as drug therapy for depression (see Chapter 13).
- Typical antipsychotic drugs (see Chapter 13), such as chlorpromazine (Thorazine), used to treat schizophrenia or to prevent vomiting
- Anticholinergic drugs such as atropine and scopolamine. Atropine has varied uses, such as treatment of bradycardia and to prepare the eye for certain eye examinations; scopolamine is effective in the treatment of motion sickness.
- Selected skeletal muscle relaxants, particularly cyclobenzaprine (Flexeril) and orphenadrine (Norflex)

OTC = over-the-counter.

EFFECTS AND DOSAGE

Skeletal muscle relaxants relieve muscle spasms and, as a result, they also relieve the accompanying pain and increase the patient's range of motion. No single muscle relaxant is recognized as superior to the others in muscle relaxant properties, and thus the selection of muscle relaxant depends largely on its adverse effect profile and the preference of the physician and/or the patient. For example, drugs with pronounced anticholinergic effects should not be used in patients with glaucoma. Several skeletal muscle relaxants, along with their typical adult oral maintenance dosage for treating muscle spasms, are listed in Table 8-1.

Several adverse effects and related cautions are common among the skeletal muscle relaxants (Box 8-2). For example, because all of these drugs function through CNS depressant effects, they all cause drowsiness and dizziness. Consequently, patients being treated with these drugs must be cautious when driving a motor vehicle. Alcohol and other CNS depressants (see Table 8-2) must also be avoided because the depressant effects from other drugs are enhanced when used concurrently with muscle relaxants. Liver and kidney function may also be diminished by skeletal muscle relaxants, with the risk increasing as the duration of therapy and dosage increases. Consequently, these organs are sometimes monitored to detect early signs of compromised function. The potential for hypersensitivity reaction is also a caution regarding treatment with most of these drugs. Hypersensitivity reactions can range from a dermatological rash to anaphylaxis.

The centrally acting skeletal muscle relaxants have the potential to cause physical dependence, although diazepam (Valium) and carisoprodol (Soma) are particularly noteworthy in this respect. The incidence of dependence increases as higher doses are used for a longer time. Both of these medications are classified as Schedule IV controlled substances. These drugs should be slowly discontinued to avoid withdrawal syndrome.

Some adverse effects are more unique to one or 2 drugs listed in Table 8-1. For example, chlorzoxazone (Parafon Forte) and methocarbamol (Robaxin) have the unusual characteristic of discoloring the urine. There is no symptom associated with this effect, but patients should be informed so they are not alarmed at the change. As already mentioned, a response unique to cyclobenzaprine (Flexeril) and orphenadrine (Norflex) are the anticholinergic adverse effects.

Diazepam (Valium) is a member of the chemical category of drugs called benzodiazepines. The term *benzodiazepine* refers to a portion of the chemical structure that these drugs have in common. There are over a dozen benzodiazepines. As a group, these compounds have many uses, such as to treat insomnia, anxiety, alcohol withdrawal syndrome, various seizures, and muscle spasms. Although each of the benzodiazepines may be

---

BOX 8-2

SUMMARY OF ADVERSE EFFECTS RELATED TO SKELETAL MUSCLE RELAXANTS

- Drowsiness
- Dizziness
- Diminished liver and kidney function
- Hypersensitivity reaction
- Physical dependence (centrally acting skeletal muscle relaxants)
- Anticholinergic effects

---

effective to some degree for these uses, some drugs in this group are significantly more effective for one or more of these therapeutic uses than others. Consequently, not all benzodiazepines are approved by the US Food and Drug Administration for each of these uses. All benzodiazepines have an abuse potential and thus are controlled substances (Schedule IV), and all cause CNS depression and thus produce drowsiness. Examples of benzodiazepines and the therapeutic category for selected drugs are listed in Table 8-2.

CHAPTER SUMMARY

Skeletal muscle relaxants have CNS depressant effects that may contribute to their mechanism of action. Use of these drugs relieves symptoms associated with muscle spasm and improves use of the affected muscles but may also cause adverse effects such as drowsiness, dizziness, diminished liver function, hypersensitivity, and anticholinergic effects. The potential for enhanced adverse effects exists if other drugs are used concurrently that also cause CNS depression or anticholinergic effects. Examples of such drugs include alcohol, antihistamines in cold remedies, anticonvulsants, antianxiety drugs, opioid analgesics, and benzodiazepines.

ROLE OF THE ATHLETIC TRAINER

As always, the athletic trainer can play a role in ensuring that the patient adheres to the proper dosage regimen and is aware of common adverse effects. Among the skeletal muscle relaxants, the most common adverse effects are drowsiness and dizziness. The potential for enhanced drowsiness exists if the skeletal muscle relaxant is combined with any of the other CNS depressants. Drug-induced drowsiness and dizziness are especially significant problems in patients competing in sports that require exceptional balance, such as gymnastics or cycling. Drowsiness is also a safety concern (eg, while driving a motor vehicle). Anticholinergic adverse effects are also problematic, and the potential exists for enhanced responses of this type due to the concurrent use of more than one drug that causes anticholinergic effects. Therefore, the athletic trainer can be sure that the patient is aware of the drugs that may exacerbate these problems (see Table 8-2 and Box 8-1), including OTC drugs that contain antihistamines or alcohol. Consequently, by understanding these drug interactions, the athletic trainer may help prevent undesirable effects and should refer the patient to a physician when such drug combinations exert an excessive adverse response.

CASE STUDY

Last weekend at the conference invitational gymnastics meet, Michelle injured her back while doing her floor exercise routine. The physician at the invitational examined her and provided Michelle with muscle relaxants to reduce her back muscle spasms. Today is the first day you have seen Michelle since the team returned home. Michelle indicates that she is still taking the medication the physician gave her and is feeling better but finds she is having a hard time staying awake in her classes and has noticed she has constipation, something she usually doesn't worry about. She is wondering if these are the result of the pain she suffered last weekend. How should you answer Michelle's questions?

BIBLIOGRAPHY

Browning R, Jackson JL, O'Malley PG. Cyclobenzaprine and back pain: a meta-analysis. *Arch Intern Med.* 2001;161:1613-1620.

Chou R, Peterson K, Helfand M. Comparative efficacy and safety of skeletal muscle relaxants for spasticity and musculoskeletal conditions: a systematic review. *J Pain Symptom Manage.* 2004;28(2):140-175.

See S, Ginzburg R. Skeletal muscle relaxants. *Pharmacotherapy.* 2008;28(2):207-213.

Witenko C, Moorman-Li R, Motycka C, et al. Considerations for the appropriate use of skeletal muscle relaxants for the management of acute low back pain. *P T.* 2014;39(6):427-435.

CHAPTER 9: ADVANCE ORGANIZER

Foundational Concepts

- Disease Process
- Classifications
- Inhalers and Spacers
- Pulmonary Functional Tests
- Section Summary

Drugs for Treating Asthma

- Quick-Relief Drugs
  - β_2-Agonists
  - Anticholinergics
  - Systemic Corticosteroids
- Long-Term Therapy
  - Inhaled Corticosteroids
  - Long-Acting β-Agonists
  - Mast Cell–Stabilizing Drugs
  - Leukotriene Modifiers
  - Methylxanthines
    Immunomodulators
- Section Summary

Role of the Athletic Trainer

9

Drugs for Treating Asthma

Chapter Objectives

At the end of this chapter, the reader will be able to:

- Recall the goals of asthma therapy and the interventions that aid in achieving therapy goals

- Explain why asthma therapy adherence is problematic and the interventions that can be implemented to improve therapy adherence

- Describe the disease process that results in the chronic inflammation of the airway and how acute exacerbations of asthma occur

- Explain a categorical classification system for asthma based on severity and summarize a therapeutic management approach for each category of severity

- Recall the advantages and disadvantages of metered dose inhalers (MDIs)

- Explain how the use of a spacer with an MDI can improve the likelihood of better drug delivery to the lungs

- Compare and contrast the 3 types of inhalers available for asthma treatment

- Explain the procedure for correct MDI technique

- Recall the problems associated with inhaler and spacer use and how to overcome them

- Explain the use of nebulizers, forced expiratory spirometer tests, and peak flow meters in the management of asthma

- Make recommendations regarding asthma therapy based on peak flow meter readings

- Identify drug categories used for quick-relief and long-term therapy for asthma

- Describe the mechanism of action for quick-relief and long-term therapy drug categories for treating asthma

- Recognize the adverse effects for quick-relief and long-term asthma medications

- Summarize the role of the athletic trainer for patients who are on an asthma drug therapy regimen

There is an arsenal of over 20 drugs in 6 different pharmacological categories that are available to combat asthma. These drugs are used to treat the more than 25 million people in the United States who have asthma. Although there are many drugs available to treat asthma, the approach to drug therapy management can be simplified by dividing asthma drugs into 2 major therapeutic groups: drugs used to obtain quick relief of acute asthma attacks (rescue therapy) and drugs to obtain long-term control to reduce the occurrence of acute attacks. Athletic trainers can have a significant impact on the therapeutic outcomes by helping patients to understand the rationale for using both of these therapeutic groups of drugs, to be compliant with the

Houglum JE, Harrelson GL, Seefeldt TM.
Principles of Pharmacology for Athletic Trainers, Third Edition (pp 147-166).
© 2016 Taylor & Francis Group.

ABBREVIATIONS USED IN THIS CHAPTER

AIA. aspirin-induced asthma	**HFA.** hydrofluoroalkane
ALT. alanine aminotransferase	**LT.** leukotriene
CNS. central nervous system	**MDI.** metered dose inhaler
COX. cyclooxygenase	**NAEPP.** National Asthma Education and Prevention Program
DPI. dry powder inhaler	
EIB. exercise-induced bronchoconstriction	**NSAID.** nonsteroidal anti-inflammatory drug
FEV$_1$. forced expiratory volume in 1 second	**OTC.** over-the-counter
	PEF. peak expiratory flow
FDA. Food and Drug Administration	**PFM.** peak flow meter
	PG. prostaglandin
FVC. forced vital capacity	**t½.** half-life
GI. gastrointestinal	**TI.** therapeutic index
IgE. immunoglobulin E	

dosage regimen, to properly use inhalers, and to monitor the effectiveness of drug therapy.

This chapter will provide basic information concerning the asthma disease process, pharmacological information relative to asthma drugs, therapy guidelines for use of these drugs to treat asthma, and suggestions as to how the athletic trainer may assist the patient to obtain better therapeutic outcomes from the asthma therapy and thus improve his or her performance.

For the athlete, control of asthma means being able to compete without being hindered by the disease or by the therapy. This is also among the points that the National Asthma Education and Prevention Program (NAEPP) uses to define asthma control, as published in 2007 by the National Heart, Lung, and Blood Institute in *Expert Panel Report 3: Guidelines for the Diagnosis and Management of Asthma*. Box 9-1 lists the points that define asthma control as reported in this document.

Achieving control of asthma requires cooperation and communication between the patient and the health care team. Consequently, it is important that patients and health care professionals be active participants in the therapy process. The components of care to achieve and maintain control of asthma are also listed in Box 9-1.

Pinpointing the appropriate medications and dosages is often a difficult task in asthma treatment. The severity of the disease differs among patients, and thus the therapy should be tailored for each patient. Therefore, it is important for the patient to accurately communicate to the physician the frequency and severity of the symptoms and to monitor the disease. Even when the appropriate drugs and dosages are prescribed, patient adherence with therapy is a significant problem because asthma is a chronic disease that necessitates long-term therapy, often with multiple drugs and/or multiple dosage units per day. Adherence is a problem in all subpopulations of asthmatics; overall, approximately 50% of all asthmatics adhere to prescribed therapy. Inadequate prescribing of drug therapy adds to the number of patients receiving inadequate treatment for asthma. Consequently, suboptimal drug prescribing and poor adherence by patients are significant problems associated with asthma therapy.

Various substances can trigger asthma reactions, and these triggers differ among patients. An obvious strategy is to avoid or minimize exposure to these triggers, but there are many potential triggers, and avoidance of exposure to these triggers may be difficult. Appropriate monitoring can also help avoid the onset of some asthma attacks and can also provide information useful to evaluate the effectiveness of therapy. Keeping asthma patients involved daily with these and other aspects of their disease requires active participation of health care professionals who can provide information and education to the patient. If patients know not only the "how," but also the "why" regarding treatment and monitoring, it may help them be persistent in the long-term management of asthma.

FOUNDATIONAL CONCEPTS

There are several pharmacologic categories of drugs available to treat asthma. To understand the logic for using these drugs, it is helpful to understand the mechanism of the disease process, the symptoms of the disease, and the terminology used to classify the severity of the disease. Knowledge of the proper use of inhalers, spacers, and peak flow meters is also useful because these devices are important aspects of asthma management.

Disease Process

Asthma is a chronic inflammatory disease of the airways. The inflammation results in obstruction of the airways from bronchoconstriction, edema, and excessive mucus production. Symptoms include wheezing, coughing, and shortness of breath. The patient may experience a feeling of chest tightness. As the extent of inflammation increases, the severity of the symptoms typically also increases. Another characteristic of chronic inflammation is that it causes bronchial hyperresponsiveness to a variety of stimuli. This results in acute exacerbations of the inflammation with enhanced symptoms of wheezing, shortness of breath, and difficulty breathing, which can last for a few days. Although patients differ regarding their response to these stimuli, examples of stimuli

---

Box 9-1

ASTHMA THERAPY GOAL AND COMPONENTS OF CARE FOR SUCCESSFUL ASTHMA CONTROL

GOAL: CONTROL OF ASTHMA

- Prevent chronic and troublesome symptoms (eg, coughing or breathlessness in the night, in the daytime, or after exertion)

- Maintain (near) normal pulmonary function

- Maintain normal activity levels (including exercise and other physical activity and attendance at school or work)

- Require infrequent use (≤ 2 days/week) of inhaled short-acting β_2-agonist for quick relief of symptoms (not including prevention of EIB)

- Meet patients' and families' expectations of and satisfaction with asthma care

- Prevent recurrent exacerbations of asthma and minimize the need for emergency department visits or hospitalizations

- Prevent loss of lung function; for children, prevent reduced lung growth

- Provide optimal pharmacotherapy with minimal or no adverse effects

COMPONENTS OF CARE FOR ACHIEVING AND MAINTAINING ASTHMA CONTROL

- Assessing and monitoring the asthma to initiate therapy and make timely adjustments

- Forming a partnership between the patient and clinician for effective education regarding the nature and management of the disease

- Controlling environmental factors and comorbid conditions that affect asthma

- Using the appropriate medications at the appropriate dosage

Adapted from National Institutes of Health, National Heart, Lung, and Blood Institute. National Asthma Education and Prevention Program (NAEPP). Summary Report 2007 of the Expert Panel Report 3: Guidelines for the diagnosis and management of asthma.

---

include typical allergens (eg, dust mites, pollen, animal dander), exercise, tobacco smoke, cold temperatures, viral infections, nonsteroidal anti-inflammatory drugs (NSAIDs), food additives (eg, sulfite preservatives), and comorbid conditions such as chronic sinusitis and gastroesophageal reflux.

The complete mechanism that results in chronic inflammation and the accompanying hyperresponsiveness is not clear, although an antibody-antigen response is responsible for the allergen-mediated inflammation and may participate in the mechanism for other stimuli as well. For the allergen-mediated response, immunoglobulin E (IgE) plays a major role by attaching to mast cells in the respiratory tract and to circulating basophils. Attachment of IgE to these cells initiates the release of chemical mediators.

> *Immunoglobulins (Ig) are also called* antibodies *and are a part of the immune system. There are 5 classes of immunoglobulins, IgE being one of them. Antibodies bind to foreign substances in the body, referred to as* antigens, *as one of the first steps in the process to get rid of the antigen.*

Regardless of the initiating cause, there are many inflammatory chemical mediators that participate in the response. To understand the mechanism of action of several asthma medications, it is of particular importance to understand the process of mediator production through arachidonic acid metabolism (Figure 9-1). As discussed in Chapter 6, arachidonic acid metabolites are produced in virtually all cells. However, with respect to asthma pathophysiology, the products of the pathway catalyzed by 5-lipoxygenase play a key role. As Figure 9-1 illustrates, during an inflammatory response phospholipase A2 is activated in the lung mast cell and causes the release of arachidonic acid inside the cell. Arachidonic acid can be the substrate for COX to synthesize prostaglandins (PGs) or for 5-lipoxygenase to synthesize the leukotrienes (LT). LTC_4 synthase catalyzes the first step in the conversion of LTA_4 to produce LTC_4, which is then released by the mast cells and eventually converted to LTD_4 and LTE_4. The LTs activate LT receptors, which causes vasodilation, increased vasopermeability, mucus secretion, edema, and marked bronchoconstriction. Regarding these effects, LTC_4 and LTD_4 are the

Figure 9-1. Biosynthesis pathways of arachidonic acid metabolites. Arachidonic acid is released from membrane-bound sites by the action of phospholipase A_2. If the arachidonic acid reacts with COX, it is converted to PGs; if it reacts with 5-lipoxygenase, it is converted to LTs. In either case, the arachidonic acid metabolites are released by the cell and will combine with the respective receptor on other cells to contribute to the symptoms of asthma. The sites of action are shown for the corticosteroids, LT modifiers, and mast cell stabilizing drugs. • — Indicates reaction catalyzed by enzyme as designated. X — Indicates reaction inhibited by drug as designated. (Adapted from Houglum JE. Asthma medications: basic pharmacology and use in the athlete. *J Athl Train.* 2000;35:179-187.)

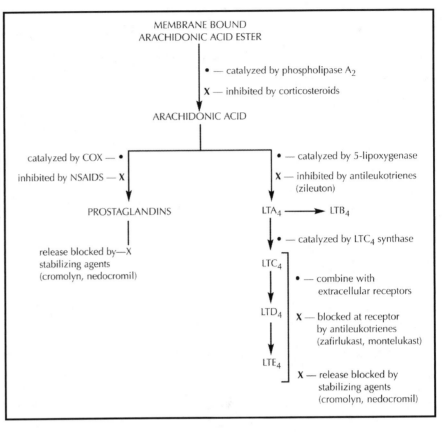

most potent; LTE_4 is significantly less potent. Some cell types convert LTA_4 to LTB_4, which attract eosinophils and neutrophils to the site. Besides mast cells, other cell types such as macrophages, neutrophils, eosinophils, and T lymphocytes also contribute to the inflammatory process by producing arachidonic acid metabolites and other chemical mediators, including histamine, platelet-activating factor, and cytokines, which contribute to the inflammatory process. Use of anti-inflammatory drugs interrupts one or more aspects of this process to decrease the damaging effects of chronic inflammation. Although the PGs contribute to the inflammatory response, they play a mixed role regarding the effect on bronchial smooth muscle, causing relaxation or constriction depending on the specific PG.

Classifications

The specific drug therapy and dosages needed to control the symptoms of asthma vary from patient to patient, depending primarily on the severity of the disease. The NAEPP has established guidelines for classifying asthma severity based on results of lung function tests and the frequency of symptoms prior to treatment (Table 9-1). The classifications of asthma severity are intermittent, mild persistent, moderate persistent, and severe persistent. The least severe classification, intermittent, exists if the patient has no more than 2 days per week with symptoms, no more than 2 nights' sleep interrupted with symptoms

per month, no interference with normal activity, the need for short-acting β_2-agonist no more than twice per week, normal lung function indicators, and less than 2 exacerbations per year that require oral corticosteroid therapy. The most serious asthma classification, severe persistent, exists if the daytime symptoms occur throughout the day; nighttime symptoms occur every night; short-acting β_2-agonists are needed several times per day; normal activity is extremely limited; forced expiratory volume in 1 second (FEV_1) is less than 60%; and exacerbations occur 2 or more times per year. All of the persistent categories require daily medication; only the intermittent category does not (Table 9-2).

Although the categorization of asthma severity is useful, patients sometimes have symptoms that overlap categories. For example, a patient may have daily symptoms (moderate persistent) but nighttime symptoms of 3 to 4 per month (mild persistent). Patients should be placed in the category of greatest severity for treatment purposes.

The NAEPP has established guidelines for drug therapy (see Table 9-2) based on the classifications of asthma severity. The guidelines recommend that all patients use a quick-relief bronchodilator, and all patients with persistent asthma also use daily anti-inflammatory medication for long-term control of inflammation. As the severity classification increases, the guidelines call for an increase in dose and/or the addition of another long-term-control drug to the therapy. When therapy is initiated,

TABLE 9-1

CLASSIFYING ASTHMA SEVERITY AND RECOMMENDED STEPS FOR INITIATING TREATMENT[a]

COMPONENTS OF SEVERITY	CLASSIFICATION OF ASTHMA SEVERITY			
	Intermittent	*Mild Persistent*	*Moderate Persistent*	*Severe Persistent*
Symptoms	≤2 days/week	>2 days/week but not daily	Daily	Throughout the day
Nighttime awakenings	≤2 times/month	3 to 4 times/ month	>1 time/week but not nightly	Often 7 times/week
SABA use for symptoms control (not for EIB)	≤2 days/week	>2 days/week but not daily, and not more once/day	Daily	Several times per day
Interference with normal activity	None	Minor limitation	Some limitation	Extremely limited
Lung function	Normal FEV_1 between exacerbations FEV_1 >80% predicted FEV_1/FVC normal	FEV_1 >80% predicted FEV_1/FVC normal	FEV_1 >60% but <80% predicted FEV_1/FVC reduced 5%	FEV_1 <60% predicted FEV_1/FVC reduced >5%
Exacerbations requiring oral corticosteroid	0 to 1 per year	≥2 per year	≥2 per year	≥2 per year
Recommended Step for Initiating Treatment	Step 1	Step 2	Step 3 and consider short course of oral corticosteroids	Step 4 or 5 and consider short course of oral corticosteroids

[a]In youths aged ≥12 years and adults not taking long-term control medications.

EIB = exercise-induced bronchoconstriction; FEV_1 = forced expiratory volume in 1 second; FVC = forced vital capacity; SABA = short-acting β_2-agonist.

Assign severity to the most severe category in which any feature occurs.

Adapted from National Institutes of Health, National Heart, Lung, and Blood Institute. National Asthma Education and Prevention Program (NAEPP). Full Report of the Expert Panel: Guidelines for the diagnosis and management of asthma (EPR-3) 2007.

however, aggressive therapy is recommended to control the symptoms, followed by an approach of a gradual decrease in drug therapy (*stepdown*) to determine the least amount of medication necessary to maintain control. Once the lowest level of treatment required to maintain control is achieved, classification of asthma severity can be gauged based upon which step of the NAEPP Stepwise Approach for Managing Asthma is needed for control:

- If step 1 therapy is needed, severity is intermittent.
- If step 2 therapy is needed, severity is mild persistent.
- If step 3 or 4 therapy is needed, severity is moderate persistent.
- If step 5 or 6 therapy is needed, severity is severe persistent.

In addition to the NAEPP classifications of severity of asthma, the following additional terminology identifies asthma based on some characteristics other than severity:

- *Chronic asthma* is the disease generally referred to as *asthma*. It includes the chronic inflammatory condition already discussed.

- An *acute asthma attack* (*exacerbation*) is a sudden onset of symptoms that is generally caused from the hyperresponsiveness associated with chronic asthma condition. The onset of the acute attack may be due to exposure to known allergens or pollutants or from some unknown factor. The acute inflammatory response causes bronchoconstriction, excessive mucus production, and edema, resulting in the symptoms described previously (eg, wheezing, coughing, shortness of breath, difficulty breathing).

TABLE 9-2

STEPWISE APPROACH FOR MANAGING ASTHMA IN YOUTHS AGED ≥ 12 YEARS AND ADULTS

Intermittent Asthma	Persistent Asthma: Daily Medications
	Consult with asthma specialist if step 4 care or higher is required. Consider consultation at step 3.

Step 6

Preferred:
High-dose ICS+LABA= oral corticosteroid AND consider omalizumab for patients who have allergies

Step 5

Preferred:
High-dose ICS+LABA AND consider omalizumab for patients who have allergies

Step 4

Preferred:
Medium-dose ICS+LABA

Alternative:
Medium-dose ICS+either LTRA, theophylline, or zileuton

Step 3

Preferred:
Low-dose ICS+LABA or medium-dose ICS

Alternative:
Low-dose ICS+either LTRA, theophylline, or zileuton

Step 2

Preferred: Low-dose ICS

Alternative: Cromolyn, LTRA, nedocromil, or theophylline

Step 1

Preferred:
SABA PRN

Step up if needed (first check adherence, environmental control, and comorbid conditions)

Assess control

Step down if possible (and asthma is well controlled at least 3 months)

Each step: Patient education, environmental control, and management of comorbidities.

Steps 2 to 4: Consider subcutaneous allergen immunotherapy for patients who have allergic asthma (see notes).

- SABA as needed for symptoms. Intensity of treatment depends on severity of symptoms; up to 3 treatments at 20-minute intervals as needed. Short course of oral systemic corticosteroids may be needed.

- Use of SABA >2 days/week for symptom relief (not prevention of EIB) generally indicates inadequate control and the need to step up treatment.

EIB=exercise-induced bronchospasm; ICS=inhaled corticosteroid; LABA=long-acting inhaled β_2-agonist; LTRA=leukotriene receptor antagonist; SABA=inhaled short-acting β_2-agonist.

If alternative treatment is used and response is inadequate, discontinue it and use the preferred treatment before stepping up.

Clinicians who administer omalizumab should be prepared and equipped to identify and treat anaphylaxis that may occur.

Adapted from National Institutes of Health, National Heart, Lung, and Blood Institute. National Asthma Education and Prevention. Program (NAEPP). Full Report of the Expert Panel: Guidelines for the diagnosis and management of asthma (EPR-3) 2007.

These symptoms may be mild enough to ameliorate spontaneously, may necessitate treatment with quick-relief (ie, rescue) medication, or may be severe enough to require emergency medical attention. Duration of an acute attack may be a few days.

- *Exercise-induced bronchoconstriction* (EIB) exists in 70% to 90% of patients with chronic asthma. Some patients may have EIB but do not have asthma-related symptoms at any other times. Onset of EIB symptoms typically occurs during exercise and for

20 to 60 minutes after exercise, with the maximum bronchoconstriction occurring within the first 5 to 15 minutes after exercise. Some patients experience a subsequent refractory period of 2 to 4 hours in which additional exercise results in less broncho-constriction. The refractory period may be a result of mast cell mediators being depleted. As with chronic asthma, EIB symptoms can include wheezing, coughing, and shortness of breath. The loss of water and/or heat from the lungs during exercise may contribute to the cause of EIB; avoiding exercise in cool, dry environments may reduce EIB.

- *Aspirin-induced asthma* (AIA) occurs in 4% to 20% of patients with chronic asthma, depending on the subpopulation; the incidence increases with age and severity of chronic asthma. There is cross-hyperresponsiveness with the other NSAIDs so that patients who are sensitive to aspirin are likely to be sensitive to other NSAIDs. There is less cross-reaction with acetaminophen, although as the dose increases above 650 mg, the likelihood of some cross-reaction increases. Even so, the symptoms of bronchoconstriction are typically milder with acet-aminophen than with aspirin.

- *Nocturnal asthma* refers to symptoms of chronic asthma that interrupt sleep. Some patients experience more frequent occurrences of nocturnal asthma than others. The cause is unknown but may be due to varying exposure to some allergens due to changes in nighttime ventilation, nighttime change in hormone levels, or other physiological changes such as gastro-esophageal reflux. The existence of nocturnal asthma can be a sign of inadequate asthma control.

- *Atopic asthma* occurs from IgE-mediated inflammatory response. IgE are antibodies located on the surface of mast cells in the airways. Patients with atopic reactions produce IgE as a result of exposure to common allergens such as cat dander, house-dust mites, cockroaches, fungal spores, and various pollens. When these antigens combine with the IgE, the mast cell releases chemical mediators such as LTs, PGs, and histamine. For many patients, atopic asthma is a significant component of the hyperresponsiveness associated with chronic asthma.

Inhalers and Spacers

Many asthma drugs are most effectively administered through inhalation because it quickly places the drug at the desired site of action, the lung. Because topical drug administration includes the mucous membranes, inhalation is considered topical application. Some pharmacokinetic parameters are eliminated by using inhalation, such

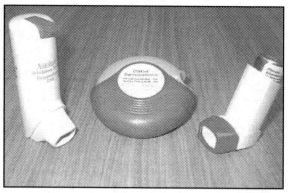

Figure 9-2. Examples of breath-actuated MDI (left), DPI (center), and MDI (right). (Reprinted with permission from Houglum JE. The basics of asthma therapy for athletes. *Athletic Therapy Today.* 2001;6[5]:16-21. © 2001 Human Kinetics, Inc.)

as gastrointestinal (GI) absorption, the first-pass effect, and systemic distribution to achieve the therapeutic effect.

A common method for delivering asthma drugs by inhalation is by using an MDI. The drug is in a pressurized container with a metering valve to control the amount of drug released during each use (Figure 9-2). A propellant is used to force the metered amount of drug from the inhaler each time the device is actuated. The drug exists as a solution or a suspended micronized powder in the inhaler but is released from the inhaler as an aerosol for delivery into the patient's mouth. As the patient inhales deeply in a coordinated fashion with the actuation of the inhaler, the drug reaches the lung. Advantages of this method of drug delivery are that the drug is delivered more directly to the tissue, there are fewer systemic adverse effects, and a quicker response is obtained compared with the oral route.

There are also some disadvantages to the use of MDIs (Box 9-2). The primary concerns are that, even with good technique, generally less than 20% of the drug reaches the lung. Although this problem is somewhat accounted for in the canister dosage, inhalation technique can significantly vary the amount of drug reaching the lung. Proper technique requires the patient to follow a set of directions and requires a certain amount of skill to coordinate the activation of the MDI and the inhalation of the aerosol. Besides the potential for poor technique, another disadvantage of inhaler use is the inconvenience; carrying MDI devices can be somewhat cumbersome, and using an inhaler is significantly bothersome for some patients compared with oral medications.

Spacers (Figure 9-3) can be used with the MDI to compensate for some of the disadvantages of inhaler use. Some spacers are hollow tubes that are attached to the MDI so that the drug is propelled into the spacer and thus travels through the spacer before being inhaled by the patient. More useful are the spacer devices that have a one-way valve that opens during inhalation. These are more specifically called *valved holding chambers* because they hold the MDI puff briefly

---

Box 9-2

SUMMARY OF ADVANTAGES AND DISADVANTAGES OF METERED DOSE INHALERS

ADVANTAGES

- Some pharmacokinetic parameters are eliminated by using inhalation, such as GI absorption, the first-pass effect, and systemic distribution, to achieve the therapeutic effect.

- The drug is delivered more directly to the tissue.

- There are fewer systemic adverse effects.

- Quicker response is obtained compared with the oral route.

DISADVANTAGES

- Requires proper technique to be effective.

- Even with good technique, less than 20% of the drug reaches the lung.

- Inconvenient because the MDI devices can be cumbersome and bothersome to use compared with taking oral medications.

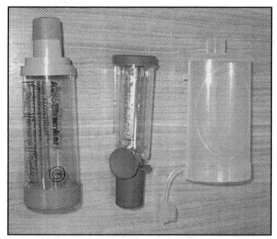

Figure 9-3. Examples of spacers, including valved holding chambers (left, center). (Reprinted with permission from Houglum JE. The basics of asthma therapy for athletes. *Athletic Therapy Today.* 2001;6[5]:16-21. © 2001 Human Kinetics, Inc.)

---

before inhalation, and the one-way valve prevents the patient from exhaling into the device. This allows the patient an extra 1 to 2 seconds before inhalation is necessary, making it easier for the patient to coordinate the activation of the inhaler with inhalation and thus improving the likelihood of better delivery of drug to the lung. It is primarily the smaller particles that have a chance of reaching the lung because they travel the farthest from the force of the propellant and are more readily carried into the lung during inhalation. Although some of the drug is exhaled, most of the remaining particles are the larger particles and, without the use of a spacer, they are deposited in the oropharynx. However, as the drug travels through the spacer, the particles of drug lose momentum so that fewer of the larger particles reach the patient's mouth. This provides a particular advantage when using inhaled corticosteroid because the deposit of these drugs in the oropharynx contributes to hoarseness and oral candidiasis infections (thrush). These adverse effects can also be minimized by rinsing the mouth with water and spitting after use of inhaled corticosteroids.

The propellants used in MDIs have historically been chlorofluorocarbons. These are the same type of gases that were discontinued as refrigerants in air conditioners and refrigerators and, as of the end of 2008, have all been discontinued in MDIs in the United States because of environmental policies. Each inhaler with the new propellants,

hydrofluoroalkanes, requires approval by the FDA because a change in propellant necessitated additional safety and efficacy studies. The spray of the hydrofluoroalkane delivery also tastes different and feels less forceful compared with chlorofluorocarbon propellants.

Dry powder inhalers (DPIs) are also used for delivery of asthma medications to the lungs. DPIs provide an alternative to the use of pressurized gases. As the patient inhales deeply, the process of inhalation through the inhaler draws the powdered drug into the lungs. The drug is contained in a capsule or other package form that the inhaler breaks open during use to allow the powder to be inhaled. The patient must be able to inhale deeply to provide enough suction to draw the drug into the lungs and thus DPI inhalers should not be used as treatment for acute asthma exacerbations. DPIs eliminate the need to coordinate inhalation with actuation of the propellant, which is a significant hindrance to adequate disease control in the elderly and very young patients, particularly. DPIs cannot be used with a spacer.

A third type of inhaler is the breath-actuated MDI. The technique to operate this inhaler is somewhat of a cross between an MDI and a DPI; a propellant is used to expel the drug, but it is not activated until the patient inhales. The breath-actuated MDI uses a lever to cock the mechanism, and the mechanism is released when the patient inhales through the mouthpiece. The breath-actuated MDI eliminates the need to coordinate the inhalation with actuation of the inhaler but, like DPIs, breath-actuated inhalers cannot be used with a spacer.

Regardless of the type of inhaler used, good technique is important to obtain adequate delivery of the drug to the lungs. The step-by-step procedure for good inhalation technique varies for MDIs compared with breath-actuated MDIs and DPIs. The procedure for use of typical MDIs is listed in Box 9-3.

Insufficient inhaler technique and poor adherence with prescribed therapy are common reasons for diminished therapeutic effectiveness and potentially diminished athletic performance and/or participation. Poor technique when using inhaled corticosteroids also leads to an increased incidence of hoarseness, cough, and oral fungal infection. Table 9-3 lists the trade names of some MDI and DPI devices; these are not trade names of the drugs but only the inhalation devices used to deliver the drugs.

Besides achieving appropriate technique, there are some other, but relatively minor, problems associated with inhaler use. For example, the nondrug components of inhaled suspensions can cause coughing. Inhalers and spacers must be kept clean to prevent accumulation of drug after repeated use. Moisture can cause problems for DPI by preventing the drug particles from flowing effectively, and cold temperatures can decrease the efficiency of the propellant gas in MDIs.

Nebulizers (Figure 9-4) are devices used to deliver drug to the lungs, but these devices are larger than MDIs and DPIs. They are used primarily in hospitals and clinics or in homes if the patient is unable to use inhalers. A few milliliters of liquid drug are placed in the nebulizer. An aerosol is created from the liquid by using either a stream of compressed air (jet nebulizer) or vibration (ultrasonic nebulizer) mechanism. The aerosol is inhaled by the patient by breathing normally through a mouthpiece during a 10- to 15-minute nebulizer treatment. Alternatively, the patient can breathe deeply and slowly with breath-holding to increase efficiency of drug delivery. Use of a face mask rather than a mouthpiece is less effective in delivering drug to the lungs because the nasal passage prevents some of the drug from reaching the lungs. The advantage of a nebulizer vs an MDI is that there is no actuation to coordinate with inhalation.

Pulmonary Function Tests

Pulmonary function tests provide a means of quantifying air flow to the lungs and thus are an objective measure of the severity of the asthma at the time of measurement (eg, during an acute exacerbation) and can be used as a means of diagnosis and monitoring of pulmonary disease. FEV_1 is one such test (Figure 9-5). The FEV_1 is determined using a forced expiratory spirometer and is a measure of the volume of air that can be exhaled in the first second after maximal inspiration. When compared with the normal values, the FEV_1 can be used to assess the severity of the asthma and, as indicated in Table 9-1, is one of the criteria used by NAEPP. The FEV_1 can be combined with other parameters, such as forced vital capacity (FVC). The FVC is the total volume of air that can be exhaled and is also used to classify asthma severity. The ratio of FEV_1/FVC is sometimes a more sensitive indicator of severity and asthma control.

The peak expiratory flow (PEF) is another pulmonary function test and is conducted using a peak flow meter

BOX 9-3
PROCEDURE FOR USING A TYPICAL METERED DOSE INHALER

STEP	ACTION
1	Prepare the MDI according to directions on container (eg, suspensions must be shaken before use to obtain a consistent dose with each use).
2	Hold inhaler upright, tip head back slightly to facilitate flow of drug into the lungs.
3	Exhale slowly.
4	Place the inhaler (or spacer with inhaler attached) in mouth and seal lips securely around the mouthpiece of the inhaler (or spacer).
5	Press down on the inhaler to release the medication and at the same time take a slow, deep inhalation.
6	Hold the breath for about 10 seconds before exhaling.
7	If another puff is needed of a quick-relief inhaler, wait about 1 minute before taking the second puff. This will give time for the first puff to begin working and may improve the effectiveness of the second puff.
8	When using a corticosteroid, rinse mouth out with water.

(PFM). PEF is the maximum flow rate of forced expiration that the patient can achieve at that time. This is the most commonly used pulmonary function test by patients because PFMs are hand-held devices (Figure 9-6) that are easy to use and inexpensive. During a 2- to 3-week period when the patient's asthma is well controlled, the patient's personal best PEF is determined so that subsequent values can be compared as a percentage of the personal best. Daily results from the PFM can be plotted to determine effectiveness of long-term therapy. The same PFM should be used each day for the most consistent results. If PEF decreases, it can be indicative of an imminent acute attack and the patient can make adjustments in therapy before the symptoms become prominent. The plan for adjusting therapy should be pre-established with the physician so that the patient knows what actions to take, particularly when acute symptoms occur. For example, if the patient's personal best PEF is 600 and the patient begins to experience acute symptoms of bronchoconstriction, the patient uses the rescue medication as prescribed, checks PEF, and then takes the following actions as pre-established with the physician:

TABLE 9-3			
INHALER DEVICES USED FOR ASTHMA THERAPY			
INHALER TRADE NAME	DRUG	TYPE	COMMENTS
Aerolizer	formoterol	DPI	Breath-actuated, single-dose capsule
Diskus	fluticasone and salmeterol	DPI	Breath-actuated
Flexhaler	budesonide	DPI	Breath-actuated
Twisthaler	mometasone	DPI	Breath-actuated
Ventolin HFA	albuterol	MDI	Propellant contains HFAs
DPI = dry powder inhaler; HFA = hydrofluoroalkane; MDI, metered dose inhaler.			

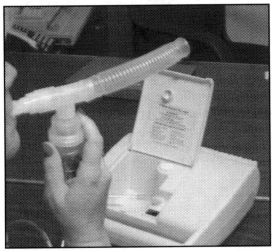

Figure 9-4. Example of a nebulizer.

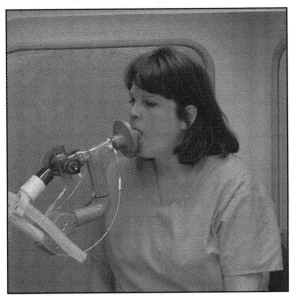

Figure 9-5. Measurement of forced expiratory volume using a spirometer.

- If flow is >480 (>80% of personal best), maintain existing quick-relief therapy as directed by the physician and recheck PEF after each quick-relief dosage.

- If flow is 300 to 480 (50% to 80% of personal best), use additional rescue medication as predetermined and continue to monitor PEF until symptoms subside and PEF is at least 80% of personal best, and contact physician as soon as possible.

- If flow is <300 (<50% of personal best), use additional rescue medication immediately and go to the emergency department.

The exact plan of action may be different for each patient, but the point is that the patient should have a pre-established written plan so that the PFM values can be used to appropriately adjust therapy. The athletic trainer must be aware of this plan. The NAEPP recommends patients with moderate or severe persistent asthma, a history of severe acute exacerbations, or poorly controlled asthma to have a written action plan and use the PFM routinely to monitor the disease and the effectiveness of therapy.

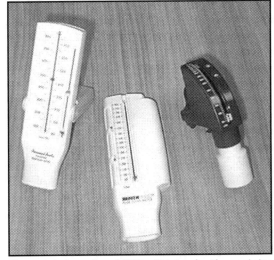

Figure 9-6. Examples of PFMs. (Reprinted with permission from Houglum JE. The basics of asthma therapy for athletes. *Athletic Therapy Today.* 2001;6[5]:16-21. © Human Kinetics, Inc.)

Section Summary

Asthma is a chronic disease, and it is an inflammatory disease. Consequently, for persistent asthma, treatment requires daily anti-inflammatory therapy to reduce the incidence of acute attacks and to decrease the long-term effects of chronic inflammation. Patients with chronic asthma are hyperresponsive to various allergens such as house dust-mites, cockroaches, pollen, animal dander, and cigarette smoke. The production and release of many chemical mediators, including the LTs through the lipoxygenase pathway of arachidonic acid metabolism, causes bronchoconstriction, mucus production, and edema, resulting in difficulty breathing, coughing, and wheezing. Most patients with chronic asthma also have EIB, which can cause these symptoms during exercise and immediately following exercise if not appropriately treated.

The severity of asthma is usually classified as intermittent, mild persistent, moderate persistent, and severe persistent based on the frequency of symptoms prior to treatment and the results of pulmonary function tests. One test that the patient can use to monitor impairment and the potential risk for exacerbation is the PEF, which can be conveniently measured using a PFM. The use of a PFM is encouraged, especially for patients with moderate and severe persistent asthma, a history of severe exacerbations, or poorly controlled asthma.

Many asthma medications are administered as inhalants, typically using MDIs and DPIs. MDIs use a propellant to force the drug into the lung when the inhaler device is actuated. For adequate delivery of drug to the lungs, the use of an MDI necessitates a slow inhalation process at the same time the inhaler is actuated. The breath-actuated inhaler does not require the same degree of coordination because the metered dose is not released by the propellant until the patient inhales. The drug from DPI enters the lung as a result of the force of the inhalation and does not use a propellant. If proper technique is used, the MDI delivers sufficient drug to the lungs. If the patient cannot adequately coordinate slow inhalation with actuation, the DPI and breath-actuated MDI are alternatives. A problem with inhalers is that much of the drug is deposited in the back of the throat, which can contribute to increased incidence of hoarseness and thrush with inhaled corticosteroid use. Spacers can be used with MDIs to decrease the amount of drug deposited in the throat and increase the amount delivered to the lungs. Spacers are chambers into which an MDI is actuated so that the drug must travel through the chamber before it is inhaled. Larger particles of drug are not propelled far enough to make it out of the chamber, so most of the drug that makes it into the airways is the smaller particles.

Poor adherence with therapy and improper inhalation technique are significant causes of poor therapeutic outcomes. The athletic trainer can assist the patient in understanding the necessity for daily adherence with therapy and can provide instruction regarding proper inhalation technique, as well as other educational information, to improve therapeutic outcomes.

DRUGS FOR TREATING ASTHMA

From a therapy standpoint, there are 2 main components of asthma to contend with: diminishing the chronic inflammation that is characteristic of the disease and treating acute flare-ups that occur with varying frequency and severity among patients with asthma. Drugs used to treat chronic asthma are referred to as *long-term control medications*, whereas drugs used to treat acute flare-ups are *quick-relief* or *rescue medications*. These 2 components of drug therapy are connected in the sense that patients with poorly controlled chronic asthma have a higher incidence of acute reactions and thus require more frequent use of quick-relief medication at higher doses.

From a pharmacological standpoint, there are 2 general categories of drugs that are used to treat the chronic and acute aspects of asthma: bronchodilators and anti-inflammatory medications. In each general category, there are also subcategories of drugs based on the pharmacological mechanism of action. Table 9-4 depicts this categorization and groups of drugs in each category that are discussed in this chapter. The bronchodilators act on the bronchial smooth muscle to cause it to relax, thus causing a larger airway opening. Anti-inflammatory drugs may act by several mechanisms, but one prime focus is to inhibit the effects of the LTs and other inflammatory chemical mediators.

Quick-Relief Drugs

The purpose of these drugs is to treat an existing acute attack (ie, *rescue therapy*) or to prevent an imminent attack, such as before exercise. Consequently, these drugs are not taken on a routine daily schedule but rather on an as-needed basis (ie, prn). The two types of quick-relief drugs are the systemic corticosteroids and the bronchodilators, which include the β_2-agonists and anticholinergic drugs. According to NAEPP, every asthma patient should have a quick-relief inhaled β_2-agonist readily available.

β_2-Agonists

The most effective drugs for treatment of an acute asthma attack are the short-acting β_2-agonists administered by inhalation. Short-acting refers to the duration of action, but these drugs also have a short onset of action. There are long-acting (longer duration of action) bronchodilators available, but they should not be used for quick-relief therapy because they have a slower onset of action. Long-acting β_2-agonists are discussed in the section on drugs used for long-term control. The predominant adrenergic receptor in

TABLE 9-4

CATEGORIZATION OF ASTHMA MEDICATIONS

BY THERAPEUTIC USE	BY PHARMACOLOGICAL ACTIVITY
Quick-relief therapy:	Bronchodilator drugs:
• Short-acting β_2-agonists by inhalation	• Short-acting β_2-agonists by oral or inhalation
• Systemic corticosteroid by oral or parenteral	• Long-acting β_2-agonists by inhalation
• Anticholinergics by inhalation	• Anticholinergics by inhalation
Long-term therapy:	• Methylxanthines by oral
• Corticosteroids by inhalation	Anti-inflammatory drugs:
• Long-acting β_2-agonists by inhalation	• Corticosteroids by systemic or inhalation
• LT modifiers by oral	• LT modifiers by oral
• Mast cell stabilizers by inhalation	• Mast cell stabilizers by inhalation
• Methylxanthines by oral	• Immunomodulator by injection

LT = leukotriene.

the bronchial smooth muscle is the β_2-receptor. Other tissues such as skeletal muscle and liver also have β_2-receptors, whereas the heart and kidney have β_1-receptors. Agonists that combine with β_2-receptors cause bronchodilation in the lung, contraction (tremor) of skeletal muscle, and glycogenolysis and *gluconeogenesis* in the liver, which causes increased blood glucose. An advantage of using β_2-agonists by inhalation is that not only does the drug reach the site of action quickly, but also the principle adverse effects of β_2-agonists (ie, muscle tremor and hyperglycemia) are minimized. Regardless, muscle tremor tends to diminish with continued use, and hyperglycemia is very transient because the pancreas releases more insulin to compensate, although the diabetic may require an adjustment in insulin dosage. The performance-enhancing effects of β_2-agonists are discussed in Chapter 16.

The adrenergic receptor type of prime importance in the heart muscle and kidney is the β_1-receptor. Activation of these receptors causes tachycardia and elevated blood pressure due to increased renin release by the kidney. Although the β_2-agonists are selective for the β_2-receptor, this selectivity is not absolute and some β_1-activity is possible, especially as the dose of the β_2-agonist increases. Consequently, β_2-agonists can exert some β_1-activity, causing elevated heart rate and blood pressure, but these too are minimized by using inhalation rather than oral β_2-agonists. Because there are several selective β_2-agonists that are effective bronchodilators for asthma treatment, there is no therapeutic rationale for using nonselective β-agonists (eg, isoproterenol, epinephrine) because they will readily combine with β_1-receptors to cause a greater likelihood for adverse effects.

There has been some controversy as to whether frequent, daily use of β_2-agonists decreases the bronchodilator effectiveness of these drugs. It has been shown that chronic use of β_2-agonists can lead to a decrease in the number of β_2 receptors expressed by the cell. A decrease in the number of receptors leads to a reduction in the response to the agonist drug. An increase in the dose may be required if tolerance develops. Because these β_2-agonists have a short duration of action, there is no therapeutic advantage to using them on a scheduled, daily basis.

Short-acting β_2-agonists are the drugs of choice for treatment of acute attacks (rescue therapy) on an as-needed basis. When these drugs are used by inhalation, onset of action occurs within 5 minutes. Duration of action varies considerably but typically is 2 to 6 hours, with somewhat shorter duration being more likely if the drug is used for protection during exercise. These drugs react directly with bronchial smooth muscle to cause bronchodilation, regardless of the cause of the bronchial constriction. The usual dose is one to 2 puffs as needed for relief, preferably with about 1 minute between the puffs. This time between puffs allows for some bronchial dilation to occur from the first puff and may enhance the effectiveness from the second puff. To prevent EIB, one to 2 puffs 5 to 15 minutes before exercise should offer sufficient protection for 2 to 4 hours. Administration of β_2-agonists by inhalation can be repeated during exercise, but the routine use of these additional doses during exercise is indicative of poor control of chronic asthma and thus long-term therapy should be re-evaluated.

The β_2-agonists are equally effective in producing bronchodilation at their respective therapeutic doses; the main

		TABLE 9-5	

ADULT DOSAGES OF SELECTED QUICK-RELIEF MEDICATIONS

GENERIC NAME	TRADE NAME	CATEGORY	DOSAGE FORM; TYPICAL ADULT DOSAGE
albuterol	Proventil, Ventolin	β_2-agonist, SA	MDI; 2 puffs (90 mcg each) every 4 to 6 hours prn
levalbuterol	Xopenex	β_2-agonist, SA	MDI; 2 puffs (45 mcg each) every 4 to 6 hours prn
methylprednisolone	Medrol	corticosteroid	oral; 40 to 60 mg/day for 3 to 10 days
pirbuterol	Maxair	β_2-agonist, SA	MDI; 2 puffs (200 mcg each) every 4 to 6 hours prn
prednisolone	Prednisolone	corticosteroid	oral; 40 to 60 mg/day for 3 to 10 days
prednisone	Prednisone	corticosteroid	oral; 40 to 60 mg/day for 3 to 10 days
MDI = metered dose inhaler; SA = short-acting; prn = as needed for relief.			

difference is the duration of action. Typical adult dosages for β_2-agonists are shown in Table 9-5.

Anticholinergics

Anticholinergic drugs are less effective than β_2-agonists for quick relief of acute attacks. Rather than stimulating β-adrenergic receptors for bronchodilation, anticholinergic drugs inhibit cholinergic receptors of the parasympathetic nervous system to cause bronchodilation. Anticholinergics are most effective in patients whose symptoms are due to excessive cholinergic stimulation. However, it is not possible to identify these patients prior to treatment.

Although there are many anticholinergic drugs, most are older drugs (eg, atropine) that have too many adverse effects. Ipratropium (Atrovent) is the only anticholinergic currently used to treat asthma. Although not free from adverse effects, ipratropium by inhalation has fewer adverse effects (eg, dry mouth, throat irritation, bad taste) but should not be used by patients who are allergic to peanuts.

Recall from Chapter 8 that anticholinergic drugs typically cause several adverse effects such as urinary retention, blurred vision, sedation, and constipation.

Significant therapeutic effects occur within 5 minutes after inhalation of ipratropium, and additive effects are obtained when combined with β_2-agonists; consequently, ipratropium plus albuterol (Combivent, DuoNeb) is available as a combination inhaled or nebulized product. Ipratropium is used as a component of therapy to treat acute asthma, either by MDI or nebulizer, but is not included in NAEPP guidelines for long-term therapy of chronic asthma and has limited effectiveness to prevent EIB.

Systemic Corticosteroids

Systemic corticosteroids are used orally or by the parenteral routes to treat severe symptoms associated with an acute exacerbation (see Table 9-5). The mechanism for these drugs is discussed later in this chapter, but in short, they inhibit the inflammatory response. A short course of therapy (3 to 10 days) is useful when short-acting β_2-agonists alone are not sufficient. Significant adverse effects are minimized with these short bursts of therapy. Some patients may experience mood changes, and diabetics may observe a loss of glucose control. Significant adrenal suppression rarely occurs, and thus discontinuation of the short therapy can be abrupt.

In situations where the acute exacerbations last longer and the use of systemic corticosteroids is continued, a tapering of the corticosteroid dose may be necessary.

Recall from Chapter 6 that adrenal suppression can occur as a result of extended systemic therapy with corticosteroids. This relatively constant exposure to the corticosteroids can cause the adrenal gland to decrease production of corticosteroid (ie, adrenal insufficiency) that may last for weeks to months after the corticosteroid drug has been discontinued. The extent of adrenal insufficiency depends on the daily dosage and the duration of corticosteroid therapy. The symptoms of adrenal insufficiency range from mild (nausea) to life threatening. To avoid these symptoms after extended corticosteroid therapy, the dosage should be tapered according to established protocols. Abrupt withdrawal of extended corticosteroid therapy may also cause an exacerbation of the disease being treated.

Long-Term Therapy

The purpose of long-term therapy is to reduce the incidence of acute exacerbations of the disease. Several categories of drugs are available for this purpose: corticosteroids, mast cell–stabilizing drugs, LT modifiers, methylxanthines, and long-acting β_2-agonists. All of these drugs

TABLE 9-6			
ADULT DOSAGES OF SELECTED LONG-TERM CONTROL MEDICATIONS			
GENERIC NAME	**TRADE NAME**	**CATEGORY**	**DOSAGE FORM; TYPICAL ADULT DOSAGE**
albuterol	VoSpire ER	β_2-agonist, LA	Oral extended release; 4 to 8 mg every 12 hours
beclomethasone	QVAR	Corticosteroid	MDI; 2 puffs (40 to 80 µg each) twice/day
budesonide	Pulmicort	Corticosteroid	DPI; 2 inhalations (90 to 180 µg each) twice/day
budesonide + formoterol	Symbicort	Corticosteroid + β_2-agonist, LA	MDI; 2 inhalations (80 to 160/4.5 µg, respectively) twice/day
ciclesonide	Alvesco	Corticosteroid	MDI; 1 puff (80 µg each) twice/day
flunisolide	AeroSpan	Corticosteroid	MDI; 2 puffs (80 µg each) twice/day
fluticasone	Flovent	Corticosteroid	MDI; 2 puffs (44, 110, 220 µg each) twice/day DPI; 2 inhalations (50, 100, 250 µg each) twice daily
fluticasone + salmeterol	Advair	Corticosteroid + β_2-agonist, LA	DPI; 1 inhalation (100, 250, or 500/50 µg, respectively) twice/day
mometasone	Asmanex	Corticosteroid	DPI; 1 inhalation (220 µg each) once or twice/day
mometasone + formoterol	Dulera	Corticosteroid + β_2-agonist, LA	MDI; 2 puffs (100 or 200/5 µg each) twice daily
montelukast	Singulair	Anti-LT	Oral tablets; 10 mg once/day
theophylline	Theo-Dur	Methylxanthine	Oral extended release; 300 mg twice/day
zafirlukast	Accolate	Anti-LT	Oral tablets; 20 mg twice/day
zileuton	Zyflo, Zyflo CR	Anti-LT	Oral tablets; 600 mg 4 times/day or 1200 mg extended release 2 times/day
LA = long-acting; LT = leukotriene; MDI = metered dose inhaler; DPI = dry powder inhaler.			

except the long-acting β_2-agonists function principally by inhibiting the inflammatory process.

Inhaled Corticosteroids

Corticosteroids by inhalation are the mainstay of long-term therapy. They do not significantly affect acute bronchoconstriction, but when used on a daily regimen they are very effective at reducing inflammation. This subsequently reduces the frequency and severity of acute attacks, improves control of nocturnal asthma, and provides protection from symptoms of EIB. Pharmacologically, corticosteroids are anti-inflammatory drugs with multiple mechanisms of action. Corticosteroids inhibit infiltration of leukocytes, inhibit the synthesis of cytokines, increase the response of the β-receptor to β-agonist stimulation, and decrease LT production by inhibiting phospholipase (see Figure 9-1).

Table 9-6 includes several corticosteroids used by inhalation for long-term asthma therapy. These drugs have approximately equal effectiveness at equipotent doses, although the duration of action differs so that some corticosteroids (eg, budesonide and fluticasone) require fewer doses per day. One reason for poor adherence to therapy is the cumbersome nature of taking many doses per day of the corticosteroid. A product that requires fewer doses per day is therefore generally considered an advantage. According to NAEPP, an inhaled corticosteroid is the preferred therapy for patients of all ages with persistent asthma. The dosage of corticosteroid can be increased with increased asthma severity. However, adding a long-acting β_2-agonist to low-dose inhaled corticosteroid is more effective in decreasing the frequency of exacerbations than doubling the corticosteroid dose. Unlike quick-relief medications, which are used as needed, corticosteroids and other long-term medications must be taken on a regular daily schedule and may require up to 3 months of daily therapy before the maximum benefit with continued therapy is achieved.

The potential adverse effects with inhaled corticosteroids can be categorized as local and systemic effects.

Although inhalation delivers sufficient drug to the lung for the therapeutic effect, most of the inhaled dose ends up in the oral cavity. The amount of corticosteroid that is deposited in the mouth and throat plays a major role in causing the local effects. These are primarily hoarseness, cough, and oral fungal (candidiasis) infection (thrush). The cough is likely due to additives in the MDI and may be reduced by using a DPI. The hoarseness and fungal infections are indicative of the amount of drug deposited in the mouth and throat. These effects can be minimized by using a spacer and by rinsing the mouth out with water after each use.

The systemic effects of inhaled corticosteroids are caused by the portion of the dose that is swallowed and the amount of drug that is absorbed into the blood from the lung. The systemic effects are minimized at lower dosages of inhaled corticosteroid use. The systemic effects of prime concern include growth suppression in children, decreased bone mineralization, and increased risk for cataracts. Although low to medium doses of inhaled corticosteroids may cause a small change in initial growth rate, the final adult height is generally unaffected. The benefit from inhaled corticosteroid use is generally greater than the potential effect on linear growth. When low-dose inhaled corticosteroid therapy is not effective, other long-term therapy (eg, long-acting β-agonist, LT modifier) is preferred in conjunction with inhaled corticosteroids rather than increasing the inhaled corticosteroid dose. The exception is in children aged 0 to 4 years, in which medium-dose inhaled corticosteroid is preferred first.

Regarding bone mineralization, low to medium doses of inhaled corticosteroids have no significant effect. Some reduction in bone mineralization correlating with dose of inhaled corticosteroid may occur in women, although the correlation with increased risk of bone fractures has not been established. Supplements of calcium and vitamin D should be considered in adults, especially for menopausal women. High cumulative lifetime doses of corticosteroids to treat asthma may increase the incidence of cataracts. The potential long-term significance of the systemic effects of inhaled corticosteroid use must be evaluated in comparison with the long-term benefit of acceptable control of chronic asthma for each patient.

Long-Acting β-Agonists

As with the short-acting β$_2$-agonists, the long-acting β$_2$-agonists (see Table 9-6) are effective by inhalation, cause bronchodilation, and lack significant anti-inflammatory activity. However, their onset of action is slower than short-acting agonists, and thus they cannot be used for rescue therapy. Another means of obtaining a longer-acting β-agonist effect is to use extended-release oral tablets of short-acting β-agonists. The oral products are more convenient for the patient than inhalants but have the disadvantage of having more significant systemic adverse effects, including tachycardia and muscle tremors. Although more cumbersome to administer, inhaled long-acting β$_2$-agonists provide more direct contact with the target tissue and fewer adverse effects than oral β-agonists and therefore are used much more frequently.

Long-acting β$_2$-agonists by inhalation can be administered as often as every 12 hours. They can be added to therapy as an alternative to increasing corticosteroid dosage but should not be used alone as the only long-term control asthma medication. Because it may be too cumbersome and inconvenient for some patients to add a third inhaler to the corticosteroid and quick-relief medications, fixed-dose combinations are available that contain varied doses of a corticosteroid and a fixed dose of a long-acting β$_2$-agonist; this provides the convenience of one inhaler to simultaneously administer both drugs. The addition of a long-acting β$_2$-agonist to inhaled corticosteroid therapy decreases the incidence of acute asthma exacerbations better than either drug alone and is more effective than merely doubling the dose of the inhaled corticosteroid.

Long-acting β$_2$-agonists are effective in reducing the use of short-acting β$_2$-agonists and decreasing nocturnal asthma. Long-acting β$_2$-agonists may improve protection from EIB but are not preferred as frequent use for this purpose because this may disguise poorly controlled persistent asthma (see also adverse effects). The long-acting β$_2$-agonist should not be used more frequently than twice per 24 hours; therefore, if the drug is being used twice per day as long-term therapy, it should not be used as an additional dose prior to exercise.

The most significant adverse effect with the long-acting β$_2$-agonists is the rare occurrence of a fatal acute asthma episode. This is a paradoxical effect of unknown cause. Consequently, the benefit of improved control must be weighed against the potential for increased risk of severe exacerbation before a long-acting β$_2$-agonist is added to therapy. The increased risk for asthma-related death is also the reason why long-acting β$_2$-agonists should not be used alone as the only long-term control medication in a patient.

Mast Cell–Stabilizing Drugs

Mast cell–stabilizing drugs are inhibitors of the inflammatory process but are less effective than corticosteroids. Cromolyn and nedocromil are the 2 mast cell–stabilizing drugs currently available. These drugs are equally effective but only by inhalation. They are not effective as rescue therapy to treat acute attacks because they take 1 to 2 weeks to show noticeable improvement of chronic asthma, take about 4 weeks to achieve maximal effect, and do not produce bronchodilation. These drugs have a low incidence of long-term adverse effects and are virtually nontoxic. They are not preferred therapy but may provide an alternative to inhaled corticosteroids in children with mild persistent asthma or may be added to corticosteroid therapy to improve control of mild persistent asthma (Step

2; see Table 9-2). Mast cell–stabilizing drugs are effective to treat allergen-induced hyperresponsiveness and nocturnal asthma. They can also be used about 15 minutes prior to exercise to prevent EIB either alone or in combination with β_2-agonists when the use of a β_2-agonist alone is insufficient to prevent EIB.

As with the corticosteroids, there may be multiple mechanisms of action for mast cell–stabilizing drugs, but a likely contributor to the mechanism is the ability of these drugs to inhibit the release of inflammatory mediators from bronchial mast cells. A stabilizing effect on the cell membrane prevents the release from the cell of inflammatory chemical mediators such as LTs, PGs, and cytokines.

Cromolyn and nedocromil are generally used 2 to 4 times per day. Adverse effects include minor throat irritation, which can be minimized by drinking water immediately after use, and a bad taste and headache associated with the use of nedocromil for some patients. The bad taste may require discontinuation of the drug in some patients.

Leukotriene Modifiers

The LTs are a group of chemical mediators principally produced during inflammation through the 5-lipoxygenase pathway from arachidonic acid (see Figure 9-1). LTC_4, LTD_4, LTE_4 are collectively referred to as the *cysteinyl LTs* (cys-LTs) because cysteine is part of the chemical structure. The cys-LTs are synthesized from LTA_4 and are agonists for the cys-LT receptor, activation of which initiates bronchoconstriction. Another LT, LTB_4, which is also synthesized from LTA_4, contributes to the inflammatory response as a chemotactic mediator but is not a cys-LT and thus does not combine with the cys-LT receptor.

The LT modifiers (also called *anti-LTs*) are subdivided according to which of 2 mechanisms define their activity. LT-receptor antagonists combine directly with the cys-LT receptor to inhibit the effect of the cys-LTs; montelukast (Singulair) and zafirlukast (Accolate) are LT-receptor antagonists. LT-synthesis inhibitors are competitive inhibitors of 5-lipoxygenase and thus decrease the production of all the LTs; zileuton (Zyflo) is a LT-synthesis inhibitor.

The LT modifiers are used orally, not by inhalation, and are for long-term therapy, not for quick relief. As evident from their mechanism, LT modifiers are anti-inflammatory drugs, not bronchodilators. They improve lung function, decrease the frequency of need for rescue medication, and may decrease the incidence of asthma exacerbations. Although LT modifiers are less effective than low-dose inhaled corticosteroids, they provide an oral alternative in patients unable to use inhalation therapy, such as young children. They are used in combination with corticosteroids to allow for a reduction in corticosteroid dose. The LT modifiers may reduce bronchoconstriction after exercise, but they should not be used as the only therapy for EIB; pretreatment with a short-acting β_2-agonist should be maintained. The NAEPP includes anti-LTs as an alternative

to therapy for persistent asthma as part of Step 2, 3, and 4 therapies in youths aged 12 years or older and adults, and as a part of either preferred or alternate therapy for Steps 2 to 6 (see Table 9-1) for ages 0 to 11 years old.

A peculiarity with the use of LT modifiers is that some patients are responders and some are not. The reason for this difference among patients is unclear, but the extent to which the LTs contribute to the asthma symptoms may differ from patient to patient. For those patients in whom these arachidonic acid metabolites contribute significantly to the asthma response, LT-modifying drugs will have a larger impact. The contribution of the pathway may be a result of the extent to which the genes are expressed for the enzymes in the lipoxygenase pathway. In general, it appears that patients who experience aspirin-induced asthma also respond well to LT modifier therapy.

The LT modifiers have relatively few adverse effects, although headache is one of the more common complaints. The most significant concern is the potential for liver damage with zileuton and zafirlukast. An elevated blood level of liver enzymes, particularly alanine aminotransferase (ALT), is indicative of liver damage. Consequently, treatment with zileuton requires monitoring of liver function by measuring blood ALT levels each month for the first 3 months and then routinely but less frequently thereafter. Patients on zileuton or zafirlukast should be aware that the symptoms of liver toxicity include jaundice, fatigue, right upper-quadrant abdominal pain, nausea, lethargy, pruritus, and flu-like symptoms. The patient should discontinue the drug and contact the physician if these symptoms occur. Neuropsychiatric adverse effects, including mood changes, depression, suicidal thoughts, and hallucinations, have been reported with all 3 LT modifiers.

> *Recall that ALT is a liver enzyme that is released into the blood when liver cells are damaged. Therefore, an increase in the blood ALT level implies liver damage.*

The incidence of Churg-Strauss syndrome is rare but has been noted with the use of LT-receptor antagonist in adults. This syndrome involves vasculitis that primarily affects the respiratory tract during its early stages and can progress to become life threatening. Most reported cases involved patients who had been receiving systemic corticosteroid therapy that was reduced after LT-receptor antagonist therapy was added. This association with the reduced corticosteroid therapy suggests that the syndrome may have existed prior to anti-LT therapy but was being masked by the anti-inflammatory effect of corticosteroids.

Zileuton (Zyflo) inhibits 5-lipoxygenase and thus reduces the production of all of the LTs. It is approved for use as long-term therapy in adults and children older than 12 years. Zileuton is rapidly absorbed after oral administration regardless of the presence of food. Because of its relatively short half-life (2 to 3 hours), the usual zileuton dosage is 4 times per day or twice per day for controlled-release tablets. As mentioned previously, ALT levels must be monitored throughout treatment but particularly during the first 3 months of therapy. Zileuton is metabolized by cytochrome P450 isozymes and inhibits the metabolism of other drugs, notably theophylline and warfarin, which are also metabolized by the same isozymes. The relatively short duration of action, the necessity to monitor for liver toxicity, and the potential for drug interaction are significant disadvantages of zileuton.

Recall from Chapters 2 and 3 that drug metabolism by cytochrome P450 (CYP450) isozymes are quite common and that drug interactions involving these isozymes occur when one drug inhibits the metabolism of other drugs. In this case, zileuton, warfarin, and theophylline are metabolized by the same CYP450 isozyme. Zileuton inhibits the metabolism of theophylline and warfarin and therefore will increase the effect of the theophylline and warfarin, which may necessitate a reduction in the dosage of these 2 drugs.

Zafirlukast (Accolate) is effective as a long-term antiasthma medication for adults and children. It is absorbed from the GI tract, but the absorption is reduced significantly by the presence of food. To optimize absorption, zafirlukast should be taken 1 hour before or 2 hours after a meal. Zafirlukast can also increase the effect of warfarin and may necessitate a reduction in warfarin dosage. Liver toxicity is a potential adverse effect. The half-life is longer than zileuton and requires only twice-daily dosing.

Montelukast (Singulair) is an effective LT-receptor antagonist. The absorption from the GI tract is not affected by food. It is available as a chewable tablet and is approved for use in children with asthma. Montelukast has several differences compared with zileuton and zafirlukast: it does not have significant potential for drug interactions with theophylline and warfarin, liver toxicity has not been reported, and the dosing schedule is once per day.

Methylxanthines

The only methylxanthine used therapeutically to treat asthma is theophylline. Other methylxanthines of some notoriety are caffeine and, to a lesser extent, theobromine (a component of chocolate), which are best known for their central nervous system stimulant effects. Of the methylxanthines, theophylline has the most significant bronchodilator activity. There are likely multiple mechanisms that contribute to this activity, 2 of which are the inhibition of adenosine receptors and the inhibition of phosphodiesterases.

Adenosine is a compound that indirectly causes bronchoconstriction, possibly by enhancing the effect of inflammatory chemical mediators. Phosphodiesterases are enzymes that terminate the activity of the cyclic AMP (adenosine monophosphate) and cyclic GMP (guanosine monophosphate); therefore, inhibition of phosphodiesterases enhances the activity of the cyclic AMP and GMP. Cyclic AMP and cyclic GMP are second-messenger molecules inside the cell that initiate many regulatory processes of the cell, including contraction and relaxation of smooth muscle.

Theophylline used to be a primary therapy for treatment of chronic asthma. However, it has significant drawbacks that have caused it to be used much less frequently than other more effective asthma medications that have become available (eg, corticosteroids, LT modifiers, mast cell–stabilizing agents, and β_2-agonists). One disadvantage of theophylline is the significant toxicity that necessitates blood-level monitoring to maintain the blood concentration of theophylline within a relatively narrow therapeutic window (see Chapter 3). Another disadvantage is the moderate degree of therapeutic effectiveness compared with newer drugs. Theophylline decreases the incidence of acute attacks, including nocturnal asthma; prevents EIB; and is an alternative to corticosteroid therapy for children. Nonetheless, one or more of the newer drugs provides these same benefits with less concern for toxicity.

Theophylline is used orally and is available in immediate- and sustained-release formulations, but considerable interpatient variability in absorption exists among patients taking the sustained release formulations. Dosage is calculated on a milligram per kilogram per day basis. Initial adverse effects include nausea, vomiting, nervousness, and insomnia, but these effects usually dissipate with continued use. Theophylline has a low therapeutic index; blood concentrations modestly above the normal therapeutic range have resulted in seizures, arrhythmias, and death. At the other end of the therapeutic window, levels below the normal range result in significantly reduced effectiveness, hence the need to adjust dosage based on routine monitoring of blood levels. Adding to the problem are the changes in the pharmacokinetics due to factors such as cigarette smoking, changes in kidney function from disease or age, and drug interactions.

Immunomodulators

Omalizumab (Xolair) is the only drug in this category that has demonstrated effectiveness when added to high-dose corticosteroid therapy plus long-acting β_2-agonist therapy to treat severe persistent asthma. NAEPP recommends it to be considered for youths aged 12 years or older and adults in Step 5 and 6 (see Table 9-2) if other preferred therapy is insufficiently effective.

Omalizumab attaches to IgE to decrease the ability of IgE to bind to mast cells and basophils, thus decreasing the release of chemical mediators from these cell types following exposure to allergens such as dust mites, pollen, and animal dander. Studies have documented an improvement in lung function and reduction in asthma exacerbations with the addition of omalizumab to inhaled corticosteroid therapy.

Administration of omalizumab is by subcutaneous injection once every 2 or 4 weeks. Of significant concern is that 0.1% to 0.2% of patients treated with omalizumab have experienced anaphylactic reaction, most within 2 hours but some later following injection. Consequently, clinicians who administer the drug must be prepared to monitor the patient for anaphylaxis and be equipped with appropriate treatment. Patients should be informed regarding the risk of anaphylaxis as well as the symptoms and treatment if it occurs.

Section Summary

Drug therapy for chronic asthma can be grouped broadly as drugs for quick relief and drugs for long-term therapy. Quick-relief drugs are used to treat existing acute attacks or to prevent exercise-induced attacks. Long-term therapy is used to decrease symptoms of chronic asthma, including the incidence of acute exacerbations of the disease. With the exception of corticosteroids, drugs that are used for long-term therapy are not used for quick relief and vice versa. Even in the case of corticosteroids, inhalation therapy is the mainstay of long-term therapy, whereas a short course of systemic therapy is the primary mode of administration to treat acute exacerbations.

For quick relief, inhaled short-acting β_2-agonists, such as albuterol (Proventil), are the most frequently used. These drugs have few adverse effects when used by inhalation and have an almost immediate onset of action. Systemic corticosteroids can be used for a few days to reduce the duration and severity of an acute exacerbation but do not provide the immediate bronchodilation effect obtained from short-acting β_2-agonists. When used several minutes before exercise, short-acting β_2-agonists are also effective in preventing EIB. Although administration of short-acting β_2-agonists by inhalation can be repeated during exercise, the routine use of these additional doses during exercise is indicative of poor control of chronic asthma and warrants a re-evaluation of long-term therapy.

Long-term therapy is effective when used on a regular, daily basis and is not effective in treating an acute attack. The intent of long-term therapy is to diminish the impairment of asthma and decrease the risk of exacerbations. This encompasses a reduction of the incidence of acute attacks not only during the day but also symptoms associated with nocturnal asthma and EIB. Improved control of chronic asthma is reflected in part by the reduced frequency with which quick-relief medication is needed during the day, at nighttime, and during exercise after the initial pre-exercise dose. Besides the inhaled corticosteroids, other long-term medications include the inhaled mast cell–stabilizing drugs, inhaled long-acting β_2-agonists, immunomodulators, and oral LT modifiers. Theophylline is also available orally but is used less frequently than the other agents because of the greater potential for significant adverse effects. Every patient with persistent asthma (mild to severe) should be using a long-term asthma-control medication. Corticosteroids are the drugs of choice for all ages, although a LT modifier or mast cell–stabilizing drug is the alternative used for mild persistent asthma. As the severity of asthma increases, either the dose of corticosteroid is increased and/or another long-acting drug is added to therapy. LTs, mast cell–stabilizing drugs, and, although discouraged for frequent use, long-acting β_2-agonists also help prevent the symptoms associated with EIB.

ROLE OF THE ATHLETIC TRAINER

Because asthma is a chronic disease, drug therapy is long term, and so is the need to monitor the effectiveness of drug therapy. Most asthmatics have EIB, which may hamper athletic performance if it is not adequately controlled. Because the most frequent causes of inadequate therapeutic outcomes are poor adherence with prescribed therapy and/or improper use of inhalers, spacers, or PFMs, the athletic trainer can play a key role in ensuring that drug therapy is optimized. The NAEPP Expert Panel Report 3 recommends that education regarding asthma be integrated into all points of care where health professionals interact with patients. In that regard, the 2 principal areas for involvement by the athletic trainer are patient education and monitoring of asthma drug use and effectiveness. Some noteworthy points are as follows:

- If the patient does not know which medication is for long-term use and which is for quick relief, it raises doubt as to whether the patient is using the medications properly. Because the quick-relief β_2-agonists and the long-term corticosteroid therapy are both used by inhalation, the patient could be confused concerning their relative use. However, as the functions of these 2 drugs and the dosing schedule for each are vastly different, a clear understanding of the proper use of the drugs is imperative to achieve suitable results. For example, the patient should understand that the long-term medication provides no protective benefit if used immediately prior to exercise. Similarly, use of the long-term medication, such as inhaled corticosteroid, is much less effective if used sporadically. It is important to use the corticosteroid daily, even when there are no asthma symptoms. Doses are not to be skipped just because the patient feels better. Based on data from other patient populations, it is reasonable to expect that if athletes understand the proper use and purpose of the asthma medications, they will have improved adherence and enhanced effectiveness from the asthma therapy.

- Besides understanding the purpose of each drug, proper inhalation technique affects the effectiveness of these drugs. Even with good technique, only about 20% of inhaled drug reaches the lung. Besides having good overall inhalation technique as described earlier in this chapter (see Box 9-3), patients must exhibit other aspects of proper inhalation:

  - The patient should have good coordination of inhaler actuation with inhalation. If not, either additional instruction and/or a valved holding chamber may be useful.

  - If the patient bends over to discretely take a puff of quick-relief medication, the amount of drug delivered to the lungs will be reduced. This may be the reason for additional puffs being required during exercise.

  - To decrease the incidence of fungal infection, the patient can decrease the deposit of corticosteroid in the mouth and throat through the use of a spacer and by rinsing the mouth out with water after inhalation of each corticosteroid dose.

  - If a portion of the drug or propellant mist does not enter the mouth, the patient is likely not placing the inhaler properly in the mouth; possibly the teeth are partially blocking the flow of drug.

- If the patient uses more than one 200-puff canister of quick-relief medication per month, asthma control is generally considered to be poor, and reevaluation of long-term therapy is likely necessary. Other criteria have been recommended by the NAEPP to classify the severity of asthma (see Table 9-1) and to use as a guide to the stepwise approach for managing asthma (see Table 9-2). Treatment should be aggressive enough to gain control of the symptoms, and then the patient can be monitored and drug therapy gradually reduced to the least medication necessary to maintain control of the symptoms.

- The use of a quick-relief medication 5 to 15 minutes before exercise is an effective means to control EIB. If symptoms develop during exercise, additional puffs can be used. However, regular additional doses of quick-relief medication during exercise may be because the chronic asthma is inadequately controlled. A reassessment of long-term control therapy

is recommended. The goal is to achieve a level of asthma management so that the disease has no impact on the patient's performance. To that end, it may be necessary to increase the inhaled corticosteroid dosage or add a long-acting β_2-agonist, a LT modifier, or mast cell stabilizer. The athletic trainer must be aware of the action plan and should notify the physician who will modify the treatment.

- If a patient has AIA, the athletic trainer should be alert to the fact that there are many over-the-counter (OTC) medications that contain NSAIDs. Consequently, symptoms from AIA may occur if the patient is self-medicating or if NSAID-containing medications are used in the athletic training room. There are many brand name and generic NSAID products. The athlete should always check the active ingredients on the OTC drug label to determine if the active ingredient is an NSAID. Additionally, some cold and sinus remedies also contain NSAIDs (eg, Dristan Sinus, BC Sinus-Cold, and Advil Cold & Sinus). Although not considered a NSAID, acetaminophen does cause some degree of cross-reaction in asthmatics with AIA. About one-third of asthmatics with AIA experience some degree of bronchoconstriction when treated with 1000 to 1500 mg of acetaminophen, although the symptoms are generally milder than with aspirin. Also, doses of less than 650 mg of acetaminophen result in only a small risk of bronchospasm. The ingredients of OTC products should be checked carefully for the amount of acetaminophen or content of any amount of NSAIDs.

- The patient should avoid the factors that initiate symptoms. The precipitating factors vary among asthmatics, but potential factors include allergens from pets, house-dust mites, fungal spores, viral infection, tobacco smoke, pollens, volatile chemicals, and comorbid conditions such as chronic sinusitis and gastroesophageal reflux. Avoiding causative agents may improve the level of control of chronic asthma and reduce acute exacerbations. For example, depending on the causative agent, the patient could exercise in an indoor, air-conditioned facility rather than outdoors during peak pollen season, require family members that smoke to do so outdoors, avoid contact with cats or dogs, or obtain appropriate treatment for contributing physiological conditions.

- Use of a PFM can be helpful for patients who have moderate or severe persistent asthma. Use of a PFM provides a means of determining current status of airflow, anticipating the need for change in quick-relief medication, evaluating the improvement of airflow as a result of therapy, and making a decision as to course of action if airflow is reduced. To obtain the most effective use of a PFM, it is necessary to use it routinely, first to establish the patient's personal best and then to monitor airflow as a percentage relative to the personal best. Results from a PFM provide a quantitative value as to the extent of airflow obstruction. A plan should be established with the physician, especially for patients with moderate to severe asthma or a history of severe exacerbations. The patient and athletic trainer should know what adjustments must be made if airflow drops below predetermined levels.

- Knowing when, where, and how to exercise can help reduce symptoms of asthma:

  o Patients who are hyperresponsive to pollen should avoid outdoor exercise during midday when pollen counts are usually higher. Alternatively, it may be more advantageous to switch exercise routines to an air-conditioned indoor environment during peak pollen season.

  o Exercise in cooler, drier air increases the likelihood of EIB, even following pretreatment with drugs; exercise in warmer, moist air decreases the likelihood of EIB symptoms.

  o Submaximal warm-up activity for 15 to 30 minutes may delay symptoms of EIB.

There are several actions that athletic trainers can take to assist the patient in maximizing the effectiveness of asthma drug therapy and minimizing the effect of asthma on athletic performance. These actions focus on monitoring the effectiveness of therapy and providing education to the patient regarding the use and effects of asthma drugs and devices.

Case Study

This is your first year as an athletic trainer at a 4A high school. Although you have worked at smaller schools, this is your first job at a larger-division school. You want to be sure you are prepared for the coming year, so you go over the medical records of the school's athletes. Out of the 250 athletes, you realize that you have 20 athletes with chronic asthma and 3 athletes with EIB. You realize that the best way to manage these student-athletes and assure good monitoring of their asthma is to develop a plan of care for asthma. You also want to create a record of each

person's PFM results for PEF and his or her daily results so you can anticipate problems before they arise. For best-care practice, you will need to know each person's rescue drug used when he or she needs quick relief for an acute attack and where it is kept. You know that the most commonly used rescue drug includes short-acting β_2-agonists, but you are not as familiar with the long-term drugs that control inflammation. You realize that because you can only recall that these long-term drugs are taken either orally or using an inhaler, you need to refresh yourself on the various medications before practices start in 2 weeks. What classes of medications are used for chronic control of asthma? What adverse effects could be expected with each class?

Bibliography

Curtiss FR. More evolution of the evidence in asthma disease management—SMART versus GOAL clinical trials debate the cost-benefit of LABA while the value of leukotriene modifiers, particularly montelukast, is uncertain. *J Manag Care Pharm*. 2006;12(4):343-346.

Fanta CH. Asthma. *N Engl J Med*. 2009;360:1002-1014.

Heaten PC, Guo JJ, Hornung RW, et al. Analysis of the effectiveness and cost benefit of leukotriene modifiers in adults with asthma in the Ohio Medicaid population. *J Manag Care Pharm*. 2006;12(1):33-42.

Helenius I, Lumme A, Haahtela T. Asthma, airway inflammation and treatment in elite athletes. *Sports Med*. 2005;35(7):565-574.

Houglum JE. Asthma medications: basic pharmacology and use in the athlete. *J Athl Train*. 2000;35:179-185.

Houglum JE. Asthma medications: basic pharmacology and use in the athlete. *Athl Ther Today*. 2001;6:16-21.

Lee JH, Cassard SD, Dans PE, Wheelock C, Ober JD. Evaluating asthma medication use before and after an acute asthma-related event. *J Manag Care Pharm*. 2001;7:303-308.

Miller MG, Weiler JM, Baker R, Collins J, D'Alonzo G. National Athletic Trainers' Association position statement: management of asthma in athletes. *J Athl Train*. 2005;40(3):224-245.

National Institutes of Health, National Heart, Lung, and Blood Institute. National Asthma Education and Prevention Program (NAEPP). Full Report of the Expert Panel: Guidelines for the diagnosis and management of asthma (EPR-3) 2007. http://www.nhlbi.nih.gov/files/docs/guidelines/asthgdln.pdf. Accessed July 21, 2015.

National Institutes of Health, National Heart, Lung, and Blood Institute. National Asthma Education and Prevention Program (NAEPP). Summary Report 2007 of the Expert Panel Report 3: Guidelines for the diagnosis and management of asthma. http://www.nhlbi.nih.gov/guidelines/asthma/asthsumm.pdf. Accessed July 21, 2015.

Oppenheimer J, Nelson HS. Safety of long-acting beta-agonists in asthma: a review. *Curr Opin Pulm Med*. 2008;14(1):64-69.

Rottier BL, Rubin BK. Asthma medication delivery: mists and myths. *Paediatr Respir Rev*. 2013;14(2):112-118.

CHAPTER 10: ADVANCE ORGANIZER

Foundational Concepts

The Common Cold

- Allergic Rhinitis
- Heat-Related Illnesses
- Section Summary

Nondrug Approaches

Drug Therapy

- Antihistamines
  - First- and Second-Generation Antihistamines
  - Uses for Allergies and Colds
  - Adverse Effects and Drug Interactions
  - Other Uses for Antihistamines
- Anticholinergics
- Nasal Decongestants
  - Uses for Allergy and Colds
  - Adverse Effects and Drug Interactions
- Corticosteroids
- Mast Cell–Stabilizing Drugs
- Leukotriene Modifiers
- Expectorants
- Antitussive Agents
- Analgesics
- Ophthalmic Products
- Antibiotics
- Allergen Immunotherapy
- Section Summary

Role of the Athletic Trainer

10

Drugs for Treating Colds and Allergies

CHAPTER OBJECTIVES

At the end of this chapter, the reader will be able to:

- Describe the pathophysiology for the common cold and allergic rhinitis

- Differentiate between the signs and symptoms of the common cold and allergic rhinitis

- Explain how over-the-counter (OTC) products used to treat the common cold and allergies can contribute to a heat-related illness

- List several steps that can be taken to reduce the incidence of common colds and allergic rhinitis from occurring and/or spreading

- Identify OTC medications for colds and allergic rhinitis that are combination products, and choose the appropriate medication based on the patient's signs and symptoms

- Explain the therapeutic use of antihistamines

- Recall the adverse effects and common drug interactions for antihistamines and nasal decongestants

- Differentiate between first- and second-generation antihistamines

- Explain the mechanism of action for antihistamines and nasal decongestants

- Explain the use of corticosteroids, mast cell–stabilizing drugs, and leukotriene (LT) modifiers in the treatment of allergic rhinitis

- Differentiate between an expectorant and antitussive

- Recall the adverse effects for expectorants and antitussives

- Explain the role of analgesics in the treatment of cold symptoms

- Explain why antibiotics are not the medication of choice for treating the common cold and allergic rhinitis

- Summarize the role of the athletic trainer for patients who are taking medications for colds or allergic rhinitis

The common cold is one of the most frequent acute illnesses. Allergic rhinitis, affecting approximately 20% of the adult population, is one of the most frequent chronic illnesses in the country. These conditions have some similarities in pathology and symptoms as well as aspects of drug therapy, but they also have some important differences that will be discussed in this chapter. Consumers spend billions of dollars annually on OTC medications to treat colds and allergies. These diseases cost additional billions for prescription medications, hospital expenses, and lost

Houglum JE, Harrelson GL, Seefeldt TM.
Principles of Pharmacology for Athletic Trainers, Third Edition (pp 169-185).
© 2016 Taylor & Francis Group.

ABBREVIATIONS USED IN THIS CHAPTER

CNS. central nervous system	**MAOI.** monoamine oxidase inhibitor
COX. cyclooxygenase	**NSAID.** nonsteroidal anti-inflammatory drug
FDA. Food and Drug Administration	**OTC.** over-the-counter
GI. gastrointestinal	**PG.** prostaglandin
IgE. immunoglobulin E	**Rx.** prescription
LT. leukotriene	**t½.** half-life

work productivity. The frequent use of OTC medications to treat colds and allergies creates enhanced potential for adverse effects, drug interactions, and use of medications that may affect athletic performance. On the other hand, effective use of drug therapy, coupled with nondrug measures, can minimize the effect of colds and allergies on the patient's athletic participation.

FOUNDATIONAL CONCEPTS

This section discusses the pathophysiology, causes, and symptoms of allergic rhinitis and the common cold. Several of these characteristics are similar for these 2 illnesses, but many are different. A comparison of the characteristics for the common cold and allergic rhinitis is shown in Table 10-1.

THE COMMON COLD

The common cold is caused by any one of more than 200 viruses. Two of the most common offenders are rhinoviruses and coronaviruses. The virus is passed from an infected person to a second person through airborne nasal discharge or, more commonly, from direct contact with the infected person's hand or an object recently handled (or sneezed on) by that person. Once the virus is on the second person's hand, it can be readily transferred to the upper respiratory tract by direct contact with the nasal passage or eyes. Some viruses can remain viable for a few hours on inanimate objects or on the hands. The virus attaches to the human cell and eventually uses the biochemical process of the human cell to make more copies of itself. The mechanisms by which viruses infect human cells and propagate are much different from the mechanisms of bacteria and fungi; thus antibacterial and antifungal drugs have no effect for the treatment of the common cold. Consequently, antibiotics (see Chapter 5) should not be used to treat these viral infections.

There are many categories of viruses and many specific viruses within the categories. Rhinoviruses are one example of a virus category for which more than 100 specific viruses have been identified. Rhinoviruses are the most frequent cause of the common cold. There are several other categories of viruses that can cause the symptoms of the common cold (eg, coronaviruses*).*

The viral infection of a common cold causes the release of various inflammatory mediators (eg, prostaglandins, LTs, kinins) that result in increased mucous secretions and increased permeability and dilation of the blood vessels in the nasal passage, all of which contribute to nasal stuffiness. Cholinergic stimulation through acetylcholine release is also a significant contributor. Histamine plays a minor role in these events. Symptoms begin 24 to 72 hours after exposure to the virus and vary in severity depending on the specific virus. Symptoms typically begin with sore throat, followed by rhinorrhea, nasal congestion, headache, body aches, occasional sneezing, and finally a cough that may persist longer than other symptoms. The common cold is usually self-limiting, lasting 7 to 10 days. Drug therapy can alleviate some of the discomfort associated with the infection but there is no cure for the common cold, hence the adage, "If you don't treat a cold it will last 7 to 10 days, but if you treat a cold it will last only 7 to 10 days."

When the neurotransmitter released by the parasympathetic fiber is acetylcholine, the response is referred to as a cholinergic response. *The acetylcholine combines with the cholinergic receptor located on the surface of the cell to cause the response—in this case, increased mucus production.*

Complications sometimes develop as a result of a cold, and these complications may extend the ramifications of the cold beyond 10 days. Two of the more common complications are ear infections, especially in children, and sinus infections. These occur as a result of inefficient drainage in the ear or sinuses, respectively. When these infections are bacterial in origin, they can be treated with antibiotics. Sometimes symptoms of other illnesses are mistaken for the common cold. For example, development of fever or nasal congestion and sneezing that lasts beyond 10 to 14 days may be indicative of allergic rhinitis or the development of a bacterial upper respiratory infection. A severe or persistent sore throat may imply a streptococcal infection. Another complication is exacerbation of asthma symptoms, a significant complication because breathing is already difficult. Treatment of asthma (see Chapter 9) may need to be more aggressive until the viral infection subsides.

	TABLE 10-1	
CHARACTERISTICS OF THE COMMON COLD AND ALLERGIC RHINITIS		
CHARACTERISTIC	**COMMON COLD**	**ALLERGIC RHINITIS**
Cause	Virus	Hypersensitivity to allergens
Communicable	Yes	No
Coughing	Yes	No
Curative drug therapy	No	No
Duration	7 to 10 days	Seasonal or perennial
Histamine involvement	Minor	Major
LT, PG involvement	Yes	Yes
Nasal congestion	Yes	Yes
Nasal itching	No	Yes
Ocular inflammation	Infrequent	Frequent
Onset of symptoms	Gradual	Rapid
Potential for complications	Yes	Yes
Prevention strategies	Hand washing, avoid crowds during cold season	Avoid allergens as much as possible
Rhinorrhea	Yes	Yes
Sneezing	Occasional, forceful	Frequent, light
Sore throat	Yes	No
Therapy focus	Antihistamines, decongestants, expectorants, analgesics, antitussives	Antihistamines, decongestants, corticosteroids, LT modifiers, ophthalmics
LT= leukotriene; PG = prostaglandin.		

Allergic Rhinitis

Allergic rhinitis is a hypersensitivity reaction in response to inhaled allergens. These allergens are also called *antigens* because they attach to IgE antibodies to initiate an allergic response. The extent of the hypersensitivity response will depend on the genetic predisposition of the patient and the extent of exposure to the allergen. There are 2 categories of allergic rhinitis: seasonal and perennial. Seasonal rhinitis (also called *hay fever*) is caused by inhalation of outdoor allergens, primarily pollen (eg, from weeds, trees, grasses) but also mold spores from decaying vegetation. Concentration of various pollens in the air changes with seasons and from one part of the country to another, but fluctuations also occur within each day. On the other hand, perennial rhinitis does not fluctuate with the seasons because it results primarily from contact with indoor allergens. House-dust mites, molds, pet dander, and cockroaches are common allergens. Consequently, symptoms of perennial rhinitis may exist sporadically or continuously depending on exposure to these allergens. The occurrence of seasonal allergic rhinitis is much more prevalent than perennial, affecting around 40 million people in the United States.

Recall from Chapter 9 that IgE is a type of immunoglobulin *(ie, antibody) that combines with specific foreign substances (ie, antigens) that enter the body. The IgE are located on mast cells in the airways and on circulating basophils. When the antigen combines with the IgE, it causes the release of inflammatory chemical mediators from the mast cells and basophils. People with allergies have a lot of IgE specific for commonly encountered antigens such as pollen.*

Because allergic rhinitis is an IgE-mediated response, an initial exposure to the allergen is necessary, causing the production of IgE antibodies against that allergen (Figure 10-1). The IgE antibodies attach to mast cells located in the mucosa of the nasal passage (Figure 10-2). Upon additional exposures to the allergen, the allergen binds to the IgE, which results in the release of inflammatory mediators such as histamine, prostaglandins, LTs, platelet-activating factor,

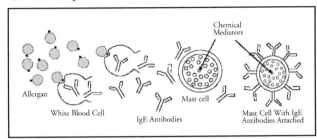

Figure 10-1. Sensitization to an allergen. (Adapted from Dishuck J, Harrelson GL. Management and treatment of allergic rhinitis and sinusitis. *Athletic Therapy Today.* 2001;6:6-10.)

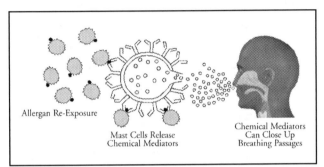

Figure 10-2. Allergic rhinitis IgE-mediated response to an allergen(s). (Adapted from Dishuck J, Harrelson GL. Management and treatment of allergic rhinitis and sinusitis. *Athletic Therapy Today.* 2001;6:6-10.)

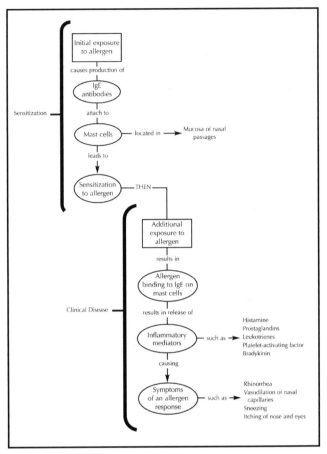

Figure 10-3. Manifestation of allergy symptoms.

and bradykinin (Figure 10-3). Histamine plays a major role in causing the symptoms of allergic rhinitis by combining with H_1 receptors. The initial symptoms (early-phase reaction) occur within minutes of exposure to the allergen and are largely due to the release of these mediators. Early-phase symptoms include rhinorrhea, vasodilation of nasal capillaries, sneezing, and itching of the nose and eyes. Nasal congestion results from the increased mucus production and vasodilation. Activation of the parasympathetic cholinergic response also contributes to the mucus production. The patient tends to sniff frequently; experience more frequent, but less severe, sneezes compared with a cold; and push the nose upward with the hand to alleviate the itching.

Initial symptoms subside within 1 to 2 hours, but a late-phase response can occur several hours after exposure to allergens and results from the accumulation of inflammatory cells (eg, basophils, eosinophils, mononuclear cells) at the nasal mucosa. The presence of these cells contributes to sneezing, rhinorrhea, nasal congestion, and enhanced responsiveness to additional allergens, possibly due to the increased number of IgE-containing cells available to react with various allergens.

Allergic rhinitis is a significant chronic disease, significant not only from the standpoint of frequency of occurrence in the population, but also regarding the impact on the patient. Persistent symptoms during allergy season can interfere with sleep, cause fatigue, affect social interaction, decrease performance at work, decrease ability to con-

centrate and learn in school, and limit ability to exercise. Overall quality of life can be notably diminished.

Heat-Related Illnesses

The topics in this chapter do not include the treatment of heat-related illness, but these conditions are worth mentioning because some drugs discussed in this chapter can contribute to the occurrence of heat-related illnesses (eg, heat cramps, heat exhaustion, and heatstroke). These conditions result from an excessive loss of fluid and electrolytes or, in the case of heatstroke, the inability to adequately cool the body core temperature. Heatstroke is the most dangerous of these conditions and is a medical emergency. Any drug that increases loss of fluid or electrolytes or diminishes the normal cooling mechanisms of the body will have the potential to contribute to heat-related illnesses. Chapter 12 discusses diuretics and β-adrenergic blockers, which are prescription drugs that can contribute to heat-related illness. The current chapter discusses commonly used OTC products used without medical supervision to treat the common cold and allergies. An adverse effect of some of these OTC drugs is that they can contribute to heat-related illness. Categories of drugs that can contribute to heat-related illness are as follows:

Box 10-1	
WAYS TO REDUCE THE INCIDENCE OF THE COMMON COLD AND ALLERGIC RHINITIS	
COLD	**ALLERGIC RHINITIS**
• Minimize the time spent in crowded locations • Cover the nose and mouth when coughing and sneezing • Wash hands frequently	• Use weather channels to determine pollen count • Limit outdoor activity during seasonal allergy seasons • Keep windows closed and use air conditioning • If possible, get rid of known allergen(s) • Dust and vacuum frequently • Use of a floor covering other than carpet can help reduce symptoms • Use air filters that are designed to remove particulate matter

- α-Adrenergic agonists (nasal decongestants) constrict peripheral blood vessels and thus decrease the heat dissipated through these vessels.

- Antihistamines and other drugs that have anticholinergic effects (see Box 8-1) can decrease sweating and thus decrease a major cooling mechanism.

- Diuretics increase urine production and thus increase fluid loss.

- β-blockers decrease blood supply to skin, thus diminishing a cooling mechanism.

Section Summary

The common cold is caused by viruses that could infect anyone, whereas allergic rhinitis is a hypersensitivity reaction that affects genetically susceptible individuals. Both illnesses cause an inflammatory response and an array of symptoms. For the common cold, these symptoms are usually self-limiting, whereas allergic rhinitis can be either seasonal or persist all year, with severity of symptoms ranging from mild to severe. Although a few of the symptoms of the common cold and allergic rhinitis are similar (eg, rhinorrhea and nasal congestion), there are many characteristics that differentiate these illnesses. Table 10-1 compared the characteristics of these illnesses. Quick onset of symptoms, an itchy nose, watery eyes, and persistent sneezing are hallmark characteristics of allergic rhinitis and are among the characteristics that differentiate it from the common cold. Some drugs discussed in this chapter can decrease the effectiveness of the body's cooling mechanisms and thus contribute to the occurrence of heat-related illnesses.

NONDRUG APPROACHES

Exposure to viruses is an everyday occurrence, but there are some steps that can be taken to reduce the incidence and possibly the morbidity once infection with the common cold occurs (Box 10-1). Because one major means of transmission is by inhalation of airborne viruses, staying away from the coughing and sneezing of cold sufferers seems obvious but is easier said than done. Crowded locations such as school or work cannot be totally avoided during the cold season, but minimizing time spent in crowded shopping malls or restaurants may be helpful. Covering coughs and sneezes is also obvious but not always practiced by cold sufferers. Because the transfer of the cold virus often occurs by contact with the hands and then transferred to the recipient's eyes and nose, frequent hand washing can reduce infection.

When the symptoms of a cold appear, maintaining moisture in the throat and nasal passage helps reduce cough, throat soreness, and congestion. Increasing fluid intake reduces the viscosity of mucus so it is easier to move the mucus out of the throat and nasal passage. Sucking on hard candy can keep the throat moist and reduces the discomfort of a sore throat. Keeping the air moist with a vaporizer or humidifier is also helpful to maintain mucus viscosity and decrease throat dryness. As a nondrug measure to facilitate easier breathing, nasal strips are available that are applied on the nose to physically enlarge the nasal passage. The strips are also available with menthol, which may contribute to congestion relief.

Just as it is impossible to avoid exposure to all common cold viruses, it is also impossible for a person with allergic rhinitis to avoid contact with all allergens. There are several ways to minimize exposure (see Box 10-1). Seasonal allergy sufferers can limit their outdoor activity and use indoor exercise routines as much as possible during peak allergy season. Yard work can be limited to the time of day with the lowest pollen count, using weather channels to determine the pollen count. Windows can be kept closed and air conditioning used to reduce pollen indoors.

For the person with perennial allergic rhinitis, an obvious preventative measure is to get rid of the known allergens. Often this is associated with a family pet or house dust, which are not always easy to avoid. Nonetheless, minimizing exposure is the key. Pets can be restricted to certain rooms; not allowing them in the bedroom is helpful. Dust and vacuum frequently to reduce house mites as well as pet allergens. Because house-dust mites concentrate in carpets, use of floor covering other than carpet can reduce this allergen. Use of high-efficiency air filters on the furnace that are designed to efficiently remove particulate matter can remove pet allergens, pollens, and mold spores.

DRUG THERAPY

There are several categories of drugs used to treat colds and allergic rhinitis. Some of these are used to treat both colds and allergies (antihistamines, decongestants); some are used primarily to treat colds (antitussives, expectorants), and some to treat allergies (corticosteroids, LT modifiers, mast cell stabilizers). The latter group is also among the categories of drugs used to treat asthma, although the target tissue for allergic rhinitis is the nasal passage rather than the bronchial tissue, and thus nasal sprays are used rather than inhalers for administration of corticosteroids and mast cell stabilizers. The reason for this commonality of therapeutic agents is that the disease processes for both allergic rhinitis and asthma have symptoms that, at least in part, result from the release of inflammatory mediators produced from arachidonic acid (see Chapter 9). Also, IgE-mediated involvement is a component to the asthma disease process for many asthmatics. Not surprisingly, many patients with asthma also have symptoms of allergic rhinitis. The presence of these coexisting diseases complicates the drug therapy somewhat because both the nasal and bronchial symptoms must be treated.

There is what seems to be an endless array of products on the market to treat the common cold and allergic rhinitis. Table 10-2 lists some brand-name OTC combination products. A glance through this table reveals that not only are there numerous combinations available, but the names are confusing because many sound similar and the product name often gives little indication of the contents. Consider, also, that the patient has more than 250 brand-name combination OTC allergy and cold/flu products from which to choose, plus numerous generic brands. With all of these product names and combinations, it is easy to imagine that patients are confused about which product to select to self-medicate their symptoms.

Although use of a combination product can be more convenient, use of these products also lends to an enhanced potential for adverse effects that could be avoided. For example, a patient who needs an antitussive to treat a nonproductive cough at the end of a bout with the common cold may not need a decongestant or analgesic any longer but may select Alka-Seltzer Plus Cold & Cough Liqui-Gels to put an end to the cough. Depending on the patient, the phenylephrine and acetaminophen could cause adverse effects that would have been avoided with a single-entity product that contains only an antitussive (eg, Delsym 12 Hour Cough Relief).

Antihistamines

Histamine is a mediator released primarily by mast cells and basophils, which store the histamine for quick release following the binding of an allergen to the IgE on the cell's surface. Histamine is found in several other tissues, including bronchial, intestinal, skin, and cerebral spinal fluid. Once released, histamine combines with the histamine receptor on the surface of other cells to initiate a response within that cell. Three histamine receptors have been identified: H_1, H_2, and H_3. The H_3 receptors are located in the central nervous system (CNS), but their function is not clearly understood and there are no drugs clinically available that are known to specifically block these receptors. The H_2 receptors are primarily found on stomach cells; activation causes an increased production of stomach acid. Drugs that inhibit the H_2 receptor (H_2 blockers) have been available since the mid-1970s and are used to treat ulcers (see Chapter 11). The H_1 receptors are found in the respiratory tract and near peripheral blood vessels. Antihistamines that block the H_1 receptor were on the market for decades prior to H_2 blockers and thus, historically, any reference to antihistamines without specifying the receptor type is generally understood to be referring to antihistamines that block the H_1 receptor. The remaining discussion of antihistamines in this chapter is in reference to H_1 antihistamines.

First- and Second-Generation Antihistamines

There are 2 categories of antihistamines (H_1): first generation and second generation. First-generation antihistamines have been available since the 1940s. The second-generation antihistamines were introduced in the 1980s; however, the second-generation antihistamines that were first introduced have since been withdrawn from the market due to the occurrence of cardiac arrhythmias, an adverse effect not observed with more recent second-generation antihistamines. Of the second-generation antihistamines that are currently on the market, the first was approved by the US Food and Drug Administration (FDA) in 1993. Examples of frequently used first-generation antihistamines are diphenhydramine (Benadryl, 25 to 50 mg/adult dose) and chlorpheniramine (Chlor-Trimeton, 4 mg/adult dose). The most prominent adverse effect with these drugs is sedation. The second-generation antihistamines are less lipophilic and therefore do not cross the blood-brain barrier as readily as the first-generation compounds. Consequently, the primary characteristic that differentiates

TABLE 10-2

SELECTED OVER-THE-COUNTER COMBINATION PRODUCTS FOR TREATMENT OF COLDS AND ALLERGIES[a]

TRADE NAME	ANTIHISTAMINE	DECONGESTANT	ANTITUSSIVE	ANALGESIC	EXPECTORANT
Dimetapp Children's Cold & Allergy Syrup	brompheniramine 1 mg	phenylephrine 2.5 mg			
Children's Triaminic Multi-Symptom Fever and Cold Suspension	chlorpheniramine 1 mg	phenylephrine 2.5 mg	dextromethorphan 5 mg	acetaminophen 160 mg	
Allerest PE Allergy and Sinus Relief Tablets	chlorpheniramine 4 mg	phenylephrine 10 mg			
Coricidin HBP Cough and Cold Tablets	chlorpheniramine 4 mg		dextromethorphan 30 mg		
Alka-Seltzer Plus Cold & Cough Liqui-Gels	chlorpheniramine 2 mg	phenylephrine 5 mg	dextromethorphan 10 mg	acetaminophen 325 mg	
Contac Cold & Flu Night Caplets	chlorpheniramine 2 mg	phenylephrine 5 mg		acetaminophen 500 mg	
Tylenol Cold Multi-Symptom Nighttime Liquid	doxylamine 6.25 mg	phenylephrine 5 mg	dextromethorphan 10 mg	acetaminophen 325 mg	
Robitussin Nighttime Cold + Flu Liquid-Filled Capsules	doxylamine 6.25 mg		dextromethorphan 15 mg	acetaminophen 325 mg	
Dristan Cold Multi-Symptom Formula Tablets	chlorpheniramine 2 mg	phenylephrine 5 mg		acetaminophen 325 mg	
Claritin-D 24 Hour Tablets	loratidine 10 mg	pseudoephedrine 240 mg			
Allegra-D 24 Hour Tablets	fexofenadine 180 mg	pseudoephedrine 240 mg			

(continued)

TABLE 10-2 (CONTINUED)

SELECTED OVER-THE-COUNTER COMBINATION PRODUCTS FOR TREATMENT OF COLDS AND ALLERGIES[a]

TRADE NAME	ANTIHISTAMINE	DECONGESTANT	ANTITUSSIVE	ANALGESIC	EXPECTORANT
Sudafed PE Pressure+Pain Caplets		phenylephrine 5 mg		acetaminophen 325 mg	
Vicks DayQuil Cold and Flu Liquicaps		phenylephrine 5 mg	dextromethorphan 10 mg	acetaminophen 325 mg	
Tylenol Cold Head Congestion Severe Caplets		phenylephrine 5 mg		acetaminophen 325 mg	guaifenesin 200 mg
Robitussin Cough & Chest Congestion DM Liquid – Filled Capsules			dextromethorphan 10 mg		guaifenesin 200 mg
Robitussin Daytime Cold+Flu Liquid-Filled Capsules		phenylephrine 5 mg	dextromethorphan 10 mg	acetaminophen 325 mg	
Advil Cold & Sinus Caplets		pseudoephedrine 30 mg		ibuprofen 200 mg	
Alka-Seltzer Severe Sinus Congestion and Cough Capsules		phenylephrine 5 mg	dextromethorphan 10 mg	acetaminophen 325 mg	
Mucinex DM Tablets			dextromethorphan 30 mg		guaifenesin 600 mg
Maximum Strength Mucinex D Tablets		pseudoephedrine 120 mg			guaifenesin 1200 mg
Children's Triaminic Day Time Cold and Cough Syrup		phenylephrine 2.5 mg	dextromethorphan 5 mg		

[a]Values indicated per ingredient represent mg per dosage unit (eg, tablet, capsule), per 5 mL for children's liquid products, and per 15 mL for other liquid products.

	GENERIC	TRADE	DOSAGE	OTC/RX
First-generation	brompheniramine	Bromax	Tablets, liquid	OTC/Rx
	carbinoxamine	Palgic	Extended-release tablets, immediate-release tablets, solution	Rx
	chlorpheniramine	Chlor-Trimeton Allergy	Extended-release tablets, immediate-release tablets, liquids	OTC/Rx
	clemastine	Tavist Allergy	Tablets, syrup	OTC
	dexchlorpheniramine	generic	Syrup	Rx
	diphenhydramine	Benadryl	Capsules, tablets, liquids, injectable	OTC/Rx
	promethazine	Phenergan	Tablets, solution, injectable	Rx
Second-generation	azelastine	Astelin, Astepro	Spray	Rx
	cetirizine	Zyrtec Allergy	Tablets, syrup	OTC
	desloratadine	Clarinex	Tablets, syrup	Rx
	fexofenadine	Allegra	Tablets, suspension	OTC
	levocetirizine	Xyzal	Tablets, solution	Rx
	loratadine	Claritin, Alavert	Tablets, syrup	OTC
	olopatadine	Patanase	Spray	Rx

TABLE 10-3

EXAMPLES OF FIRST- AND SECOND-GENERATION ANTIHISTAMINES

OTC = over-the-counter; Rx = prescription.

the first-generation from second-generation compounds is the significantly reduced incidence of sedation with the second-generation antihistamines. Examples of second-generation antihistamines, which are sometimes referred to as *nonsedating antihistamines*, are fexofenadine (Allegra, 180 mg/day adult dose) and loratadine (Claritin, 10 mg/day adult dose). Other examples of first- and second-generation antihistamines are listed in Table 10-3.

The first-generation antihistamines have long been available OTC. In 2002, loratadine was the first of the second-generation products available OTC. One argument for this shift to OTC status was the fact that second-generation antihistamines have a lower incidence of adverse effects than first-generation antihistamines, which are already used as OTC products to treat allergic rhinitis.

All antihistamines are available as oral medications except azelastine (Astelin) and olopatadine (Patanase), which are nasal sprays (see Table 10-3). Some antihistamines are also available in liquid form as syrups or elixirs, and some come in extended-release dosage forms. It should be noted that certain antihistamines are available as ophthalmic formulations; these products are intended to be administered to the eye for treatment of allergic

conjunctivitis. Diphenhydramine is available in many dosage forms, including topical formulations intended to be applied to the skin. These products are discussed later in this chapter.

Uses for Allergies and Colds

Histamine is considered a major contributor to the symptoms of allergic rhinitis, and, consequently, antihistamines are a mainstay of therapy. Antihistamines decrease the rhinorrhea, itchy nose and eyes, and sneezing associated with allergic rhinitis. They do not decrease nasal congestion significantly. This may be because other mediators also contribute to nasal congestion and, during the late-phase response, the accumulation of immune cells contributes to nasal congestion. Antihistamines are more effective when present prior to the release of histamine; therefore, daily use of these drugs as a preventative, or at least 1 to 2 hours prior to exposure, is more effective than use after symptoms occur.

Histamine does not play a significant role in the symptoms of the common cold. Nonetheless, antihistamines are somewhat effective in reducing mucus production and drying the nasal passage, but the mechanism of action is not due to histamine antagonism. As discussed next, one adverse effect of antihistamines, particularly the first-generation antihistamines, is to cause anticholinergic effects. One cholinergic response is mucus production, and thus inhibition of this process becomes a benefit when treating the common cold, hence the inclusion of a first-generation antihistamine in many OTC cold products. However, the drying effect on the respiratory tract is a disadvantage when sinus drainage or movement of mucus out of the bronchial tree (ie, expectoration) is desired. Consequently, first-generation antihistamines should be used with caution in patients with lower respiratory tract diseases (eg, asthma and chronic bronchitis).

> *Recall from Chapter 8 that anticholinergic effects include blurred vision, constipation, urinary hesitancy, dry mouth, and decreased sweating.*

Adverse Effects and Drug Interactions

The adverse effect profile for the first-generation antihistamines is more notable than for the second-generation compounds. Sedation and anticholinergic effects are the prime concern. Some first-generation antihistamines have a greater sedative effect (eg, diphenhydramine, promethazine, carbinoxamine, clemastine) than others (eg, chlorpheniramine, brompheniramine, dexchlorpheniramine). Not only is drowsiness a potential hazard while driving a vehicle, but it can also negatively affect performance at work, in school, and in athletics. Even if the person does not feel drowsy, cognitive abilities, including the ability to operate a motor vehicle, can be diminished. Because reaction time and perception are affected, athletic performance could also be affected. Drowsiness at nighttime can be an advantage to facilitate sleep; however, diminished cognitive function can continue even the next morning. Concomitant use of other CNS depressants (eg, opioid analgesics, some anticonvulsants, antianxiety agents, and alcohol) will exacerbate the sedative properties. In some children and elderly patients, antihistamines can cause paradoxical CNS stimulation that results in insomnia, nervousness, irritability, and tremors. The incidence of sedation for the second-generation antihistamines varies from lower incidence at recommended doses (cetirizine, Zyrtec) to nonsedating even at higher-than-recommended doses (fexofenadine, Allegra).

Anticholinergic adverse effects are also more predominant with first-generation than with second-generation antihistamines. Again, there is some variation in the extent of these effects among the many first-generation compounds; for example, brompheniramine, dexchlorpheniramine, and chlorpheniramine have less of these adverse effects than diphenhydramine, promethazine, clemastine, and carbinoxamine. The anticholinergic effects include dry mouth, urinary retention, blurred vision, tachycardia, reduced sweating, and constipation. These effects may be quite tolerable for most patients, but patients with preexisting conditions such as cardiovascular disease, narrow-angle glaucoma, or urinary retention should avoid the first-generation products. Similarly, decreased sweating is not likely to be of significant consequence for most patients, but it may be a contributing factor in the development of heatstroke in a predisposed patient who is exercising heavily in a hot, humid environment. The potential problems associated with the anticholinergic effects can be made worse if the antihistamine is combined with other drugs that also have anticholinergic effects (eg, drugs for motion sickness, certain groups of antidepressant drugs, gastrointestinal antispasmodics, typical antipsychotic drugs, and some drugs to treat Parkinson's disease).

Another adverse effect associated with first-generation antihistamines is that they can cause photosensitization in some patients, making them more prone to sunburn. Caution is advised with use in all patients; the use of sunscreens and appropriate protective clothing is recommended until the patient's response is determined.

Other Uses for Antihistamines

Besides being used to treat the common cold or allergic rhinitis, some antihistamines have other therapeutic uses. Histamine causes redness of the skin (urticaria) and itching (pruritus) as a result of atopic dermatitis (IgE-mediated hypersensitive response after systemic absorption of an allergen), contact dermatitis (eg, poison ivy), or eczema. Some antihistamines such as diphenhydramine, hydroxyzine (Vistaril), and promethazine (Phenergan) are used topically and/or orally for treatment of dermatitis.

The prominent sedative properties of diphenhydramine (Nytol, Sominex) and doxylamine (Unisom) are used as an advantage to market antihistamines as OTC sleep aids. These agents are effective for short-term use to treat insomnia. Some morning hangover is common and is a disadvantage because it may diminish the person's effectiveness in morning activities such as driving, completing tasks at work, or exercising/playing sports.

Some antihistamines are effective at preventing motion sickness and the nausea and vomiting associated with adverse effects of drugs. Drug-induced gastric irritation and motion sickness causes the release of acetylcholine, which stimulates the vomiting center in the CNS. Therefore, the anticholinergic effect of antihistamines, especially when given prior to the offending drug or motion, can prevent the nausea and vomiting. Prescription and OTC agents are available, such as promethazine (Phenergan), meclizine (Bonine), dimenhydrinate (Dramamine), and diphenhydramine.

> *Scopolamine, an anticholinergic drug, not an antihistamine, is also useful to treat motion sickness and is available as a patch (Transderm Scop) for transdermal absorption.*

Anticholinergics

Because the anticholinergic effect of antihistamines can be advantageous in the treatment of the common cold and allergic rhinitis, it is not surprising that a drug in the anticholinergic category is available for treatment of these illnesses. Ipratropium (Atrovent) is available by prescription as a nasal spray. Systemic anticholinergics tend to have numerous adverse effects and thus are not used for these illnesses, but the spray minimizes the systemic adverse effects. Typical dosing is frequent—2 sprays per nostril 3 to 4 times per day—and thus a disadvantage. The drug should not be used in patients who are allergic to peanuts because ipratropium may cause an allergic response. The inhaler dosage form of ipratropium is used to treat asthma and chronic obstructive pulmonary disease (see Chapter 9).

Nasal Decongestants

Dilation of peripheral blood vessels in the nasal passage contributes significantly to nasal congestion. Decongestants are α-adrenergic agonists; they activate the α-receptors on the peripheral blood vessels of the nasal passage to cause constriction of those blood vessels and a decrease in mucosal edema. Because these drugs combine with one of the same receptors as the neurotransmitters of the sympathetic nervous system, and thus mimic these neurotransmitters, the nasal decongestants are also referred to as *sympathomimetics*.

> *Adrenergic refers to drugs that combine with the same receptors as the adrenergic neurotransmitters (norepinephrine and epinephrine), which are released by activation of the sympathetic nervous system. Therefore, α-adrenergic agonists combine specifically with the alpha-type of adrenergic receptor.*

Uses for Allergy and Colds

Decongestants are used to relieve nasal stuffiness associated with the common cold and allergic rhinitis, both seasonal and perennial. One decongestant, phenylpropanolamine, was popular until 2000 when the FDA advised the removal of phenylpropanolamine from the market because of increased risk for hemorrhagic stroke in women taking these drugs. Subsequently, the oral decongestant used in almost all OTC decongestant products became pseudoephedrine; it is available alone (Sudafed) and in many combination products (see Table 10-2) for the treatment of colds and allergies. It is available in several oral dosage forms, including capsules, tablets, syrups, and extended-release products. However, because pseudoephedrine can be used to make methamphetamine, a 2006 federal law required that all OTC medications that contain pseudoephedrine be kept behind the pharmacy counter so that customers must ask for them, show identification, and sign for the product prior to purchase. As a result of this inconvenience, the decongestant component of many oral OTC products has been switched by the pharmaceutical manufacturer from pseudoephedrine to phenylephrine (see Table 10-2).

> *Phenylpropanolamine was also used in weight-loss products (ie, diet pills). Such use in OTC products had been controversial for years and contributed to the overall incidence of hemorrhagic stroke. Considering that nondrug measures of diet and exercise can achieve weight loss, the risk of adverse effects from adrenergic agonists may outweigh the potential benefits for this use.*

Pseudoephedrine is absorbed readily from the gastrointestinal tract. Onset of action is less than 30 minutes, and duration is about 4 hours. It does not have to be used prior to onset of nasal decongestion and thus can be used as needed or on a regularly scheduled basis. Phenylephrine is generally considered less effective than pseudoephedrine as a decongestant, has a higher incidence of cardiovascular adverse effects, and has a shorter half-life than pseudoephedrine.

Several decongestants are available for topical use as nasal sprays, inhalers, or drops. Nasal decongestants are more effective, faster acting, and produce fewer CNS stimulant and other systemic effects than oral decongestants. Nonetheless, their use should be limited to 3 to 5 days because of the potential to cause rebound congestion. Examples are tetrahydrozoline (Tyzine), levmetamfetamine (Vicks Vapo Inhaler), phenylephrine (Neo-Synephrine 4-Hour), and oxymetazoline (Afrin 12-Hour Original, Neo-Synephrine 12-Hour).

As with other OTC products, the names are sometimes confusing because a few companies have several products that use the same brand name and are slight variations from one another in content or duration of action. For example, the following all contain 0.05% oxymetazoline as the decongestant: Afrin 12-Hour Original Pump Mist, Afrin 12-Hour Original, Afrin Severe Congestion with Menthol, Afrin No-Drip 12-Hour, and Afrin No-Drip 12-Hour Severe Congestion with Menthol. Selection depends primarily on personal preference.

Adverse Effects and Drug Interactions

The most common adverse effect from pseudoephedrine or phenylephrine is CNS stimulation that may cause insomnia, agitation, tremor, headache, or restlessness. Pseudoephedrine is marketed as a nondrowsy cold and allergy medication. Some products have pseudoephedrine in combination with first-generation antihistamines (see Table 10-2) as a means to counter the sedative properties of the antihistamine. Additional adrenergic effects can cause tachycardia, peripheral vasoconstriction, and altered glucose metabolism. The incidence of tachycardia and vasoconstriction is greater with phenylephrine and can be of significance to patients who have existing hypertension or heart disease because these effects can exacerbate the disease. Consequently, oral decongestants should not be used in patients with these diseases and should be used with caution in patients with diabetes mellitus because of the potential to alter insulin requirements. Caution is also warranted even when topical nasal decongestants are used in patients with diabetes mellitus or cardiovascular disease. The peripheral vasoconstriction action of nasal decongestants can decrease the effectiveness of the body's natural cooling mechanism; therefore, these drugs should be used with caution in patients who are in an environment conducive to heatstroke (eg, hot, humid, poor air circulation, heavy exercise).

Decongestants applied topically as intranasal sprays and drops generally have milder systemic effects. However, local adverse effects, such as local irritation and rebound congestion, are significant problems. Rebound congestion is a potential adverse effect with the use of decongestants applied topically to the nasal mucosa. The incidence of rebound congestion increases when nasal sprays and drops are used for more than 3 to 5 days. In this condition, congestion becomes worse, and the effectiveness and duration of action of the decongestant diminishes with continued use of the decongestant. Patients with rebound congestion have a tendency to continue using the nasal decongestant in an effort to relieve the congestion, thus perpetuating the problem. If rebound congestion occurs, the topical nasal decongestant can be discontinued in one nostril at a time, and normal saline nasal spray used in that nostril to soothe the irritated mucosa. Use of an oral decongestant may also minimize the discomfort. It takes 1 to 2 weeks for the nasal mucosa to return to normal. Other potential problems associated with nasal decongestants are primarily local effects (eg, nasal burning, stinging, and dryness of the mucosa). These local effects and the potential for rebound congestion with nasal sprays and drops make them less useful for perennial allergic rhinitis in which long-term therapy is needed.

In terms of drug interactions, the one with the most devastating potential is the combination of any decongestant, including topical products, with monoamine oxidase inhibitors (MAOIs). Decongestants should not be used in patients who are using an MAOI or have used an MAOI within the previous 3 weeks because hypertensive crisis can result. Another interaction is the combination of oral decongestants with caffeine. Use of caffeine is prevalent in soft drinks and coffee (see Table 16-3) and has CNS and cardiovascular effects similar to pseudoephedrine. These effects are additive when both drugs are used together; therefore, this combination can be particularly hazardous to patients with existing hypertension. The combination of caffeine and ephedrine has demonstrated a prolonged exercise time to exhaustion compared with placebo or either drug alone.

> MAOIs *are a group of drugs that are categorized therapeutically as antidepressant drugs (see Chapter 13), although they also have some other uses. MAOIs inhibit the inactivation of sympathomimetics, enhancing their activity and causing a potentially dangerous exaggerated hypertensive response. Examples of MAOIs are phenelzine (Nardil) and tranylcypromine (Parnate).*

Corticosteroids

Topical use of corticosteroids as nasal sprays has become a primary therapy for control of allergic rhinitis. By inhibiting the production of inflammatory mediators (see Chapter 9), corticosteroids reduce all of the major symptoms of allergic rhinitis (eg, runny nose, itching, sneezing, and nasal congestion). They also reduce infiltration of inflammatory cells and inhibit symptoms of the late-phase reaction. The onset of action is slower for nasal corticosteroids than for antihistamines or decongestants. Some benefit is observed within 1 to 3 days, but maximal effect may take 2 to 3 weeks. Use of these corticosteroid products is most effective to prevent symptoms, and thus it is beneficial to use them for 2 to 4 weeks prior to anticipated exposure as well as during exposure.

Adverse effects of nasal corticosteroids are relatively minor. Nasal irritation, headache, and pharyngitis occur in some patients. Localized infection of the nasal passage occurs on rare occasions but necessitates discontinuation of the corticosteroid and/or treatment with an antibacterial agent. Significant systemic effects are rare.

Nasal corticosteroid products are available as aqueous sprays or as aerosol canisters with propellants. The aqueous sprays produce less drying and are less irritating to the nasal mucosa than the aerosols but produce more of a taste. Dosage regimens vary from 1 to 4 times per day, depending on the specific product and the response obtained. After a few weeks of therapy, the effectiveness should be assessed and the dosage regimen adjusted so that the lowest effective dosage is used. Table 10-4 lists some nasal products and typical adult dosage. All of the intranasal corticosteroids require a prescription except for triamcinolone and fluticasone. In 2013, the FDA approved intranasal triamcinolone (Nasacort Allergy 24 Hour) for OTC use. The following year, intranasal fluticasone (Flonase) was changed to OTC status. These OTC products are available at the same strength and dose as the previous prescription products.

Oral corticosteroids are also used as short-term therapy (ie, up to 1 week) when symptoms are severe. An example of a typical regimen would be 20 mg of prednisone once daily for 7 days. As with use of systemic corticosteroids for any purpose, consideration should be given to other existing diseases that may be adversely affected by the corticosteroid (eg, hypertension, ulcers, and diabetes mellitus) (see Chapter 6).

TABLE 10-4			
CORTICOSTEROID INTRANASAL PRODUCTS[a]			
GENERIC NAME	TRADE NAME	DOSAGE FORM	TYPICAL ADULT DOSAGE (SPRAYS/NOSTRIL)
beclomethasone	Beconase AQ	Spray	1 to 2 bid
budesonide	Rhinocort Aqua	Spray	1 once/day
ciclesonide	Omnaris	spray	2 once/day
flunisolide	Nasarel	Spray	2 bid to tid
fluticasone	Flonase	Spray	2 once/day
mometasone	Nasonex	Spray	2 once/day
triamcinolone	Nasacort AQ	Spray	1 to 2 once/day
bid = twice per day; tid = 3 times per day.			
[a]All products are prescription only except triamcinolone and fluticasone.			

Mast Cell–Stabilizing Drugs

As with the corticosteroids, the mast cell–stabilizing drugs are also used to treat asthma as well as allergic rhinitis (see Chapter 9). Their mechanism of action is to inhibit the release of inflammatory mediators from mast cells. Cromolyn (NasalCrom) is available OTC as a nasal spray for treatment of allergic rhinitis. As with inhalation products for treatment of asthma, use of the nasal spray for rhinitis takes several days for a noticeable improvement, takes a few weeks or more for maximal effect, has a dosage regimen of multiple doses per day, and is most effective if dosing begins prior to onset of symptoms and then continues on a regular daily schedule. The advantages of cromolyn are the OTC availability and the lack of systemic adverse effects. The disadvantages are the frequent dosing schedule (3 to 6 times per day) and that the effectiveness is less than the corticosteroids. Nasal irritation occurs in some patients.

Leukotriene Modifiers

LTs are mediators released during the inflammatory response that contribute to symptoms of asthma (see Chapter 9) and to the early- and late-phase symptoms of allergic rhinitis. LT modifiers inhibit the effect of LTs by one of 2 mechanisms: inhibition of the enzyme that produces them or competitive inhibition of the LT receptor. For example, montelukast (Singulair) blocks the LT receptor. Montelukast was originally approved for asthma therapy but became available to treat seasonal allergic rhinitis in 2003. Adverse effects are infrequent but include headache and upper respiratory tract infection (eg, ear infection). The recommended dosage is the same as for treatment of asthma: 1 tablet orally per day at a dose of 4, 5, or 10 mg, depending on the age of the patient. Because the dosage form and regimen are the same for the treatment of allergic rhinitis and asthma, the drug can be of potential benefit in patients with both of these diseases, but montelukast has been shown to be less effective than corticosteroid nasal spray in these patients.

Expectorants

An expectorant is a drug that decreases the viscosity of lower respiratory tract secretions so that they can be moved out of the respiratory tract more efficiently by coughing (ie, productive cough). The most commonly used expectorant is guaifenesin, either alone (Mucinex, 600 to 1200 mg every 12 hours) or in combination with many cold and cough remedies (see Table 10-2). For example, Mucinex DM and Robitussin Cough and Chest Congestion DM both contain guaifenesin. However, there is some question as to the usefulness of guaifenesin in these combination products for several reasons:

- An infection with the common cold (without complications) typically affects only the upper respiratory tract and the cough is nonproductive.

- Although recommended OTC dosages (200 to 400 mg every 4 hours) of guaifenesin are usually void of adverse effects, the extent of therapeutic effectiveness at these dosages is somewhat uncertain. High doses can cause vomiting, headache, drowsiness, and diarrhea.

- Use of first-generation antihistamines with expectorants is counterproductive regarding expectorant action because the anticholinergic action can dry mucous secretions and thus make the mucus more difficult to expectorate. Similarly, the combination of an expectorant with a cough suppressant is counterproductive.

Nondrug measures to facilitate expectorant activity are to stay well-hydrated and to keep the air humidified.

Antitussive Agents

A frequent symptom of the common cold is coughing. *Antitussive agents* are cough suppressants. These drugs act in the CNS to increase the threshold for coughing. Cough is a reflex intended to mobilize mucus out of the respiratory tract and therefore should not be suppressed if it is productive. However, an antitussive is warranted when a cough interferes with sleep, is unproductive, or is contributing to an irritated and sore throat. Usually viral respiratory infections are nonproductive. A rule of thumb is that it is appropriate to treat dry, hacking coughs with antitussives and to treat productive coughs with an expectorant. Suppression of a productive cough could hinder the body's ability to fight the infection. Because the intended purpose of an expectorant is to move secretions from the respiratory tract, in some cases the combination of antitussives with expectorants in the same product could be counterproductive.

The most common nonopioid antitussive is dextromethorphan. Characteristics of dextromethorphan are that it does not cause respiratory depression at therapeutic doses, it is available OTC, and it is effective at 10 to 30 mg every 4 to 8 hours. Dextromethorphan has a low incidence of adverse effects at normal antitussive doses, but it can add to the CNS depressant effects of other drugs (eg, alcohol, antihistamines) and should not be used in combination with MAOIs. It should be noted that although dextromethorphan is the most common OTC antitussive, there is concern that it has some abuse potential at higher doses. There are many reports of abuse, particularly among younger teens and pre-teens who do not have alcohol or other drugs readily available. Dextromethorphan remains OTC because scientific studies must be completed to confirm the abuse and physical dependence potential. Diphenhydramine also has antitussive properties; the first-generation antihistamines in combination with a decongestant are recommended for cough caused by the common cold. However, these agents have several adverse effects, particularly sedation, that need to be considered when selecting a medication.

The most frequently used opioid antitussive is codeine (see Chapter 7). Hydrocodone is also effective but has a higher abuse potential. Codeine is more effective than dextromethorphan to treat severe cough. Usual adult dosages are 10 to 20 mg codeine every 4 to 6 hours. Codeine can produce euphoria and drug dependence, but the likelihood is small at antitussive doses. Codeine can suppress respiration and thus should be used with caution in patients with respiratory disease such as asthma or emphysema. Respiratory depression is the cause of death in overdose situations; an opioid analgesic antagonist, naloxone (Narcan), can be used to reverse this effect. Constipation is a common adverse effect. Codeine cough syrups are controlled substances (Schedule V) and are available in mixtures containing various other drugs to treat colds. The laws of some states allow limited purchase of codeine-containing cough medications without a prescription.

In addition to systemic antitussive agents, cough drops are also used to relieve cough. These products contain menthol, which has some local anesthetic action to suppress the cough and to soothe a sore throat. Sucking on hard candy also soothes the throat and offers relief.

Analgesics

Analgesics are often used as part of the treatment regimen for the common cold; in fact, they are a component of many cough and cold remedies (see Table 10-2). Relief of sore throat or headache pain is often the impetus for the use of analgesics, although they may also be used to reduce fever (antipyretic). Acetaminophen and ibuprofen (see Chapter 7) are the analgesics of choice for pain accompanying a cold. Aspirin is not recommended for children and teenagers because of the risk of Reye's syndrome when aspirin is used in conjunction with a viral infection. Most cough and cold remedies with an analgesic/antipyretic component have been reformulated to use acetaminophen. Normal adult dosages of acetaminophen range from 500 to 1000 mg, with a daily maximum of 4000 mg.

As an alternative to systemic analgesics, relief of sore throat can be attained through topically applied throat sprays or lozenges. Examples of local anesthetics that are components of lozenges are dyclonine (Sucrets), menthol (Hall's Mentho-Lyptus), or both menthol and benzocaine (Cepacol Extra Strength). Camphor and menthol vapors have some antitussive and anesthetic action and thus are used as creams and ointments (Vicks VapoRub) for topical application to the chest and/or throat. A nondrug measure to relieve sore throat is merely to keep the throat moist by sucking on hard candy.

Ophthalmic Products

Itching, watering, and redness of the eyes compose the ocular inflammation (allergic conjunctivitis) that is a significant component of allergic rhinitis for many patients. The systemic use of antihistamines or decongestants can help alleviate these symptoms. There are also many ophthalmic products available for treating these ocular inflammation symptoms. These products include drugs in the categories of corticosteroids, antihistamines, decongestants, mast cell stabilizers, and nonsteroidal anti-inflammatory drugs. Examples of ophthalmic products for treatment of allergic rhinitis are provided in Table 10-5. Each product is applied directly to the eye, most often as drops. Adverse effects are usually local in nature, such as stinging or burning of the eyes and blurred vision.

Drugs for Treating Colds and Allergies 183

TABLE 10-5

SELECTED OPHTHALMIC PRODUCTS TO TREAT OCULAR SYMPTOMS OF ALLERGIC RHINITIS

DRUG CATEGORY	GENERIC NAME	TRADE NAME	OTC/RX
Antihistamines	azelastine	Optivar	Rx
	emedastine	Emadine	Rx
	olopatadine	Patanol	Rx
Corticosteroids	dexamethasone	Maxidex	Rx
	loteprednol	Lotemax	Rx
	prednisolone	Pred Forte	Rx
Mast cell stabilizers	nedocromil	Alocril	Rx
	pemirolast	Alamast	Rx
NSAIDs	ketorolac	Acular	Rx
	diclofenac	Voltaren	Rx
Ophthalmic decongestants	naphazoline	Naphcon A, Clear Eye Redness Relief	OTC
	oxymetazoline	Visine L.R.	OTC
	tetrahydrozoline	Visine	OTC

NSAIDs = nonsteroidal anti-inflammatory drugs; OTC = over-the-counter; Rx = prescription.

Antibiotics

Antibiotics are mentioned here to emphasize that they are effective only against bacteria and that neither the common cold nor allergic rhinitis is caused by bacterial infection. Many people have the mistaken impression that they should get "a shot of penicillin" to treat their cold when in fact antibiotics have no impact on viruses. However, some patients develop complications of bacterial infections as the symptoms of a cold or allergic rhinitis linger. Sinusitis and ear infections, especially in young children, are examples of bacterial complications that should be treated with antibiotics.

Allergen Immunotherapy

As described in the Foundational Concepts section, an allergen is a substance that initiates an allergic response. The concept of allergen immunotherapy involves desensitization of a patient to an allergen by exposing the patient to a small amount of the antigen and then gradually increasing it over time. This helps to build tolerance to the antigen. After the dose of the antigen has been increased to its optimal amount, maintenance doses of the antigen are given to maintain tolerance. Allergen immunotherapy is used for allergies to specific antigens. Traditionally, this treatment has involved subcutaneous injection of the antigen ("allergy shots"). However, the FDA has recently approved 3 sublingual tablet formulations of antigens to use in allergen immunotherapy. The first product approved is called Oralair and is a mixture of pollen allergens from 5 grasses. Two additional products have since been approved. Grastek is approved for the treatment of allergic rhinitis in those sensitive to grass pollen, and Ragwitek is approved for ragweed allergies. The sublingual administration will be more convenient for patients because they can self-administer the therapy instead of requiring a visit to the prescriber's office. It should be noted that there is a risk for an allergic reaction to the allergen when it is administered. This can occur with both subcutaneous and sublingual allergen immunotherapy. For this reason, it is recommended that patients wait at the prescriber's office for 30 minutes after receiving an allergy shot. It is also recommended that the first dose of the sublingual therapy be given at the prescriber's office. The patient can then self-administer the therapy at home. A prescription for an epinephrine auto-injector is recommended in patients receiving the sublingual therapy in case there is a serious allergic reaction (see Chapter 3). Sublingual allergen immunotherapy should also not be used in patients with severe or uncontrolled asthma, and patients who are having active asthma symptoms should not take the tablet.

Section Summary

Second-generation antihistamines, decongestants, oral LT modifiers, and nasal corticosteroids, used individually or in combination, have been the mainstay of treatment for seasonal and perennial allergic rhinitis. Severe allergic rhinitis may require a few days of oral corticosteroids.

Sedation and diminished cognitive performance are the most problematic adverse effects associated with the first-generation antihistamines.

The second-generation antihistamines do not readily cross the blood-brain barrier and thus have significantly reduced incidence of these adverse effects. Both groups of antihistamines are effective in blocking the H_1 receptor in the nasal passage and thus decreasing the occurrence of sneezing, rhinorrhea, and itching. Nasal corticosteroids inhibit the inflammatory response, including the impact of prostaglandins and LTs. Topical use of corticosteroids in this fashion is the most effective therapy for allergic rhinitis and usually lacks systemic adverse effects. Other drugs such as pseudoephedrine (a decongestant), montelukast (a LT modifier), or cromolyn (a mast cell stabilizer) can also be used to help alleviate the symptoms of allergic rhinitis.

First-generation antihistamines are used to treat the common cold, not because of the histamine-blocking ability, but because of the anticholinergic effects that are attributed to these drugs. Anticholinergic response inhibits nasal secretions and causes a drying of the nasal passage. Decongestants are also frequently a part of the OTC regimen to treat a cold. These drugs constrict the blood vessels in the nasal passage to open the airways. However, because they also constrict other peripheral blood vessels and affect glucose metabolism, decongestants should be used cautiously in patients with hypertension, heart disease, or diabetes. Expectorants (decrease viscosity of secretions), antitussives (inhibit cough), and analgesics (relief of sore throat pain) are among the other OTC drugs that are available to treat the common cold. Opioid antitussives are more effective than OTC antitussives but also have adverse effects not observed with OTC antitussives such as constipation and respiratory depression.

ROLE OF THE ATHLETIC TRAINER

As is the case for many other diseases, inadequate therapy for allergic rhinitis can hinder the patient's athletic performance for longer than necessary. Although the duration of a cold is relatively short and self-limiting, serious complications can develop, which can significantly delay the patient's return to normal activity level. Because both allergic rhinitis and the common cold are often self-medicated with OTC medication by the patient, the potential exists for adverse effects from the OTC medication and/or drug interactions with other medications that the patient is taking to treat other conditions. The role of the athletic trainer should focus on whether the patient is taking the medications as prescribed (ie, right dose at the right time) and whether the patient is experiencing sufficient response so that the negative impact of the disease and the therapy are minimized. The following are examples of therapy considerations that the athletic trainer should be cognizant of:

- Does the patient adhere to the dosage regimen prescribed by the physician? If effectiveness of therapy is not optimal, poor adherence to therapy is often the reason.

- Is the patient experiencing symptoms that could be attributed to adverse drug effects? If symptoms are not readily explained by a diagnosed disease, suspect the drug therapy. Either the adverse effects of individual drugs or the drug interactions from combinations of drugs may be the cause. The most common adverse effects are drowsiness from first-generation antihistamines and CNS stimulation with decongestants. If the patient feels lethargic, use of these antihistamines during the day may be the cause. If the patient is not sleeping well at night, use of decongestants too close to bedtime may be the cause. The athletic trainer should not discount the fact that the magnitude of the adverse responses vary from person to person and may be enhanced by drug interactions.

- Is the patient competing at the level where nasal decongestants would be banned substances? (See Chapter 17.)

- Is the patient taking appropriate actions to avoid allergens that are contributing to the allergic rhinitis?

- If nasal corticosteroids are part of the therapy, is the patient using appropriate technique to administer the nasal spray? Appropriate technique is to first clear the nasal passage of mucus, tilt the head slightly forward, place the tip of the nasal spray into one nostril and point the tip away from the nasal septum while holding the bottle upright, block the other nostril, spray while breathing in slowly through the nose (with mouth closed), hold breath for a few seconds, and then exhale through the mouth.

- Are the symptoms of a common cold lingering too long? If the symptoms are getting worse instead of better after 7 to 10 days, if sinus headache is reoccurring, or if fever develops that was not present earlier, complications may have developed that require medical attention.

- Is the patient taking OTC combination products to treat cold or allergy symptoms that include more drugs than necessary? Single-component products are available so that a decongestant is used only when congestion is present, an analgesic is included only when pain relief is desired, etc.

- Is the patient who will be training in conditions that have a significant risk of heat-related illnesses also taking any drugs (OTC or prescription) that may contribute to these illnesses, particularly systemic decongestants and first-generation antihistamines? If such therapy cannot be modified without adding risk of exacerbation of existing disease, extra precautions should be taken (eg, lighter clothing, better air circulation, exercising during the cooler part of the day, and ensuring adequate fluid and electrolyte intake) to avoid heat-related illnesses.

For the athletic trainer, key roles regarding drug therapy are to be watchful that the therapy is appropriately effective and to educate the patient regarding appropriate use of the medications. The starting point for the athletic trainer is to know what to look for and what questions to ask. If the symptoms of allergic rhinitis or common cold do not respond adequately to therapy, or if the therapy causes problematic adverse effects, there is likely to be a negative impact on the patient's athletic performance.

CASE STUDY

It seems that the university's wrestling team benefited from the exceptionally long break the coach gave them over the Christmas holidays because they all seem eager to continue the remaining part of the season in earnest.

However, Sam, the team's 74-kg class wrestler, appears uncomfortable and less energetic. He reports that over break he contracted an upper respiratory tract infection. Sam started taking an OTC medication to relieve his runny nose when he first felt the onset of the cold. He states that it seems to be helping, but he is feeling more tired since starting the medication. What is a possible explanation for Sam's symptoms?

BIBLIOGRAPHY

Chelladurai Y, Lin SY. Effectiveness of subcutaneous versus sublingual immunotherapy for allergic rhinitis: current update. *Curr Opin Otolaryngol Head Neck Surg.* 2014;22(3):211-215.

Cooper RJ. Over-the-counter medicine abuse—a review of the literature. *J Subst Use.* 2013;18(2):82-107.

Pray WS, Pray GE. Allergic rhinitis: nonprescription treatment options. *US Pharm.* 2011;36(7):14-19.

Pray WS, Pray GE. Proper use of nonprescription nasal sprays. *US Pharm.* 2014;39:8-11.

Simons FER, Simons KJ. Histamine and H_1-antihistamines: celebrating a century of progress. *J Allergy Clin Immunol.* 2011;128(6):1139-1150.

Sur DK, Scandale S. Treatment of allergic rhinitis. *Am Fam Physician.* 2010;81(12):1440-1446.

Trangsrun AJ, Whitaker AL, Small RE. Intranasal corticosteroids for allergic rhinitis. *Pharmacotherapy.* 2002;22(11):1458-1467.

CHAPTER 11: ADVANCE ORGANIZER

Foundational Concepts

- Key Aspects of Gastrointestinal Physiology
- Disorders of the Gastrointestinal Tract
  - Heartburn and Gastroesophageal Reflux Disease
  - Peptic Ulcer Disease
  - Constipation
  - Diarrhea
  - Irritable Bowel Syndrome
  - Inflammatory Bowel Disease
  - Hemorrhoids
  - Exercise-Induced Problems
- Section Summary

General Nondrug Considerations

- Gastroesophageal Reflux Disease
- Peptic Ulcer Disease
- Constipation
- Diarrhea
- Irritable Bowel Syndrome
- Inflammatory Bowel Disease
- Hemorrhoids
- Section Summary

Gastrointestinal Drugs

- Proton-Pump Inhibitors
- H_2-Receptor Antagonists
- Comparison of H_2-Receptor Antagonists and Proton-Pump Inhibitors
- Combination Therapy to Treat *Helicobacter pylori*–Associated Ulcers
- Antacids
- Physical Barriers
- Misoprostol
- Laxatives
  - Bulk-Forming Laxatives
  - Stool Softeners
  - Osmotic Laxatives
  - Stimulant Laxatives
- Antidiarrheal Agents
  - Opioids
  - Absorbents
  - Bismuth Subsalicylate
- Drugs for Treating Irritable Bowel Syndrome
- Drugs for Treating Inflammatory Bowel Disease
- Drugs for Treating Hemorrhoids
- Section Summary

Role of the Athletic Trainer

Drugs for Treating
Gastrointestinal Disorders

CHAPTER OBJECTIVES

At the end of this chapter, the reader will be able to:

- Explain the normal gastrointestinal (GI) physiological process and how drugs can affect this process

- Explain the function of the proton pump in maintaining stomach acidity and how drugs affect the proton pump

- Explain the pathophysiology and identify the signs and symptoms of gastroesophageal reflux disease (GERD), heartburn, and peptic ulcer disease (PUD) and recall how these conditions can be exacerbated

- Explain the pathophysiology, signs and symptoms, and causes of constipation, diarrhea, irritable bowel syndrome (IBS), inflammatory bowel disease (IBD), and hemorrhoids

- Summarize the effects of exercise on GI pathological conditions

- Suggest nondrug interventions for the treatment of GERD, PUD, constipation, diarrhea, IBS, IBD, and hemorrhoids

- Explain how proton-pump inhibitors (PPIs) and H_2-receptor antagonist drugs affect GERD, PUD, and heartburn

- Compare and contrast PPIs and H_2-receptor antagonist categories of drugs

- Describe a drug therapy regimen for the treatment of *Helicobacter pylori* (*H pylori*)–associated ulcers

- Summarize the mechanism of action, dosing regimen, and adverse effects of medications that are considered physical barriers in the treatment of GERD and PUD

- Identify the different types of laxatives and recall their uses, mechanisms of action, dosing regimens, and potential adverse effects

- Identify common antidiarrheal medications and recall their mechanisms of action, dosing regimens, and potential adverse effects and drug interactions

- Identify the medications available to treat IBS and explain their mechanisms of action

- Explain the mechanisms of action for drugs used to treat IBD and recall their potential adverse effects

- Identify 8 categories of hemorrhoid medications and recall their mechanisms of action and potential adverse effects

- Summarize the role of the athletic trainer for patients who are self-medicating for GI symptoms or are on a physician-prescribed formal GI drug therapy regimen

Houglum JE, Harrelson GL, Seefeldt TM.
Principles of Pharmacology for Athletic Trainers, Third Edition (pp 187-208).
© 2016 Taylor & Francis Group.

ABBREVIATIONS USED IN THIS CHAPTER

AIDS. acquired immuno-deficiency syndrome	**IBS.** irritable bowel syndrome
ANC. acid-neutralizing capacity	**LES.** lower esophageal sphincter
CNS. central nervous system	**NSAID.** nonsteroidal anti-inflammatory drug
COX. cyclooxygenase	**OTC.** over-the-counter
FDA. Food and Drug Administration	**PG.** prostaglandin
	PGI$_2$. prostacyclin
GERD. gastroesophageal reflux disease	**PPI.** proton-pump inhibitor
GI. gastrointestinal	**PUD.** peptic ulcer disease
H$_2$RA. histamine-receptor antagonist	**t½.** half-life
IBD. inflammatory bowel disease	

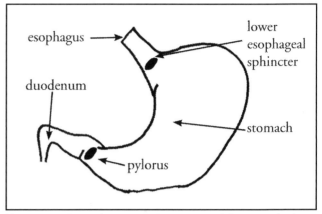

Figure 11-1. Stomach anatomy. During normal function, the lower esophageal sphincter prevents reflux of gastric acid and other contents into the esophagus, and the pylorus prevents unnecessary flow of gastric acid into the duodenum and prevents entry of bile acids into the stomach. (Adapted from Lichtenstein GR. *The Clinician's Guide to Inflammatory Bowel Disease.* Thorofare, NJ: SLACK Incorporated; 2003.)

FOUNDATIONAL CONCEPTS

The esophagus, stomach, and small intestine have several mechanisms to protect those tissues from being damaged and to keep them functioning properly. Due to the harsh environment of acidity and digestive enzymes, an inappropriate diet, ingestion of certain drugs and chemicals, or the aging process, these mechanisms are compromised and result in GI disorders. A brief discussion of the GI disorders will be helpful to understand the mechanism of action and logic of drug therapy. The focus areas of this section are the causes and symptoms of these disorders. Common terminology is also defined.

Key Aspects of Gastrointestinal Physiology

From the mouth, the esophagus empties into the stomach (Figure 11-1), where the acidity can result in a pH range of 1 to 5, depending on stomach contents. The lower esophageal sphincter provides a barrier between the stomach and the esophagus. This sphincter is usually constricted but relaxes during swallowing to allow the food to pass into the stomach. Because the esophagus does not have the same protective mechanisms as the stomach, one purpose of the sphincter is to prevent stomach acid and digestive enzymes from coming in contact with the esophageal tissue.

Gastric acid (hydrochloric acid) is released at a relatively low, baseline rate when food or other stimuli are not present. This baseline rate fluctuates, with greater production at night. The presence of food in the stomach causes the release of gastrin and acetylcholine, the latter also

There are many GI disorders, with an array of varied characteristics. Characteristics range from acute to chronic (traveler's diarrhea vs GERD); mild to incapacitating (heartburn vs IBS); fairly well understood to complex and poorly understood (PUD vs IBD); and few therapy choices to many choices (diarrhea vs PUD). Consequently, it is beyond the intent of this book to discuss every GI disorder and appropriate therapy. The intent of this chapter is to give the athletic trainer an overview of the most common GI disorders, their etiology, and the information regarding the most commonly used drugs for treatment of GERD, PUD, constipation, diarrhea, IBS, IBD, and hemorrhoids.

Many patients do not seek medical assistance for proper diagnosis and treatment of GERD, PUD, constipation, and diarrhea because, in part, there are many over-the-counter (OTC) medications available to treat these disorders. Because these are drugs that the athlete, like the general population, will be using with the least oversight by a health care professional, they are the focus of this chapter. The athletic trainer may be in a position to be the health care professional to provide some oversight in the form of basic advice regarding nondrug measures that may help alleviate symptoms and the appropriate use and potential effects from the drug therapy, or to refer athletes with GI disorders to the appropriate health care professional for additional care.

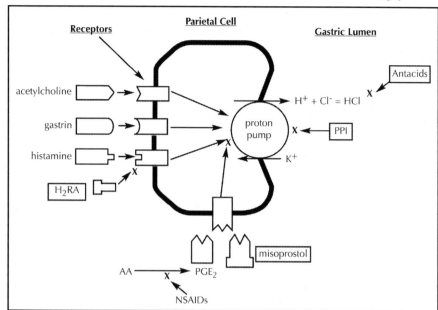

Figure 11-2. Production and inhibition of gastric acid. The parietal cell of the stomach is the source of acid production as it pumps protons (H⁺) into the gastric lumen to form hydrochloric (HCl) acid. Acetylcholine, gastrin, and histamine bind to their respective receptors located on the surface of the parietal cell membrane, initiating a sequence of events inside the cell culminating in the secretion of protons by the proton pump. In a similar fashion, PG E$_2$ (PGE$_2$; see Chapter 6) binds to its receptor but causes a decrease in acid production as a mechanism to prevent excessive acid secretion. The drugs used to affect acidity are designated in ☐ and their site of action designated by X. Proton pump inhibitors (PPIs), H$_2$-receptor antagonists (H$_2$RAs), and PGE$_2$ receptor agonists (misoprostol) decrease acid production, whereas antacids neutralize the acid after it is released. The site of action of NSAIDs is also shown, which inhibit the protective effects of endogenous PGE$_2$. AA = arachidonic acid.

being released in response to the sight and smell of food. Histamine is also released by specialized stomach cells. The parietal cells of the stomach have receptors for histamine (H$_2$ receptors), acetylcholine, and gastrin. The binding of any of these 3 compounds to their respective receptor on the parietal cells (Figure 11-2) activates a process called the *proton pump* (also known as the H$^+$, K$^+$-ATPase), which actively transports hydrogen ions (protons = H$^+$) into the stomach to combine with chloride ions to form hydrochloric acid. There are several mechanisms that help prevent excessive acid production. Two such mechanisms are the production of prostaglandins (PGs) E$_2$ (PGE$_2$) and I$_2$ (PGI$_2$); PGE$_2$ inhibits acid secretion from parietal cells, and PGI$_2$ increases secretion of protective mucus and bicarbonate buffer from epithelial cells.

One role of stomach acid in digestion is to activate the digestive enzyme pepsin. Pepsinogen is the inactive form of pepsin; it is produced by stomach cells and released into the stomach in response to autonomic regulation. The acidic pH of the stomach catalyzes the conversion of pepsinogen to pepsin.

When food leaves the stomach, it enters the duodenum, the first segment of the small intestine, where most of the digestion and absorption of food (and drugs) occurs. The pyloric sphincter prevents intestinal enzymes and bile from entering the stomach and minimizes gastric acid movement into the small intestine. Damage to the duodenal mucosa can occur if gastric acid regularly passes into the duodenum. In the large intestine, normal bacterial flora has an important role because these bacteria break down waste products and produce some vitamins that are absorbed into the bloodstream. There are also a small number of potentially pathogenic bacteria and yeast present in the colon, but, under normal circumstances, their numbers are too small to present a significant problem. Serious problems (diarrhea is a common symptom) can occur if these pathogens are allowed to increase in number because of disease, diet, or drugs.

> *Drugs that combine with the acetylcholine receptor and have an action like acetylcholine are called* cholinergic drugs. *Because acetylcholine activates the parasympathetic nervous system, cholinergic drugs are also called* parasympathomimetics.

Peristalsis moves the contents through the small and large intestines. Mucus is produced to protect and lubricate the intestinal tract; local irritation and stress increase mucus production. The rhythmic movement of the intestinal smooth muscle and mucus secretion are increased by parasympathetic innervation and decreased by the sympathetic system. Consequently, cholinergic drugs will increase the rate at which the contents move through the intestine. If movement of intestinal contents is too fast, there is insufficient absorption of water and other intestinal contents from the intestine, and diarrhea results. Inhibition of the parasympathetic system (ie, anticholinergic drugs) causes constipation. Other mechanisms can also alter the normal absorption rate of water, electrolytes, and dietary contents and thus cause diarrhea or constipation. These include a change in the amount or type of bacteria in the intestinal flora, the presence of poorly absorbed substances (eg, magnesium ions), or inflammatory intestinal disease.

Disorders of the Gastrointestinal Tract

The GI disorders discussed in this section are primarily limited to those for which treatment is discussed later. The

---

Box 11-1

Protective Stomach Mechanisms for Gastric Acid

- Secretion of the mucous barrier
- Secretion of the bicarbonate buffer
- Ability to repair damaged mucosal tissue
- Production of PGs

---

pathophysiology and mechanism of disease are discussed to an extent to facilitate an understanding of the approach to drug therapy.

Heartburn and Gastroesophageal Reflux Disease

Heartburn, also called *acid indigestion*, results from the contact of gastric acid, and to some extent bile and pepsin, with the esophageal mucosa. Heartburn feels like a burning chest pain primarily located behind the sternum, but it may move upward toward the neck. GERD is a chronic condition that exists when heartburn occurs regularly (ie, more than twice a week) and can be associated with significant complications. Reflux of acid may cause spontaneous regurgitation of gastric contents to the throat, which can initiate bronchial constriction in patients with asthma. Because heartburn and GERD are often self-treated, it is difficult to accurately determine the incidence rate, but up to 40% of adults experience heartburn symptoms at least once a month.

Repeated reflux for an extended period can result in reflux esophagitis or erosive esophagitis, which is associated with progressive inflammation and erosion of the esophageal mucosa. Barrett's esophagus can occur due to years of reflux; this is a premalignant change in epithelial cells of the esophagus that significantly increases the risk for esophageal cancer. Barrett's esophagus occurs in approximately 10% to 20% of patients with chronic GERD and is a risk factor for esophageal cancer development.

The basic cause of heartburn is that the lower esophageal sphincter is inefficient in preventing the reflux of stomach contents into the esophagus; eventually, the presence of gastric acid and pepsin causes damage to esophageal tissue. A dysfunction of the pyloric sphincter can also allow some bile acid to enter the stomach and contribute to GERD symptoms.

The reflux of gastric acid, pepsin, and bile into the esophagus is most often due to spontaneous and transient relaxation of the sphincter. Reflux may also occur because of increased intra-abdominal pressure during straining, bending over, coughing, or eating or during pregnancy. Certain foods and drugs can directly irritate the esopha-

geal mucosa, increase gastric acid production, or decrease the lower esophageal sphincter pressure, thereby decreasing sphincter effectiveness. Examples are chocolate, coffee, carbonated beverages, fatty foods, orange and tomato juice, tomato-based foods, spicy foods, garlic, onions, peppermint, spearmint, caffeine (from any source), anticholinergics, alcohol, aspirin, and other nonsteroidal anti-inflammatory drugs (NSAIDs). Fatty foods and large meals delay gastric emptying and increase the likelihood of reflux in patients who experience GERD. Factors that tend to protect the esophagus, such as the saliva buffering that coats the esophagus, diminish with age, and therefore damage to the esophagus occurs more often in the elderly. Hiatal hernia can also be the cause of GERD. This condition exists when the stomach partially sits in the chest cavity because of a weakness in the diaphragm. The severity of GERD depends on the amount and frequency of acid refluxing into the esophagus as well as the ability of the saliva to neutralize the acid. Long-term GERD can cause complications, including ulcers, cancer, or narrowing of the esophagus, which interferes with swallowing. Some people experience symptoms of GERD primarily at night when they are lying down. In this position, it is easier for reflux to occur because gravity is not opposing the reflux, and during this time there is less saliva being swallowed to act as a buffer.

Peptic Ulcer Disease

Peptic ulcers are chronic erosion of the mucosa of the stomach (gastric ulcer) or small intestine (duodenal ulcer). PUD affects a significant number of Americans, with approximately 500,000 people diagnosed annually; however, the incidence and complications of PUD have been declining. Abdominal pain is the most common symptom and may include burning or cramping, although some patients are asymptomatic. Pain often begins 1 to 3 hours after eating and is alleviated by food or antacids. Many patients have pain that awakens them from sleep. The most significant life-threatening problems associated with peptic ulcers are GI bleeding and perforation.

Gastric acid contributes to the cause of the peptic ulcer as well as the pain. There is usually an increased production of gastric acid associated with duodenal ulcers. However, the ulcerogenic effect of gastric acid occurs after one or more of the normal protection mechanisms have been compromised (Box 11-1). The defense mechanisms are compromised most frequently by use of NSAIDs or by *H pylori* infection. There is also a significant causal relationship from cigarette smoking, but much less convincing correlation exists to directly connect diet and psychological stress as contributors.

Over half the people in the world may be infected with *H pylori*, a gram-negative bacterium that has the ability to live between the mucous layer and the epithelial cells of the stomach. Transmission is by fecal-to-oral route such as through contaminated food or water. Mouth-to-mouth transfer is also possible. Peptic ulcer eventually develops in approximately 15% of the population infected with *H pylori*, but almost every person with non–NSAID-induced PUD is infected with *H pylori*, and elimination of *H pylori* significantly reduces the incidence of ulcer recurrence.

H pylori has the ability to buffer hydrochloric acid in the organism's immediate vicinity and to cause damage to gastric mucosa by release of various enzymes and other factors produced by the organism. Other ramifications of the infection are increased gastric acid secretion associated with duodenal ulcers and an altered immune response to the infection, which may contribute to the damage of gastric epithelial cells. Infection with *H pylori* is the most common cause of duodenal and gastric ulcers.

NSAIDs are among the most commonly used prescription and OTC drugs and are the drugs most frequently associated with causing peptic ulcers. Repeated use of NSAIDs is the most common cause of PUD, particularly gastric ulcers, in patients not infected with *H pylori*. Risk factors that increase the occurrence of complications from NSAID use are listed in Box 11-2. NSAIDs cause ulcers through topical irritation due to the acidic nature of most of these drugs, especially aspirin, and due to the systemic effect on PG synthesis. Additionally, these drugs may slow the healing process in existing peptic ulcers and contribute to GI bleeding because of their ability to inhibit platelet aggregation.

> *Recall from Chapter 6 that synthesis of PGs, thromboxanes, and prostacyclin (as a group referred to as eicosanoids) require the activity of an enzyme called cyclooxygenase (COX) and that there are 2 forms of the COX enzyme: COX-1 and COX-2. COX-1 is produced in virtually all tissues so that an appropriate level of eicosanoids exists to regulate normal functions. COX-2 is also produced for this purpose in some tissues, but the activity of COX-2 is greatly increased in response to pain and tissue injury. PG production by stomach cells is a protection mechanism against the effects of stomach acid; NSAIDs diminish the protectant effect by inhibiting COX, particularly COX-1.*

> *Recall from Chapter 6 that TXA_2 causes platelet aggregation but NSAIDs inhibit TXA_2 production in platelets. Aspirin has a more pronounced effect than other NSAIDs regarding this effect.*

Constipation

The "normal" frequency of bowel movements varies from one person to another, and therefore the definition of

---

Box 11-2

RISK FACTORS THAT INCREASE THE OCCURRENCE OF PEPTIC ULCER COMPLICATIONS FROM NONSTEROIDAL ANTI-INFLAMMATORY DRUGS

- Higher daily dosage
- Longer duration of daily use
- Advanced age of the patient, history of peptic ulcer
- Concurrent use of corticosteroids or anticoagulants

---

constipation is not universal. Nonetheless, constipation is generally considered to exist if there are less than 3 bowel movements per week, if stools are hard and dry, if straining is necessary for bowel evacuation, or if there is a feeling of incomplete bowel evacuation. Although it occurs at any age, the incidence of constipation increases among those older than 65 years, with about one-third of this population reporting constipation as a problem. Constipation is a symptom, not a disease itself.

The cause of constipation can be associated with endocrine diseases such as diabetes mellitus or hypothyroidism. The incidence of drug-induced constipation is most significant with the use of drugs that have anticholinergic effects (eg, tricyclic antidepressants and antihistamines), opioid analgesics, and calcium- or aluminum-containing antacids. Lifestyle, primarily related to diet and exercise, influences bowel regularity. Dietary fiber increases the bulk of the fecal mass and stimulates peristalsis. Exercise increases abdominal muscle tone and facilitates the effect of gravity on bowel function. Sufficient water intake is also an important aspect to prevent dry, hard stools that can cause constipation. Water depletion from exercise must also be considered. As people get older, changes in diet, exercise, muscle tone, and therapeutic drug regimens may all be contributing factors to constipation. Another cause of constipation related to lifestyle is merely a conscious effort to prevent a bowel movement because of inconvenient timing (ie, busy lifestyle).

Besides a diminished frequency of bowel movements, other symptoms of constipation can include headache, back pain, and abdominal discomfort. Further complications from constipation are primarily due to the need to strain during a bowel movement. Such an effort can eventually result in hemorrhoids, and patients with existing heart problems or hypertension can exacerbate those conditions while straining.

Diarrhea

Diarrhea is an increased frequency of bowel movements or decreased consistency of stool compared with the norm for that person. Two bowel movements per day could be normal for one person but considered diarrhea for another. As with constipation, diarrhea is not a disease but rather a symptom of an underlying condition. Most episodes of diarrhea are self-limiting, but severe or chronic cases can be fatal, usually due to dehydration. Acute diarrhea usually lasts 1 to 3 days but could extend as long as 2 weeks. Chronic diarrhea lasts for a few weeks or more and requires more extensive medical attention to diagnose the cause, to monitor the patient's hydration and nutritional status, and to treat appropriately with both drug and nondrug measures. The focus of this discussion will be acute diarrhea.

The intestine absorbs almost 9 L of fluid per day, most of it from the small intestine. Diarrhea occurs because of a change in the normal processes of absorption or secretion of water and electrolytes from the intestine or a decrease in time to travel through the intestinal tract (ie, increased motility), which prevents fluid reabsorption. If the amount of water in the colon exceeds the amount that can be reabsorbed, diarrhea will result. This can occur for several reasons. Some illnesses such as acquired immunodeficiency syndrome (AIDS), IBD, and IBS have diarrhea as a symptom. Some drugs cause diarrhea by directly affecting the intestinal content of water and electrolytes (eg, antacids containing magnesium), disrupting the normal bacterial flora (eg, antibiotics, especially broad spectrum such as tetracyclines), damaging GI epithelial cells (eg, some anticancer drugs), or increasing GI motility with cholinergic agonists such as bethanechol (Urecholine), which is used to treat urinary retention. Some undigested foods have a laxative effect, such as foods that are very fatty or have high roughage content. Patients who are lactose intolerant will experience diarrhea from lactose-containing foods (ie, dairy products).

Patients with lactose intolerance lack the digestive enzyme lactase. Therefore, lactose remains in the GI tract and becomes a nutrient for bacterial flora. Byproducts of enhanced bacterial metabolism cause cramps and diarrhea.

However, most cases of diarrhea are caused by bacterial, protozoal, and viral infections, often through contaminated food or water. For example, traveler's diarrhea is usually caused by various bacteria; the major causative agent differs from country to country. In the United States, *Campylobacter*, *Salmonella*, and *Escherichia coli* are often pinpointed as causative bacteria in food contamination. Some bacteria cause diarrhea by producing toxins, whereas others directly affect the intestinal mucosal cells. Damage to epithelial intestinal cells decreases the absorption of solutes to cause an osmotic effect (ie, an increase in water content) in the GI tract. An inflammatory response to the infection decreases water absorption and increases mucus release into the intestinal lumen.

Most viral-induced diarrhea is from the 24-hour flu-type viruses that produce a sudden onset of diarrhea, which lasts 24 to 48 hours. *Giardia lamblia* is a common cause of protozoal diarrhea. It is transmitted by ingestion of fecal material from contaminated streams or lakes and is also prevalent among day care centers.

Symptoms of acute diarrhea include frequent, watery stools; abdominal cramps; fever; vomiting; and weakness. Symptoms may occur within hours or take a few days, depending on the cause. For example, infection with *Salmonella* will initiate symptoms within 12 to 24 hours and *E coli* 8 to 72 hours, whereas it takes 2 to 4 days for the onset of symptoms from *Campylobacter* and 1 to 3 weeks for *Giardia*. Symptoms from most infectious diarrhea are self-limiting and last a few days, although *Giardia* may persist if not treated adequately. The most common complication of diarrhea is dehydration. Symptoms of mild dehydration are dry mouth and thirst. If dehydration progresses, additional symptoms may include dry mucous membranes, increased pulse, rapid breathing, lethargy, and confusion.

Irritable Bowel Syndrome

IBS is a common disorder in which the colon, for no apparent reason, is more sensitive to stimuli than normal. As a result, diet, hormones, and nerve impulses have an enhanced impact on the contraction of the large intestinal smooth muscle. For example, psychological or emotional stress (eg, anxiety and depression) and foods (eg, dairy products, onions, beans, broccoli, chocolate, alcohol, caffeine, dietary fat, artificial sweeteners, and herbal teas) are common triggers. Onset of symptoms is often early adulthood and is typically initiated during a stressful event. For some patients, symptoms improve and disappear; for others they persist. There is no known underlying disease that causes the symptoms of IBS, nor does IBS eventually progress to another disease.

The most common symptoms of IBS are abdominal cramps and pain; gassiness; bloating; and either diarrhea, constipation, or diarrhea alternating with constipation. The diarrhea results from the increased frequency and force of smooth muscle contraction, and the constipation is caused by spasms that delay movement through the colon. The frequency and extent of these symptoms vary among patients from mild to disabling. Diagnosis is primarily based on the elimination of other causes of the symptoms.

Inflammatory Bowel Disease

IBD is a term that refers to 2 similar diseases: Crohn's disease and ulcerative colitis. As the name implies, a major characteristic of these diseases is inflammation. IBD can affect people of all ages, but the onset of symptoms is usually between ages 15 and 25 years, and the incidence is approximately 5 per 100,000 population. Crohn's disease usually involves the small and large intestines but can affect any part of the digestive tract. All layers of the intestinal wall can be affected, and the lesions are not continuous (ie, not confined to one area). Ulceration of intestinal tissue causes significant damage. Ulcerative colitis involves inflammation of the colon and rectum. Inflammation does not involve the full thickness of the bowel wall, and the affected area is continuous. The cause of these diseases is unknown, but it is likely that genetic factors predispose patients to an autoimmune mechanism; for example, antibodies produced in response to a microbial infection are antibodies of a genetically determined structure that happen to also attack the patient's normal cells in the GI tract.

The symptoms of IBD include painful abdominal cramps and pain, fever, diarrhea, rectal bleeding, anemia, and weight loss. There are different levels of severity (mild, moderate, severe), and the severity fluctuates over time for any given patient. However, in all cases, these diseases have pronounced symptoms and potential for complications involving other tissues (eg, eyes, joints, liver, and skin). The nature of these diseases necessitates that the patient be under the direct and careful supervision of a physician. Drug therapy is a necessary part of treatment, but dietary modification and management of the resulting emotional stress are also parts of the treatment approach. When drug therapy cannot control the symptoms, surgery is indicated to remove the affected portion of intestine. Surgery is usually curative for ulcerative colitis where the affected area is confined, but recurrence is the norm for Crohn's disease.

Hemorrhoids

Hemorrhoids are painful swelling of hemorrhoidal blood vessels at the anus. The vessels involved may be venous or arterial and may be internal or external; some patients have a combination of internal and external. Many factors have been attributed to the cause of hemorrhoids. Among these are pregnancy, constipation, diarrhea, straining with stool, heavy lifting with straining, prolonged sitting or standing, and heredity.

Mild symptoms of hemorrhoids include bleeding, itching, burning, and inflammation. More severe symptoms are increased bleeding, anal pain, protrusion outside the anal canal of hemorrhoidal or rectal tissue, seepage of fecal material, or blood clot formation within the blood vessel. Bleeding can occur with external hemorrhoids and usually occurs with internal hemorrhoids, typically after defecation. Chronic blood loss can cause anemia. Symptoms similar to hemorrhoids are also a part of other anorectal diseases (eg, polyps and cancer); therefore, accurate diagnosis is necessary. There are many OTC products available to treat the various symptoms associated with hemorrhoids, but large or protruding hemorrhoids are often surgically removed.

Exercise-Induced Problems

Some GI symptoms may be a result of, or exacerbated by, exercise. For example, diarrhea is a common problem among athletes, particularly participants in endurance sports. For long-distance runners, the persistent jarring of the intestinal tract during long-distance running or the diminished blood supply to the GI tract while the demand for blood to skeletal muscles is increased may play a role in causing diarrhea. Running may also aggravate preexisting IBS in some patients. Diarrhea among early-morning runners is a relatively common complaint. GERD occurs more frequently during exercise than at rest. Symptoms of GERD increase with increasing intensity of exercise, and exercise with more jarring is more problematic. Eating just before exercising can also contribute to symptoms of GERD.

Section Summary

Gastric acid is produced by the stomach and transported into the lumen by a proton-pump mechanism (see Figure 11-2). Gastrin, acetylcholine, and histamine increase the release of gastric acid. The lower esophageal sphincter protects the esophagus from the damage by gastric acid. When the sphincter does not function properly, gastric acid can reflux into the esophagus and irritate the gastroesophageal mucosa, causing occasional heartburn or GERD if it occurs frequently. GERD-associated erosive esophagitis can also develop. Citrus fruits and juices, carbonated beverages, coffee, caffeine, alcohol, fatty and spicy foods, and NSAIDs exacerbate GERD symptoms. The most common symptom is chest pain located behind the sternum. Exercise, such as running that involves jarring of the abdominal organs, and exercising soon after eating can contribute to GERD symptoms.

PUD encompasses gastric and duodenal ulcers. Chronic use of NSAIDs and the presence of *H pylori* are the 2 causative agents linked to most PUD. Gastric acid contributes to cause and symptoms of PUD. Abdominal pain is a common symptom, especially 1 to 3 hours after eating. The potential for GI bleeding and perforation are also serious concerns.

Acute constipation is a common GI disorder, and although adverse effects of drugs are sometimes the cause, proper diet, exercise, and adequate fluid intake can prevent the problem in many situations. On the other hand, diarrhea may be caused by food, infection, drugs, or long-distance running in some athletes. Diarrhea and constipation are also among the most common symptoms of IBS, along with bloating, gassiness, and cramps. Patients with IBS are very sensitive to stimuli that cause these symptoms; common stimuli include certain foods and stress.

IBD refers to Crohn's disease and ulcerative colitis. Inflammation of various portions of the intestine, possibly due to an autoimmune mechanism, causes diarrhea, cramps, and pain. Other tissues (eg, eyes, joints, liver, and

---

Box 11-3

NONDRUG MEASURES THAT CAN ASSIST IN THE TREATMENT OF GASTROESOPHAGEAL REFLUX DISEASE

- Avoid foods that exacerbate symptoms, such as spicy foods, coffee, caffeine, citrus juices, and tomato juice, which have a direct irritant effect on damaged esophageal tissue; fatty foods, alcohol, chocolate, peppermint, and spearmint, which decrease lower esophageal sphincter; and carbonated beverages, which contribute to acidity, increase pressure in the stomach, and contribute to reflux through belching.

- Stop smoking cigarettes.

- Elevate the head of the bed 6 to 8 inches by raising the legs at the head of the bed or by placing supports under the mattress. This improves clearance of acid from the esophagus and adds the benefit of gravity. Merely adding pillows does not help. Lying on the left side rather than the right side may be helpful.

- Avoid large meals or lying down within 3 hours after eating (eg, eating before bedtime).

- Minimize anything that increases abdominal pressure, such as obesity, straining during bowel movements, and tight-fitting clothing.

- Eliminate as much as possible the use of drugs that have anticholinergic effects (eg, antihistamines, tricyclic antidepressants, and opioid analgesics), which will delay the movement of food from the stomach.

- Use a large amount of liquid when taking drugs that have a direct mucosal irritating effect, such as NSAIDs, tetracycline antibiotics, iron, potassium supplements, and oral bisphosphonates such as alendronate (Fosamax) and risedronate (Actonel), which are used to treat osteoporosis; this helps to move the drug through the esophagus quicker.

- Avoid vigorous exercise for 2 to 3 hours after eating.

---

skin) may also be involved. Drug therapy, diet, and stress management are part of therapy, but surgery is an option if these are insufficiently effective.

Hemorrhoids result from the swelling of hemorrhoid vessels and can cause itching, burning, anal pain, and bleeding. Factors that precipitate hemorrhoids include pregnancy, poor bowel habits, heavy lifting and straining, sitting and standing for prolonged periods, and heredity.

GENERAL NONDRUG CONSIDERATIONS

There are a few nondrug measures that can be taken to help alleviate and reduce the recurrence of symptoms from the GI disorders discussed in this chapter. A change of lifestyle to incorporate these measures may be the most difficult aspect of therapy for some patients.

Gastroesophageal Reflux Disease

Treatment is aimed at alleviating the immediate symptoms, decreasing the frequency and/or acidity of the reflux, promoting healing of the esophageal mucosa, and preventing

recurrence. Sometimes a combination of approaches is warranted to eliminate symptoms and facilitate healing. There are several nondrug measures that should be implemented to assist in accomplishing these treatment goals (Box 11-3).

Peptic Ulcer Disease

PUD is not a self-care disease. Patients who have symptoms related to PUD should first obtain appropriate diagnosis. If use of NSAIDs is not a contributor to PUD, then infection with *H pylori* is likely. Tests are available to confirm the presence of the organism. The treatment regimen will vary depending on the etiology of the disease. Eradication of *H pylori* is the principal effort in treating PUD caused by this infection, whereas diminishing the effect of NSAIDs and inhibiting gastric acid production is the focus of therapy for NSAID-induced PUD. In either case, prescription drugs are a part of the most effective drug regimen. However, regardless of the underlying cause, the goal for treating PUD is to alleviate pain, facilitate healing, and prevent recurrence of the disease. Some specific nondrug measures that are helpful in accomplishing these treatment goals include eliminating the use of NSAIDs, avoiding foods that aggravate the patient's symptoms (eg, alcohol, caffeine, carbonated beverages, and spicy foods), and eliminating cigarette smoking. If use of NSAIDs cannot be eliminated, then either lowering the dose or switching to an NSAID that is more selective for COX-2 (see Table 6-4) may decrease the problem. The use of corticosteroids in combination with NSAID therapy increases the risk of PUD and exacerbates existing PUD. Therefore, this combination should be avoided in patients with PUD, and other patients using these drugs concurrently should be monitored for PUD. The evidence is not clear whether oral corticosteroid therapy alone contributes to PUD, but caution warrants that patients on corticosteroid therapy be watchful for the symptoms of PUD.

Constipation

There are several classes of drugs that are effective in the treatment of constipation, but therapy should also include lifestyle changes that can help alleviate the problem. Among these lifestyle changes are adequate fiber and fluid intake. Adult daily fiber intake should be 20 to 30 g. This can be achieved through high-fiber foods such as bran cereals, fruits (especially apricots, dates, apples, prunes, and raisins), vegetables (especially green beans, peas, corn, broccoli, and carrots), and legumes. Plenty of fluid intake, primarily water, is also important, although the amount necessary varies depending on factors such as daily fluid loss (eg, sweating) and kidney function. Regular exercise can also help to maintain normal bowel function. Not to be overlooked is the contribution of drug therapy to the cause of constipation. In some cases, a change in therapy may be possible without sacrificing therapeutic outcomes (eg, switching from aluminum-containing antacid to one containing both aluminum and magnesium, or switching from a first-generation to a second-generation antihistamine for treatment of allergies).

As noted later in this chapter, magnesium has a laxative effect, whereas aluminum has a constipating effect. Also, recall from Chapter 10 that first-generation antihistamines may have anticholinergic adverse effects, which include constipation.

Diarrhea

Acute mild to moderate diarrhea is by definition self-limiting and can usually be readily managed by combining drug therapy with nondrug measures. The goals of therapy are to relieve the symptoms and prevent fluid and electrolyte loss. However, patients with severe or chronic diarrhea should seek medical assistance so that the underlying cause can be determined and treated. This includes patients who experience diarrhea along with repeated vomiting, high fever, abdominal pain, or blood in the stool.

Regular diet may be suitable for patients with diarrhea, although avoiding foods rich in fat, simple sugar, spices, or caffeine may be advantageous because these could contribute to diarrhea. A priority in dietary management is to prevent depletion of fluids and electrolytes. Oral rehydration products are available that contain sodium and other electrolytes along with a low concentration of glucose (2.5%). The active transport of glucose during absorption from the GI tract also facilitates the absorption of sodium and water. However, the use of high concentrations of glucose (> 10%) and other simple sugars can have an osmotic diarrhea effect and thus cause additional problems. Sports drinks that do not have high glucose concentrations (eg, Gatorade, Powerade, All Sport) may be used as a rehydration solution for mild diarrhea in older children and adults, especially if additional sodium is provided (eg, crackers).

If the cause of acute diarrhea can be identified, then removal of the causative agent is obviously a part of nondrug measures. For example, if the cause is lactase deficiency, then identifying and removing the source of lactose is appropriate. Diarrhea from the use of antibiotics, NSAIDs, or other drugs may warrant a change in drug therapy or reduction of the dosage.

Irritable Bowel Syndrome

The focus of nondrug treatment is management of diet, eating habits, and stress. Keeping a diary of foods eaten and symptoms experienced may help pinpoint specific foods that are exacerbating the disease. Introducing gas into the intestine can also contribute to symptoms, and therefore it may be helpful to eliminate carbonated beverages and chewing gum (which causes swallowing of air). Smaller rather than larger meals can also reduce cramping and diarrhea. Patients with constipation as a predominant symptom should increase dietary fiber and fluid intake. Other approaches that are effective in reducing symptoms are stress management and relaxation, including exercise.

Inflammatory Bowel Disease

The most notable nondrug measure for patients with IBD is to maintain proper nutrition. Inflammation of the GI tract can diminish the digestion and absorption of food in that portion of the digestive tract. Obviously, patients who have had surgical removal of affected portions of the GI tract will have a similar problem. Dietary supplements are generally sufficient to satisfy the nutritional needs. Among the supplements, iron may be needed if blood loss has been significant, and folic acid should be given with sulfasalazine therapy because this drug diminishes absorption of folic acid. Patients with severe IBD may require parenteral nutrition.

Hemorrhoids

Because poor bowel habits can contribute to hemorrhoids, improvement in these habits is a good starting point for treatment. Avoiding constipation, diarrhea, straining with stool, and prolonged sitting on the toilet are all helpful. To prevent constipation, the patient may need to modify dietary habits, such as increasing fiber and fluid intake, and add exercise. Patients should also avoid heavy lifting or straining. Taking these actions will not alleviate existing symptoms but may reduce further aggravation of these symptoms. Use of a sitz bath for several minutes 2 to 3 times per day may provide some symptomatic relief.

Section Summary

Not surprisingly, diet and eating habits have an impact on the occurrence of symptoms for each of the diseases or conditions that affect the GI tract. Therefore, a common recommendation among the nondrug measures for treating these conditions is dietary modification. Fatty or spicy food, onions, coffee, alcohol, chocolate, citrus juices, and carbonated beverages are among the foods that can exacerbate symptoms of GERD. Many of these same foods are problematic for patients with PUD. Patients with constipation should increase the amount of high-fiber foods in their diets and enhance their fluid intake. On the other hand, diarrhea requires the patient to guard against fluid and electrolyte loss. Certain foods may exacerbate symptoms of IBS, but the causative foods differ somewhat from patient to patient. Patients can monitor their diet along with occurrence of symptoms to identify the foods that should be avoided. For IBD, rather than avoiding foods, nutritional supplementation is of greatest diet-related concern.

Drugs can also adversely affect these diseases. Drugs such as NSAIDs, tetracycline antibiotics, potassium, iron supplements, and oral bisphosphonate drugs can irritate the mucosa of the esophagus and enhance the pain associated with GERD. NSAIDs are also the major contributor to the drug-induced symptoms of PUD. Many drugs have the potential to cause constipation or diarrhea. In particular, drugs that have anticholinergic adverse effects and calcium- and aluminum-containing antacids can contribute to constipation; NSAIDs and some antibiotics are potential causes of drug-induced diarrhea.

GASTROINTESTINAL DRUGS

Most approaches to therapy for GERD and PUD are to neutralize the existing acidity of gastric acid, inhibit the secretion of the acid, physically block the effect of the acid on tissue, or increase the natural protective effects of mucus. Drugs that inhibit the secretion of gastric acid or chemically neutralize the acidity will cause an increase in gastric pH, which is an important factor to facilitate healing, and decrease the activation of pepsinogen to pepsin. The longer the time during the day that the pH is maintained above 4, the better the esophageal healing rate from GERD-induced damage. Chronic constipation and diarrhea may be caused from an underlying disease, and thus a key part of treatment involves treating the underlying disease. However, acute mild constipation and diarrhea may be idiopathic and self-limiting and respond adequately to OTC medications.

Not surprisingly, the site of action of many of the GI drugs discussed in this chapter is within the GI tract; many are not appreciably absorbed, and thus their systemic effects are somewhat minimal. Even the GI drugs that work through a systemic mechanism (PPIs and histamine-receptor antagonists [H_2RA]) have relatively few prominent adverse effects. Consequently, discussions of the pharmacological effects are relatively brief.

Proton-Pump Inhibitors

PPIs are the most effective therapy for treatment of GERD, erosive esophagitis, and PUD and for maintenance therapy of GERD. These drugs inhibit the H^+, K^+-ATPase (see Figure 11-2). This ATPase is an enzyme that secretes protons (ie, acidity) into the stomach in exchange for K^+ and is therefore called the proton pump. As shown in Figure 11-2, the mechanism by which acetylcholine, gastrin, and histamine increase acidity is by activating the proton pump. Therefore, the effects of acetylcholine, gastrin, and histamine on acid secretion are inhibited by PPIs. These drugs irreversibly inhibit the ATPase enzyme and thus have a longer duration of action.

All PPIs are inactivated by gastric acid, and thus the oral products contain an enteric coating that is dissolved in alkaline pH, causing them to be rapidly absorbed from the small intestine. To ensure that the coating protects the drug, these products should not be crushed or chewed. Dosing is preferable about 15 to 60 minutes before a meal because PPIs only inhibit actively secreting proton pumps. For most patients, dosing prior to breakfast is advisable, although it may be advantageous for patients bothered particularly by nighttime symptoms to take the dose before the evening meal. PPIs have half-life of approximately 1 to 2 hours; however, their effect lasts much longer because they have an irreversible effect on the proton pump, making dosing once per day effective. Adult doses are shown in Table 11-1.

The incidence of adverse effects from PPIs is relatively low, and the effects are usually mild but can include headache, dizziness, nausea, constipation, or diarrhea. These drugs are metabolized by cytochrome P450 enzymes and thus have the potential to decrease the metabolism rate (ie, increase the effect) of several drugs, including warfarin

TABLE 11-1

PROTON-PUMP INHIBITORS—TYPICAL ADULT ORAL DOSAGE REGIMENS[a]

GENERIC NAME	TRADE NAME	PEPTIC ULCER DISEASE[b]	GERD	GERD WITH EROSIVE ESOPHAGITIS	GERD MAINTENANCE
dexlansoprazole	Dexilant	na	30 mg	60 mg	30 mg
esomeprazole[c]	Nexium	20 to 40 mg	20 mg	20 to 40 mg	20 mg
lansoprazole[d]	Prevacid	15 to 30 mg	15 mg	30 mg	15 mg
omeprazole[c]	Prilosec	20 to 40 mg	20 mg	20 mg	20 mg
pantoprazole	Protonix	na	na	40 mg	40 mg
rabeprazole	Aciphex	20 mg	20 mg	20 mg	20 mg

na = not approved for this use by the FDA.

[a]All dosages are once per day, and except for maintenance therapy, duration is 4 to 8 weeks.

[b]Includes prevention and treatment of NSAID-induced ulcers and eradication of *H. pylori* infection.

[c]Also available OTC at 20 mg/day for 14-day treatment of frequent (≥twice/week) heartburn.

[d]Also available OTC at 15 mg/day for 14-day treatment of frequent (≥twice/week) heartburn.

(an anticoagulant), phenytoin (an anticonvulsant), and benzodiazepines (antianxiety drugs).

Because the PPIs are well tolerated, 3 PPIs (omeprazole, lansoprazole, and esomeprazole) have reached OTC status. These drugs are available as once-per-day treatments for frequent (2 or more days per week) heartburn and are meant to be taken as 14-day courses of treatment. In addition, several combination products containing PPIs are available. For example, omeprazole is available in combination with the antibiotics clarithromycin and amoxicillin for treatment of ulcers caused by *H pylori*. Esomeprazole is available in combination with the NSAID naproxen; esomeprazole is found in this combination to reduce the risk for a naproxen-induced ulcer.

> *Recall from Chapter 2 that* cytochrome P450 (CYP450) *is a group of enzymes that are located in the liver and metabolize drugs.*

H₂-Receptor Antagonists

H₂RAs, also known as *H₂-blockers*, are competitive antagonists to histamine receptors on the stomach parietal cells (see Figure 11-2). Therefore, these drugs suppress gastric acid secretion and are effective in treating mild heartburn, GERD, and PUD. The H₂RAs are most effective in inhibiting basal and nocturnal gastric acid secretion as compared with the secretion stimulated by food or other triggers.

The H₂RAs can be used alone or combined with antacids. Table 11-2 provides examples and dosages for the H₂RAs. Lifestyle changes, along with a couple of weeks of treatment

with these drugs, are usually sufficient to alleviate symptoms of mild heartburn. Increased dosages and a longer treatment period are required to treat GERD. For example, dosages for ranitidine (Zantac) can range from 75 mg per day for up to 2 weeks for mild heartburn to 600 mg per day for up to 12 weeks for erosive esophagitis or moderate to severe GERD. In general, the higher dosage regimen and more frequent dosing interval provide better healing rates. Not surprisingly, patients with less severe GERD experience higher healing rates when comparing any given dosage regimen.

The H₂RAs are all absorbed orally, and some metabolism occurs in the liver, but kidney excretion is the major means by which drug action is terminated. The incidence of adverse effects (eg, headache and diarrhea) is low for the H₂RAs and, as a result, they are available OTC for self-care of heartburn or mild GERD. These drugs are approximately equally effective, and thus selection can be based on personal preference and/or cost. The one exception is regarding cimetidine (Tagamet), which, compared with the other H₂RAs, has a higher incidence of drug interactions, especially at higher doses. Cimetidine inhibits cytochrome P450 and can therefore increase the effect of other drugs that are also substrates for these enzymes. Examples include warfarin (an anticoagulant), phenytoin (an anticonvulsant), and benzodiazepines (antianxiety drugs).

Comparison of H₂-Receptor Antagonists and Proton-Pump Inhibitors

Therapy with PPIs is a more effective treatment for moderate to severe GERD than treatment with H₂RAs. After 4 weeks of therapy, healing rates are approximately 80% and

TABLE 11-2					
H₂-RECEPTOR ANTAGONISTS—TYPICAL ADULT ORAL DOSAGE REGIMENS					
GENERIC NAME	TRADE NAME	HEARTBURN	GERD	PEPTIC ULCER DISEASE	PEPTIC ULCER MAINTENANCE
cimetidine	Tagamet	200 mg prn 1 to 2 times/day	400 mg qid or 800 mg bid	800 mg hs or 300 mg qid or 400 mg bid	400 mg hs
famotidine	Pepcid	10 to 20 mg prn 1 to 2 times/day	20 mg bid	40 mg hs or 20 mg bid	20 mg hs
nizatidine	Axid	75 mg prn 1 to 2 times/day	150 mg bid	300 mg hs or 150 mg bid	150 mg hs
ranitidine	Zantac	75 mg prn 1 to 2 times/day	150 mg bid	300 mg hs or 150 mg bid	150 mg hs
bid = twice per day; hs = at bedtime; prn = as needed; qid = 4 times per day.					

50% for PPIs and H₂RAs, respectively. Healing rates increase after 8 weeks of therapy but are still higher for PPIs. Patients with severe GERD who are placed on maintenance therapy to prevent relapse have a lower incidence of relapse with PPIs than patients taking H₂RAs. The short-term use of an H₂RA at bedtime as an addition to PPI therapy has been effective to resolve nighttime symptoms of GERD, which sometimes occur due to increased nocturnal secretion rates.

Both of these categories of drugs are effective for treatment of PUD or as maintenance therapy for patients with recurrent ulcer symptoms. All of the H₂RAs are approximately equally effective in the treatment of PUD, as are all of the PPIs in comparison with each other. However, healing rates are somewhat higher, and relapse rates lower, with PPIs compared with H₂RAs. A PPI is generally recommended as a component of the 3-drug regimen to treat *H pylori*–associated ulcer. PPIs are also the preferred treatment of gastric ulcers induced by NSAIDs or if NSAID therapy must be continued despite the gastric or duodenal ulcer. As preventative therapy for patients taking NSAIDs and who are at risk for PUD (ie, elderly, PUD history, high-dose NSAID, and concurrent use of corticosteroids or anticoagulants), PPIs or misoprostol is preferred. Use of H₂RAs may prevent NSAID-induced duodenal ulcers, but higher doses are necessary to reduce the incidence of gastric ulcers, which occur more frequently than duodenal ulcers from NSAID use.

Combination Therapy to Treat Helicobacter pylori–Associated Ulcers

Many combinations of drugs and varied dosage regimens have been used to treat ulcers associated with *H pylori*. The intent of therapy is to treat immediate symptoms of PUD and to eradicate the infection as a means of preventing relapse. Several different combinations of drugs and varied

dosage regimens have demonstrated eradication rates of more than 80%. Use of just one drug does not achieve the same eradication rate nor is it as effective in preventing reoccurrence. For example, patients with *H pylori*–associated PUD who are treated with H₂RAs alone have a recurrence rate of more than 85% within 1 year, whereas patients treated with *H pylori* eradication therapy have a recurrence rate of approximately 20%. Although 2-drug regimens demonstrate a marked improvement in eradication rates compared with one-drug regimens, a variety of 3-drug regimens are considered superior. The use of 4-drug regimens has also been effective but introduces another layer of potential adverse effects and increases the likelihood of poorer compliance to therapy; however, it is an option if there is relapse following a 3-drug regimen.

Table 11-3 lists a few of the many multiple-drug regimens that are used. These combinations each include one or more antibiotics and a PPI. For example, frequently used combinations include a PPI, clarithromycin, and either amoxicillin or metronidazole. The 3-drug regimens that include clarithromycin are preferred in most situations. Chapter 5 discusses general principles regarding the use and effects of antibiotics, including specific aspects of therapy with penicillins and tetracyclines. Metronidazole is used to treat various protozoal infections but is also effective against anaerobic bacteria, including *Helicobacter*. Some adverse effects associated with the use of this antibiotic are nausea, vomiting, diarrhea, and a bad taste in the mouth. Bismuth has antibacterial effectiveness against *H pylori* and is a component of several multiple-drug regimens.

Antacids

The purpose of antacids is to neutralize some of the existing gastric acid and thus increase the gastric pH. Antacids are used for treatment of PUD, heartburn, and mild GERD, although they are less effective than H_2RAs and PPIs to treat these conditions. The ability to neutralize acid is expressed as milliequivalents of acid-neutralizing capacity (ANC). A dose of 40 to 80 mEq ANC is a reasonable starting dose. Typically, dosing is after meals and at bedtime; duration of use should not exceed 2 weeks.

The advantage of antacids is that they have a quick onset of action (5 to 15 minutes). The disadvantages of antacids are that they are significantly less effective in the treatment of GERD and PUD compared with other available drugs, have a short duration of action (less than 1 hour on an empty stomach), and have the potential for several adverse effects and drug interactions. The duration of action can be extended to 1 to 3 hours by use within 1 hour after eating, which delays gastric emptying and increases the time of contact with gastric acid. Nonetheless, the short duration requires frequent dosing to maintain continuous relief and eliminates the possibility of effective suppression of gastric acid throughout the nighttime. Despite the significant disadvantages and the availability of more effective drugs, antacids remain popular for self-care of heartburn, GERD, and PUD. One of the more practical uses for these drugs is as an addition to acid-suppression therapy (ie, H_2RAs or PPIs) on an as-needed basis to provide relief of acute symptoms between doses of acid-suppression therapy. Larger doses of some of these same products are used as laxatives.

Antacids are available as OTC products in many dosage forms, including suspensions, chewable tablets, and powders. The antacid components in these products are one or more salts of aluminum, magnesium, calcium, or sodium—the most common being aluminum hydroxide, magnesium hydroxide, calcium carbonate, and sodium bicarbonate (Table 11-4). As is often the case when there are so many similar OTC products available, the brand names can be confusing and even misleading. For example, Maalox Regular Strength Chewable Tablets contain calcium carbonate, whereas Maaalox Advanced Regular Strength Liquid contains aluminum and magnesium hydroxide.

Aluminum, magnesium, calcium, and sodium differ in their ANCs, durations of action, and adverse effects. Aluminum salts decrease smooth muscle motility and thus cause constipation. Aluminum hydroxide has the lowest ANC but one of the longer durations of action. On the other hand, magnesium salts that enter the small intestine draw water into the intestine (osmotic effect) to cause diarrhea. Because aluminum causes constipation and magnesium causes diarrhea, these 2 are combined in many antacid products (see Table 11-4) in an effort to balance these effects; in reality, some diarrhea is often experienced. Some aluminum and magnesium are absorbed from the GI tract but are excreted by the kidney; thus, accumulation of these ions is generally not a problem unless the patient has diminished kidney function.

TABLE 11-3

EXAMPLES OF DRUG REGIMENS[a] TO ERADICATE *H. PYLORI*

	DRUG COMBINATION	DAILY DOSAGE
1.	amoxicillin	1000 mg bid
	clarithromycin	500 mg bid
	lansoprazole[b]	30 mg bid
2.	metronidazole	500 mg bid
	clarithromycin	500 mg bid
	omeprazole[b]	20 mg bid
3.	bismuth subsalicylate	525 mg qid
	metronidazole	250 mg qid
	tetracycline	500 mg qid
	omeprazole[b]	40 mg bid

bid = twice per day; qid = 4 times per day.
[a]Duration of treatment is 7 to 14 days.
[b]Any of the other PPIs can be used instead.

Calcium carbonate and sodium bicarbonate have more ANC than aluminum and magnesium salts. However, when either of these 2 antacids reacts with gastric acid, they form carbon dioxide, which can cause belching and abdominal distention, both of which can increase esophageal reflux. Most of the calcium is not absorbed and can cause constipation. On the other hand, sodium bicarbonate is absorbed into the bloodstream. As with aluminum and magnesium salts, the calcium and sodium bicarbonate that are absorbed generally do not pose a problem. The exception is use of sodium bicarbonate, which can cause metabolic alkalosis in patients with reduced kidney function. The large sodium content may also be detrimental to patients who are trying to restrict their sodium intake. Therefore, sodium bicarbonate is not a preferred antacid and should not be used for an extended time.

The major potential for drug interactions is a result of the ability of the aluminum, magnesium, and calcium ions to bind to some drugs when they physically come in contact with them in the GI tract. The increase in gastric pH can also alter the solubility and absorption of some drugs and thus reduces their bioavailability. Examples are the binding of aluminum, magnesium, and calcium ions to tetracycline antibiotics to diminish their absorption, and the increase in gastric pH that reduces the absorption of some NSAIDs (including aspirin). To avoid these problems, a general rule of thumb is that antacids should be used 2 hours before or after oral administration of other drugs.

TABLE 11-4

SELECTED ANTACIDS

TRADE NAME	ALUMINUM HYDROXIDE[a]	MAGNESIUM HYDROXIDE[a]	CALCIUM CARBONATE[a]	SODIUM BICARBONATE[a]
Alka-Seltzer Heartburn Relief Chews	–	–	750	–
Alka-Seltzer Heartburn + Gas Relief Chews[b]	–	–	750	–
Alternagel	600	–	–	–
Concentrated Phillips' Milk of Magnesia	–	800	–	–
Extra Strength Alka-Seltzer Effervescent Tablets[c]	–	–	–	1985
Maalox Advanced Maximum Strength Liquid[b]	400	400	–	–
Maalox Advanced Maximum Strength Chewable Tablets[b]	–	–	1000	–
Maalox Advanced Regular Strength Liquid[b]	200	200	–	–
Maalox Regular Strength Chewable Tablets	–	–	600	–
Mylanta Ultimate Strength Liquid	500	500	–	–
Mylanta Supreme Liquid	–	135	400	–
Mylanta Regular Strength Liquid[b]	200	200	–	–
Mylanta Maximum Strength Liquid[b]	400	400	–	–
Original Alka-Seltzer Effervescent Tablets[d]	–	–	–	1916
Original Phillips' Milk of Magnesia	–	400	–	–
Phillips' Chewable Tablets	–	311	–	–
Tums Regular Strength Chewable Tablets	–	–	500	–
Tums Extra Strength Chewable Tablets	–	–	750	–
Tums Ultra Strength Chewable Tablets	–	–	1000	–

[a]Content represents mg per dosage form or per 5 mL liquid.
[b]Also contains simethicone to reduce gas.
[c]Also contains aspirin 500 mg.
[d]Also contains aspirin 325 mg.

Physical Barriers

Sucralfate (Carafate) is more frequently used to treat peptic ulcers than GERD. It is the aluminum salt of sulfated sucrose. The acid environment of the stomach causes the sucralfate molecules to react with each other and become a viscous, sticky substance. The sucralfate adheres to epithelial cells to form a physical barrier of protection, especially in areas of damaged mucosa. Sucralfate also inhibits pepsin, binds to bile acids, and stimulates production of PGs. Administration is recommended 1 hour prior to meals so that it is in sufficient contact with gastric acid and does not adhere to food components rather than to stomach epithelial cells and ulcer craters. Frequent dosing is required (4 times per day) because the maximum duration of action is only 6 hours; a course of therapy is typically 4 to 8 weeks. As with antacids, sucralfate should be used 2 hours or more apart from other drugs to prevent potential drug interactions in

		TABLE 11-5		
		EXAMPLES OF OVER-THE-COUNTER LAXATIVES		
CLASSIFICATION	**GENERIC NAME**	**TRADE NAME**	**DOSAGE FORM**	**ONSET (HR)**
Bulk-forming	methylcellulose	Citrucel	Powder	12 to 72
	polycarbophil	FiberCon	Tablets	12 to 72
	psyllium	Metamucil	Powder	12 to 72
Osmotic	magnesium citrate solution	generic	Solution	1 to 3
	magnesium hydroxide	generic milk of magnesia	Suspension	1 to 3
	polyethylene glycol solution	MiraLax	Solution	3 to 4
	sodium phosphate	Fleet Phospho-soda	Solution	1 to 3
	sodium phosphates	Fleet	Enema	< 1
	glycerin	generic	Suppository	< 1
Stimulant	bisacodyl	Dulcolax	Tablets	6 to 10
	bisacodyl	Fleet Bisacodyl	Enema	< 1
	bisacodyl	Dulcolax	Suppository	< 1
	senna	Ex-Lax	Tablets	6 to 10
Stool softener	docusate	Colace	Capsules	12 to 72
	docusate	Enemeez	Enema	< 1

the GI tract. Even with this 2-hour separation, the bioavailability of some drugs (eg, tetracycline, digoxin, ketoconazole, and the fluoroquinolone antibiotics) may be diminished; use of a different drug to treat PUD or GERD may be advisable for patients taking these other medications. Some patients experience constipation from the aluminum. Most of the sucralfate is excreted through the GI tract, and thus systemic adverse effects are minimized.

Alginic acid is another agent that forms a physical barrier that may add protection from gastroesophageal reflux. Alginic acid is used in combination with various antacid combination products (eg, Gaviscon Tablets). When taken with a full glass of water, it forms viscous foam that floats and provides a protective barrier to prevent reflux through the lower esophageal sphincter. This mechanism only works when the patient is in the upright position.

Misoprostol

Misoprostol (Cytotec) is a synthetic derivative of PG E_1 (PGE$_1$; see Chapter 6) and is used in conjunction with NSAID therapy to reduce the incidence of NSAID-induced ulcers. This drug adds back the protective effects of PGs that the NSAIDs remove through inhibition of the COX-1 enzyme (see Figure 11-2). Misoprostol is a potent compound and hence the dosages are small: 400 to 800 mcg per day with food. Adverse effects can be significant and include diarrhea, nausea, and abdominal cramps. A reduced dos-

age may be necessary in some patients to alleviate adverse effects. Misoprostol can cause uterine contractions and thus is contraindicated during pregnancy or in patients in whom conception is a possibility.

Laxatives

The major categories of laxatives are bulk forming, stool softeners, osmotic laxatives, and stimulant laxatives (Table 11-5). Selection of the appropriate laxative depends on the circumstances of the constipation. For example, a bulk-forming laxative is more appropriate than a stimulant laxative for most patients with the need for more frequent use of a laxative. On the other hand, an osmotic laxative is more appropriate than a bulk laxative when a relatively quick evacuation of the bowel is desired. Some laxatives are also available for rectal administration as enemas (liquid applied into the rectum) or suppositories, which are usually cylinder- or cone-shaped semisolids made of a substance that melts at body temperature. Rectal administration offers an advantage if oral administration is undesirable (eg, due to nausea); however, there is some discomfort to the patient. Because the laxative reaches the colon immediately, the onset of action is shorter compared with oral administration (minutes vs hours). Patients with frequent or chronic constipation should see their physician to determine the cause and the appropriate treatment of the constipation. It should be noted that there are other agents used for specific causes of constipation. For example, 2 opioid antagonists, methylnaltrexone and alvimopan, are used to block the constipating effects of the opioid analgesics.

Bulk-Forming Laxatives

Bulk-forming laxatives are generally nondigestible plant products such as psyllium (Metamucil) or semisynthetic cellulose material such as methylcellulose (Citrucel). These laxatives swell when in contact with fluid, forming a substance of gel consistency that stimulates peristalsis and travels readily through the GI tract, moving other intestinal contents with it at the same time. Consumption of at least 8 ounces of fluid per dose is important. Bulk-forming laxatives are the agents of choice for most patients with constipation and usually initiate a response in 12 to 72 hours. Systemic effects are rare because the laxative is not absorbed into the bloodstream. Bulk-forming laxatives can interfere with the absorption of some drugs (eg, tetracyclines, warfarin, and aspirin) when administered within 1 to 2 hours of the drug due to physical or chemical binding of the drug to the nonabsorbable laxative.

Stool Softeners

Stool softeners, such as docusate (Colace), are also called emollient laxatives. They are surfactants in that they reduce the surface tension to allow oil and water to mix, which results in softening of the stool and facilitates movement. Onset of action is 12 to 72 hours after oral use. These laxatives may be more useful in preventing constipation than treating it.

Mineral oil is usually categorized as a lubricant laxative because it coats the stool to facilitate easier movement; however, it also helps to keep the stool soft. It is not a preferred laxative and is the only lubricant laxative of practical use. Potential problems associated with use of mineral oil are aspiration into the lungs, anal leakage, and a decreased absorption of fat-soluble vitamins.

Osmotic Laxatives

Osmotic laxatives are agents that draw water into the intestinal lumen, which increases peristalsis. One group of osmotic laxatives is the saline laxatives. These are ions that are not appreciably absorbed from the GI tract, such as magnesium, sulfate, phosphate, and citrate. The onset of action is within 1 to 6 hours, and they are useful for an acute laxative effect rather than routine management of constipation. Laxative doses of magnesium hydroxide are larger than the antacid doses. Some magnesium ions are absorbed and can therefore lead to toxic levels of magnesium in the blood, especially in patients with reduced renal function. Abdominal cramps and nausea are potential adverse effects. Sodium is also absorbed following use of sodium phosphate laxatives. The increase in sodium can worsen disease symptoms in patients with heart failure and

therefore should not be used in these patients. There are also concerns about reduced kidney function with use of sodium phosphate laxatives. Because of this, the US Food and Drug Administration (FDA) has released warning statements about not using sodium phosphate laxatives with certain medications, such as angiotensin-converting enzyme inhibitors, or in patients with preexisting kidney disease. As with antacid use, saline laxatives should be taken apart from other oral drug administration to avoid the potential for reduced absorption of the other drug.

Other examples of osmotic laxatives, but not saline type, are lactulose (Constilac) and polyethylene glycol (MiraLax). Lactulose is by prescription only and is a disaccharide that is not absorbed from the small intestine but is converted to organic acids in the large intestine, which then have an osmotic action to draw water into the lumen. Onset of action is 1 to 2 days, and abdominal discomfort is common. Polyethylene glycol is not readily absorbed and retains water in the intestine. It is recommended only for short-term use.

Glycerin is another osmotic laxative but is often referred to as a hyperosmotic because it has a local irritant effect along with the osmotic effect. It is absorbed orally and thus is not effective as a laxative by that route but is frequently used as a rectal suppository or enema. It causes a bowel movement in less than 1 hour and may cause a burning sensation during administration. Glycerin suppositories have been used for years in children and adults.

Stimulant Laxatives

The mode of action of the stimulant laxatives is a direct effect on the intestinal smooth muscle to increase motility. They may also cause an increase of water and electrolyte secretion into the intestine. Examples are senna (Ex-Lax) and bisacodyl (Dulcolax); both are available OTC and have an onset of action of 6 to 10 hours. They are not recommended for daily use but can be used occasionally for acute constipation or to evacuate the bowel prior to diagnostic procedures of the GI tract or prior to surgery. Abdominal cramps, which can be severe, are a common adverse effect of all of the stimulant laxatives.

Antidiarrheal Agents

There are only a few drugs available to provide symptomatic relief of diarrhea (they do not resolve the underlying cause of the diarrhea). The exception may be bismuth subsalicylate, which has an antibacterial effect useful in the treatment of traveler's diarrhea.

Opioids

The principal opioids used to treat diarrhea are loperamide (Imodium), diphenoxylate (Lomotil), and difenoxin (Motofen).

Diphenoxylate (Lomotil) and difenoxin (Motofen) have similar effects because one is the metabolite of the other. The metabolism of diphenoxylate is an example of an active drug being converted by the liver to an active metabolite (see Chapter 2). In this case, the liver converts the active diphenoxylate to the active difenoxin:

diphenoxylate $\longrightarrow$ difenoxin

The antidiarrheal effect of these opioids is a result of their ability to combine with the μ-opioid receptor (see Chapter 7) on the GI smooth muscle, causing a decrease in motility. Although other opioids also diminish GI motility, these 3 drugs do not penetrate the CNS as readily as other opioids and therefore have significantly less potential for abuse and physical dependence. Among these 3 opioids, loperamide has the least abuse potential and thus is the only one that is not a controlled substance; difenoxin and diphenoxylate are Schedule IV and V (see Table 1-7), respectively. A small amount of atropine (an anticholinergic) is added to diphenoxylate and difenoxin products to deter the use of higher doses for abuse purposes.

Because loperamide is very effective and has a low incidence of adverse effects, it is available OTC and thus is the most commonly used of the opioid antidiarrheal drugs. It is used to treat acute nonspecific diarrhea (eg, traveler's diarrhea) as well as chronic diarrhea from various causes. For OTC use, the total daily dose should not exceed 8 mg. Loperamide is readily absorbed orally and is available in several dosage forms. Adverse effects can include drowsiness, dry mouth, nausea, vomiting, and constipation.

Although other opiates (eg, paregoric, opium tincture) are effective in the treatment of diarrhea, they also have a higher incidence of adverse effects, potential for abuse, and they are controlled substances. Consequently, these products have a lower preference for use to treat diarrhea.

Absorbents

These compounds are nonselective in their ability to absorb other compounds and may be effective to treat nonspecific acute diarrhea. Polycarbophil (Fiber-Lax) and psyllium (Metamucil) are generally considered laxatives but may also be useful for mild diarrhea. Although the mechanism is not clearly understood, these products absorb water and may improve the viscosity of the stool. They have no known systemic toxicity, but they may interfere with the absorption of some drugs if used concomitantly.

Bismuth Subsalicylate

Bismuth subsalicylate (Pepto-Bismol) is effective to treat mild, nonspecific diarrhea as well as mild-to-moderate traveler's diarrhea. The mechanism of its antidiarrheal action is not clear. The acidity of the stomach converts the bismuth subsalicylate to salicylic acid and bismuth oxychloride. The salicylic acid may have some local anti-inflammatory activity before it is absorbed into the blood. The bismuth remains in the GI tract, where it has an anti-inflammatory and antibacterial effect. This antibacterial action contributes to the therapeutic effectiveness for treating bacteria-induced diarrhea (eg, traveler's diarrhea) and is the reason for use in the multidrug regimen for the treatment of *H pylori*–induced peptic ulcers (see Table 11-3).

Generally, bismuth subsalicylate is very safe and can be used up to 8 times per day at the recommended dose. It can also be used 4 times per day to prevent traveler's diarrhea; hence, it is a widely used OTC antidiarrheal product. Nonetheless, it does have several potential adverse effects and drug interactions. Patients for whom use of aspirin is a precaution should not use bismuth subsalicylate. This would include patients who have aspirin-induced asthma or are taking warfarin (an anticoagulant) and children who have a viral infection such as the flu. Bismuth subsalicylate may also inhibit the absorption of other drugs given concurrently. Sulfides produced by bacteria in the mouth and intestine form bismuth sulfide, which causes a harmless darkening of the tongue and stool in some patients.

Drugs for Treating Irritable Bowel Syndrome

The use of antidiarrheal agents and laxatives are a mainstay of drug treatment for IBS, although treatment of coexisting depression or pain also has beneficial outcomes in many patients. Of the antidiarrheal agents, loperamide (Imodium) is used most often because it is available OTC and has a low incidence of adverse effects. When constipation is a predominant symptom of IBS, bulk-forming laxatives are preferred, such as psyllium (Metamucil) or methylcellulose (Citrucel). If a bulk-forming laxative does not alleviate the problem, docusate (Colace) or an osmotic laxative (see Table 11-5) may be added.

Abdominal pain and depression are significant problems for some patients. Antidepressants (see Chapter 13) are often effective for these patients. Besides their antidepressant effect, these drugs also alleviate pain associated with IBS, an effect that is independent of the antidepressant effect. The mechanism for the pain relief is not clear. Although the tricyclic antidepressants have an anticholinergic effect that may contribute to the relief of bowel spasms, the benefit cannot be totally attributed to the anticholinergic effect. Examples of tricyclic antidepressants are imipramine (Tofranil), desipramine (Norpramin), and amitriptyline (Elavil). Tricyclic antidepressants should be used with caution in patients for whom anticholinergic effects are problematic (eg, glaucoma, cardiovascular disease, and urinary retention).

TABLE 11-6

EXAMPLES OF DRUGS USED TO TREAT INFLAMMATORY BOWEL DISEASE

GENERIC NAME	TRADE NAME	CATEGORY
adalimumab	Humira	Anti-inflammatory antibody
azathioprine	Imuran	Immunosuppressant
balsalazide	Colazal	Anti-inflammatory salicylate
budesonide	Entocort EC	Anti-inflammatory corticosteroid
certolizumab	Cimzia	Anti-inflammatory antibody
cyclosporine	Gengraf	Immunosuppressant
golimumab	Simponi	Anti-inflammatory antibody
infliximab	Remicade	Anti-inflammatory antibody
mercaptopurine	Purinethol	Immunosuppressant
mesalamine	Asacol	Anti-inflammatory salicylate
metronidazole	Flagyl	Antibiotic
natalizumab	Tysabri	Anti-inflammatory antibody
olsalazine	Dipentum	Anti-inflammatory salicylate
prednisone	Deltasone	Anti-inflammatory corticosteroid
sulfasalazine	Azulfidine	Anti-inflammatory salicylate

Some more specific drugs are FDA approved for treatment of severe IBS. Alosetron (Lotronex) is specific for diarrhea-predominant IBS in women; the drug is not effective in men. It is an orally effective drug that increases absorption of water and sodium, decreases abdominal pain, and increases the time for movement through the intestinal tract. Although effective, alosetron is potentially dangerous because it can cause ischemic colitis (restricted blood flow to the intestine), serious complications from constipation, and death. Consequently, this drug can only be used with close association and active involvement of the patient, pharmacist, and physician. A specific protocol of patient information and monitoring by physician and pharmacist is required. The patient must discontinue use of the drug and contact his or her physician if constipation occurs.

Two agents are available for use in constipation-predominant IBS. Lubiprostone (Amitiza) is approved for use in women older than 18 years with constipation-predominant IBS. It works by activating chloride channels and increasing fluid in the intestine. The increased fluid in the intestine softens the stool and therefore relieves the constipation. Linaclotide (Linzess) is approved for treatment of constipation-predominant IBS in adult patients. It also increases fluid in the intestine, although it works through a different mechanism than lubiprostone. Diarrhea is a potential adverse effect with both of these agents.

Drugs for Treating Inflammatory Bowel Disease

The seriousness and complexity of IBD (ulcerative colitis and Crohn's disease) requires that the drug therapy change as the symptoms change. Examples of drugs used to treat IBD are shown in Table 11-6. Therapy can be complex and include various anti-inflammatory agents, immunosuppressive therapy, and antibiotics. Additional drug therapy may also be necessary to treat systemic complications of the disease such as arthritis. No drug cures IBD, but the primary goal of therapy is to bring about remission, which may last a few years in some cases.

Mesalamine (Asacol) or one of its various chemical derivatives is frequently used to treat mild to moderate ulcerative colitis and Crohn's disease involving the colon. Mesalamine is a derivative of salicylic acid, and 5-ASA is a synonym. Other derivatives of 5-ASA are olsalazine (Dipentum), balsalazide (Colazal), and sulfasalazine (Azulfidine). Mesalamine is available in oral dosage forms as well as enemas and suppositories for rectal administration. The anti-inflammatory activity of 5-ASA is primarily in the large intestine. The mechanism of action is unknown, although inhibition of cyclooxygenase and/or lipoxygenase may play a part. Sulfasalazine has the most prominent adverse effect potential and includes headache, nausea, and fatigue. Patients should also know that sulfasalazine causes the urine to turn orange-yellow, a harmless effect. This drug may increase the patient's sensitivity to the sun. Sulfasalazine inhibits the absorption of folic acid and therefore folic acid supplements are necessary during therapy. Mesalamine and balsalazide have fewer adverse effects than sulfasalazine. Diarrhea is common with olsalazine.

The anti-inflammatory action of corticosteroid therapy is useful in treatment of moderate to severe ulcerative colitis and Crohn's disease. Oral corticosteroids such as prednisone (Deltasone) are effective for moderate to severe IBD, and rectally administered corticosteroids are useful when the affected area is at or near the rectum. Even with a short course of therapy (7 to 10 days), some adverse effects of corticosteroids can be expected, such as insomnia, mood changes, and nervousness. When the desired response is obtained, the corticosteroid is discontinued by tapering the dose. If corticosteroids cannot be tapered off without a relapse, surgery becomes a consideration.

Severe ulcerative colitis or Crohn's disease requires more aggressive therapy, including parenterally administered corticosteroid at higher doses, and thus hospitalization. Mesalamine derivatives are not effective to treat severe IBD. Cyclosporine (Gengraf), an immunosuppressive drug, is useful for treatment of ulcerative colitis and Crohn's disease that are unresponsive to corticosteroids. Drugs that are antibodies that block the inflammatory cascade are also available. Additional immunosuppressive drugs and antibiotics that may be used to treat severe Crohn's disease are listed in Table 11-6. Use of these drugs may allow a reduction in corticosteroid dosage yet achieve remission.

Mesalamine or one of its derivatives is standard treatment to maintain remission of IBD, although success is greater for ulcerative colitis patients. Azathioprine (Imuran) and mercaptopurine (Purinethol) are used to maintain remission in patients who do not respond to mesalamine or its derivatives. Corticosteroids are not effective in maintaining remission or changing the course of either disease. Consequently, dosage of corticosteroid should be tapered off when remission is obtained.

Drugs for Treating Hemorrhoids

The goal of treatment is to alleviate the symptoms of pain, itching, burning, and inflammation. There are several categories of drugs that are used to accomplish relief of these symptoms. Drugs in each category are available in OTC anorectal products, creams, ointments, suppositories, solutions, and moist pads. By using topical dosage forms, the compounds are placed directly at the site of the problem. Although systemic effects are minimized when prescribed frequency of use is not exceeded, adverse effects are not eliminated because some systemic absorption occurs for several of these compounds.

A list of the categories of hemorrhoid treatments follows, including a short description of their effects and generic names of some of the compounds in the category. Use of a bulk-forming laxative or stool softener may also be necessary to avoid constipation in some patients. Table 11-7 lists examples of products that contain these compounds.

- *Corticosteroids* are effective in reducing inflammation, itching, and swelling. Hydrocortisone is the most commonly used topical corticosteroid, and at 0.25% and 1% concentrations, it is the only one available OTC. Hydrocortisone is low potency, and topical use does not cause systemic adverse effects.

- *Local anesthetics* provide temporary relief of itching, burning, and pain by blocking nerve impulses. Allergic reactions may occur; therefore, patients should be instructed to discontinue the product if redness, swelling, and pain do not diminish or

TABLE 11-7		
EXAMPLES OF ANORECTAL PRODUCTS FOR TREATMENT OF HEMORRHOIDS		
TRADE NAME	**ACTIVE INGREDIENTS**	**DOSAGE FORM**
Analpram-HC[a]	Hydrocortisone acetate, pramoxine HCl	Cream
Anusol HC[a]	Hydrocortisone	Cream
Anusol HC[a]	Hydrocortisone acetate	Suppository
Preparation H	Petrolatum, glycerin, phenylephrine, pramoxine	Cream
Preparation H	Mineral oil, petrolatum, phenylephrine	Ointment
Preparation H	Phenylephrine, witch hazel	Cooling gel
Preparation H	Cocoa butter, phenylephrine	Suppository
Preparation H	Witch hazel	Medicated wipes
Proctocort[a]	Hydrocortisone	Cream
Proctocort[a]	Hydrocortisone acetate	Suppository
Tronolane	Zinc oxide, pramoxine	Cream
Tucks	Witch hazel	Pads
Tucks	Pramoxine	Spray
Tucks	Topical starch	Suppository
Tucks	Mineral oil, pramoxine, zinc oxide	Ointment
[a]By prescription only; all others are OTC.		

become worse. Examples are benzocaine, benzyl alcohol, dibucaine, pramoxine, and tetracaine.

- *Astringents* relieve irritation and inflammation, decrease mucus, and coagulate protein in skin, thus protecting underlying tissue. Examples are calamine, zinc oxide, and witch hazel (*Hamamelis* water).

- *Vasoconstrictors* reduce swelling by constricting blood vessels and relieve local itching by slight anesthetic effect. Vasoconstriction occurs through an β-adrenergic effect (see Chapter 12) similar to the mechanism of nasal decongestants (see Chapter 10). Similar precautions and adverse effects exist for the use of vasoconstrictors for hemorrhoids as for nasal decongestants (eg, nervousness, tremor, precaution in patients with hypertension, diabetes mellitus). Examples are pseudoephedrine and phenylephrine.

- *Protectants* form a physical barrier on the skin, lubricate tissues to prevent irritation, and prevent loss of water from the tissue. Little or no systemic absorption occurs. Examples are aluminum hydroxide gel, lanolin, mineral oil, zinc oxide, cocoa butter, shark liver oil, bismuth salts, lanolin, petrolatum, glycerin, and hard fat.

- *Counterirritants* produce a feeling of cooling, tingling, or warmth and distract from pain and itching. Examples are menthol and camphor. Menthol can produce an allergic reaction; therefore, patients should be instructed to discontinue the product if redness, swelling, and pain do not diminish or become worse.

- *Keratolytics* increase the rate of sloughing of epidermal surface cells so that medications may be more accessible to the underlying tissue. Examples are alcloxa and resorcinol.

Section Summary

Treatment of GERD focuses on neutralizing gastric acid or decreasing acid production. In either case, the amount of acid available for reflux into the esophagus is decreased, thus giving the esophageal mucosa time to heal. From the standpoint of healing rates, PPIs are the most effective therapy; examples are esomeprazole (Nexium) and omeprazole (Prilosec). PPIs have few and usually mild adverse effects. The H_2RAs such as ranitidine (Zantac) and famotidine (Pepcid) are an option for treatment of GERD but are less effective than PPIs. All H_2RAs are available by prescription and OTC for treatment of heartburn. The effectiveness among the PPIs is comparable, as is the effectiveness among the drugs in the H_2RA category. These 2 categories of drugs exert their effect via systemic action; therefore, they must be absorbed into the bloodstream to reach their target sites in the specialized cells of the stomach. All of the drugs in these 2 categories are absorbed readily after oral administration.

Antacids are also used to treat GERD by virtue of their ability to neutralize gastric acid. However, although they have a quick onset of action, these drugs are less effective and have a shorter duration of action than either the PPIs or the H_2RA. Antacids can be used as an adjunct to other therapy. Among the more prominent problems associated with antacids is the potential for diarrhea with magnesium salts (Phillips' Chewable) and constipation with aluminum (Alternagel) and calcium (Tums) salts.

Treatment for PUD depends on the cause. If PUD is linked to the presence of *H pylori*, then combination therapy to eradicate the bacteria is appropriate. Many effective combinations of antibiotics (eg, amoxicillin, clarithromycin, and tetracycline) and PPIs (eg, omeprazole) have been identified. If the PUD is NSAID induced, removing the NSAID or reducing the dosage is appropriate, along with the use of drug therapy to treat PUD. PPIs and H_2RAs are effective for treatment and maintenance therapy of PUD, although healing rates are higher for PPIs. Misoprostol (Cytotec), a synthetic PG derivative, and the PPIs are available to prevent PUD in patients who are at risk for PUD but must be maintained on NSAIDs.

Antacids (eg, Mylanta liquid, Maalox tablets) are less effective than PPIs or H_2RAs but are sometimes added to therapy. Sucralfate (Carafate) is also available. When used prior to meals, sucralfate offers protection by forming a viscous barrier between the epithelial cells and the gastric acid. Antacids and sucralfate may interfere with bioavailability of other drugs if administered concomitantly.

Acute constipation can be treated with any one of several categories of laxatives. Exercise, dietary fiber, and adequate fluid intake can all help prevent constipation. To treat constipation, dietary fiber can be added in the form of bulk-forming laxatives such as psyllium (Metamucil). Osmotic laxatives, such as milk of magnesia, are also effective and act by drawing water into the GI tract. For both types of laxatives, it is important that sufficient water be ingested at the time of the laxative dose. Bulk-forming laxatives take longer to act (12 to 72 hours) compared with osmotic laxatives (1 to 6 hours). Other mechanisms for laxative action are stool softeners and stimulants. Stool softeners, such as docusate (Colace), allow water to more readily mix with GI contents to keep the stool softer so it passes through the GI tract more readily; onset is 12 to 72 hours. Stimulant laxatives have a quicker onset (6 to 10 hours) but are not recommended for frequent use. They increase GI motility by acting on the smooth muscle; bisacodyl (Dulcolax) and senna (Ex-Lax) are examples. Enemas and suppositories have the shortest onset of action (less than 1 hour).

Treatment of severe or chronic diarrhea necessitates determination of the underlying cause. Management of acute mild to moderate diarrhea usually involves treatment of symptoms and maintenance of fluids and electrolytes. Loperamide (Imodium) is an OTC opioid and is a very effective and frequently used antidiarrheal agent. It acts on the smooth muscle to decrease GI motility. Drowsiness, dry mouth, nausea, and vomiting are potential adverse effects. Absorbent compounds are not absorbed systemically and so have few adverse effects. Bismuth subsalicylate (Pepto-Bismol) is also frequently used, although the mechanism of action is not clear. It is particularly effective for bacteria-induced diarrhea. The salicylate content is released when in contact with gastric acid, and thus it should not be used in patients who must avoid aspirin.

The focus of drug therapy for IBS is management of diarrhea or constipation. Loperamide is most frequently used for diarrhea; bulk-forming laxatives such as psyllium are recommended for constipation. Tricyclic antidepressants are effective in relieving abdominal pain as well as depression in some patients with IBS and these symptoms.

Treatment of IBD is more complex than IBS. Use of a salicylate derivative such as mesalamine (Asacol) is useful to treat ulcerative colitis and Crohn's disease. A corticosteroid such as prednisone (Deltasone) is often effective as additional therapy for these diseases when of mild to moderate severity. Patients with severe IBD are hospitalized for treatment with higher doses of a corticosteroid and use of antibiotics or immunosuppressant drugs such as cyclosporine (Gengraf). Once remission is obtained, the aggressive therapy is discontinued and corticosteroid therapy is tapered off. Mesalamine or one of its derivatives is most often used to maintain remission; corticosteroids are not effective for this purpose. Crohn's disease is typically less responsive to drug therapy than ulcerative colitis, in part because Crohn's disease can recur in any part of the digestive tract, whereas ulcerative colitis is limited to the rectum and colon.

The goal of therapy for hemorrhoids is to relieve the symptoms of itching, burning, pain, and inflammation. Many OTC products are available, often with several compounds present in one product that attempt to alleviate these symptoms through various mechanisms. Using compounds that are local anesthetics, vasoconstrictors, counterirritants, physical protectants, or corticosteroids are among the approaches to relieve symptoms.

ROLE OF THE ATHLETIC TRAINER

There are a few unique aspects related to the symptoms and treatment of GI disorders that may affect the role of the athletic trainer. Many drugs are available OTC to treat various GI disorders and therefore patients will self-diagnose and self-medicate, which may lead to inappropriate treatment. For example, a patient who is using an OTC H_2RA to treat persistent and recurring symptoms of PUD may require *H pylori* eradication treatment rather than continued H_2RA use, or a patient may be trying to treat erosive esophageal GERD with heartburn doses of an OTC H_2RA. A patient who is concerned about persistent diarrhea may have an underlying GI condition or may be experiencing adverse effects from a drug such as an antibiotic. The athletic trainer should encourage the patient to obtain accurate diagnosis, especially when symptoms persist or reoccur.

Another problem with self-diagnosis is that the patient may observe some symptoms (eg, gastric pain) but not properly assess the significance of other symptoms. The athletic trainer should be aware that patients with weight loss, bleeding, anemia, and difficulty swallowing should be referred to a physician because these are signs of more severe stages of GERD, PUD, and lower GI disorders. In addition, chest pain below the sternum that occurs on exertion or that radiates to the jaw or arm should not be interpreted as GERD but requires immediate medical attention.

Once the patient is properly diagnosed and treated, the athletic trainer can encourage the patient to comply with therapy. If the therapy includes several doses per day of more than one drug, such as for *H pylori* eradication treatment, it takes diligence to maintain the proper daily regimen throughout the entire course of therapy. For treatment of GERD and PUD, the dosage regimen and duration of treatment have a significant impact on the outcome.

Knowledge of nondrug measures related to GI disorders can allow the athletic trainer to provide additional useful information to the patient. For example, is the patient who is periodically bothered by constipation consuming sufficient water and fiber? Is a patient who is complaining of diarrhea consuming coffee or foods with high sugar content before running, or is there too much fiber in the diet? Patients with GERD should be advised to not exercise vigorously too soon after eating, and patients with PUD or GERD should be advised to avoid the most frequently used drugs: alcohol, caffeine, and nicotine (tobacco).

Fortunately, most of the drugs used to treat GI disorders have relatively few systemic adverse effects. Nonetheless, the potential for such adverse effects or drug interactions should not be overlooked. New complaints that arise even a few weeks after the addition of drug therapy could be the result of an adverse effect or drug interaction. The patient can be encouraged to seek consultation with a pharmacist or physician for a review of the patient's drug therapy to determine the likelihood that the new complaints are drug related.

Because GI disorders are a very common group of disorders, and because OTC products are numerous and readily accessible for the treatment of these disorders, opportunities exist for the athletic trainer to provide useful assistance and advice to the patient regarding GI disorders and related therapy. The goal, after accurate diagnosis, is to attain proper management of the disease through appropriate drug therapy, as well as through nondrug measures, so that GI disorders do not hinder the patient's athletic performance.

CASE STUDY

During the team's road trip to the annual tristate weekend tournament, the women's softball coach, Coach Peggy, admits to you that she has had "stomach problems" for the past year. She stopped eating the Mexican food she loves and is making a point of eating a healthy breakfast of toast and orange juice. She also sucks on peppermint drops because she thought the mint would calm her stomach, but none of these steps have stopped her heartburn problem. Coach Peggy says it is worst at night when she tries to go to sleep. You tell her that she may have GERD and advise her on things to avoid eating and drinking. You advise her to see her physician for diagnosis, assessment of complications, and medication therapy. Coach Peggy asks you what medications are available. How would you respond to this question?

BIBLIOGRAPHY

Anastasi JK, Capili B, Chang M. Managing irritable bowel syndrome. *Am J Nurs.* 2013;113(7):42-52.

Katz PO, Gerson LB, Vela MF. Guidelines for the diagnosis and management of gastroesophageal reflux disease. *Am J Gastroenterol.* 2013;108:308-328.

Kozuch PL, Hanauer SB. Treatment of inflammatory bowel disease: a review of medical therapy. *World J Gastroenterol.* 2008;14(3):354-377.

Krinsky DL, Ferreri SP, Hemstreet B, Hume AL, Newton GD, Rollins CJ, Tietze KJ. *Handbook of nonprescription drugs. An integrated approach to self-care.* 18th ed. Washington, DC: American Pharmacists Association; 2015.

Love BL, Johnson A, Smith LS. Linaclotide: a novel agent for chronic constipation and irritable bowel syndrome. *Am J Health Syst Pharm.* 2014;71:1081-1091.

O'Connor A, Gisbert J, O'Morain C. Treatment of *Helicobacter pylori* infection. *Helicobacter.* 2009;14(Supplement 1):46-51.

Pray WS. Updates in nonprescription therapy for heartburn and GERD. *US Pharm.* 2009;34(10):52-55.

Villoria A, Garcia P, Calvet X, Gisbert JP, Vergara M. Meta-analysis: high-dose proton pump inhibitors vs. standard dose in triple therapy for *Helicobacter pylori* eradication. *Aliment Pharmacol Ther.* 2008;28(7):868-877.

CHAPTER 12: ADVANCE ORGANIZER

Foundational Concepts

- Autonomic Nervous System Receptors
- Hypertension
  - Blood Pressure–Controlling Mechanism
  - Lifestyle Modification
  - Pharmacologic Therapy
- Angina Pectoris
  - Chronic Stable Angina
  - Variant Angina
  - Unstable Angina
- Myocardial Infarction
- Heart Failure

Drug Therapy

- Diuretics
- Angiotensin-Converting Enzyme Inhibitors
- Angiotensin II Receptor Blockers
- Direct Renin Inhibitors
- Calcium Channel Blockers
- β-Blockers
- Organic Nitrates
- Vasodilators
- Digoxin
- Section Summary

Therapy Strategies

- Hypertension
- Angina
- Myocardial Infarction
- Heart Failure
- Section Summary

Role of the Athletic Trainer

12

Drugs for Treating Hypertension and Heart Disease

CHAPTER OBJECTIVES

At the end of this chapter, the reader will be able to:

- Explain the function of the 2 subdivisions of the autonomic nervous system—sympathetic and parasympathetic—and how they affect physiological processes

- Recall and describe the 3 major types of cholinergic receptors

- Differentiate between sympathomimetic and parasympathomimetic types of drugs

- Explain the blood pressure thresholds for initiating treatment, the blood pressure goals, and the classes of medications recommended as initial therapy for hypertension

- Explain the important role that the renin-angiotensin-aldosterone system plays in regulating blood pressure

- Recall lifestyle modifications that can lower blood pressure and explain their therapeutic benefits

- Describe the pathophysiology of angina, myocardial infarction (MI), and heart failure

- Differentiate the 3 types of angina

- Explain the uses, mechanisms of action, physiological effects, adverse effects, and drug interactions

of β-blockers, diuretics, angiotensin-converting enzyme (ACE) inhibitors, angiotensin receptor blockers (ARBs), direct renin inhibitors, calcium channel blockers (CCBs), organic nitrates, and vasodilators in the treatment of cardiovascular conditions

- Describe various considerations in the overall treatment plan for cardiovascular disease that can affect the effectiveness of drug therapy

- Summarize the role of the athletic trainer for patients who are on drug therapy for cardiovascular diseases

This chapter presents a discussion about drugs used to treat several of the most prevalent serious cardiovascular diseases. Heart disease is the leading cause of death in the United States. These are also diseases for which exercise can improve symptoms and/or progression of the disease. Although just one of these diseases may be diagnosed (eg, hypertension, angina, heart failure, MI), there is a connection among them. For example, chronic hypertension increases the risk for angina, heart failure, and MI; the presence of angina increases the risk for MI; and MI is one cause of heart failure. In this chapter, the drugs used to treat these conditions are discussed by pharmacological category (eg, β-blockers, CCBs) and then reviewed briefly by therapeutic category (eg, antihypertensives, drugs for heart failure). The complexity of the therapeutic regimen sometimes used

Houglum JE, Harrelson GL, Seefeldt TM.
Principles of Pharmacology for Athletic Trainers, Third Edition (pp 211-235).
© 2016 Taylor & Francis Group.

ABBREVIATIONS USED IN THIS CHAPTER

ACE. angiotensin-converting enzyme

ACEI. ACE inhibitor

ARB. angiotensin receptor blocker

CCB. calcium channel blocker

CHD. coronary heart disease

CNS. central nervous system

COPD. chronic obstructive pulmonary disease

DRI. direct renin inhibitor

GI. gastrointestinal

HDL. high-density lipoprotein

LDL. low-density lipoprotein

MAO. monoamine oxidase

MAOI. monoamine oxidase inhibitor

MI. myocardial infarction

NSAID. nonsteroidal anti-inflammatory drug

t½. half-life

TI. therapeutic index

to treat these diseases, along with the array of potential adverse effects and drug interactions, creates a challenge for the athletic trainer. However, a few useful principles are reiterated that can guide the athletic trainer in assisting patients who are receiving therapy for hypertension and heart disease.

FOUNDATIONAL CONCEPTS

Endogenous control mechanisms to maintain proper blood pressure and cardiac function require the intricate involvement of neurotransmitters from the autonomic nervous system and CNS and the release of numerous hormones. The mechanisms of action of these neurotransmitters and hormones are also the sites of action for drugs used to treat hypertension and heart disease. A discussion of some of these mechanisms is included in this section as a basis for understanding the cause of the disease (or symptoms) and the rationale for treatment regimens.

Autonomic Nervous System Receptors

The autonomic nervous system is the part of the peripheral nervous system that automatically controls body functions such as blood flow to organs and tissues, heart rate, respiration, digestive processes, and blood pressure. It has 2 subdivisions: the parasympathetic and sympathetic systems. Usually a tissue response initiated by these 2 subdivisions will have opposite effects, so that, for example, activation of the parasympathetic system decreases heart rate, whereas activation of the sympathetic system increases

heart rate. Each of these subdivisions is a 2-neuron fiber system (Figure 12-1). The first neuron (preganglionic fiber) begins in the spinal cord and terminates at the site of specialized nerve tissue called a *ganglion*. The cell body of the second neuron (postganglionic fiber) begins at the ganglion and ends at the tissue being innervated, typically smooth muscle or cardiac muscle. A small space (synapse) separates the pre- from the postganglionic fiber. The terms *sympathetic* and *parasympathetic* are anatomical terms; their differentiation is determined by several anatomical characteristics, such as the length of the pre- vs postganglionic fiber and the origin of the neuron from the spinal cord. The terms *cholinergic* and *adrenergic* are pharmacologic terms that indicate the neurotransmitter released at the site.

Each nerve fiber releases a neurotransmitter. The preganglionic fibers of the sympathetic and parasympathetic systems release acetylcholine into the synapse at the ganglion. Acetylcholine is also released at the parasympathetic postganglionic fiber. Consequently, the parasympathetic system is referred to as the *cholinergic* nervous system. The neurotransmitter released at the tissue site by most of the sympathetic postganglionic fibers is norepinephrine. Another name for norepinephrine is noradrenaline; hence, the sympathetic system is also referred to as the *adrenergic* nervous system. When a neurotransmitter is released, it combines with the corresponding receptor, activates a transduction mechanism within the cell, and ultimately causes a tissue response (eg, smooth muscle contraction or relaxation).

> *Recall from Chapter 3 that transduction mechanisms are a sequence of reactions within the cell that are initiated as a drug or hormone combines with the appropriate receptor located on the surface of the cell.*

Most tissues are innervated by sympathetic and parasympathetic fibers, and, as previously mentioned, activation of these 2 fiber types typically has opposite effects on the tissue. Table 12-1 lists the responses from the autonomic nervous system on selected tissues. Note that, in general, the stimulation of the parasympathetic system initiates processes that conserve energy or conduct "housekeeping" types of functions. These include digestion of food and increased rate of excretory functions. In contrast, stimulation of the sympathetic system results in preparation for energy expenditure or for fight-or-flight functions. These include increased heart rate and decreased intestinal motility. In addition, a sympathetic preganglionic-like fiber innervates the adrenal gland to stimulate the release of epinephrine into the bloodstream. Release of epinephrine is increased because of excitatory response. Epinephrine causes increased heart rate, dilation of bronchial smooth muscle, and increased glycogen conversion to glucose (glycogenolysis). Although there is a low level of neurotransmitter release occurring all the time in each tissue, one

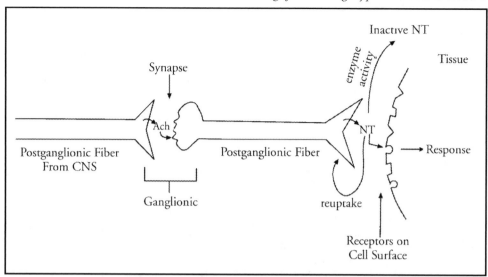

Figure 12-1. A nerve impulse from the central nervous system (CNS) travels along the preganglionic fiber, resulting in the release of the neurotransmitter acetylcholine (Ach) at the ganglion. Ach is the neurotransmitter at the ganglion for the sympathetic and parasympathetic fibers. Acetylcholine combines with the nicotinic receptor on the postganglionic fiber. The combination of the Ach with the nicotinic receptor causes the nerve impulse to be continued along the postganglionic fiber, which causes a neurotransmitter (NT) to be released at the site where the nerve fiber innervates the tissue. For sympathetic nerves, NT = norepinephrine (NE); for parasympathetic nerves, NT = acetylcholine. There are many types of receptors on the surface of each cell of the tissue. The NT binds to receptors for which it has an affinity, initiating a response inside the cell. The receptors to which NE binds are α- and β-receptors, and drugs that combine with these receptors are called adrenergic drugs. The receptors to which Ach binds are called muscarinic receptors and drugs that combine with this receptor are called cholinergic drugs. The binding of the NT (or agonist drug) to the receptor causes a response in the tissue; the binding of an antagonist drug (blocker) prevents the NT from binding to the receptor, and hence prevents the response from the NT. Termination of action of the NT occurs by the reuptake of the NT into the nerve terminal or by inactivation of the NT by specific enzyme activity (eg, cholinesterase for ACh and monoamine oxidase [MAO] for NE). Drugs that inhibit these inactivating enzymes or reuptake mechanisms will prolong and/or intensify the effect of the NT, thereby indirectly mimicking the NT activity.

subdivision of the autonomic nervous system dominates in each tissue (ie, it provides the autonomic tone for that tissue). As examples, sympathetic tone dominates in the cardiovascular system, whereas parasympathetic tone predominates in the digestive system.

The type of receptors that exist at any site will determine the response observed from neurotransmitters and from drugs that mimic neurotransmitters. There are 2 major types of adrenergic receptors: alpha (α) and beta (β). There are 2 major subtypes of these receptors (α_1, α_2 and β_1, β_2). Table 12-1 shows the type of receptor that predominates in various tissues. Key tissue responses to especially note are the peripheral vasoconstriction (eg, skin and mucosa) due to α_1-receptor activation, increased heart rate and force of contraction due to activation of β_1-receptors in the heart, and dilation of the bronchi due to β_2-receptor activation in the bronchial smooth muscle. Activation of the α_2-receptors serves to inhibit the release of additional norepinephrine. Although α_2-receptors exist at some tissue sites, the action of drugs at these sites is minimal. However, some drugs (not discussed) are agonists at the α_2-receptor in the CNS that decrease sympathetic outflow (ie, reduce the sympathetic response from CNS to the periphery), resulting in bradycar-

dia and vasodilation, which are antihypertensive responses. An example is clonidine (Catapres).

There are 3 major types of cholinergic receptors: muscarinic, nicotinic ganglionic, and nicotinic neuromuscular (Box 12-1). The nicotinic receptors are so named because nicotine is an agonist at these receptors. Although there are some drugs that act as agonists or antagonists at the nicotinic ganglionic receptor, the use of these drugs is limited because they affect both the sympathetic and parasympathetic systems and thus tend to have numerous adverse effects. Drugs that combine with the nicotinic neuromuscular receptor are also limited, but antagonists are used as skeletal muscle relaxants during surgery. Drugs that combine with the muscarinic receptor, located in the tissue innervated by the postganglionic parasympathetic fiber, are used to increase (agonists) or decrease (antagonists) the response of the parasympathetic nervous system. The terms *cholinergic* and *anticholinergic* are generally reserved for drugs that act at the muscarinic receptor site. Although drugs that act at the nicotinic receptors also either mimic or block the effects of acetylcholine at these sites, such drugs are usually specified as neuromuscular or ganglionic to differentiate them from the cholinergic muscarinic drugs.

		TABLE 12-1	
RESPONSES OF TISSUES TO AUTONOMIC NERVOUS SYSTEM ACTIVATION			
TISSUE	**ADRENERGIC RECEPTOR**	**ADRENERGIC ACTIVATION (SYMPATHETIC ACTIVATION)**	**CHOLINERGIC ACTIVATION (PARASYMPATHETIC ACTIVATION)**
Eye	α_1	Pupil dilation	Pupil constriction
Heart	β_1	Increased heart rate	Decreased heart rate
		Increased contractility	Decreased contractility
		Increased conduction velocity	Decreased conduction velocity
Blood vessels	α_1	Constriction in skin, mucosa, gastrointestinal	–
	β_2	Dilation in skeletal muscle	–
	β_2	Dilation in liver, heart, lungs	–
	β_1, β_2	Dilation in kidney	–
Kidney	β_1	Increased renin secretion	–
Bronchial muscle	β_2	Relaxation	Contraction
Intestinal motility	β_1	Decreased	Increased
Intestinal secretion		–	Increased
Urinary bladder	β_2, β_3	Relaxation	Contraction
Urinary sphincter	α_1	Contraction	Relaxation
Skeletal muscle	β_2	Increased glycogenolysis and increased contractility	–
Liver	α_1, β_2	Increased glycogenolysis and gluconeogenesis	–
Salivation	α_1	Increased (slightly)	Increased
Pancreas	α_1	Decreased insulin secretion	–
	β_2	Increased insulin secretion (slightly)	–
Fat cells	$\beta_1, \beta_2, \beta_3$	Increased lipolysis	–
– Indicates no effect or may not be physiologically significant.			

	BOX 12-1
SUMMARY OF THE 3 MAJOR TYPES OF CHOLINERGIC RECEPTORS	
Muscarinic	Located in the tissue innervated by the postganglionic parasympathetic fiber, these are used to increase or decrease the response of the parasympathetic nervous system. The terms *cholinergic* and *anticholinergic* are generally reserved for drugs that act at this receptor site.
Nicotinic ganglionic	Drugs that combine with this receptor are limited because they affect both the sympathetic and parasympathetic systems and thus tend to have numerous adverse effects.
Nicotinic neuromuscular	Drugs that combine with this receptor are also limited but some antagonists are used as skeletal muscle relaxants during surgery.

Termination of receptor response occurs because of 2 general mechanisms: neurotransmitter reuptake back into the nerve terminal that released it and inactivation by enzymes (see Figure 12-1). Examples of enzymes are cholinesterase, which inactivates acetylcholine, and monoamine oxidase (MAO), which inactivates norepinephrine. Inhibition of these enzymes by drugs will cause the neurotransmitter to have a more intense and longer duration of action. For example, drugs that are MAOIs can have an adverse effect of increased blood pressure because they increase the effect of norepinephrine at peripheral blood vessel sites.

> *Recall from Chapter 7 (see also Chapter 13) that MAOIs are drugs used to treat depression. These drugs are not first-line agents because they are notorious for adverse effects and drug interactions. Examples are phenelzine (Nardil) and tranylcypromine (Parnate).*

Drugs that mimic the sympathetic or parasympathetic nervous systems are referred to as sympathomimetics and parasympathomimetics, respectively. The mechanisms for mimicking these autonomic responses may be direct (receptor agonists) or indirect by inhibiting reuptake or inhibiting enzymatic inactivation of the neurotransmitter. Albuterol (Proventil) is an example of a direct β-agonist (see Chapter 9), whereas MAOIs are indirect-acting sympathomimetics.

Hypertension

An estimated 74 million people in the United States have high blood pressure. Hypertension increases the risk for stroke, angina, MI, heart failure, and kidney disease. Therefore, control of hypertension has obvious benefits in decreasing morbidity and mortality from these complications. Hypertension is more common among the elderly.

The diagnosis and treatment of hypertension are guided by statements that summarize the research in blood pressure management and provide recommendations based on the strength of research findings. The Joint National Committee (JNC) hypertension guidelines have been the most widely used for diagnosis and treatment. The most recent hypertension guideline was released in 2014 by the JNC 8 panel.[1] These guidelines provide 9 recommendations for the initiation of antihypertensive drug therapy. Normal blood pressure is defined as systolic blood pressure ≤ 120 mm Hg and diastolic blood pressure ≤ 80 mm Hg. The blood pressure thresholds for initiation of drug therapy are included in Table 12-2. For the general population of patients aged 60 years and older, drug therapy should be initiated if the systolic blood pressure is ≥ 150 mm Hg or if the diastolic blood pressure if ≥ 90 mm Hg. For patients younger than 60 years, the systolic blood pressure threshold is dropped to ≥ 140 mm Hg. This is also the recommended threshold for patients aged 18 years and older with diabetes mellitus or chronic kidney disease.

TABLE 12-2		
BLOOD PRESSURE THRESHOLDS FOR INITIATING DRUG THERAPY		
PATIENT AGE (YR)	**SYSTOLIC PRESSURE (MM HG)**	**DIASTOLIC PRESSURE (MM HG)**
≥ 60	≥ 150	≥ 90
< 60	≥ 140	≥ 90

Adapted from 2014 Evidence-Based Guidelines for the Management of High Blood Pressure in Adults. Report from the Panel Members Appointed to the Eighth Joint National Committee (JNC 8). *JAMA*. 2014;311(5):507-520.

Blood Pressure–Controlling Mechanisms

If the hypertension is known to be caused by the existence of a specific condition (eg, renal disease, adrenal tumor, pregnancy), it is *secondary hypertension*; if the cause is unknown, it is called *primary* or *essential hypertension*. Approximately 95% of patients have essential hypertension. It is presumed that most hypertension is multifactorial in origin, being caused by a combination of several environmental and genetic factors. Any factor that increases peripheral vascular resistance will contribute to elevated blood pressure. These factors include increased peripheral vasoconstriction, obesity, and elevated fluid volume. An alteration in any of the many mechanisms that control blood pressure can contribute to hypertension. Some of these controlling mechanisms are listed in Box 12-2.

> *Some classes of medications can also cause increased blood pressure, including oral decongestants, nonsteroidal anti-inflammatory drugs, and corticosteroids.*

The renin-angiotensin-aldosterone system plays an important role in regulating blood pressure. Renin is an enzyme that is released by the kidney in response to a decrease in blood flow to the kidneys, drop in blood pressure, diminished sodium and water retention, or increased sympathetic response through stimulation of β_1-adrenergic receptors on certain renal cells. Renin converts plasma angiotensinogen to angiotensin. Angiotensinogen is a glycoprotein that is continuously produced by the liver. Angiotensin I is a peptide composed of 10 amino acids. Another enzyme, ACE, catalyzes the conversion of angiotensin I to angiotensin II, which combines with angiotensin II receptors (Figure 12-2). ACE is present in cells of blood vessels and is therefore readily available to catalyze the formation of angiotensin II.

Angiotensin II has several effects that contribute to an increase in blood pressure and blood volume. It causes

---

Box 12-2

CONTROLLING MECHANISMS FOR BLOOD PRESSURE

- The central and sympathetic nervous systems contribute to the regulation of blood pressure. Excessive sympathetic response enhances the vasoconstricting effect through stimulation of the α_1-receptor on the arterioles and venules and increases heart rate and contractility through stimulation of β_1-receptors. On the other hand, stimulation of α_2-receptors in the CNS inhibits sympathetic outflow to decrease blood pressure.

- Calcium channels are pores on the surface of the cell membrane of the heart muscle, arteries, and arterioles. When the pores open, calcium ions are allowed into the cell, which leads to contraction of the vascular smooth muscle and cardiac muscle. In the heart muscle, activation of β_1-receptors leads to influx of calcium through the calcium channels, resulting in increased heart rate and force of contraction.

- Baroreceptors are an endogenous blood pressure–sensing mechanism in the walls of some larger arteries. In response to rapid reduction in blood pressure, a feedback system stimulates the sympathetic nervous system to increase peripheral vasoconstriction and heart rate. An alteration of the effectiveness of these baroreceptors through disease, age, or genetics can contribute to hypertension.

- Excessive dietary intake of sodium increases blood pressure in some patients.

- Potassium plays a role in normal blood pressure maintenance to the extent that a deficiency of these ions can contribute to hypertension.

- Some medications cause increased blood pressure as an adverse effect by increasing peripheral vasoconstriction, increasing CNS sympathetic outflow, or increasing fluid volume. Examples include chronic alcohol use, corticosteroids, estrogens, MAOIs, antidepressants, NSAIDs, oral contraceptives, oral decongestants, and weight-loss drugs.

- An abnormal renin-angiotensin-aldosterone system can result in increased sodium and water retention and/or increased vasoconstriction.

Figure 12-2. Effects of ACE on the renin-angiotensin system.

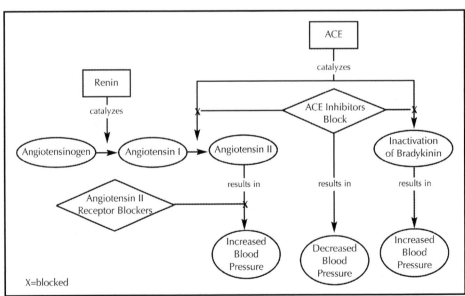

vasoconstriction by direct action on blood vessels and by the indirect action of increasing CNS sympathetic outflow and releasing epinephrine from the adrenal medulla. Angiotensin II also increases sodium and water retention by a direct action on the kidney and by indirect action through the release of aldosterone from the adrenal glands.

Aldosterone is a mineral corticosteroid that causes reabsorption of sodium and water by the renal tubule. As blood pressure begins to increase, the amount of renin released by the kidney decreases. In addition, angiotensin II acts as a feedback mechanism by inhibiting renin release. In summary, an increase in renin activity will increase angiotensin II, which increases blood pressure by vasoconstriction and increased blood volume.

Besides the effect on the renin-angiotensin system, ACE also catalyzes the inactivation of bradykinin. This peptide hormone has vasodilation properties that contribute to reducing blood pressure. Therefore, inhibiting ACE will decrease blood pressure by diminishing the effect of renin and by increasing the effect of bradykinin.

Although hypertensive patients may be asymptomatic, treatment of hypertension is important because chronic hypertension increases the risk for stroke, coronary heart disease (CHD), congestive heart disease, angina, MI, transient ischemic attacks, retinopathy, and renal damage. Therefore, control of hypertension decreases the occurrence of these conditions.

Lifestyle Modifications

All patients with elevated blood pressure should adopt lifestyle modifications as a part of therapy; these lifestyle modifications should be continued even when drug therapy is started (Box 12-3). These modifications can lower blood pressure and can decrease the amount of antihypertensive medication needed to control the blood pressure. Among these modifications is eliminating cigarette smoking and limiting daily alcohol consumption. Alcohol consumption and cigarette smoking increase blood pressure. Excess body weight contributes to hypertension; therefore, weight reduction should be a goal for patients above their desirable body weight; even a loss of 10 pounds can reduce blood pressure. Weight loss should be accomplished by a combination of diet management to reduce caloric intake and exercise.

A reduction in dietary salt intake can also reduce blood pressure in some patients. Processed food contributes to most of the salt intake for the average American diet. Limiting the total daily intake of sodium chloride (table salt) to no more than 2.4 g is helpful. Other dietary recommendations are to decrease total fat, particularly saturated fat intake, and maintain adequate dietary potassium. Potassium may protect against hypertension and improve blood pressure in hypertensive patients; however, a 2013 statement on lifestyle modifications found that there was insufficient evidence to support that increased dietary potassium reduces blood pressure.[2] Diuretic therapy, a common class of medications used in hypertension management, can cause depletion of potassium, and it is therefore important for these patients to be cognizant of their potassium intake. Selected fresh fruits and vegetables are among foods that are good sources of potassium (Table 12-3). The DASH (Dietary Approaches to Stop Hypertension) diet is a nutrition plan that has been specifically developed as a lifestyle medication to lower blood pressure in patients with hypertension. This diet encourages intake of healthy foods such as fruits, vegetables, lean meats, and low fat dairy products. It is also rich in nutrients such as potassium and calcium and low in sodium.

BOX 12-3

SUMMARY OF LIFESTYLE MODIFICATIONS TO LOWER BLOOD PRESSURE

- Eliminate cigarette smoking
- Limit daily alcohol consumption
- Reduce weight in patients who are over their desirable body weight
- Reduce dietary salt intake
- Decrease total fat intake
- Maintain adequate dietary potassium
- Regular aerobic exercise of mild to moderate intensity

There is no concrete recommendation regarding the use of caffeine-containing beverages and the impact on hypertension. Although it is clear that the administration of caffeine causes an acute increase in blood pressure, the relationship between caffeinated drinks and blood pressure is unclear. Some studies have shown no effect, whereas others have shown a positive or negative effect. Variables among these studies include whether coffee, tea, soft drinks, or caffeine tablets were used; whether men or women were the subjects; study length; how much caffeinated beverage was consumed; and whether the subjects in the study were regular drinkers of caffeinated beverages prior to the study. It has been suggested that other components of the diet and the genetics of the subject (rate of caffeine metabolism) also contribute to the varied research findings.

Exercise can have a positive effect on hypertension. Regular aerobic exercise of mild to moderate intensity lowers blood pressure in patients with essential hypertension. The molecular mechanism for this antihypertensive effect has not been pinpointed, but it is likely that a reduction in cardiac output and/or peripheral resistance results. Moderately intense exercise, such as 30 to 45 minutes of brisk walking several days per week, can lower blood pressure. The initial exercise routine should be low intensity and short duration with a progressive increase in both parameters. The initial level and intensity of exercise as well as the target goal will vary depending on the severity of the hypertension, patient's age, and existence of other complicating diseases (eg, CHD, diabetes mellitus).

Pharmacologic Therapy

Medication therapy plays a central role in the management of hypertension. As previously discussed, the blood pressure thresholds for initiation of drug therapy are described in Table 12-2. With initiation of drug therapy and lifestyle modifications, the goal of therapy is to reduce the

Table 12-3

Approximate Potassium Levels in Foods

FOOD	< 250 MG PER SERVING[a]	250 TO 500 MG PER SERVING[a]	> 500 MG PER SERVING[a]
Apple	✓		
Apple juice		✓	
Apricots		✓	
Asparagus	✓		
Avocado			✓
Banana		✓	
Beans, baked/franks		✓	
Beans, kidney			✓
Beans, lima			✓
Beans, navy			✓
Blueberries	✓		
Broccoli		✓	
Cantaloupe		✓	
Carrots, cooked		✓	
Cauliflower, raw		✓	
Chicken		✓	
Corn	✓		
Dates			✓
Grapefruit juice		✓	
Ham		✓	
Hamburger		✓	
Hot dog	✓		
Kiwi		✓	
Milk, skim		✓	
Orange juice		✓	
Peach	✓		
Peanuts			✓
Peas	✓		
Pineapple juice		✓	
Pizza slice, pepperoni	✓		
Potato, baked + skin			✓
Potato, sweet		✓	
Raisins			✓
Rice	✓		
Salmon		✓	

(continued)

TABLE 12-3 (CONTINUED)			
APPROXIMATE POTASSIUM LEVELS IN FOODS			
FOOD	< 250 MG PER SERVING[a]	250 TO 500 MG PER SERVING[a]	> 500 MG PER SERVING[a]
Shrimp	✓		
Soup, split pea/ham		✓	
Soup, tomato		✓	
Soybean nuts			✓
Tomato		✓	
Tomato juice			✓
Tuna	✓		
Yogurt, plain			✓
[a]Serving size is 3 oz entree, 1 cup, 8 fluid oz, or per each where appropriate.			

blood pressure to below these treatment initiation thresholds. It should be noted that there are additional guidelines that recommend lower blood pressure goals in patients with specific disease states, such as diabetes mellitus.

When initiating antihypertensive therapy, most patients will be placed on a single medication. If the response to the initial medication is not satisfactory, the guidelines recommend 2 strategies. The first strategy is to increase the dose of the first medication to the maximum dose and then add a second medication if the patient is still not at goal. The second strategy is to add a second medication prior to maximizing the dose of the first medication. In some patients, initiating therapy with 2 medications may be the best strategy. There are several classes of medications used in the treatment of hypertension, but 4 classes of medications are preferred for initial therapy as well as for the additional medications in an antihypertensive regimen. These classes of medications are recommended because of their effectiveness in lowering blood pressure and improving cardiovascular outcomes as well as their side effect profile. Thiazide diuretics, ACE inhibitors (ACEIs), ARBs, and CCBs are the recommended classes of medications for hypertension treatment. There are specific medications recommended for particular patient groups; for example, ACEIs and ARBs are recommended for patients with chronic kidney disease. The medication recommendations from the 2014 hypertension treatment guidelines are outlined in Table 12-4.[1]

Angina Pectoris

Angina is a type of CHD in which the coronary arteries are not able to supply sufficient oxygen to the heart muscle. Consequently, angina is also referred to as *ischemic heart disease*. The major symptom of angina is a sudden pain that originates behind the sternum and radiates to the left shoulder and arm. Pain or discomfort may also be felt in the neck and jaw. Pain occurs when the demand for oxygen to the heart muscle increases beyond what the coronary arteries can supply. There are 3 forms of angina pectoris: chronic stable, variant, and unstable (Box 12-4).

Chronic Stable Angina

Chronic stable angina, also called *exertional angina*, is the classic angina and is the most common form of angina (more than 7 million Americans). Atherosclerosis of one or more of the coronary arteries causes partial occlusion of the affected coronary arteries and thus restricts the amount of blood (hence oxygen) that can flow through those arteries. At rest, there is sufficient oxygen reaching the heart muscle, but when the demand increases (eg, due to exercise), a portion of the heart does not receive enough oxygen to satisfy the demand, and pain results. The pain from exertional angina gradually subsides when the patient stops the exertion and rests. In contrast to an angina attack, if an artery becomes completely blocked, an MI results, the pain lasts 20 to 30 minutes, and heart muscle cells that do not receive oxygen die if blood flow is not restored within a few hours.

Drugs to treat exertional angina are intended to increase the amount of oxygen reaching the heart muscle and/or decrease the demand for oxygen; the focus of nondrug measures is to accomplish the same thing. Loss of excess weight, smoking cessation, treatment of existing hypertension and hyperlipidemia, and a program of regular exercise are among the key nondrug and adjunct measures.

Variant Angina

Variant angina (also called *Prinzmetal angina* or *vasospastic angina*) also results in insufficient blood flow through a coronary artery but is caused from a coronary artery spasm. This spontaneous contraction of the smooth muscle of the artery causes reduced blood flow beyond

TABLE 12-4

MANAGEMENT OF BLOOD PRESSURE IN ADULTS

PATIENT POPULATION	GOAL BLOOD PRESSURE (MM HG)	RECOMMENDED MEDICATIONS[a]
Non-Black patients aged ≥60 yr (no diabetes mellitus or chronic kidney disease)	< 150/90	Thiazide diuretic, ACEI, ARB, CCB
Non-Black patients aged <60 yr (no diabetes mellitus or chronic kidney disease)	< 140/90	Thiazide diuretic, ACEI, ARB, CCB
Black patients aged ≥60 yr (no diabetes mellitus or chronic kidney disease)	< 150/90	Thiazide diuretic, CCB
Black patients aged <60 yr (no diabetes mellitus or chronic kidney disease)	< 140/90	Thiazide diuretic, CCB
Non-Black patients with diabetes mellitus, no chronic kidney disease	< 140/90	Thiazide diuretic, ACEI, ARB, CCB
Black patients with diabetes mellitus, no chronic kidney disease	< 140/90	Thiazide diuretic, CCB
Patients with chronic kidney disease, with or without diabetes mellitus	< 140/90	ACEI, ARB (can consider a thiazide diuretic or CCB in black patients with no protein in the urine)

ACEI=angiotensin-converting enzyme inhibitor; ARB=angiotensin receptor blocker; CCB=calcium channel blocker.

[a]Lifestyle modifications are recommended for all patients, and these modifications should continue once medications are initiated.

Adapted from 2014 Evidence-Based Guidelines for the Management of High Blood Pressure in Adults. Report from the Panel Members Appointed to the Eighth Joint National Committee (JNC 8). *JAMA.* 2014;311(5):507-520.

Box 12-4

SUMMARY OF THE 3 FORMS OF ANGINA PECTORIS

ANGINA TYPE	DESCRIPTION	THERAPY FOCUS
Chronic stable	Also called exertional angina Due to partial occlusion of ≥1 coronary artery, which is benign at rest but results in chest pain with increased activity due to the insufficient flow of oxygen to the heart	Drug and nondrug interventions are intended to increase the amount of oxygen reaching the heart muscle and/or decrease the demand for oxygen.
Variant	Also called Prinzmetal angina or vasospastic angina Results from insufficient blood flow through a coronary artery but is caused by a coronary artery spasm	Drug focus is to increase oxygen supply rather than to specifically reduce demand because the cause is not a result of increased demand
Unstable	Condition in which there is a change in the severity of pain or pattern of angina compared with what the patient has experienced	Drug therapy focus is to increase oxygen delivery to the heart muscle, decrease demand for oxygen, and alleviate persistent pain

that point and hence symptoms similar to chronic stable angina. However, Prinzmetal angina symptoms can occur at any time, not specifically associated with exercise. The focus of drug therapy is to increase oxygen supply rather than to specifically reduce demand because the cause is not a result of increased demand.

Unstable Angina

Unstable angina is a condition in which there is a change in the severity of pain or pattern of angina compared with what the patient has experienced previously (eg, if a patient with chronic stable angina experiences more frequent angina attacks, begins experiencing attacks even at rest, or if the intensity of the anginal pain increases noticeably compared with prior experiences). This suggests a change in the CHD status, such as the occurrence of coronary emboli. The onset of unstable angina is a medical emergency because the risk for death is greater than that with stable angina. The focus of drug therapy is to increase oxygen delivery to the heart muscle, decrease demand for oxygen, and alleviate persistent pain.

Myocardial Infarction

CHD is the leading cause of death among men and women in the United States, and MI leads this list. As with angina, MI is an ischemic heart disease in that occlusion of a coronary artery prevents sufficient blood from reaching a portion of the heart muscle. However, with MI, the ischemia is persistent and progresses to cause death of some myocardial cells. The location and number of cells that die will determine the extent of loss of myocardial function. An MI is an emergency situation, and immediate goals include reducing myocardial oxygen demand, restoring coronary blood flow, preventing additional damage, and minimizing complications (eg, ventricular dysrhythmia and heart failure). Because an acute MI is an emergency and drug therapy is handled by emergency medical personnel and physicians, no discussion is included regarding therapy. The athletic trainer should realize that any patient who has symptoms of MI should immediately receive medical attention. Symptoms include chest pain or pressure, nausea, vomiting, profuse sweating, numbness or tingling in the arm, and shortness of breath.

Existence of atherosclerotic plaques, leading to thrombus formation and platelet aggregation, is the cause of the vast majority of MI. Not surprising, therefore, is that hyperlipidemia and hypertension are among the risk factors for MI, as are smoking and history of angina. Consequently, part of the drug therapy regimen includes treatment of these conditions.

Initial treatment of acute MI includes immediate cessation of activity to decrease oxygen demand and providing supplemental oxygen. For rapid thrombolytic therapy, aspirin should be chewed and swallowed (325 mg) as soon as possible after the onset of MI symptoms unless the patient has an allergy to aspirin. Morphine is the analgesic of choice because its cardiovascular effects reduce myocardial oxygen demand. Other therapies that are helpful in patients within the first few hours after an MI are β-blockers, ACEIs, and either angioplasty or thrombolytic therapy such as alteplase (Activase), which is a drug that breaks apart an existing thrombus.

Heart Failure

Approximately 5 million Americans have heart failure. The incidence of heart failure increases with age, with more than 70% of the patients being older than 60 years. The 5-year survival rate is about 50%. The essence of the problem is that the heart cannot pump with enough force to adequately supply blood to the tissues. Factors that contribute to heart failure include hypertension, CHD, diabetes mellitus, valvular disease, obesity, high blood cholesterol, alcohol abuse, and the process of aging.

Heart failure develops over years. As failure begins, the ventricles fail to eject all of the blood and therefore the diastolic filling also increases. The heart enlarges due to excess blood in the chambers. When the heart muscle stretches, the compensating mechanism causes an automatic increase in contractility to increase cardiac output. There are limits, of course, to the compensatory mechanism, which are exceeded as heart failure continues. Other compensatory mechanisms also occur, such as an increased sympathetic tone and decreased parasympathetic effect. These autonomic nervous system effects cause increased heart rate and contractility, which helps to increase cardiac output. Constriction of the blood vessels also occurs, which helps to maintain blood pressure to tissues but also increases the return of blood to the heart and increases the arterial pressure that the heart must pump against.

The renin-angiotensin system is also activated during heart failure, which increases angiotensin II and aldosterone levels. Aldosterone increases sodium and water retention; angiotensin II adds to an enhanced sympathetic tone by constricting systemic arterioles and veins to increase blood pressure. Decreased blood flow to the kidneys also contributes to water retention and eventual edema. As months or years of elevated aldosterone and angiotensin II

TABLE 12-5

NEW YORK HEART ASSOCIATION FUNCTIONAL CLASSIFICATION OF HEART FAILURE

Class I	Patient has no limitation of ordinary physical activity from undue fatigue, dyspnea, or palpitation.
Class II	Patient has slight limitation of physical activity. Normal physical activity produces fatigue, dyspnea, palpitations, or angina.
Class III	Patient has marked limitation of physical activity. There are no symptoms when patient is at rest, but even mild activity causes symptoms.
Class IV	Patient experiences symptoms at rest and increased discomfort occurs with any physical activity.

persist, it contributes to other aspects of the pathophysiology. For example, aldosterone increases the deposition of collagen within the heart, leading to cardiac fibrosis and eventual diminished function of the heart. This scenario of physiological changes eventually results in pulmonary and peripheral edema. Other primary symptoms of the condition include fatigue, exercise intolerance, shortness of breath, and tachycardia. The aldosterone antagonists are used in the management of heart failure because of their ability to block the negative effects of aldosterone in the heart.

Heart failure is a progressive disease, and, consequently, there is a range of severity of these symptoms among patients. Heart failure is also referred to as *congestive heart failure* because of the pulmonary and peripheral edema, but the term is being used less frequently because some patients do not have symptoms of this fluid congestion. A widely used system of classifying patients regarding the severity of heart failure is the New York Heart Association Functional Classification (Table 12-5). In this classification, Class I heart failure is the least severe and Class IV the most severe.

Treatment of heart failure includes drug therapy, limiting sodium and excess fluid intake, reducing alcohol intake, losing excess weight, and exercising, depending on the severity of heart failure. Regarding the exercise, note that patients with Class I and II heart failure (see Table 12-5) are physically active. In fact, low-intensity aerobic exercise on a regular basis has been demonstrated to improve symptoms and the quality of life in patients with stable heart failure. For safety reasons, patients need to progress slowly in an individualized exercise program and may require supervision during early stages of the exercise program.

DRUG THERAPY

Drug therapy for cardiovascular diseases generally requires long-term therapeutic regimens, often with multiple-drug therapy to achieve desired therapeutic outcomes, along with routine monitoring of the disease to assess the effectiveness of the therapy. Some therapy is intended to alleviate acute symptoms, whereas the focus of other therapy is to minimize the long-term effects of the disease. It may also be necessary in some patients to use other drugs to treat an underlying disease such as dyslipidemia, diabetes mellitus, or alcoholism. Consequently, it is likely that patients will be on multiple-drug therapy for the cardiovascular disease, thus enhancing the likelihood of adverse effects and drug interactions.

Diuretics

Diuretics are drugs that increase the excretion of sodium (Na^+) and chloride (Cl^-) ions. The amount of sodium chloride (NaCl) in the body is the major factor that determines the extracellular fluid volume, which then contributes to blood pressure. The more NaCl, the more extracellular fluid volume (and thus blood volume) and the higher the blood pressure. Accumulation of extracellular fluid in any tissue constitutes edema. The major uses of diuretics are to reduce edema and treat hypertension. Regarding these uses, there are 3 major categories of diuretics: thiazide diuretics, loop diuretics, and potassium-sparing diuretics (Table 12-6).

These categories of diuretics differ in their specific site of action in the nephron of the kidney (Figure 12-3)—loop diuretics in the Henle's loop, thiazide diuretics in the early distal convoluted tubule, and potassium-sparing diuretics in the late distal convoluted tubule and collecting duct. Besides increasing the excretion of Na^+ and Cl^-, diuretics affect the exchange of other ions, potassium (K^+) being the one of prime concern. Thiazide and loop diuretics increase the excretion of K^+, whereas, as evident from the name, potassium-sparing diuretics prevent loss of K^+. The potassium-sparing diuretics have only a weak diuretic effect but are useful in combination with either a thiazide or loop diuretic to prevent hypokalemia (low blood potassium). The thiazide diuretics are the diuretics of first choice for treatment of hypertension. A decrease in blood volume through diuresis is likely the mechanism for the initial antihypertensive activity of thiazide diuretics. However, blood volume returns to nearly the initial level with continued use. A reduction in peripheral vascular resistance occurs with long-term use of thiazide diuretics. The loop diuretics induce a more pronounced diuretic effect and are therefore used when enhanced fluid removal is needed (eg, heart failure).

TABLE 12-6

SELECTED DIURETICS

CATEGORY	GENERIC NAME	TRADE NAME	DOSAGE RANGE[a] (TOTAL MG/DAY)
Thiazide	chlorthalidone	Hygroton	12.5 to 25
	hydrochlorothiazide	Hydrodiuril	12.5 to 50
	indapamide	Lozol	1.25 to 2.5
	methyclothiazide	Enduron	2.5 to 5
	metolazone	Zaroxolyn	1.25 to 10
Loop	bumetanide	Bumex	0.5 to 2
	furosemide	Lasix	20 to 80
	torsemide	Demadex	2.5 to 20
Potassium-sparing	amiloride	Midamor	5 to 20
	eplerenone[b]	Inspra	50 to 100
	spironolactone[b]	Aldactone	25 to 100
	triamterene	Dyrenium	100 to 300

[a]Adult oral dosage range for treatment of hypertension/edema.
[b]Also categorized as aldosterone antagonist.

Technically, the terms thiazides *and* thiazide diuretics *refer to a group of diuretics that share a specific chemical structure and therefore also a common mechanism of action. Subsequent to the initial use of this term, several other diuretics with the same mechanism of action but without the thiazide structure were introduced. These diuretics are often jointly grouped as thiazides and related diuretics or thiazide-type diuretics. Because the differences are primarily in the chemical structure rather than pharmacological properties, for simplicity these 2 groups are referred together as* thiazide diuretics *in this text.*

Of the potassium-sparing diuretics, amiloride (Midamor) and triamterene (Dyrenium) prevent potassium loss by directly inhibiting sodium-potassium exchange through sodium channels in the distal tubule. However, spironolactone (Aldactone) and eplerenone (Inspra) produce their effects by inhibiting aldosterone, which then promotes sodium excretion and potassium retention. In addition, the aldosterone antagonism decreases cardiac remodeling, a process that changes the shape, size, and effectiveness of the heart because of cardiac injury. Angiotensin II and aldosterone play a significant role in initiating the remodeling process, which contributes to the progression of heart failure. Consequently, spironolactone and eplerenone are

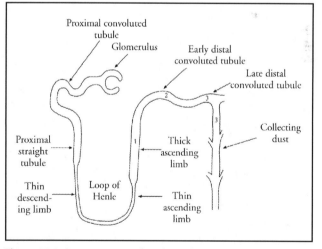

Figure 12-3. Representation of nephron showing the sites of diuretic action. 1 = site of action of loop diuretics, 2 = site of action of thiazide diuretics, and 3 = sites of action of potassium-sparing diuretics.

used for the treatment of moderate to advanced heart failure and increase survival in these patients.

Diuretics are effective orally and may be used to treat edema associated with acute and chronic conditions, including heart failure; thiazide diuretics are also among the first-line treatment options recommended for hypertension. The onset of diuretic action of the thiazide and loop diuretics is within 1 hour after oral ingestion. The potassium-sparing diuretics are not very water soluble and are therefore absorbed more slowly from the gastrointestinal tract. Thiazide diuretics are usually the first choice to achieve diuresis, whereas loop diuretics have the potential to produce greater fluid loss when necessary. Thiazide diuretics are filtered at the glomerulus to reach their tubular site of action. Loop diuretics reach their tubular site by active transport and are therefore more effective in patients with heart failure because these patients typically have reduced glomerular filtration rate.

Concerning adverse effects, a major concern with long-term use of thiazide and loop diuretics is to prevent hypokalemia. Depending on the dose of diuretic and duration of therapy, patients using loop or thiazide diuretics may be advised to eat foods rich in potassium (see Table 12-4) or use potassium supplements. Alternatively, a potassium-sparing diuretic can be used concurrently with the loop or thiazide diuretic. Symptoms of hypokalemia include muscle fatigue and cramps, with eventual cardiac dysrhythmias. Because thiazide or loop diuretics are used to treat heart failure, and because digoxin is used to treat heart failure (see below), it is noteworthy that hypokalemia will cause toxicity from lower doses of digoxin. Consequently, potassium levels are monitored more closely for patients receiving digoxin and a diuretic.

Hyperkalemia is a concern with the use of potassium-sparing diuretics; therefore, potassium supplements should not be used with potassium-sparing diuretics. ACEIs also have a potassium-sparing effect and are therefore generally not used in combination with potassium-sparing diuretics. The aldosterone antagonist diuretic spironolactone (Aldactone) is chemically related to the androgens and progestins and thus may cause gynecomastia and sexual dysfunction in men, whereas women may experience deepening of the voice, hirsutism, and menstrual irregularities. However, eplerenone (Inspra) has a lower incidence of these adverse effects but has a higher risk for hyperkalemia and is thus contraindicated in patients with impaired kidney function.

Adverse effects with thiazide and loop diuretics include increased plasma levels of low-density lipoprotein (LDL) cholesterol, total cholesterol and total triglycerides, hyperglycemia, and sexual dysfunction. These are primarily a concern with higher doses of these diuretics (eg, 100 mg/day of hydrochlorothiazide). Use of NSAIDs with thiazide and loop diuretics can diminish the effectiveness of the diuretics. The mechanism for this is likely to include the NSAID inhibition of the prostaglandin (PG)-mediated improvement of renal blood flow, fluid excretion, and/or vasodilation. Athletic trainers should also note that diuretics can be abused or misused by athletes as performance-enhancing drugs or masking agents (see Chapter 16).

Angiotensin-Converting Enzyme Inhibitors

ACEIs are effective drugs for the treatment of hypertension, heart failure, and MI. By inhibiting ACE, these drugs decrease the production of angiotensin II and therefore diminish the effect of angiotensin II on vasoconstriction and aldosterone release. ACEIs also prevent the breakdown of bradykinin, which, among other actions, increases the release of vasodilating PGs (ie, ACEIs prolong bradykinin's effect, which increases PG-mediated vasodilation). The result of ACEIs is arterial and venous vasodilation, decreased systemic vascular resistance, increased sodium and water excretion, increased potassium retention, and increased blood flow to the kidney.

There are many ACEIs on the market (Table 12-7). Captopril (Capoten) was the first to receive US Food and Drug Administration (FDA) approval. All are effective antihypertensives, with no particular clear-cut advantage of any one drug. Their effectiveness and preferred adverse effect profile have placed them as first-line therapy for hypertension and heart failure.

The ACEIs differ somewhat in their degree of oral absorption and potency, but recommended dosing accommodates for these differences. The activity of most ACEIs is primarily terminated by renal excretion of the active drug, and therefore dosage adjustment may be necessary if renal impairment exists. Most of the ACEIs are administered orally as a prodrug and thus rely on the liver to metabolize the drug to the active form. Captopril (Capoten) and lisinopril (Zestril) are exceptions. Because activation of the prodrug depends on liver function, diminished liver function can decrease the conversion of the prodrug to the active form. Typical oral dosing is 1 to 2 times per day.

The ACEIs are effective alone or in combination with diuretics or β-blockers to treat hypertension or heart failure but are not effective for treating angina. The vasodilation and reduced blood volume are major contributors to the antihypertensive effect. Unlike β-blockers, ACEIs do not affect the automatic cardiac and baroreceptor responses and therefore do not cause significant exercise intolerance. They also do not cause sexual dysfunction, fatigue, bronchoconstriction, hypokalemia, or hyperglycemia as do β-blockers or diuretics. The lack of these effects provides an advantage for the use of ACEIs for the treatment of hypertension in patients who also have diabetes mellitus or asthma. The potassium retention aspect of ACEIs is an advantage to prevent hypokalemia when combined with thiazide diuretics. In fact, use of potassium supplements and potassium-sparing diuretics should be avoided with ACEIs unless blood tests reveal the existence of hypokalemia. The antihypertensive effect of ACEIs is greater in some patients than others. Patients with high renin blood levels respond better to ACEIs, but patients with normal renin levels may also respond, presumably due to a decreased rate of bradykinin inactivation, a higher level of angiotensin II produced in local tissue sites, or greater tissue responsiveness to normal angiotensin II levels.

ACEIs have become an important part of the therapy for heart failure. Therapy with these drugs relieves symptoms and delays progression of the disease. Use of ACEIs

TABLE 12-7

RENIN-ANGIOTENSIN SYSTEM BLOCKERS

CATEGORY	GENERIC NAME	TRADE NAME	DOSAGE RANGE[a] (TOTAL MG/DAY)
Angiotensin-converting enzyme inhibitors	benazepril	Lotensin	10 to 40
	captopril	Capoten	50 to 200
	enalapril	Vasotec	5 to 40
	fosinopril	Monopril	10 to 40
	lisinopril	Zestril	10 to 40
	moexipril	Univasc	7.5 to 30
	perindopril	Aceon	4 to 8
	quinapril	Accupril	10 to 40
	ramipril	Altace	2.5 to 20
	trandolapril	Mavik	1 to 4
Angiotensin II receptor blockers	azilsartan	Edarbi	40 to 80
	candesartan	Atacand	8 to 32
	eprosartan	Teveten	400 to 800
	irbesartan	Avapro	150 to 300
	losartan	Cozaar	25 to 100
	olmesartan	Benicar	20 to 40
	telmisartan	Micardis	20 to 80
	valsartan	Diovan	80 to 320
Direct renin inhibitor	aliskiren	Tekturna	150 to 300
Aldosterone antagonists	spironolactone	Aldactone	25 to 100
	eplerenone	Inspra	50 to 100

[a]Adult oral dosage range for treatment of hypertension.

provides a multipronged approach: dilation of arterioles improves cardiac output; venous dilation reduces pulmonary and peripheral edema; inhibition of aldosterone increases sodium and water excretion to reduce edema; and inhibition of the angiotensin II-mediated effect on cardiac remodeling and dilation of arterioles to the kidneys improve renal function, which also reduces edema.

Treatment of MI is another approved use of some ACEIs; their use for acute MI decreases mortality. Therapy is begun immediately and may be continued long term if necessary.

Although most patients generally tolerate ACEIs well, some adverse effects can be problematic. A persistent dry cough occurs in 5% to 20% of patients, which may require discontinuation of the ACEI. The cough develops, at least in part, from the accumulation of bradykinin. It occurs more frequently in women than men and dissipates over several days after discontinuation of the ACEI. For patients being treated for heart failure with ACEIs, pulmonary edema should be eliminated as the cause of the cough before the ACEI is discontinued; diuretic therapy should diminish the cough if pulmonary edema is the origin.

Another bradykinin-linked adverse effect is angioedema, a rare condition in which rapid swelling in the nose, throat, and larynx may lead to death if not treated; it occurs more frequently in people of African descent. Other adverse effects that may warrant discontinuation of therapy are skin rashes, loss of taste, and taste disturbances that occur in 4% to 10% of patients. First-dose hypotension is common with ACEIs, especially in patients who are sodium or volume depleted or in patients on diuretics. Consequently, patients should be started with a low-dose ACEI and diuretics should be discontinued 2 to 3 days prior to initiating ACE inhibitor therapy. ACEIs have complex effects on kidney function. In patients with chronic kidney disease, ACEIs can help protect the kidneys. However, use of these medications can cause acute declines in kidney function in some patients; because of this, they should not be used in patients with certain kidney conditions such as bilateral renal artery stenosis. Drugs that directly affect the renin-angiotensin-aldosterone system should not be used during pregnancy due to the potential for major congenital malformations or death.

Drug interactions with ACEIs occur with antacids and NSAIDs. Antacids can interfere with the absorption of ACEIs and should not be taken concurrently. NSAIDs can decrease the antihypertensive effect by inhibiting the bradykinin-induced antihypertensive (ie, vasodilation) effects. Concurrent use of diuretics with an ACEI may cause first-dose hypotension. To prevent hyperkalemia, potassium supplements and potassium-sparing diuretics should be avoided with ACEIs unless hypokalemia is identified.

Angiotensin II Receptor Blockers

ARBs comprise a category of drugs that became available after the ACEIs, obtaining FDA approval in 1995. In contrast to ACEIs, which decrease the production of angiotensin II, ARBs combine with the receptor site to prevent the response of angiotensin II after it has been produced. Therefore, ARBs have pharmacological effects similar to ACE inhibitors: vasodilation and increased sodium and water excretion through suppression of aldosterone release. However, ARBs do not affect bradykinin metabolism; therefore, the incidence of some adverse effects is significantly reduced in comparison with ACEIs.

There are several ARBs approved for treatment of hypertension (see Table 12-7). They have approximately equal antihypertensive effectiveness. The dose-response curve (see Chapter 3) for these drugs is quite flat, which means that increasing the dose does not cause much increase in response. The pharmacokinetics are somewhat dissimilar for the drugs within this category (half-life [t½] ranges from 2.5 to 24 hours); major routes of plasma clearance of active drug vary from liver metabolism to bile excretion and renal elimination; and depending on the drug, liver metabolism results in the drug being converted from inactive to active, from active to inactive, or from active to more active.

For treatment of hypertension, ARBs are as effective as ACE inhibitors in lowering blood pressure and are first-line agents. Angiotensin II receptor blockers provide an alternative to the ACE inhibitors for patients who experience the bothersome cough. ARBs have been effective in the treatment of heart failure and to treat MI.

Adverse effects from ARBs are minimal. In comparison with ACEIs, the cough, angioedema, first-dose hypotension, and taste disturbances are reduced or nonexistent with ARBs. Hyperkalemia is only a concern if ARBs are combined with potassium-sparing diuretics or potassium supplements or in patients with renal disease. The effects

on kidney function and pregnancy are similar to those of the ACE inhibitors.

Direct Renin Inhibitors

Aliskiren (Tekturna) is the first direct renin inhibitor to be approved by the FDA for the treatment of hypertension (see Table 12-7). This drug affects the renin-angiotensin-aldosterone system by combining directly to renin, thus inactivating the renin. By reducing the amount of renin activity, the amount of angiotensinogen being converted to angiotensin I is reduced, which ultimately reduces the amount of angiotensin II. Aliskiren is approved for the management of hypertension, but it is not included as a first-line medication in the treatment guidelines.

Adverse effects from aliskiren are relatively low. Bradykinin levels are not increased, and thus the incidence of cough associated with aliskiren is low. Hyperkalemia also is not common. As with other inhibitors of the renin-angiotensin-aldosterone system, aliskiren should not be used during pregnancy. Patients with type 2 diabetes mellitus appear to be at increased risk for adverse effects from aliskiren; for this reason, aliskiren should not be used in combination with an ACEI or an ARB in a diabetic patient.

Calcium Channel Blockers

Calcium channels are the gates that control the flow of calcium into the cells of arterial smooth muscle and cardiac muscle. Influx of calcium results in contraction of these muscle cells, which causes peripheral vasoconstriction, increased heart rate and force of contraction, and cardiac arteriole vasoconstriction. Blocking these channels with CCBs causes the opposite effects: peripheral vasodilation, decreased heart rate and force of contraction, and dilation of arterioles of the heart. There are 2 types of CCBs: those that affect the calcium channels of the heart and vascular muscle and those that are selective for only vascular smooth muscle.

The CCBs are approved for treatment of hypertension (Table 12-8), and some are approved for treating chronic stable and vasospastic angina. They are absorbed readily after oral administration, but first-pass liver metabolism significantly diminishes the amount of active drug that reaches the active site. Typical dosages account for the first-pass effect, but patients with liver dysfunction may need a lower dosage due to a diminished impact on first-pass metabolism. Elderly patients may also require dosage adjustment due to diminished hepatic function.

Peripheral arteriole vasodilation reduces blood pressure. Dilation of the arterioles of the heart increases blood and oxygen to the heart muscle, coupled with the reduced arterial blood pressure, is of obvious benefit in treating angina. The effect on heart rate and contractility reduces the oxygen demand on the heart and is beneficial for treating both hypertension and angina. Rapid vasodilation can occur with

TABLE 12-8		
CALCIUM CHANNEL BLOCKERS		
GENERIC NAME	TRADE NAME	DOSAGE RANGE[a] (TOTAL MG/DAY)
amlodipine[b]	Norvasc	2.5 to 10
diltiazem[b,c]	Cardizem LA, others	120 to 360
felodipine	Plendil	2.5 to 10
isradipine	DynaCirc CR	5 to 20
nicardipine[b]	Cardene SR	60 to 120
nifedipine[b]	Procardia XL, others	60 to 120
nisoldipine	Sular	20 to 40
verapamil[b,c]	Calan SR, others	120 to 480

[a]Adult oral dosage range for treatment of hypertension.
[b]Also approved for treatment of chronic stable and vasospastic angina.
[c]Besides blocking calcium channels in vascular smooth muscle, also blocks calcium channels in the heart = nonselective.

TABLE 12-9		
β-BLOCKERS		
GENERIC NAME	TRADE NAME	DOSAGE RANGE[a] (TOTAL MG/DAY)
acebutolol[b]	Sectral	200 to 400
atenolol[b]	Tenormin	25 to 100
betaxolol[b]	Kerlone	5 to 20
bisoprolol[b]	Zebeta	2.5 to 20
carvedilol[c]	Coreg	12.5 to 50
labetalol[c]	Normodyne	200 to 600
metoprolol[b]	Lopressor, Toprol XL	100 to 200
nadolol	Corgard	40 to 80
nebivolol[b,c]	Bystolic	5 to 40
penbutolol	Levatol	20 to 40
pindolol	Visken	5 to 60
propranolol	Inderal	40 to 320
timolol	Blocadren	20 to 40

[a]Adult oral dosage range for treatment of hypertension.
[b]Selective for β_1-receptors.
[c]Also has vasodilating properties.

CCBs, resulting in *reflex tachycardia* (a baroreceptor reflex effect), which is counterproductive for treatment of both angina and hypertension. This tachycardia is offset by cardiac effects of nonselective CCBs: verapamil (Calan) and diltiazem (Cardizem). Nifedipine (Procardia) and all of the other CCBs currently available (nifedipine-like CCBs) are much more selective for the calcium channels of vascular smooth muscle than heart muscle. Consequently, the selective CCBs do not have the cardiac effects to offset the reflex tachycardia and therefore some antihypertensive benefit is lost. Some of the nifedipine-like CCBs (also called *dihydropyridines* from their chemical structure) have a greater reflex tachycardia response than others in this group but can be combined with a β-blocker to prevent the reflex tachycardia. Alternatively, slow-release dosage forms can be used so that the drop in blood pressure is gradual, thus minimizing the baroreceptor reflex. CCBs do not have an effect on exercise tolerance.

Adverse effects are related to the vasodilation and smooth muscle relaxation effects. For example, facial flushing, headache, gingival hyperplasia, and edema of lower extremities are adverse effects common to all the CCBs. Additionally, CCBs decrease the contraction of intestinal smooth muscle, which results in constipation. Bradycardia from verapamil (Calan) and diltiazem (Cardizem) can occur but is of little consequence unless the patient also has certain heart diseases (eg, heart block, heart failure), in which case a nifedipine-like CCB is preferred because they do not affect heart muscle. Although β-blockers reduce reflex tachycar-

dia from nifedipine-like CCBs, use of β-blockers with verapamil (Calan) or diltiazem (Cardizem) should be avoided because they have similar effects on the heart and if used together will increase the potential for heart block.

β-Blockers

The number of β-blocker drugs has grown over the years to now encompass an array of more than a dozen drugs (Table 12-9). These drugs are competitive inhibitors of the β-adrenergic receptors and are also called *β-adrenergic antagonists*. Blockade of these receptors causes a variety of effects, some beneficial and some not. Most of the therapeutic and adverse effects of these drugs can be explained by the activity at specific receptor sites. Not all β-blockers exhibit these effects to the same extent, in part because some β-blockers are relatively selective for β_1-adrenergic receptors (selective blockers) and other β-blockers are nonselective, combining significantly with both β_1- and β_2-receptors. Note that the selective β-blockers may elicit some β_2 response, particularly at higher doses. The primary effect of β-blockers with a brief discussion is provided (Box 12-5).

- β-blockers slow the heart rate and the conduction velocity of the impulse. Therefore, when the level of adrenergic stimulation is low, the effect of adrenergic

Box 12-5

SUMMARY OF PRIMARY EFFECT OF β-BLOCKERS

- Decreased heart rate and force of contraction due to blockade of β_1-receptors

- β-blockers slow the rate of impulses initiated by the sinoatrial node and the conduction velocity of the impulse through the atrioventricular node

- Exercise fatigue may occur because of the β-blocker, preventing the heart from automatically increasing cardiac output

- Reduced release of renin by the kidney due to β_1-receptor blockade, reducing the impact of the renin-angiotensin system

- Bronchoconstriction from the blockade of β_2-receptors in the lung

- Inhibition of glycogenolysis in the liver and muscle cells due to β_2-receptor blockade

- Inhibition of sympathetic-induced activation of lipase in fat cells

- Decreased peripheral vascular resistance due to long-term use of β-blockers

blockade will also be low. However, when adrenergic agonist activity is high, such as during exercise or stress, the impact of an antagonist will be greater. As a result, β-blockers prevent the heart from over-exertion but also prevent the automatic increase in cardiac output, resulting in exercise fatigue.

- β-blockers slow the rate of impulses initiated by the SA node and the conduction velocity of the impulse through the AV node. Therefore, blockade of β_1-receptors is useful in treating certain tachy-dysrhythmias (abnormal rhythm in which the beats are too fast), including exercise-induced tachydys-rhythmia.

- There is a reduced release of renin by the kidney due to β_1-receptor blockade, reducing the impact of the renin-angiotensin system.

- Bronchoconstriction from the blockade of β_2-receptors in the lung occurs. This is usually of little consequence for patients with normal lung function. However, for patients with compromised lung function, this effect can be life threatening. Consequently, nonselective β-blockers are contra-indicated in patients with asthma or chronic obstruc-

tive pulmonary disease; selective β_1-blockers must be used with great caution in these patients.

- There is inhibition of glycogenolysis in the liver and muscle cells due to β_2-receptor blockade. Activation of glycogenolysis by sympathetic response (release of epinephrine from adrenal glands) mobilizes stored glucose from the liver during hypoglycemia. The epinephrine also elicits warning symptoms of hypoglycemia (eg, nervous feeling, tachycardia). Inhibition of this process by nonselective β-blockers is generally of little consequence for most patients, but it may delay recovery from hypoglycemia in patients who have insulin-dependent diabetes. β-blockers may also mask the warning symptoms of hypoglycemia; tachycardia usually accompanies hypoglycemia-induced sympathetic nervous system activation and is a warning sign of hypoglycemia but this helpful symptom is inhibited by all β-blockers.

- There is inhibition of sympathetic-induced activation of lipase in fat cells. Activation of this enzyme causes the conversion of stored triglycerides to fatty acids and results in the release of fatty acids into the blood from fat cells. Although the exact mechanism is not pinpointed and a third receptor (β_3) may be involved, nonselective β-blockers may affect the metabolism of triglycerides and fatty acids.

- There is decreased peripheral vascular resistance due to long-term use of β-blockers. The mechanism is unclear but this is beneficial for treatment of cardiovascular disease.

Primary uses for β-blockers are to treat the chronic diseases of hypertension, angina, and heart failure. Therefore, useful characteristics of these drugs are that they are orally effective and require only once- or twice-per-day dosing, due to an inherently long $t\frac{1}{2}$ or an extended-release formulation. The activity of some β-blockers is terminated primarily by liver metabolism (eg, metoprolol, propranolol, timolol), by excretion as active drug in the urine (eg, acebutolol, atenolol, nadolol), or by significant termination by both routes (eg, pindolol).

The β-blockers are approximately equally effective for treatment of hypertension and angina, and thus drug selection can be based in part on the most suitable pharmacokinetic parameters (eg, $t\frac{1}{2}$ as affected by liver and kidney function), cost, adverse effects, and existence of other diseases. These drugs are used either alone or in combination with other antihypertensive drugs. They decrease blood pressure in hypertensive, but not normotensive (having normal blood pressure), patients. The mechanism for the antihypertensive response is not clear, although a likely key factor is the ability of β-blockers to decrease peripheral vascular resistance after long-term use. Other mechanisms that may contribute to their use as antihypertensive therapy are the inhibition of the renin-angiotensin mechanism, decrease in cardiac output, and inhibition of reflex tachycardia that occurs with the use of vasodilators (see below). β-blockers are considered second-line options for treatment of hypertension.

Angina is also effectively treated with β-blockers. By decreasing the heart rate and contractility, the β-blockers decrease oxygen demand and thereby decrease the frequency and intensity of anginal attacks. These drugs are effective for preventing symptoms of stable, not variant, angina when used on a daily basis. They also provide the benefit of inhibiting reflex tachycardia caused by nitroglycerin therapy. If β-blocker therapy must be discontinued, gradual rather than abrupt withdrawal is necessary to prevent precipitation of anginal attacks or MI.

Some β-blockers are effective in the treatment of heart failure. At one time, these drugs were contraindicated in patients with heart failure, but they have been shown to slow the progression of the disease. Short-term use of β-blockers may not alleviate specific symptoms, but long-term use of the appropriate drug, beginning at a low dose, has been shown to prolong life. The ability of β-blockers to decrease the sympathetic response that is usually elevated in patients with heart failure leads to the beneficial effect in heart failure. Metoprolol (Toprol XL), carvedilol (Coreg), and bisoprolol (Zebeta) have demonstrated effectiveness for this use.

There are several other uses for selected β-blockers that are not as pertinent to this chapter but are worth noting. Such uses include preventing migraine headache, treating acute panic symptoms, inhibiting some symptoms of pheochromocytoma (a catecholamine-secreting tumor), managing certain types of dysrhythmias, treating acute MI and preventing recurrences of MI, and treating glaucoma topically. The ergogenic effects of β-blockers are discussed in Chapter 16.

Some of the significant adverse effects are specific for patients who also have a coexisting disease. Because of the potential for bronchoconstriction (even with ophthalmic preparations), β-blockers should be avoided in asthmatics or limited to β_1-selective agents (eg, metoprolol, acebutolol, atenolol) if use of a β-blocker is necessary. Note that the cardioselectivity for β_1-receptors is lost as the dose increases. Similarly, due to the ability of β-blockers to mask the symptoms of hypoglycemia and to delay the recovery of hypoglycemia by glycogenolysis, the use of β-blockers in diabetics should be used with caution and limited to β_1-selective agents. Other adverse effects that are significant in some patients include bradycardia, insomnia, sexual dysfunction, depression, nightmares, increased levels of plasma triglycerides, reduced levels of high-density lipoprotein (HDL) cholesterol, fatigue, and decreased exercise tolerance.

Organic Nitrates

Nitroglycerin is the prototype organic nitrate. Used since the 1800s, it remains the most frequently used drug to treat acute angina attacks. The principal effect of nitroglycerin is to dilate peripheral vascular smooth muscle. This primarily involves veins, although arterioles are affected to a lesser extent. Vasodilation reduces the blood returning to the heart and therefore decreases the oxygen demand by the heart, a beneficial effect in a patient experiencing stable (exertional) angina. The relaxation of vascular smooth muscle by nitroglycerin also alleviates spasms of those muscles, and hence nitroglycerin is useful for the treatment of variant angina.

Nitroglycerin is very potent (0.3 to 0.6 mg for relief of acute attack) and very lipid soluble, both attributes that are conducive to the use of sublingual and transdermal dosage forms. Regardless of the dosage form, the plasma t½ of nitroglycerin is very short (approximately 5 minutes). Sublingual administration is the most common route for treatment of acute angina with nitroglycerin. The sublingual tablets are inexpensive and dissolve very quickly under the tongue, provided the patient does not have a dry mouth. Onset of action is within 3 minutes and duration is less than 1 hour. Patients should take the first dose as soon as possible when pain begins. The patient may use 3 sublingual tablets over 15 minutes (5 minutes apart); however, the patient should seek emergency care if the first sublingual tablet does not relieve the angina pain because this may be a sign of unstable angina or MI. Sublingual tablets can be used 5 to 10 minutes prior to exertion as a short-term preventative of anginal attacks. Nitroglycerin is chemically unstable and will lose effectiveness if exposed to light and moisture. Therefore, tablets should be stored in tightly closed glass containers, protected from light and moisture, and discarded after 6 months of being opened. Sublingual tablets are not effective orally (by swallowing) because of significant first-pass metabolism.

> *Recall from Chapter 2 that the oral route refers to the drug being swallowed. Recall also from Chapter 2 that nitroglycerin taken orally is subject to the enzymes in the intestinal cells and the liver before reaching the general circulation (ie, first-pass metabolism). Therefore, if sublingual nitroglycerin tablets are swallowed, the nitroglycerin is inactivated before it can reach the site of action.*

A burning sensation under the tongue is indicative of active nitroglycerin, although some patients, especially the elderly, may lack sufficient sensation to experience the burning.

Other dosage forms for treatment of acute angina are buccal tablets and translingual spray. The buccal tablets are placed between the lip and gum or cheek and gum. These tablets provide onset within 2 minutes and have a sustained effect for 3 to 5 hours. Buccal tablets provide relief of acute attacks, but compared with sublingual tablets they provide more sustained relief for longer periods of exercise tolerance. The translingual spray provides a metered dose of nitroglycerin onto or under the tongue with onset and duration similar to sublingual tablets.

Nitroglycerin is also available in sustained-release tablets and capsules, transdermal systems, and ointments, which provide the drug for a longer time. Larger doses (2.5 to 9 mg/dosage unit) are used for the tablets and capsules, not only to provide drug for a longer time but also to accommodate for the first-pass hepatic metabolism. Onset is 20 to 45 minutes and duration is up to 8 hours. The many transdermal systems make nitroglycerin available in various patch devices and allow a continuous release of nitroglycerin. The doses of transdermal patches are designated as release rates (eg, 0.2 mg/hr); the higher the release rate, the higher the blood concentration of nitroglycerin achieved. Nitroglycerin ointment is also placed on the skin for a transdermal effect. Doses of ointment are measured as inches of ointment squeezed from the tube. The ointment is spread over an area of skin on the chest or back.

The onset of action of the sustained release and transdermal nitroglycerin products is too slow to be used to treat acute attacks, but they are used to prevent angina attacks. A significant concern regarding the daily use of nitroglycerin is the development of *tolerance*, referring to a diminished effectiveness of the nitroglycerin because of frequent or continuous exposure to the drug. Tolerance can develop after one day of continuous exposure, especially at higher doses of nitroglycerin. The cause of tolerance is not clear. To prevent tolerance, each day should include 8 to 14 hours in which no nitroglycerin (or other nitrate drug) is administered. For example, the transdermal patch could be removed at night. When the patch is reapplied, onset of action occurs in about 1 hour.

Adverse effects from daily nitroglycerin use are generally manageable. Headache is common, sometimes severe, but subsides after several days of treatment. The rapid vasodilation causes reflex tachycardia through the baroreceptor reflex. Tachycardia is counterproductive in the treatment of angina, and therefore a β-blocker or CCB that suppresses the heart (verapamil or diltiazem) can be used to prevent reflex tachycardia. Orthostatic hypotension (postural hypotension) is also a potential problem associated with vasodilation. Dizziness, with potential for fainting, occurs upon standing because of blood pooling in the veins from nitrate-induced vasodilation. This pooling prevents a sufficient transient increase in blood pressure needed upon standing. Concurrent use of alcohol or CCBs, which also have a vasodilation effect, can accentuate the orthostatic hypotension response. Use of sildenafil (Viagra) and related drugs to treat erectile dysfunction within 24 hours of nitroglycerin or any other organic nitrate can result in potentially fatal hypotension.

Other organic nitrate drugs are also available for the treatment of angina. These are available as oral, chewable, or sublingual dosage forms for prophylaxis of angina attacks and/or treatment of acute attacks. The adverse effects, potential for tolerance, and drug interactions are similar for these drugs as for nitroglycerin. Examples are isosorbide mononitrate (Imdur) and isosorbide dinitrate (Isordil). They offer no particular therapeutic advantage over nitroglycerin.

Vasodilators

As discussed in this chapter, ACEIs, CCBs, and organic nitrates all have a vasodilation component to their mechanisms of action. There are other categories of drugs that also cause peripheral vasodilation as a major component of their mechanism. These other vasodilators are used to treat hypertension, but they are not the first-line or second-line drugs for most patients because they exert a lesser impact on the symptoms or disease process or because the frequency or severity of adverse effects is more pronounced. Consequently, vasodilators as a category of drugs are only briefly mentioned here to provide a more complete picture of the drugs available to treat hypertension.

These vasodilators fall into 3 general categories: α_1-adrenergic blockers, centrally acting α_2-adrenergic agonists, and direct-acting vasodilators. The α_1-adrenergic blockers combine with the α-receptors on the peripheral blood vessels to prevent adrenergic-stimulated vasoconstriction; prazosin (Minipress) is an example. Activation of the α_2-receptor in the CNS indirectly affects the peripheral nervous system by decreasing sympathetic outflow (ie, reduces the CNS-controlled sympathetic response), thereby reducing the response at the α-adrenergic receptor. An example of a centrally acting α_2-adrenergic agonist is clonidine (Catapres). Other vasodilators do not function selectively through adrenergic receptors but instead are direct-acting vasodilators; examples include hydralazine (Apresoline) and minoxidil (Loniten).

Digoxin

Digoxin (Lanoxin) is a member of a group of drugs called *cardiac glycosides* but is the only one in this group commonly used therapeutically. The major use for digoxin is to treat heart failure. The therapeutic benefit stems primarily because of digoxin's ability to increase the force of contraction. Because of the positive inotropic response, cardiac output increases, exercise tolerance improves, urine output increases, edema decreases, and renin release is decreased, which subsequently reduces the response from angiotensin II and aldosterone. These effects help to alleviate symptoms of heart failure, but digoxin does not improve survival.

The mechanism for digoxin centers on the drug's ability to inhibit the enzyme called Na^+, K^+-ATPase. (Note: This ATPase has a different function from the one in the stomach cells discussed in Chapter 11.) Inhibition of this enzyme results in an accumulation of calcium ions within the cell, which increases the force of contraction. The concentration of potassium plays an important role in the therapeutic effect and toxic effect of digoxin. Potassium competes with digoxin for the same ATPase enzyme-binding site; therefore, an increase in potassium concentration decreases the response from of digoxin, and a decrease in potassium will increase digoxin effects. Consequently, hyperkalemia minimizes digoxin effectiveness, whereas hypokalemia can cause digoxin toxicity; both effects occur without a change in the digoxin dosage. Monitoring of potassium blood levels is therefore a part of digoxin therapy.

Two key characteristics of digoxin are that it has a low therapeutic index and that many factors affect the pharmacokinetic and pharmacodynamic parameters. Significant changes in these parameters may warrant a dosage adjustment of digoxin to maintain optimal effectiveness. As already mentioned, blood potassium levels can affect the response from digoxin. Considering that diuretics are also frequently used as a component of heart failure therapy and that some diuretics can cause hypokalemia (eg, thiazide and loop diuretics), caution is warranted to prevent a problem when diuretics and digoxin are combined.

Digoxin is excreted mostly unchanged in the urine. As urine output increases with increased cardiac output, the dose of digoxin may need adjustment as it is excreted at a faster rate. Drug interactions occur with a variety of drugs that alter the absorption or renal excretion of digoxin or change the conduction of impulses in the heart to either potentiate or antagonize the cardiac effects of digoxin. Examples of drugs that increase an effect of digoxin are erythromycin, tetracyclines, β-blockers, CCBs, and sympathomimetics. Examples of drugs that decrease an effect of digoxin are antacids and cholestyramine.

Because of the potential for the effectiveness of digoxin to be modified by drug interactions, changes in potassium blood concentration, and changes in kidney function, it is standard procedure to monitor the patient's digoxin blood concentration and/or signs of cardiac toxicity. Adverse effects that may be early signs of toxicity are anorexia, nausea, vomiting, fatigue, blurred vision, or the appearance of halos around objects. Cardiac toxicity includes a variety of dysrhythmias that can progress to heart failure. Closer monitoring of digoxin blood levels and adverse effects typically occurs at the beginning of therapy, if there is a change in dosage, if there are signs of toxicity, if symptoms of heart failure increase, or if a drug with the potential for drug interaction is added to the patient's drug therapy.

Typical dosage range for maintenance digoxin therapy is 0.125 to 0.5 mg/day in a single dose of an oral tablet. Digoxin has a long t½ (1.5 to 2 days), and consequently, it takes at least 6 days (approximately 4 t½) for a stable blood level to be obtained when initiating therapy or adjusting the dose unless a loading dose is given. Oral absorption of digoxin tablets varies from 70% to 80% among most patients. Digoxin is also available as liquid-filled soft capsules (Lanoxicaps), which provide a somewhat higher rate of absorption. The higher absorption rate necessitates a downward adjustment in dosage with the capsule compared with tablets; the major disadvantage is higher cost.

> *Recall from Chapter 3 that a loading dose is one or more doses that are higher than the maintenance dose and administered at the beginning of therapy for the purpose of more quickly achieving the desirable blood level.*

Section Summary

For the treatment of hypertension and heart disease, there are several categories of drugs with numerous examples within each category. Knowledge of the mechanisms of action of these drug categories provides a means of understanding the uses and many of the common adverse effects. The following are some key points:

- Diuretics decrease the workload of the heart by decreasing blood volume and peripheral vascular resistance. These drugs are used to treat hypertension and edema associated with heart failure. Hypokalemia is a common adverse effect associated with thiazide and loop diuretics, but the addition of potassium supplements or potassium-sparing diuretics can offset the problem. Unrelated to the diuretic effect, spironolactone is also effective in treating heart failure.

- ACEIs prevent the formation of angiotensin II and thus inhibit the peripheral vascular constriction and fluid retention effects of angiotensin II. ACEIs are useful for the treatment of hypertension, heart failure, and MI. A persistent cough is a common adverse effect that sometimes warrants discontinuation of the drug. ACEIs do not pose the problems to diabetics and asthmatics that β-blockers do, and they are useful when combined with diuretics for their potassium-sparing effect.

- ARBs have a usefulness similar to ACEIs because both categories of drugs interfere with the renin-angiotensin system. The ARBs do not cause the cough and have less significant potassium retention effects compared with ACEIs.

- CCBs decrease the contraction of myocardium and vascular smooth muscle. Selective CCBs only affect vascular smooth muscle. Because CCBs cause vasodilation, reflex tachycardia can occur with the selective CCBs unless a β-blocker is used concurrently. Uses for CCBs are primarily for treatment of hypertension and angina.

- β-blockers decrease the heart rate and force of contraction and therefore prevent the heart from overexertion. The selective β₁-blockers are more specific for the heart than nonselective β-blockers and thus have fewer adverse effects. Uses include the treatment of hypertension, angina, MI, and heart failure. The potential for significant adverse effects resides primarily with patients with coexisting diseases of asthma or diabetes mellitus. Exercise intolerance is also a common adverse effect.

- Nitroglycerin is the drug of choice for treatment of acute angina attacks. This drug reduces the oxygen demand on the heart by causing peripheral vasodilation. Sublingual tablets produce an effect within 3 minutes but are of short duration. Adverse effects are short term and commonly include a burning sensation under the tongue and headache. Transdermal and sustained-release oral dosage forms are available to prevent attacks.

- Digoxin is used to treat heart failure to relieve symptoms, although it does not improve survival. The heart more efficiently pumps blood due to the effect of digoxin, and, consequently, blood flow to the kidney also increases. Digoxin has a low therapeutic index and thus must be monitored for toxicity; hypokalemia increases the effect of digoxin and can precipitate toxic symptoms.

THERAPY STRATEGIES

Besides drug therapy, an important part of the overall treatment plan for cardiovascular diseases are the nondrug measures that can have a significant impact on the symptoms, disease progression, and effectiveness of drug therapy. These include the lifestyle modifications mentioned in the foundational concepts section of this chapter. Another nondrug measure is to promote adherence with drug therapy. As is the case with the treatment of other chronic diseases, lack of adherence is a major impediment to achieving therapeutic outcomes, contributing to inadequate control in over two-thirds of hypertensive patients. Poor adherence is particularly a problem with hypertension therapy because it often requires a multiple drug regimen, and the lack of immediate symptoms associated with hypertension diminishes the incentive to maintain therapy. Two means of improving adherence are to educate the patient regarding the potential effects of uncontrolled hypertension and to reduce the complexity of the drug regimen. Regarding the latter issue, the therapy for patients with a multiple-drug regimen should be reviewed to determine whether a switch from multiple dosing per day to once-a-day or twice-a-day dosing is appropriate. Another option is to replace therapy with the corresponding fixed-dose combinations (ie, more than one drug in the same dosage form) that are available (Table 12-10). Using combinations like these reduces the number of tablets or capsules that the patients must remember to take each day.

Another aspect of treating hypertension and heart disease is the use of drugs that can have an indirect impact on the disease. Because elevated blood lipids are risk factors contributing to cardiovascular disease, patients with hypertension or heart disease may also be taking drugs to reduce blood triglyceride and LDL cholesterol or increase the HDL cholesterol. Primary goals in treating hyperlipidemia are to reduce the LDL cholesterol and increase the HDL cholesterol. There are a variety of drugs available to accomplish these goals, including the statins (Box 12-6), which is a group of drugs. The statins decrease the synthesis of cholesterol by inhibiting an enzyme called HMG-CoA reductase; hence, these drugs are also called HMG-CoA reductase inhibitors. The statins are quite effective in reducing LDL cholesterol and triglycerides and increasing HDL cholesterol, and they have relatively few adverse effects, making them the most commonly used drugs to lower blood cholesterol levels. Use of antiplatelet therapy (eg, aspirin) or anticoagulant therapy (eg, warfarin) may also be a part of the patient's drug regimen to prevent thrombus formation, which is a potential ramification of heart disease. The use of drugs to reduce LDL cholesterol or to prevent thrombosis adds to the complexity of the dosage regimen, contributes to the adherence issues and introduces an additional layer of potential adverse effects and drug interactions. Typically, therefore, it is necessary for the patient's drug therapy to be monitored by the physician and/or pharmacist.

Because some pharmacological categories of drugs are used to treat more than one cardiovascular disease, and because multiple drug therapy is often necessary to treat hypertension and heart disease, a few aspects regarding drug therapy are provided here.

Hypertension

- The 2014 hypertension guidelines recommend 4 classes of medications for initial treatment of hypertension: thiazide diuretics, ACEIs, ARBs, and CCBs.

- Therapy with one medication is the most common strategy for initiating therapy. The dose of this medication can be increased or additional medications can be added if the patient does not reach treatment goals. In some patients, initiation of therapy with 2 medications is the preferred strategy.

- Initial doses of antihypertensive therapy should be low, particularly in elderly patients, and then doses should be increased gradually as needed. Because chronic hypertension generally does not place the patient in immediate danger, it is better to place the patient at lower risk of adverse effects as the dose is gradually increased. In addition, baroreceptor responses are less dramatic when blood pressure is gradually decreased.

- Use of specific antihypertensive drug categories may be preferred in certain patients. Examples include:

  ○ In patients of African descent, use of thiazide diuretics and CCBs is preferred.

TABLE 12-10

SELECTED FIXED-DOSE COMBINATION PRODUCTS TO TREAT HYPERTENSION

CATEGORY	DRUG COMPONENTS	TRADE NAME[a]
Diuretic + diuretic	hydrochlorothiazide + triamterene	Dyazide
	hydrochlorothiazide + spironolactone	Aldactazide
	hydrochlorothiazide + amiloride	Moduretic
Diuretic + β-blocker	chlorthalidone + atenolol	Tenoretic
	hydrochlorothiazide + metoprolol	Lopressor HCT
	hydrochlorothiazide + bisoprolol	Ziac
Diuretic + ACEI	hydrochlorothiazide + benazepril	Lotensin HCT
	hydrochlorothiazide + enalapril	Vaseretic
	hydrochlorothiazide + lisinopril	Zestoretic
	hydrochlorothiazide + moexipril	Uniretic
Diuretic + ARB	hydrochlorothiazide + losartan	Hyzaar
	hydrochlorothiazide + valsartan	Diovan HCT
	hydrochlorothiazide + candesartan	Atacand HCT
CCB + ACEI	amlodipine + benazepril	Lotrel
	verapamil + trandolapril	Tarka
	felodipine + enalapril	Lexxel
CCB + ARB	amlodipine + olmesartan	Azor
	amlodipine + valsartan	Exforge

[a]Most trade-name products are available in multiple-dosage combinations of the respective pair.

ACEI = angiotensin converting-enzyme inhibitor; ARB = angiotensin receptor blocker; CCB = calcium channel blocker.

○ In patients with chronic kidney disease, use of ACEIs and ARBs is preferred.

○ If the patient has asthma or chronic obstructive pulmonary disease, nonselective β-blockers are contraindicated; β_1-specific antagonists should also be avoided.

○ In pregnant patients, agents that inhibit the renin-angiotensin-aldosterone system should not be used.

Angina

- A goal of chronic stable angina therapy is to reduce the oxygen demand with β-blockers (preferred initial therapy) or increase oxygen supply with CCBs and organic nitrates. Treatment of variant angina is aimed at increasing cardiac oxygen supply with CCBs and organic nitrates; β-blockers are not useful because oxygen demand is not increased in variant

BOX 12-6

GENERIC AND TRADE NAMES OF STATINS USED TO TREAT HYPERLIPIDEMIA

- Atorvastatin (Lipitor)
- Fluvastatin (Lescol)
- Lovastatin (Mevacor)
- Pitavastatin (Livalo)
- Pravastatin (Pravachol)
- Rosuvastatin (Crestor)
- Simvastatin (Zocor)

angina. These drugs decrease the frequency and severity of angina but do not decrease the mortality risk (from MI). Ranolazine (Ranexa) is another agent approved for treatment of angina; however, the mechanism of action of this agent is unknown.

- Other therapy is used to decrease the risk for mortality in patients with angina. This includes antiplatelet therapy (eg, low-dose aspirin), cholesterol-lowering drugs, and antihypertensive therapy.

- Short-acting nitroglycerin tablets or spray is standard therapy for relief of an acute angina attack.

- β-blockers or CCBs that affect the heart (diltiazem, verapamil) are often used in combination with long-acting organic nitrates to offset the reflex tachycardia.

Myocardial Infarction

- Long-term treatment to prevent subsequent MI includes treatment of underlying conditions of hypertension, angina, and hyperlipidemia.

- Antiplatelet therapy with low-dose aspirin (75 to 81 mg/day), unless contraindicated, is effective in preventing recurrent MI. Larger doses have not been shown to provide an additional advantage. Specific pharmacology related to aspirin is covered in Chapters 6 and 7.

- Long-term therapy with β-blockers is standard therapy following MI except in low-risk patients and if β-blockers are otherwise contraindicated.

- ACEIs are useful after MI to prevent recurrent MI and heart failure. Depending on the symptoms and clinical evidence, patients may benefit from therapy for several weeks to indefinitely.

Heart Failure

- ACEIs, β-blockers, and spironolactone (in selected patients) improve survival and symptoms of heart failure. Digoxin and diuretics improve symptoms but do not affect survival.

- ACEIs are the cornerstone of therapy for patients with heart failure and should be a part of the drug therapy for all patients with heart failure unless a specific contraindication exists.

- Diuretics are also a standard component of therapy for patients to relieve peripheral or pulmonary edema. Diuretics are used in combination with ACEIs and β-blockers. Thiazide or loop diuretics can be used, depending on the degree of edema and the patient's renal function.

- Long-term use of β-blockers is standard therapy for patients with class II or III heart failure (see Table 12-5). Previously thought to be a contraindication for β-blocker use, patients with heart failure benefit from the decrease in sympathetic tone. Patients who also have hypertension, angina, and elevated heart rate are more likely to benefit from β-blockers, whereas patients who also have asthma, bradycardia, or hypotension are not good candidates.

- Use of ARBs is an alternative in patients who cannot tolerate adverse effects of ACEIs.

- Spironolactone (Aldactone) is a potassium-sparing diuretic but is used in lower doses as an aldosterone antagonist to treat heart failure. Recommended for patients with moderate to severe heart failure, spironolactone may be used in combination with the patient's standard care but particular care should be taken to avoid hyperkalemia in patients also receiving ACEIs.

- Digoxin (Lanoxin) does not improve survival but can be used to improve symptoms of heart failure. It can be considered as an addition to standard therapy.

Section Summary

Treatment of hypertension and heart disease often require multiple-drug therapy to obtain adequate control of symptoms and prevent progression of the disease. Combination of drugs sometimes proves useful beyond the therapeutic effect of the individual drug on the disease. For example, use of ACEIs along with diuretics not only provides 2 drugs with antihypertensive activity but the ACEIs help prevent the hypokalemia that often arises from diuretic therapy.

Although first-choice drugs have been established as part of treatment protocol (eg, diuretics, ACE inhibitors, CCBs, and ARBs for hypertension; ACE inhibitors, β-blockers, and diuretics for heart failure), selection of the drug regimen must also include a consideration for other aspects of the patient's clinical history. For example, use of nonselective β-blockers in patients with coexisting asthma or diabetes mellitus presents the potential for additional risks. If the patient is pregnant, use of ACEIs, direct renin inhibitors, and ARBs must be avoided. Thiazide diuretics would not be a choice to treat hypertension in a patient with history of allergic reactions to sulfonamide antibiotics. Consequently, coexisting diseases, other physiological conditions, history of drug use, potential drug interactions, race, and age become more important considerations when multiple drug therapy is necessary.

ROLE OF THE ATHLETIC TRAINER

As evidenced by the array of categories of drugs available for the treatment of hypertension and heart disease, the issue of therapeutic effectiveness, adverse effects, and drug interactions are considerably complex. Consequently, the role of the athletic trainer in assisting patients directly regarding drug therapy may be somewhat limited. Nonetheless, there are some points worth emphasizing, especially regarding recurrent themes that may be useful for the athletic trainer.

- If the patient is experiencing new symptoms (or adverse effects) or a change in severity of symptoms, the drug therapy should be considered as a cause. The recent addition of another drug to therapy, the occurrence of a drug interaction, or a change in adherence are possible reasons for new symptoms to appear.

- The athletic trainer should encourage the patient to comply with the prescribed therapeutic regimen. Poor adherence is a major cause of treatment failures. If the regimen seems too difficult for the patient to reasonably comply with therapy, a review of the medications by a physician or pharmacist may be useful to determine if dosage regimens can be simplified by the use of combination products or by using drugs that require fewer doses per day.

- The athletic trainer can help the patient understand the necessity for the drug therapy and the important role of nondrug measures. Educating the patient about the disease and the potential impact the therapy can have on symptoms and/or progression of the disease may improve adherence with therapy. For example, although a patient may be asymptomatic for essential hypertension, treatment is necessary to reduce the long-term consequences such as heart disease or stroke.

- A patient who is beginning an exercise regimen after being diagnosed with hypertension or heart disease is likely to require a gradual increase in exercise. The starting point for this exercise, as well as the target level of exercise, must be planned carefully to accommodate the individual's needs and abilities.

- Exercise intolerance is an anticipated effect when β-blockers are used. Not only do these drugs limit the heart's ability to properly respond to the increased demand during exercise, but β-blockers decrease the liver's ability to provide glucose to the blood. Therefore, the ability for vigorous and sustained exercise may be compromised, and thus the athletic trainer should be sure that the patient understands these limitations.

- NSAIDs can diminish the effectiveness of diuretics, β-blockers, and ACEIs. Patients should be aware that self-medicating with over-the-counter analgesic and anti-inflammatory drugs has the potential to cause this drug interaction.

CASE STUDY

Two of your largest football offensive linemen, Dan and Andrew, were put on antihypertensive medications over the summer. You were concerned about their blood pressures during spring practice because routine blood pressure readings on both of them indicated they were hypertensive, with readings in the 145/92 and 152/95 ranges, so you are pleased that they each followed up with their family physicians. Andy is now taking losartan, and Danny is taking lisinopril. You know that both of these medications affect the renin-angiotensin system, but because you are unfamiliar with the side effects, you decide to look them up in case either of the athletes reports to you with any complaints. What is the difference between these 2 medications? What adverse effects could the athletes experience?

REFERENCES

1. James PA, Oparil S, Carter BL, et al. 2014 Evidence-based guideline for the management of high blood pressure in adults. Report from the panel members appointed to the eighth Joint National Committee (JNC 8). *JAMA.* 2014;311(5):507-520.
2. Eckel RH, Jakicic JM, Ard JD, et al. 2013 AHA/ACC guideline on lifestyle management to reduce cardiovascular risk. *J Am Coll Cardiol.* 2013;63(25):2960-2984.

BIBLIOGRAPHY

Abrams J. Chronic stable angina. *N Engl J Med.* 2005;352:2524-2533.

Chintanadilok J, Lowenthal DT. Exercise in treating hypertension: tailoring therapies for active patients. *Phys Sportsmed.* 2002;30:11.

Cohen JD. Overview of physiology, vascular biology, and mechanism of hypertension. *J Manag Care Pharm.* 2007;13(5):S6-S8.

Hamer M. Coffee and health: explaining conflicting results in hypertension. *J Hum Hypertens.* 2006;20:909-912.

Yancy CW, Jessup M, Bozkurt B, et al. 2013 ACCF/AHA guideline for the management of heart failure. A report of the American College of Cardiology Foundation/American Heart Association Task Force on Practice Guidelines. *Circulation.* 2013;128:e240-e327.

CHAPTER 13: ADVANCE ORGANIZER

Foundational Concepts

- Schizophrenia
- Major Depression
- Bipolar Disorder
  - Major Depression
  - Mania
  - Hypomania
  - Mixed
- Anxiety Disorders
  - Generalized Anxiety Disorder
  - Panic Disorder
  - Social Anxiety Disorder
  - Obessive-Compulsive Disorder
  - Posttraumatic Stress Disorder
- Attention Deficit/Hyperactivity Disorder
- Insomnia
- Eating Disorders
- Section Summary

Drugs for Treating Schizophrenia

- Typical Antipsychotic Drugs
  - Adverse Effects
- Atypical Antipsychotic Drugs
  - Adverse Effects
  - Drug Interactions
- Therapy Considerations For Antipsychotic Drugs
- Section Summary

Drugs for Treating Depression

- Tricyclic Antidepressants
  - Adverse Effects
  - Drug Interactions
  - Therapy Considerations
- Selective Serotonin Reuptake Inhibitors
  - Adverse Effects
  - Drug Interactions
  - Therapy Considerations
- Monoamine Oxidase Inhibitors
  - Adverse Effects
  - Drug Interactions
  - Therapy Considerations
- Serotonin/Norepinephrine Reuptake Inhibitors
- Miscellaneous Drugs for Treating Depression
  - Bupropion (Wellbutrin)
  - Mirtazapine (Remeron)
  - Trazodone (Desyrel)
  - Vilazodone (Viibryd) and Vortioxetine (Brintellix)
  - St. John's Wort
- Section Summary

Drugs for Treating Bipolar Disorder

- Mood Stabilizers
  - Lithium (Lithonate, Lithobid)
    - Adverse Effects
    - Drug Interactions
    - Therapy Considerations
  - Valproic Acid (Depakene, Stavzor)/Divalproex Sodium (Depakote)
    - Adverse Effects
    - Drug Interactions
    - Therapy Considerations
  - Carbamazepine (Equetro, Tegretol)
    - Adverse Effects
    - Drug Interactions
    - Therapy Considerations
- Antipsychotic Drugs
- Section Summary

Drugs for Treating Anxiety Disorders

- Drugs for Treating Generalized Anxiety Disorder
  - Benzodiazepines
    - Adverse Effects
    - Drug Interactions
    - Therapy Considerations
  - Buspirone (BuSpar)
    - Adverse Effects
    - Drug Interactions
    - Therapy Considerations
  - Antidepressants
- Drugs for Treating Panic Disorder
- Drugs for Treating Social Anxiety Disorder
- Drugs for Treating Obsessive-Compulsive Disorder
- Drugs for Treating Posttraumatic Stress Disorder
- Section Summary

Drugs for Treating Attention Deficit/Hyperactivity Disorder

- Stimulant Drugs
  - Adverse Effects
  - Drug Interactions
  - Therapy Considerations
- Nonstimulant Drugs
- Atomoxetine (Strattera)
  - Centrally Acting α_2 Receptor Agonists
- Antidepressants
- Section Summary

Drugs for Treating Insomnia

- Benzodiazepines
- Other Drugs
- Section Summary

Drugs for Treating Eating Disorders

- Drug Therapy for Anorexia Nervosa
- Drug Therapy for Bulimia Nervosa
- Section Summary

Role of the Athletic Trainer

13

Drugs for Treating Psychiatric Disorders

CHAPTER OBJECTIVES

At the end of this chapter, the reader will be able to:

- Differentiate the characteristics and signs and symptoms of various types of psychiatric disorders
- Classify specific types of psychiatric disorders in a broad classification system
- Summarize the mechanism of action for drugs used to treat various types of psychiatric disorders
- Explain drug and nondrug approaches to the treatment of various types of psychiatric disorders
- Identify drugs that can be used to treat various types of psychiatric disorders, along with their adverse effects, drug interactions, and therapy considerations
- Summarize the role of the athletic trainer for patients who are on drug therapy for psychiatric disorders

FOUNDATIONAL CONCEPTS

This chapter discusses drugs that are used to treat several types of psychiatric disorders: schizophrenia, depression, bipolar disorder, anxiety, attention deficit/hyperactivity disorder (ADHD), insomnia, and eating disorders. Unlike many other diseases that rely on objective tests such as blood pressure, blood glucose, lipid levels, or the presence

ABBREVIATIONS USED IN THIS CHAPTER	
ADHD. attention deficit/hyperactivity disorder	**MI.** myocardial infarction
AN. anorexia nervosa	**NCAA.** National Collegiate Athletic Association
BN. bulimia nervosa	**NSAID.** nonsteroidal anti-inflammatory drug
CNS. central nervous system	**OCD.** obsessive-compulsive disorder
FDA. Food and Drug Administration	**OTC.** over-the-counter
GABA. gamma aminobutyric acid	**PTSD.** posttraumatic stress disorder
GAD. generalized anxiety disorder	**SAD.** social anxiety disorder
GERD. gastroesophageal reflux disease	**SNRI.** serotonin-norepinephrine reuptake inhibitor
GI. gastrointestinal	**SSRI.** serotonin reuptake inhibitor
IOC. International Olympic Committee	**t½.** half-life
MAO. monoamine oxidase	**TCA.** tricyclic antidepressant
MAOI. monoamine oxidase inhibitor	**TI.** therapeutic index

Houglum JE, Harrelson GL, Seefeldt TM.
Principles of Pharmacology for Athletic Trainers, Third Edition (pp 239-266).
© 2016 Taylor & Francis Group.

TABLE 13-1

SYMPTOMS OF SCHIZOPHRENIA

POSITIVE SYMPTOMS	NEGATIVE SYMPTOMS	COGNITIVE SYMPTOMS
Hallucinations[a]	↓ Logical conversation	↓ Attention
Delusions	↓ Motivation	Memory difficulty
Paranoia	↓ Emotional expression	↓ Task completion ability
Disordered thought/speech	Socially withdrawn	
Agitation, hyperactivity	↓ Self-care skills	
[a]Hallucinations may be auditory (most common) or visual.		

of bacteria to secure the diagnosis, the diagnosis of psychiatric disorders relies primarily upon psychological testing, use of rating scales, and careful assessment of the patient's thoughts, emotions, and actions. Although for many of these disorders the specific neurotransmitter has been identified that is produced in excessive or subnormal levels, the cause for these changes has not been pinpointed. General discussion about the disease process will help the athletic trainer understand the reason certain categories of drugs are used for treatment.

Some of the disorders discussed in this chapter can be debilitating, effectively preventing the patient from participating in athletic activity. However, these disorders exist with a broad range of severity among patients, and therefore it is possible that athletic trainers in some practice settings may encounter patients who have been diagnosed with these conditions but are being sufficiently managed to allow them to be physically active. Consequently, these disorders are included in this chapter.

Schizophrenia

Schizophrenia is a chronic psychiatric disorder in which the patient has disturbances of reality and perception, inappropriate mood, and impaired cognitive function. The cause of schizophrenia is unknown, but there is sufficient evidence to implicate a genetic predisposition coupled with any one of many external events that affects the brain's development. The risk for schizophrenia is approximately 10 times higher than the general population for a child with a parent who has schizophrenia. The incidence of schizophrenia in the United States is about 1%. It affects men and women equally. Onset usually ranges from adolescence to age 40 years. Schizophrenia is a chronic disease with no cure, although frequency of acute episodes tends to decrease as the patient ages. Life expectancy is shorter than that of the general population.

Changes in metabolic and regulatory processes have been noted in schizophrenia that include altered neurotransmitter levels. From a therapeutic standpoint, the

neurotransmitters of interest are dopamine and serotonin. Drugs that alleviate some of the symptoms of schizophrenia block specific receptors for these neurotransmitters in the central nervous system (CNS).

Although the symptoms of schizophrenia can be grouped into 3 categories (positive, negative, and cognitive), the clinical presentation varies widely from one patient to another. The term *positive symptoms* is somewhat misleading because all of the symptoms are negative relative to their impact on the patient, but positive symptoms refer to a distorted enhancement or exaggeration of a normal function. A *negative symptom* is a diminution of a normal function. Table 13-1 provides examples of these responses. Symptoms vary among patients, and although most patients have both positive and negative symptoms, positive symptoms are more prominent in younger patients and women, whereas negative symptoms are more prominent in older patients and men. Substance abuse and addiction are common comorbid conditions in patients with schizophrenia; for example, use of cigarettes is about 3 times higher among patients with schizophrenia than in the general population.

Patients with schizophrenia lose touch with reality and may hear voices that direct their actions, believe that their actions are being controlled by an external force, or believe that someone is persecuting them. Verbal and physical hostility can occur. Disordered thinking, emotional withdrawal, poor personal hygiene, and appetite and sleep disturbances are also common. Not surprisingly, these patients have difficulty maintaining jobs and relationships. Patients with schizophrenia have acute psychotic episodes where the symptoms are more pronounced. When the acute episodes abate, there are some symptoms that continue, including anxiety, suspicious nature, lack of motivation, poor judgment, and poor personal self-care, all of which contribute to poor social interaction. These residual symptoms also complicate therapy because they contribute to the patient's lack of desire to comply with drug therapy. Consequently, there is a great need to encourage patients to maintain drug therapy.

Major Depression

Major depression is a mood disorder that significantly diminishes the patient's ability to function normally. Patients who are depressed due to specific life events (eg, death of family member, loss of job) typically recover without treatment (uncomplicated depression). There are specific diagnostic criteria that define a major depressive episode, including a depressed mood nearly every day for at least 2 weeks. Drug treatment for depression is typically restricted to major depression. A life event may trigger the symptoms in some patients, whereas in other patients there is no such obvious trigger. There is a genetic component also; close relatives of patients with depressive disorders are more likely to develop depression than other patients. Depression occurs twice as frequently in women than in men. The age of onset of major depression is usually in the 20s, but it can begin at any age. Other causes of depression symptoms can be drugs, particularly some antihypertensives, and medical disorders such as myocardial infarction, diabetes mellitus, cancer, and neurologic diseases.

Diminished effects of neurotransmitters in the brain have been implicated as playing a role in the cause of major depression. Concentrations of serotonin and norepinephrine particularly have been studied. All drugs commonly used to treat depression increase the effect of one or both of these neurotransmitters, and antidepressant drugs are categorized according to their effect on these neurotransmitters. Unfortunately, the pathogenesis of the disease is more complex than merely abnormal norepinephrine and serotonin levels, and, consequently, no one drug totally remits all the symptoms of depression. In addition, the effect on the neurotransmitters occurs quickly after drug administration, but the observable effect on the depression symptoms occurs after a few weeks of therapy.

Symptoms can develop suddenly but more typically develop over days to weeks. Symptoms of a major depressive episode include depressed mood, loss of interest or pleasure in all (or almost all) activities, decreased or increased appetite, insomnia or hypersomnia, loss of energy, feelings of worthlessness or guilt, and diminished ability to concentrate or make decisions. The symptoms must occur nearly every day for most of the day for at least 2 weeks for diagnosis as a major depressive episode and must cause significant distress or impairment in social, occupational, or other important areas of functioning. Thoughts of suicide may be present, and patients should be assessed for the risk of suicide.

Bipolar Disorder

Bipolar disorder (previously known as manic-depressive illness) is a mood disorder in which the patient cycles through varying degrees of mania and depression with some periods of relatively normal mood. Frequency in the United States is about 1.5%, with occurrence being the same for men and women. Onset of symptoms can be anywhere from adolescence to mid-life, but the average age of the first bipolar episode is about 20 years. Heredity is a major risk factor for bipolar disorder, but there is a wide variation in the pattern and severity of mood episodes. There are 4 types of mood episodes: major depression, mania, hypomania, and mixed.

Major Depression

As discussed previously, patients experiencing a major depressive episode have a loss of interest or pleasure in life for 2 weeks or more. Patients with major depression are likely to have hypersomnia, weight gain, diminished psychomotor activity, and low energy level. These episodes generally occur longer than manic episodes, and women have more episodes than men.

Mania

Patients with mania have an elevated mood (euphoria), unrealistic optimism, hyperactivity, decreased need for sleep, abundance of ideas but poor attention (thoughts move quickly from one topic to another), rapid speech pattern, irritability, and elevated self-esteem. During manic episodes, patients have poor judgment and make high-risk and impulsive decisions (eg, reckless driving, illegal activities) and thus require close supervision or hospitalization. Severe episodes may result in hallucinations and delusions. These symptoms begin abruptly, increase during the first few days, last for at least one week, and impair the patient's ability to function at work and socially.

Hypomania

The symptoms of hypomania are less pronounced than manic episodes so that the patient maintains the ability to function at work and socially. Because of the increased feeling of well-being, ideas, energy, and productivity during hypomanic episodes, patients may like these episodes; however, these episodes can sometimes change to manic episodes.

Mixed

During mixed episodes, the patient experiences some symptoms of both mania and depression at the same time, or a change from one mood to another in the same day for one week or more. These patients are more susceptible to suicidal tendencies because they can have high energy but also depressive feelings such as hopelessness.

The patterns of bipolar episodes vary considerably among patients. Some patients may cycle between mania and depression with normal mood between episodes, but others may experience repeated episodes of either mania or depression before they experience the other mood. Women tend to have more depressive episodes, whereas men tend to have a more equal distribution between manic and depressive episodes. Duration of episodes can range from days to many months, and the number of episodes can vary from 4 in 10 years to 4 or more in 1 year (rapid cycling).

Anxiety Disorders

Anxiety is an emotional state that everyone has experienced to one extent or another. A stressful situation (real or imagined) that creates a sense of uncertainty can cause the person to be fearful and apprehensive of the outcome. The emotional state leads to physiological changes such as nervousness, sweating, increased heart and respiratory rates, and fatigue. In most cases, the anxiety is initiated due to a specific event or circumstance (situational anxiety); the person makes physical, mental, or emotional adjustments to the situation; and the anxiety is of short duration. Situational anxiety generally does not require drug therapy. However, patients with anxiety disorders have irrational fears, excessive anxiety that becomes debilitating, and physical symptoms that can become significant health concerns (eg, cardiovascular, respiratory, and gastrointestinal [GI] disorders). In the United States, approximately 25% of the population experiences at least one episode of an anxiety disorder during their lifetime.

As with other psychiatric disorders, the physiologic cause of anxiety disorders has not been pinpointed, but prominent theories focus on the disruption of normal response from neurotransmitters. Changes in the effects of norepinephrine, GABA, serotonin, and dopamine in selected portions of the brain have been suspected as playing a key role in contributing to the symptoms of anxiety disorders. Therefore, pharmacological interventions have focused on affecting the response from these neurotransmitters or their receptors.

There are several categories of anxiety disorders: generalized anxiety disorder (GAD), panic disorders, and social anxiety disorder (SAD). Obsessive-compulsive disorder (OCD) and posttraumatic stress disorder (PTSD) have long been considered as categories of anxiety disorders. However, a recent revision to the guidelines for diagnosis of psychiatric disorders (the *Diagnostic and Statistical Manual of Mental Disorders* [DSM-5]) has separated these disorders into separate sections to emphasize the distinctions between these conditions and other disorders associated with anxiety. In this textbook, OCD and PTSD will be discussed with the anxiety disorders because anxiety is an important symptom of these conditions and the agents used for treatment are similar to other anxiety disorders. Table 13-2 summarizes major symptoms of each anxiety disorder.

Generalized Anxiety Disorder

Patients with GAD have excessive and uncontrollable worry about several events or activities with symptoms persisting for 6 months or more. GAD is a chronic disorder in which the patient experiences periods of remission and exacerbation. Most patients with GAD eventually develop a depressive disorder, another anxiety disorder, and/or substance abuse.

Panic Disorder

The diagnostic criterion for panic disorder is recurrent, spontaneous panic attacks followed by at least one month of persistent concern that another panic attack may occur, worrying about the consequences of another attack, or a significant change in behavior because of the attack. Frequency of attacks varies considerably, ranging from daily attacks for a few consecutive days to no attacks for months. Patients tend to seek emergency help during the attack and avoid places and situations in which emergency assistance may be less available (eg, trains, buses, crowds, traveling alone). Depression, other anxiety disorders, and/ or alcohol abuse are often comorbid conditions. Panic disorder is generally a lifetime illness that begins in the late teens to 30s. The lifetime risk of suicide is greater among these patients than in the general public.

Social Anxiety Disorder

SAD is the most common anxiety disorder. The hallmark of patients with SAD is the intense but irrational fear of being negatively evaluated or scrutinized in a social interaction or performance situation to the extent that the fear interferes with the daily routine, work performance, or social life or there is considerable distress about having the fear. Patients fear that they will act in an embarrassing or humiliating fashion. Examples of these situations are speaking or eating in public, meeting new people, attending parties, acting, playing sports, dancing, being the center of attention, or entering a room when others are seated. Being exposed to the undesired situation evokes intense anxiety with symptoms such as blushing, muscle tension, diarrhea, trembling, sweating, shortness of breath, abdominal discomfort, and palpitations. Consequently, these situations are usually avoided. For some patients, the anxiety is limited to one or 2 social situations (eg, public speaking or meeting new people). Depression, other anxiety disorders, and substance abuse are common comorbid conditions. Most patients do not report their symptoms unless they seek help for a comorbid condition. SAD typically begins during the teen years, and about half of patients can identify a specific embarrassing or humiliating event that triggered the onset of their disorder. This disorder can affect the patient's social interaction and employment pursuits throughout life. Patients with SAD are more likely to be unemployed and financially dependent on others, less likely to marry, and more likely to divorce.

Obsessive-Compulsive Disorder

OCD is a chronic disorder in which patients have either obsessions and/or compulsions that consume at least one hour per day, cause significant distress, and interfere with normal daily living. An obsession is a recurrent, involuntary, persistent thought, impulse, or mental image that is unwanted, irrational, excessive, or inappropriate and causes significant distress. Examples of obsessions are persistent

Table 13-2

Symptoms of Anxiety Disorders

TYPE OF DISORDER	SYMPTOM
Generalized anxiety disorder	<ul><li>Person worries or has anxiety about several events or activities.</li><li>Person has difficulty controlling worry or anxiety.</li><li>Anxiety occurs most days for ≥6 months.</li><li>Anxiety causes restlessness, fatigue, difficulty concentrating, irritability, muscle tension, and/or sleep disturbances.</li><li>Anxiety or physical symptoms cause impairment of social, work, or other important areas.</li></ul>
Panic disorder	<ul><li>Sudden onset of intense fear (panic attack), peaking within 10 min with at least 4 of these defining symptoms: racing or pounding heart, sweating, trembling, shortness of breath, choking feeling, chest pain, nausea, dizzy or lightheadedness, detached feeling, fear of losing control, fear of dying, numbness or tingling, chills or hot flashes.</li><li>Continuing anxiety about having additional panic attacks and/or making negative changes to behavior to avoid precipitating a panic attack.</li></ul>
Social anxiety disorder	<ul><li>Marked and persistent fear of social or performance situations when person is exposed to unfamiliar people or scrutiny.</li><li>Such situations almost always provoke anxiety.</li><li>The level of anxiety experienced is excessive based on the interaction inducing the anxiety</li><li>Feared situations are avoided or endured with intense anxiety.</li><li>The anxiety significantly interferes with work, school, relationships, or normal routine.</li><li>For persons younger than 18 years, fear has lasted ≥6 months.</li></ul>
Obsessive-compulsive disorder	<ul><li>Obsessions include thoughts, impulses, or images that are intrusive, senseless, and cause anxiety or distress—not simply excessive worries about real-life problems. The person tries to ignore or neutralize with thoughts or actions and realizes the obsessions are from his or her own mind.</li><li>Compulsions include repetitive behavior that the person feels driven to perform, including repeated hand washing, arranging objects in order, counting, or repeating words silently.</li><li>Obsessions/compulsions cause distress and are time consuming.</li><li>The disorder interferes with school, work, relationships, or normal routine.</li></ul>
Posttraumatic stress disorder	<ul><li>Caused by exposure to a traumatic event; typically the person experienced or witnessed the event, but this is not always the case.</li><li>The event is persistently reexperienced by flashbacks, thoughts, hallucinations, dreams, or physiologic reactions to triggers.</li><li>Person persistently avoids reminders of the event.</li><li>Person has symptoms of generalized emotional numbing or altered mood.</li><li>May have problems with irritability, sleep, concentration.</li></ul>

thoughts about contamination (ie, germs), doubts about having completed a task (eg, locking the door), harming a loved one, or needing items in a certain order or symmetry. A compulsion is a repetitive, intentional behavior or mental act that the patient is driven to perform, often in response to an obsession or in accordance to rigid rules. Examples are repetitive hand washing, counting, checking, and touching. The patient feels that carrying out the compulsion will prevent some discomfort or a horrible event. Anxiety is experienced by the patient if prevented from performing the compulsion. The OCD patient realizes that the compulsive behavior is senseless and thus may attempt to conceal the behavior. About half of the patients with OCD also have another psychiatric disorder or a drug or alcohol abuse problem. Some OCD patients (up to 40%) have symptoms of Tourette's syndrome (involuntary motor movements such as facial tics).

Posttraumatic Stress Disorder

PTSD occurs after a person experiences a traumatic event, typically as a victim or a witness. Directly experiencing the traumatic event is not a requirement for PTSD diagnosis; "learning that the traumatic event(s) occurred to a close family member or close friend" or "experiencing repeated or extreme exposure to aversive details of the traumatic event(s)" can also trigger symptoms of PTSD.[1] Such events include severe car accidents, terrorist actions, combat, hostage situations, sexual assault, or natural disasters. The patient with PTSD persistently experiences the event through dreams, flashbacks, and other recurring thoughts. Reliving the event in this manner causes patients to avoid any situation that may remind them of the event. Patients have an emotional numbing that causes a lack of responsiveness; reduced interest in previously enjoyable activities; detachment from others; difficulty with relationships; and a sense that they may not live long, have a career, get married, or have children. PTSD is a chronic disorder, but some patients improve and have mild symptoms, whereas other patients have more severe, persistent symptoms. The pattern of the symptoms over the years is impacted by the severity and violence of the traumatic event. Most patients have comorbid major depression, other anxiety disorders, and/or substance abuse.

Attention Deficit/Hyperactivity Disorder

ADHD is the most common psychiatric disorder among children, occurring in about 3% to 5% of children, with a higher incidence in boys than in girls. Primary characteristics of the disorder are inattention, hyperactivity, and impulsivity. Some children have principally hyperactivity and impulsivity, some have principally inattention, and others have a combination. Diagnostic criteria require symptoms to be apparent by age 7 years. Inattention is manifested by the child being unable to concentrate on schoolwork, being readily distracted, not paying attention, and not completing tasks. The hyperactive child is unable to remain seated, fidgets, and runs around excessively. Impulsivity is demonstrated by calling out in class, the inability to wait their turn in group activities, and acting before thinking (eg, running into the street). These symptoms hamper learning, affect the child's self-image, and impair social interactions. Consequently, children with ADHD also have a greater likelihood to develop a learning disability, psychiatric disor-

der, and/or behavioral disorder. As ADHD patients become young adults, compared with their peers they have a higher incidence of academic problems, delinquency, school suspensions, and contact with law enforcement agencies. If the child with ADHD also develops an aggressive behavior (not part of ADHD diagnostic criteria) during the developmental period to adulthood, there is an increased incidence of criminal behavior compared with peers.

ADHD often persists into adulthood, but the symptoms are manifested in somewhat different behavior. For example, hyperactivity is more subtle and displayed as an inability to relax, excessive talking, and restlessness. Impulsiveness can be displayed as interrupting others when they are speaking, blurting out rude comments, or being moody. Inattentiveness can manifest as the inability to remain mentally focused and to constantly lose and forget things. Consequently, ADHD in the adult can have a significant impact on social and work-related activities because the patient has problems organizing time to complete tasks, forgets meetings and conversations with colleagues, has unstable moods, and speaks without thinking.

As with all other psychiatric disorders discussed in this chapter, the cause of ADHD has not been identified. There are genetic factors that play a role in the development of ADHD but also a connection with certain adverse family and social environments. Studies of the pathophysiology of ADHD indicate that these patients have a diminished response from norepinephrine and dopamine in certain parts of the brain; hence, the drug therapy enhances these neurotransmitter effects.

Insomnia

Insomnia is the most common sleep disorder. Although not generally categorized by itself as a psychiatric disorder, insomnia is mentioned here because it can be caused by several psychiatric conditions, it can lead to depression if chronic, and the category of drugs most frequently used to treat insomnia, benzodiazepines, is also discussed in this chapter.

Insomnia is the inability to get a good night's sleep. For some patients the problem is the inability to fall asleep, whereas for others it is remaining asleep throughout the night, awakening too early in the morning, or just not obtaining a restful sleep. Intermittent insomnia lasts for a few days, short-term insomnia lasts for less than 3 weeks, and chronic insomnia lasts more than 3 weeks. Sleep loss can cause drowsiness during the daytime, reduced work productivity, reduced level of concentration, automobile accidents, altered mood, and reduced level of athletic performance.

There are many causes of insomnia, ranging from jet lag to chronic medical conditions. Personal and work-related situations are common stressors that cause intermittent and short-term insomnia. Poor sleep conditions (eg, mattress quality, room conditions) can also disturb sleep. Medical conditions such as asthma, heart disease, ulcers, gastro-esophageal reflux disease, pain, and pregnancy can result in loss of sleep. Psychiatric conditions such as depression, mania, and anxiety disorders are frequently concurrent conditions accompanying chronic insomnia. Some drugs can also cause of insomnia; among them are the selective serotonin reuptake inhibitors (SSRIs) and CNS stimulants such as caffeine and nasal decongestants. If insomnia is not caused by medical conditions, life stressors, or drugs, it may be due to an inherent abnormal sleep pattern.

A normal sleep pattern is composed of 2 phases: rapid eye movement (REM) sleep and nonrapid eye movement (NREM) sleep. There are also 4 stages to NREM sleep that begin as the person becomes drowsy and progresses as the person falls into a deeper sleep. In contrast to NREM sleep, during REM sleep there is REM, brain activity, changes in respiratory and heart rate, and dreaming. During a normal sleep pattern, there are several cycles of NREM and REM sleep throughout the night.

Sleep apneas are repetitive disruptions of breathing during sleep that cause arousal from sleep as an automatic means to begin breathing again. Use of various compact and portable breathing devices is the preferred treatment. There is no drug therapy for sleep apneas, and thus these conditions are not considered further. Drugs that have CNS-depressant effects (eg, alcohol, benzodiazepines, narcotic analgesics, OTC sleep aids, antihistamines) should be avoided because they may reduce the patient's capability for automatic arousal.

Eating Disorders

Anorexia nervosa (AN) and bulimia nervosa (BN) are mental disorders in which the patient is obsessed with his or her body weight and shape and is critical of any flaws related to these characteristics. These eating disorders occur more frequently in women than in men, and onset of symptoms is typically during the teen years, although they can begin during the adult years. There appears to be a genetic predisposition to the psychological and emotional characteristics that are common among these patients, but the rising incidence of AN and BN is often attributed to the media-based emphasis on being thin, particularly in the fashion industry and by television and movie personalities. Eating disorders can also be triggered by social and psychological situations such as stressful relationships. Some athletes are at greater risk for eating disorders; female gymnasts, distance runners, figure skaters, and male wrestlers are examples.

Patients with AN achieve thinness by starving themselves and may use various methods to rid themselves of calories, such as self-induced vomiting, excessive exercising, and misuse of laxatives or diuretics. Some patients with AN participate in binge eating similar to BN patients, followed by purging behavior. Patients with AN are underweight but view themselves as being fat and have an intense fear of gaining weight. They try to hide their thinness by wearing baggy clothes or layers of clothing. Additional indications that a person may have AN are skipping meals, eating only low-calorie items, making excuses for not eating, and frequently complaining about being fat.

Patients with BN have repeated episodes (at least weekly but may be more frequent) of binge eating followed by an attempt to get rid of the calories by purging behavior (eg, vomiting or misuse of laxatives or diuretics) or by excessive exercise or fasting. The binge eating includes a large intake of calories, often by raiding the refrigerator and cupboard when alone at home, or by going to several fast food restaurants and eating alone. Eating continues even until significant discomfort occurs. These patients are close to normal weight, but because they don't have any control over their eating habits, they are preoccupied with their body weight and shape. Many patients have symptoms alternating between AN and BN.

Occurrence of other psychiatric disorders is common among patients with eating disorders, including depression, anxiety disorders, and drug and alcohol abuse. Severity of AN and BN varies among patients, but these eating disorders are unhealthy behaviors and can result in numerous medical complications such as GI problems, electrolyte disturbances, heart problems, anemia, and death.

Section Summary

Diagnosis of psychiatric disorders relies on evaluating the patient's thoughts, emotions, and actions against established criteria for these disorders. These thoughts, emotions, and actions are more intense and of longer duration than the typical changes that most people experience as a result of their life events. For most disorders, an abnormal response (either increased or decreased) from one or more neurotransmitters in specific portions of the brain have been identified as contributing to the symptomatology. Selected key characteristics of the psychiatric disorders were discussed in this chapter:

- Schizophrenia: Disordered thinking and diminished ability to distinguish reality from false reality, disconnected thoughts, and hallucinations and delusions

- Major depression: Depressed mood, diminished interest in activities previously of interest, worthless feeling, fatigue, diminished motivation, and possible thoughts of suicide

- Bipolar disorder: Cycled episodes of depression, mania, or hypomania with the manic episodes eliciting euphoria, irritability, rapid thoughts, unrealistic optimism, poor judgment, decreased sleep, and impulsive actions

- Anxiety disorders: The circumstances that cause anxiety symptoms vary among the different anxiety disorders, but in all cases the patient feels an excessive apprehension, fear, and uneasiness that can significantly impair social and work-related activities. The specific characteristics for each anxiety disorder are shown in Table 13-2.

- ADHD: Inability to focus on a single task to completion, blurting out statements inappropriately, poor organizational ability, easily distracted, inability to sit still, and excessive talking

- Insomnia: Inability to fall asleep or stay asleep throughout the night. Causes include medical conditions, drugs, psychiatric disorders, various personal or work-related stress, and inherent abnormal sleep patterns. Patients may experience intermittent insomnia (a few days), short-term insomnia (1 to 3 weeks), or chronic insomnia (more than 3 weeks).

- Eating disorders: AN and BN are mental disorders in which patients are obsessed with body weight and shape. The prime characteristic of AN is the intense fear of gaining weight, resulting in a self-image of being fat although the patient is underweight. Patients with BN go on cycles of binge eating followed by efforts to rid themselves of calories by self-induced vomiting, misuse of laxatives or diuretics, excessive exercise, or fasting. Many patients exhibit characteristics of both AN and BN, but in either case, significant health complications can result. Existence of other psychiatric disorders is common among patients with eating disorders.

DRUGS FOR TREATING SCHIZOPHRENIA

Psychosis is a general term referring to a condition in which the person has lost touch with reality and the logical flow of thought is disrupted; schizophrenia is one type of psychosis. Drugs used to treat psychosis are antipsychotic drugs. The drugs used to treat schizophrenia can be divided into 2 major categories: typical antipsychotics (also known as conventional, traditional, or first generation) and atypical antipsychotics (also known as second generation). The primary distinguishing characteristic that separates these 2 categories is that the atypical antipsychotic drugs have a lower incidence of extrapyramidal adverse effects than typical antipsychotics and have broader efficacy for the symptoms of schizophrenia, affecting the positive, negative, and cognition symptoms. Typical antipsychotic drugs reduce the positive symptoms but have little effect on the negative or cognitive symptoms. Table 13-3 lists typical and atypical drugs used to treat schizophrenia and the usual dosage range for maintenance therapy.

Antipsychotic drugs can also be categorized based on their chemical structure. Identifying these drugs by chemical classification has no therapeutic benefit to predict efficacy or adverse effect profile, but one group, the phenothiazines, is worth noting because this group was among the first antipsychotic drugs and contains the prototype (chlorpromazine), which is often used for comparison with other antipsychotic drugs; consequently, the term phenothiazines has been in common use for many decades.

Typical Antipsychotic Drugs

The typical antipsychotic drugs have equal efficacy when used in equipotent doses. They are subgrouped based on potency (ie, low, medium, high) because the adverse effect profile corresponds somewhat with these subgroups. Among the theories to describe the molecular basis for schizophrenia is the need to block the activity at the dopamine and serotonin receptors in specific locations of the brain. Typical antipsychotic drugs block receptors for acetylcholine, norepinephrine (α-receptor), histamine (H_1 receptor), and dopamine (D_2 receptor) in the peripheral nervous system and/or the CNS but have little effect on serotonin receptors.

Recall from Chapter 3 that potency is an indication of the relative dose a drug requires to produce a particular effect but is of little therapeutic consequence because drug doses can be adjusted to compensate for differences in potency.

Adverse Effects

The effects on the neurotransmitter receptors at various sites inside and outside the CNS are the primary cause for the numerous adverse effects from typical antipsychotic drugs. Table 13-4 summarizes the adverse effects. Acute dystonia, pseudoparkinsonism, akathisia, and tardive dyskinesia are referred to as *extrapyramidal symptoms* because they occur as a result of dopamine receptor blockade in the extrapyramidal portion of the brain. Tardive dyskinesia occurs months to years after therapy begins and is a late-onset adverse effect. The other extrapyramidal symptoms have an early onset, beginning days to weeks after therapy is initiated, and they have a higher incidence from high-potency typical antipsychotic drugs. Tardive dyskinesia symptoms are particularly disconcerting adverse effects because of the nature of the symptoms but also because they can be irreversible. Careful monitoring of the schizophrenia patient for extrapyramidal effects

TABLE 13-3

DOSAGE RANGE FOR ANTIPSYCHOTIC DRUGS USED TO TREAT SCHIZOPHRENIA

CATEGORY	GENERIC NAME	BRAND NAME	USUAL MAINTENANCE DOSAGE (MG/DAY)
Typical, low potency	chlorpromazine	Thorazine	200 to 600
	thioridazine	Mellaril	200 to 600
Typical, medium potency	loxapine	Loxitane	20 to 100
	perphenazine	Trilafon	8 to 32
Typical, high potency	fluphenazine	Prolixin	2 to 20
	haloperidol	Haldol	2 to 208
	thiothixene	Navane	6 to 30
	trifluoperazine	generic	4 to 20
Atypical antipsychotics	aripiprazole	Abilify	10 to 30
	asenapine	Saphris	10 to 20
	clozapine	Clozaril	150 to 600
	iloperidone	Fanapt	12 to 24
	lurasidone	Latuda	40 to 80
	olanzapine	Zyprexa	10 to 20
	paliperidone	Invega	3 to 12
	quetiapine	Seroquel	300 to 400
	risperidone	Risperdal	2 to 6
	ziprasidone	Geodon	40 to 160

is necessary when typical antipsychotic drugs are used. The atypical antipsychotic drugs have a very low incidence of extrapyramidal effects.

Other adverse effects with typical antipsychotic agents, especially the low-potency drugs, are orthostatic hypotension and sedation. Hypotension results from blockade of the α-adrenergic receptors, preventing automatic vasoconstriction of the blood vessels when rising to a seated or standing position. This adverse effect has a higher incidence among elderly patients and patients with preexisting cardiovascular disease. Orthostatic hypotension can be prevented by educating patients to rise slowly and to sit or lie down if they feel lightheaded or faint. The impact of sedation can be minimized by taking the medication at bedtime, but caution is still warranted at other times, especially while driving. Tolerance occurs to orthostatic hypotension after 2 to 3 months and to sedation after several days of therapy.

Anticholinergic adverse effects (see Chapters 8 and 10) are also common among the low-potency typical antipsychotic agents (see Table 13-4). Dry mouth and blurred vision diminish after a couple weeks of therapy. Constipation can persist, but the effect can be minimized by adequate fluid and fiber intake, exercise, and use of a laxative as needed. Regarding urinary hesitancy and retention, voiding prior to each dose of antipsychotic drug may be helpful, but reduction of the dose or change in antipsychotic drug therapy may be necessary. Anticholinergic drugs inhibit sweating, and thus problems associated with body temperature regulation can occur, especially when exercising in hot weather. Tachycardia is another anticholinergic response and is of particular concern in patients with preexisting cardiac disorders.

Other adverse effects that may occur from typical antipsychotic drugs are seizures, cardiac dysrhythmias, gynecomastia, and sexual dysfunction in men and women. Therefore, these drugs should be avoided in patients with a preexisting seizure disorder, breast cancer, or a preexisting sexual dysfunction disorder or who are taking other medications that cause cardiac dysrhythmias.

Atypical Antipsychotic Drugs

The atypical antipsychotic drugs (see Table 13-3) are the drugs of choice for treatment of schizophrenia. These drugs are effective blockers of serotonin in the CNS but have a lower

TABLE 13-4

ADVERSE EFFECTS FROM TYPICAL ANTIPSYCHOTIC DRUGS

ADVERSE EFFECT	CHARACTERISTIC	SUBGROUP WITH HIGHEST INCIDENCE[a]
Acute dystonia[b]	Onset within a few days of beginning therapy: painful muscle spasm causing neck twisting, arching back, jaw clenching, or difficulty swallowing or breathing	High potency
Pseudoparkinsonism[b]	Onset within a few days or weeks of beginning therapy: slowness of voluntary movement, drooling, shuffling gait, mask-like expression, slow speech, and tremor	High potency
Akathisia[b]	Onset within a few days to weeks of beginning therapy: inability to sit still, restless movements of rocking, shifting legs, and tapping feet	High potency
Tardive dyskinesia[b]	Onset months to years after beginning therapy; can be irreversible: abnormal involuntary movements of tongue, lips, jaw; protrusion of tongue; facial movements such as grimacing; purposeless movements of arms, legs, spine	All similar[c]
Orthostatic hypotension	Onset and duration for the first couple weeks of therapy and after dosage increases: lightheadedness or fainting when rising too quickly to a sitting or standing position	Low potency
Sedation	Onset and duration for first days of therapy; drowsiness is problematic if during daytime	Low potency
Anticholinergic	Onset and greatest intensity occurs during first couple weeks: dry mouth, urinary hesitancy, constipation, blurred near vision	Low potency

[a]Other subgroups of typical antipsychotic drugs have low to moderate incidence of these same effects.

[b]Collectively, these are referred to as *extrapyramidal adverse effects* because they occur due to the drug's impact on the extrapyramidal portion of the brain.

[c]All typical agents have similar incidence of tardive dyskinesia, which increases with dosage and duration of treatment.

affinity for dopamine receptors compared with the typical antipsychotic drugs. Because of these and other differences in blocking neurotransmitter receptors, the adverse effect profile and efficacy for atypical antipsychotics are more desirable. As with the typical antipsychotic drugs, the atypical drugs diminish the positive symptoms of schizophrenia, but they also diminish the negative and cognitive effects.

Adverse Effects

A major advantage of the atypical agents is that the incidence of extrapyramidal adverse effects (see Table 13-4) is much less than with typical antipsychotic agents. However, as with typical antipsychotic drugs, sedation and orthostatic hypotension occur with atypical antipsychotics. Atypical antipsychotics cause a higher incidence of weight gain and diabetes mellitus than typical antipsychotics. Adjustment in diet and exercise may be necessary to prevent unwanted weight gain. Patients with schizophrenia have a higher incidence of type 2 diabetes mellitus, but the use of atypical anti-

psychotic drugs increases the prevalence. The atypical drugs can also disrupt glucose regulation and aggravate preexisting diabetes mellitus. Patients with preexisting diabetes mellitus or at risk of developing diabetes mellitus (see Chapter 14) should be monitored for onset of hyperglycemia or loss of glucose control (eg, polydipsia, polyphagia, polyuria, weakness).

Table 13-5 summarizes the differences between typical and atypical antipsychotic drugs relative to the incidence of adverse effects. The incidence of adverse effects varies among the drugs within both categories of antipsychotic drugs. For example, aripiprazole (Abilify) has a low incidence of sedation, orthostatic hypotension, weight gain, and diabetes mellitus, as well as no anticholinergic effects. In contrast, clozapine (Clozaril) and olanzapine (Zyprexa) have a moderate to high incidence of these same adverse effects.

Clozapine (Clozaril) is the most effective antipsychotic drug. However, agranulocytosis is a potentially fatal adverse effect that occurs in about 1% of patients on clozapine, with greatest risk occurring within the first 6 months of therapy. Weekly blood tests are required during the first 6 months of therapy to monitor for this adverse effect. If the white blood cell count and absolute neutrophil count are stable at 6 months, the frequency of blood tests can be reduced to every other week for 6 months. If the values are still stable, monthly monitoring is completed thereafter. The potential for agranulocytosis makes clozapine a less favored choice among the atypical antipsychotic drugs, but it is used when other antipsychotic drugs have been ineffective.

Drug Interactions

Use of other drugs that also cause anticholinergic effects or sedation introduce the most common drug interactions; see Box 8-1 and Table 8-2 for examples of these drugs. Concurrent use of these drugs with typical or atypical antipsychotic drugs is likely to accentuate the anticholinergic and sedative effects. Because over-the-counter (OTC) cold remedies, sleep aids, and drugs for motion sickness can be selected by the patient without supervision, patients must be warned about the potential for enhanced sedation and anticholinergic effects. Similarly, alcohol will enhance the sedation from antipsychotic drugs and thus should be avoided.

Therapy Considerations for Antipsychotic Drugs

The goals of drug therapy for the treatment of schizophrenia are to treat acute episodes, prevent acute episodes, and provide the patient with optimal level of functioning with minimal adverse effects. Atypical antipsychotic agents are preferred (not clozapine) to begin treatment. The adverse effects should be considered in drug selection because all atypical antipsychotic agents are equally efficacious but differ regarding the prevalence of some adverse effects that could be important for some patients.

The antipsychotic drugs are used to treat acute episodes with the intent of alleviating symptoms as soon as possible. The onset of response usually occurs within 3 weeks, but optimal response may take longer. If the desired response is not achieved, the patient is switched to another antipsychotic agent. If the second agent is not effective, clozapine (Clozaril) may be an alternative. Once the patient is stabilized on a specific drug and dose, continued improvement and onset of potential adverse effects should be monitored over several months. The goal of maintenance therapy is to find the lowest dose of the right drug for the patient that minimizes relapses but alleviates symptoms. Long-term treatment (years to lifelong) is necessary depending on the occurrence of acute episodes, existence of symptoms, and history of suicide attempts.

Psychotherapy, along with social and vocational training, is useful in combination with drug therapy. Unfortunately, there is a high rate of nonadherence to drug therapy among

TABLE 13-5		
ADVERSE EFFECTS WITH ANTIPSYCHOTIC DRUGS		
	INCIDENCE OF ADVERSE EFFECTS[a]	
ADVERSE EFFECT	*Typical Drugs*	*Atypical Drugs*
Extrapyramidal	Low-high	Very low
Sedation	Yes	Yes
Orthostatic hypotension	Yes	Yes
Anticholinergic	Yes	No[b]
Seizures	Yes	No[c]
Sexual dysfunction	Yes	No
Gynecomastia/galactorrhea	Yes	No
Weight gain	Low	Low-high
Type 2 diabetes mellitus	No	Yes

[a]The incidence varies among the specific drugs within both drug categories.

[b]Except clozapine and olanzapine have significant anticholinergic effects.

[c]Except clozapine, especially at higher doses and in patients with seizure disorders.

patients with schizophrenia; only approximately one-third of patients adhere to their medications as prescribed. This may be due to the high incidence of adverse effects or because some patients are unable to recognize that they have an illness. All of the currently available typical and atypical antipsychotic agents are effective orally, but long-acting forms of some antipsychotics are also available as intramuscular injections that are administered every 2 to 4 weeks. Although injecting antipsychotic drugs poses some disadvantages, use of long-acting injectable dosage forms can help maintain a more consistent response from the drug, reduce the chance of nonadherence, and reduce the incidence of relapse.

Section Summary

Drugs used to treat schizophrenia can be categorized as either typical or atypical. The atypical antipsychotic drugs are the agents of first choice because they reduce the positive, negative, and cognitive symptoms of schizophrenia, whereas the effectiveness of typical agents is limited to the positive symptoms of the schizophrenia. The atypical agents also have the advantage of a better adverse effect profile, a much lower incidence of potentially devastating extrapyramidal effects, and fewer anticholinergic and sexual dysfunction effects. However, sedation

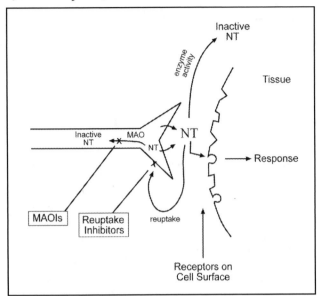

Figure 13-1. As the neurotransmitters (NT) epinephrine, serotonin, and dopamine are released from the nerve terminal, some of the NT combines with the specific receptor for that NT and some undergoes a reuptake process back into the nerve terminal where it is either released again or inactivated by monoamine oxidase (MAO). Reuptake inhibitors block (X) the reuptake process, leaving more NT available to combine with the receptor. MAOIs block (X) the activity of MAO, leaving more NT to be released from the nerve terminal.

and orthostatic hypotension can occur, and the incidence of weight gain and onset of type 2 diabetes mellitus (see Chapter 14) are greater among atypical agents. OTC cold remedies, sleep aids, motion sickness drugs, and alcohol can accentuate the anticholinergic and/or sedative adverse effects of antipsychotic agents.

Schizophrenia is a chronic disorder, and treatment may be lifelong. The intent of therapy is to minimize the occurrence of acute episodes and to normalize as much as possible the patient's social functioning, while at the same time minimizing the adverse effects from the dosage regimen. It can take weeks to observe some desired therapeutic response from antipsychotic drug therapy and months for the maximal effect. Clozapine is the most effective antipsychotic drug, but because of the potential for fatal agranulocytosis, it is only used after other antipsychotic agents (including at least one atypical agent) have been ineffective. Adherence to prescribed drug therapy is poor among patients with schizophrenia, and, consequently, relapse is common.

DRUGS FOR TREATING DEPRESSION

There are several categories of antidepressant drugs: tricyclic antidepressants (TCAs), SSRIs, monoamine oxidase inhibitors (MAOIs), serotonin-norepinephrine reuptake inhibitors (SNRIs), and a miscellaneous group of antidepressants. The primary mechanism of these drugs is to either increase the effect of serotonin or both norepinephrine and serotonin in the CNS by either blocking the reuptake of the neurotransmitter back into the nerve terminal or by blocking monoamine oxidase, an enzyme that inactivates both of these neurotransmitters (Figure 13-1). Both mechanisms increase the chance for the neurotransmitters to combine with the receptor to produce a response. An insufficient response from norepinephrine and/or serotonin is believed to contribute to major depression, but some other mechanism must also contribute because there is a considerable time gap (ie, weeks) between the almost immediate increase in neurotransmitter at the nerve terminal and the observable relief of the depression.

Antidepressant drugs are used to treat major depression, not uncomplicated depression that may result from life events. There is no means of determining which antidepressant will be effective in any given patient. If one drug is not effective after a suitable time and dosage, another drug from the same or different category can be used instead. Selection of an antidepressant is made based on the previous effectiveness of antidepressants in the patient, the potential for drug interactions, the patient's medical history, the adverse effect profile of the antidepressants, and the cost. For example, the antidepressants' adverse effect profiles vary considerably, so an antidepressant that causes hypertension, seizures, or cardiac toxicity would not be the drug of choice to treat major depression in a patient who also has hypertension, epilepsy, or cardiac dysrhythmia. Most patients need to be switched from one drug to another at least once because of inadequate therapeutic response or unacceptable adverse effects.

The intent of therapy is to resolve the acute depressive episode and to prevent relapse. Dosage of the antidepressant is gradually increased to the maintenance dosage as the patient is monitored to determine the extent of adverse effects, its effectiveness in resolving the depression, and signs of suicidal tendency, especially during the initial stages of therapy or later if drug therapy is again altered. Changes in mood for the worse or other behavioral changes (eg, hoarding toxic medications, making a will, giving away valuables) may be signs of increased suicidal tendencies. Once the desired dose and effect are attained, maintenance therapy is continued for months to years, depending on the existence of relapses during therapy and the risk for recurrent episodes.

The percentage of patients with poor adherence to antidepressant drug therapy is high, and nonadherence should be suspected as a potential cause for poor therapeutic response. Reasons for nonadherence are adverse effects, memory problems, guilty feelings, lack of understanding of the importance of daily medication adherence, poor efficacy (especially early in treatment), and cost of the medications. Intervention by health care professionals to monitor the patient's response to therapy, reinforce the need to maintain daily therapy, and provide other educational messages leads to increased adherence by patients being treated for major depression.

TABLE 13-6

DOSAGE RANGE FOR DRUGS USED FOR TREATING DEPRESSION

CATEGORY	GENERIC NAME	TRADE NAME	DOSAGE RANGE[a] (MG/DAY)
TCAs	amitriptyline	Elavil	100 to 300
	clomipramine	Anafranil	100 to 250
	desipramine	Norpramin	100 to 300
	doxepin	Sinequan	100 to 300
	imipramine	Tofranil	100 to 300
	nortriptyline	Pamelor	50 to 150
	protriptyline	Vivactil	15 to 60
	trimipramine	Surmontil	100 to 300
SSRIs	citalopram	Celexa	20 to 40
	escitalopram	Lexapro	10 to 20
	fluoxetine	Prozac	10 to 80
	fluvoxamine	Luvox	100 to 300
	paroxetine	Paxil	20 to 50
	sertraline	Zoloft	50 to 200
MAOIs	isocarboxazid	Marplan	40 to 60
	phenelzine	Nardil	45 to 90
	selegiline	Emsam	6 to 12 mg[b]
	tranylcypromine	Parnate	20 to 60
SNRIs	desvenlafaxine	Pristiq	50
	duloxetine	Cymbalta	40 to 60
	levomilnacipran	Fetzima	40 to 120
	venlafaxine	Effexor	75 to 375
Miscellaneous	bupropion	Wellbutrin	150 to 450
	mirtazapine	Remeron	15 to 45
	trazodone	Desyrel	150 to 600
	vilazodone	Viibryd	40
	vortioxetine	Brintellix	5 to 20

MAOI = monoamine oxidase inhibitor; SNRI = serotonin norepinephrine reuptake inhibitor; SSRI = selective serotonin reuptake inhibitor; TCA = tricyclic antidepressant.

[a]Usual adult oral dosage range.

[b]Administered as a transdermal patch.

Tricyclic Antidepressants

This category of antidepressants has been available for over 50 years, and these drugs were the drugs of choice for treatment of depression for much of that time. The TCAs block the reuptake of norepinephrine and serotonin, hence their therapeutic effect. Table 13-6 lists examples of TCAs and their respective dosage ranges.

Adverse Effects

Many of the adverse effects from TCAs occur because, in addition to blocking the reuptake of norepinephrine and serotonin in the CNS, the TCAs block histamine and acetylcholine receptors, as well as α-adrenergic receptors for norepinephrine in blood vessels. As a result, anticholinergic adverse effects are common with the use of TCAs (eg, dry mouth, constipation, urinary retention, blurred vision, and tachycardia). Orthostatic hypotension is also common and has the potential to cause significant harm to the patient from falls if the severity of this adverse effect is not properly monitored for potential dosage adjustment or if the patient is not instructed to rise slowly from a lying or sitting position. Sedation from histamine receptor blockade in the CNS is another common adverse effect.

TCAs can cause cardiac conduction problems, but this effect is usually limited to an overdose of TCAs or to patients with preexisting impaired cardiac conduction. Nonetheless, this potential toxicity is of significant concern because these drugs are in the hands of patients who may have suicidal tendencies. Other adverse effects include weight gain, lower seizure threshold at higher doses, sexual dysfunction, and increased sweating (although one would expect decreased sweating due to the anticholinergic properties).

The extent of these adverse effects varies among the TCAs. For example, imipramine (Tofranil) has a significantly higher incidence of orthostatic hypotension than does nortriptyline (Pamelor), whereas they both have anticholinergic effects similar to protriptyline (Vivactil), but protriptyline has less sedation than the other two.

Drug Interactions

Drugs that can cause potential problems when used during TCA therapy are drugs that affect the same receptors or neurotransmitters as the TCAs. The use of MAOIs should be avoided with TCAs because of the potential for severe hypertension as a result of an excessive response of norepinephrine on the heart and blood vessels. An enhanced effect may also occur from nasal decongestants because the uptake of these adrenergic agonists into nerve terminals is inhibited by TCAs. Drugs that cause anticholinergic effects or sedation should be used with caution because these effects are enhanced when such drugs are used concurrently with TCAs. See Box 8-1 and Table 8-2 for a listing of drugs that have anticholinergic and sedative effects; examples include antihistamines, alcohol, OTC sleep aids, and products for motion sickness.

Therapy Considerations

All of the TCAs have a long half-life (t½) and thus can be administered once per day, typically in the evening to minimize some of the adverse effects. Initial dosing is usually low and is gradually increased. Observable clinical response for all of the antidepressants is slow; usually 3 to 4 weeks for a good response and often longer for the maximal benefit. Because of the high incidence of adverse effects, the nonadherence rate is high. If the TCA being used is not producing the desired effect and nonadherence

is suspected, the blood level can be checked because the range of concentration for appropriate efficacy has been established for these drugs. The TCAs have a relatively low therapeutic index (TI), with the lethal dose being about 8 to 10 times the typical daily dose. Consequently, the supply of TCA prescribed is limited to one week at a time for patients who are at higher risk for suicide. Abrupt discontinuation of TCAs can result in withdrawal symptoms within 24 to 48 hours that include headache, chills, sweating, restlessness, nausea, diarrhea, and insomnia.

Selective Serotonin Reuptake Inhibitors

SSRIs have been available for over 20 years, fluoxetine (Prozac) being the first one on the US market; others are listed in Table 13-6. These drugs are the most commonly used category of drug to treat depression. The SSRIs are as effective as the TCAs in the treatment of major depression but have fewer adverse effects. The SSRIs block the reuptake of serotonin into the nerve terminal but lack affinity for the histamine, acetylcholine, or norepinephrine receptors.

Adverse Effects

SSRIs as a group do not have appreciable anticholinergic, sedative, orthostatic hypotensive, or cardiac conduction adverse effects compared with the TCAs. The SSRIs have some differences; paroxetine (Paxil) has some anticholinergic effects and fluvoxamine (Luvox) causes some sedation. The incidence of seizures and weight gain are also reduced with SSRIs compared with TCAs. The major adverse effects are sexual dysfunction, nausea, vomiting, and headache. Rather than sedation, a degree of CNS-stimulant effect occurs with some SSRIs, which can result in restlessness, anxiety, agitation, and insomnia. Among the adverse effects, sexual dysfunction has the highest incidence and may result in nonadherence with therapy; one option for such patients is to switch them to an antidepressant in the miscellaneous category that lacks this adverse effect. Some patients may require concomitant medication to treat insomnia.

Drug Interactions

MAOIs should not be used concurrently with SSRIs. This combination can increase serotonin levels to cause serotonin syndrome. Symptoms of this syndrome include shivering, hyperthermia, agitation, seizures, tremor, confusion, diaphoresis, tachycardia, hypertension, ataxia, nystagmus, and myoclonus. Cardiovascular collapse, coma, and death have occurred. When therapy is to be switched from an SSRI to an MAOI, a long-enough washout period must be included to accommodate for the long t½ of the SSRI. At least 2 weeks should elapse after discontinuing one and beginning the other (except 5 weeks when going from fluoxetine to an MAOI due to fluoxetine's long t½).

Therapy Considerations

All of the SSRIs can be given once per day. The SSRIs that cause CNS stimulation should be taken in the morning, except fluvoxamine (Luvox), which should be taken at bedtime. Response to SSRIs is slow, taking 4 to 6 weeks for maximum response. Unlike the TCAs, the incidence of the adverse effects is similar among the SSRIs, except for the sedative/stimulant properties. When SSRIs are discontinued, the dosage must be gradually reduced. Abrupt discontinuation can cause a withdrawal syndrome characterized by dizziness, insomnia, nausea, vomiting, diarrhea, irritability, aggression, tremors, anxiety, and headache. These withdrawal symptoms can last 1 to 3 weeks, but symptoms are reversed if SSRI therapy is restarted.

In addition to treatment of major depression, the SSRIs have been used in the management of complications related to postconcussive syndrome. Symptoms of depression, anxiety, and irritability can be treated using SSRIs. Other antidepressants have been used to manage other symptoms of postconcussive syndrome, including amitriptyline for headache and trazodone for sleep disturbances.

Monoamine Oxidase Inhibitors

MAOIs are as effective as TCAs and SSRIs in the treatment of major depression, but they are reserved for use after TCAs and SSRIs have failed to be effective, due to their potential for serious adverse effects and numerous drug interactions. MAO is an enzyme that inactivates norepinephrine, serotonin, and dopamine (monoamines) in the CNS and peripheral nervous system (see Figure 13-1). This enzyme is also prominent in the liver and small intestine and serves as a mechanism to inactivate monoamines in drugs and foods. The inhibition of MAO at the nerve terminal by MAOIs causes an increased availability of norepinephrine and serotonin for the treatment of depression.

Adverse Effects

Orthostatic hypotension is a common adverse effect of MAOIs. Anticholinergic effects also occur but with less frequency and intensity compared with TCAs. Tranylcypromine (Parnate) causes CNS stimulation, whereas the other MAOIs cause mild sedation. Sexual dysfunction can occur in men and women.

Hypertensive crisis is the adverse effect of most concern because of the potential fatal consequences. This can occur because of a drug interaction or from eating food that is high in tyramine (Box 13-1), a monoamine that increases

---

BOX 13-1

EXAMPLES OF FOODS HIGH IN TYRAMINE CONTENT

- Chocolate-containing foods and beverages in larger quantities
- Aged cheese (excludes cottage cheese, cream cheese)
- Non-fresh meat: aged meats and processed meats (hot dogs, summer sausage, pepperoni), dried meats, pickled fish, and pickled meat
- Brewer's yeast and yeast concentrates
- Wine, beer, and other malt beverages
- Soy products, fava beans, pickles, olives
- Figs, avocados, grapes, pineapples, raisins

---

the release of norepinephrine from nerve terminals. In the absence of MAOIs, tyramine is inactivated by MAO in the small intestine and liver. In the presence of MAOIs, however, a larger amount of tyramine reaches the nerve terminal to increase the release of norepinephrine, causing increased heart rate and peripheral vasoconstriction. Symptoms of hypertensive crisis are sudden-onset headache, tachycardia, stiff neck, nausea, vomiting, sweating, and rapid increase in blood pressure.

Drug Interactions

There are many drugs that interact with MAOIs. Any drug that increases the response from norepinephrine or mimics the effects of norepinephrine has the potential to cause a hypertensive episode if used concurrently with an MAOI. Drugs of this type include nasal decongestants, amphetamines and other CNS stimulants, adrenergic agonists used to treat asthma, TCAs, and SSRIs. In addition, the sedating and anticholinergic properties of MAOIs can be enhanced if other drugs are used with these same adverse effects.

Therapy Considerations

An important part of therapy with MAOIs is to provide appropriate patient education regarding orthostatic hypotension and hypertensive crisis. Patients must be given a list of foods that are rich in tyramine that must be avoided or restricted in the diet. Box 13-1 provides a selected list. Patients should also be advised that MAOIs have many potential drug interactions and that no drug (OTC or prescription) should be taken without the physician's approval. The patient should know the symptoms of hypertensive crisis.

Serotonin/Norepinephrine Reuptake Inhibitors

The SNRIs are a category of antidepressants that are similar to TCAs in their mechanism of action; they inhibit the reuptake of both serotonin and norepinephrine into the nerve terminal. However, they differ from TCAs in that they do not block cholinergic, histamine, or α-adrenergic receptors and thus show an overall pharmacological response similar to the SSRIs. Adverse effects include nausea, constipation, headache, weight loss, nervousness, sweating, insomnia, increased blood pressure, and sexual dysfunction in males and females. As with the SSRIs, abrupt discontinuation of therapy with SNRIs can cause a withdrawal syndrome within days after therapy is stopped; symptoms are nausea, headache, tachycardia, anxiety, dizziness, and agitation. MAOIs should be avoided when using SNRIs. The SNRIs are available for oral use and are given 1 to 3 times per day depending on dose and specific drug.

> *Suicidal thoughts or a suicide attempt are signs of depression. Paradoxically, antidepressants have actually been shown to increase suicide risk in certain patients. The increased risk for suicide appears to involve all of the antidepressant classes. The risk is highest in the early part of antidepressant therapy in children, adolescents, and adults younger than 25 years.*

Miscellaneous Drugs for Treating Depression

These antidepressants are drugs that do not clearly fit into any of the other categories based on the chemical structure or mechanisms of action. These miscellaneous drugs offer an alternative therapy for patients who are not responding to other antidepressants or need an antidepressant devoid of a specific adverse effect. A selection of antidepressants that fall in the miscellaneous category follows.

Bupropion (Wellbutrin)

The mechanism of action of bupropion is believed to involve inhibition of reuptake of the neurotransmitters dopamine and/or norepinephrine. The ability of bupropion to alleviate depression is similar to TCAs and requires 1 to 3 weeks for an initial response. Bupropion has CNS stimulant activity and, like some other CNS stimulants, causes appetite suppression. A major difference in adverse effect profile of bupropion compared with all other antidepressants is that bupropion causes increased sexual desire and therefore may be used to treat major depression in patients who experience sexual dysfunction with another antidepressant. Symptoms relative to the stimulant action are among the most common and include dizziness, headache, tachycardia, and insomnia.

Nausea, constipation, and dry mouth are additional common adverse effects. At higher doses, bupropion can cause seizures. Concurrent use with MAOIs may increase the risk for toxicity from bupropion. One disadvantage of bupropion is that it needs to be taken 3 times per day; however, bupropion is also available in sustained-released and extended-release products, which allow for less frequent dosing. Another US Food and Drug Administration (FDA)–approved use is to aid patients in smoking cessation.

Mirtazapine (Remeron)

Mirtazapine is another drug that does not fall into any of the other categories based on chemistry or mechanism of action. The antidepressant activity is likely from affecting the activity of multiple neurotransmitters. The most common adverse effects are somnolence (ie, state of near sleep), dizziness, increased appetite (weight gain), and increased cholesterol level. Anticholinergic effects (eg, dry mouth and constipation) are mild. Somnolence is accentuated by concurrent use of CNS depressants, including alcohol. Concurrent use with MAOIs should be avoided. The drug can be given once per day near bedtime.

Trazodone (Desyrel)

Trazodone is less effective for major depression than TCAs or SSRIs. Significant sedation is a common adverse effect that is used as an advantage by combining trazodone with other antidepressant therapy that is causing insomnia (eg, SSRIs, bupropion). Dizziness and orthostatic hypotension are also common, but anticholinergic adverse effects are not. Alcohol and other CNS depressants should be avoided. Dosage is typically 3 times per day for major depression. Therapeutic effect may take several weeks to occur.

Vilazodone (Viibryd) and Vortioxetine (Brintellix)

Vilazodone and vortioxetine are recently approved atypical antidepressants; vilazodone was approved in 2011, and vortioxetine received FDA approval in 2013. Both of these antidepressants inhibit the reuptake of serotonin. However, they differ from the traditional SSRIs in that they have additional effects on serotonin receptors. These agents share several adverse effects with the SSRIs, including sexual dysfunction and gastrointestinal adverse effects.

St. John's Wort

St. John's wort has been used to treat mild depression, especially as a self-treatment remedy. It is discussed with the herbal supplements in Chapter 15.

Section Summary

There are many antidepressant drugs, and they can be grouped into 5 categories (see Table 13-6) based on their

TABLE 13-7
DOSAGE RANGE OF MOOD-STABILIZING DRUGS

GENERIC NAME	TRADE NAME	DOSAGE RANGE[a] (MG/DAY)
lithium	Lithonate, Lithobid	600 to 1800
valproic acid/divalproex sodium	Depakene, Stavzor/Depakote	750 to 2500
carbamazepine	Equetro	400 to 1600
[a]Usual adult oral dosage range for maintenance therapy.		

chemistry and/or mechanism of action: TCAs, SSRIs, MAOIs, SNRIs, and miscellaneous drugs. If a patient does not respond sufficiently to one drug, another in the same or a different category can be used as an alternative. However, a few weeks of therapy are required to fully evaluate whether the drug is sufficiently effective. Abrupt discontinuation of TCAs can bring on cholinergic adverse effects, whereas abrupt discontinuation of SSRIs or SNRIs will initiate a withdrawal syndrome that includes dizziness, insomnia, nausea, irritability, anxiety, and headache.

The specific adverse effects vary among the categories of antidepressants, and the incidence of some of these effects can vary among the drugs within the category. Therefore, the selection of the appropriate drug for a patient includes consideration of the adverse effect profile and the patient's medical history so that the adverse effects do not exacerbate any other existing medical condition. The TCAs are noted for an array of adverse effects, including sedation, anticholinergic effects, orthostatic hypotension, weight gain, sexual dysfunction, seizures, and cardiac toxicity. Consequently, the SSRIs, which have fewer adverse effects, have replaced TCAs as the first-choice antidepressant drugs. Although MAOIs also lack many of the adverse effects of the TCAs, they interact with many drugs and have the potential to cause hypertensive crisis if foods that are high in tyramine content are ingested. The SNRIs and miscellaneous antidepressants also have some disconcerting adverse effects; however, in some cases, they are better tolerated by select patients and serve as alternative therapy in patients not responding to SSRIs.

The high incidence of drug interactions between antidepressants and OTC and prescription drugs requires that the concurrent use of all other drugs be monitored. A major concern is to avoid drugs that have pharmacological effects similar to the adverse effects of the antidepressant drug. Nasal decongestants and drugs that have anticholinergic, sedative, or hypertensive effects are generally suspect for being problematic. In addition, MAOIs have numerous drug interactions, and concurrent use of MAOIs with other antidepressants should be avoided. In general, a 2-week washout period is necessary when switching from an MAOI to another antidepressant, or 2 to 5 weeks when switching from another antidepressant to an MAOI.

The intent of antidepressant therapy is to resolve the acute depression episode and to prevent relapse through long-term continuous therapy. Dosage of the antidepressant is gradually increased to the maintenance dosage while the patient is monitored for the severity of adverse effects, the drug's effectiveness in resolving the depression, and signs of suicidal tendency. Maintenance therapy is typically continued for months to years, depending on the patient's response to therapy.

DRUGS FOR TREATING BIPOLAR DISORDER

Drugs used for treating bipolar disorder can be grouped into 2 categories: mood stabilizers and antipsychotics. The intent of therapy with these drugs is to treat the existing episode of mania, hypomania, or depression and to prevent future episodes while minimizing the adverse effects of the drug therapy. Use of multiple drugs concurrently for treatment of bipolar disorder is common. Duration of therapy varies from long term to lifetime depending on the number of episodes, the nature of the episodes, and the patient's family history.

Mood Stabilizers

Mood stabilizers (Table 13-7) are used at all stages of bipolar disorder. They are used in combination with other drugs for acute mania or depression and to prevent future episodes.

Lithium (Lithonate, Lithobid)

Lithium is an effective drug to treat acute manic episodes and to prevent recurrent episodes of mania and depression. It was the first drug approved (1970) by the FDA that was effective for the treatment of mania. The mechanism of action of lithium is not clear. The major disadvantage of this drug is the low TI. This is illustrated by comparing the effective serum concentration of maintenance therapy with lithium in adults (0.4 to 1.2 mEq/L) with the concentration that elicits early signs of toxicity (1.2 to 1.5 mEq/L). Consequently, patients taking lithium must have their lithium blood levels monitored on a regular basis.

> Recall from Chapter 3 that TI is a measure of the relative safety of the drug and is the ratio of the toxic dose for 50% of the population to the effective dose for 50% of the population (TD_{50}/ED_{50}). Using the values provided here for lithium as an approximation of the TD_{50} and ED_{50}, the range for TI = 0 to 3.75.

Adverse Effects

Some of the adverse effects occur because of lithium blood levels being too high (ie, toxicity) and some occur even when the drug is at therapeutic levels. Early adverse effects with lithium therapy include nausea, diarrhea, confusion, muscle weakness, headache, polydipsia, polyuria, and a fine hand tremor. Although many of these effects subside with continued use of the drug, other means of reducing these adverse effects is to take the lithium with food, use an extended-release dosage form, or lower the dose of lithium. Some adverse effects can be alleviated with additional drug therapy, such as antidiarrheal drugs and β-blockers to treat the diarrhea and tremors.

Long-term use of lithium can lead to renal toxicity, goiter, and hypothyroidism. Therefore, kidney function should be monitored and lithium should be used at the lowest possible effective dose. Lithium concentrates in the thyroid and has multiple, and generally reversible, effects in the thyroid gland, including reducing the release of thyroxine. Hypothyroidism can be treated with the use of thyroid hormone until the lithium is discontinued.

Signs of lithium toxicity can occur when the drug is within therapeutic levels. These early signs are fine hand tremor, GI upset, memory and concentration difficulties, thirst, and diarrhea. At higher blood levels, lithium causes coarse hand tremor, confusion, increased deep tendon reflexes, lethargy, slurred speech, and muscle fasciculations. At levels above 2.5 mEq/L, lithium causes seizures, coma, and death. Patients must be aware of the progressing signs of toxicity. Lithium is excreted in the urine, and, consequently, patients with reduced kidney function (eg, elderly patients) are at greater risk for toxicity. Concurrent use of drugs that decrease excretion of lithium also increases the risk for toxicity.

Drug Interactions

Drugs that alter kidney function have the potential to alter lithium excretion. Thiazide diuretics and angiotensin-converting enzyme inhibitors (see Chapter 12) can increase the risk of lithium toxicity because they decrease lithium excretion as they increase sodium excretion. Nonsteroidal anti-inflammatory drugs (NSAIDs) also affect kidney function (see Chapter 6) and can decrease lithium excre-

tion. Aspirin is an exception and thus can be used, as can acetaminophen, which is not an NSAID, as OTC analgesics in patients taking lithium.

Therapy Considerations

The usual daily dosage for maintenance therapy with lithium is 600 to 1800 mg/day (see Table 13-7). In an effort to decrease the intensity of adverse effects and the risk for toxicity, the daily lithium dosage is usually 2 to 4 doses per day rather than a single dose. Daily dosage for treatment of acute manic episodes is 900 to 2400 mg/day. The low TI for lithium warrants that blood levels be monitored every few days initially and every several months once the patient has been stabilized. Patients should know the symptoms of lithium toxicity and be advised to drink 2 to 3 L of water daily to avoid dehydration.

Valproic Acid (Depakene, Stavzor)/ Divalproex Sodium (Depakote)

Valproic acid was originally approved as an antiepileptic drug but has become the preferred mood-stabilizing drug. It is at least as effective as lithium in the treatment of acute manic episodes and for maintenance therapy to prevent additional bipolar episodes. Valproic acid has advantages over lithium: it has a much higher TI and fewer adverse effects and takes a shorter time to produce the therapeutic effects. As with lithium, the exact mechanism of action for the mood-stabilizing effect is not known.

Adverse Effects

Nausea, vomiting, diarrhea, indigestion, tremor, and sedation are the most common adverse effects. The GI adverse effects can be minimized by taking the drug with food, using an H_2-blocker (see Chapter 11), using an enteric-coated product (Stavzor), or using a chemically modified enteric-coated form of valproic acid called divalproex (Depakote). Dosing at bedtime can reduce the problems associated with sedation, and using a β-blocker may relieve the tremor. Other adverse effects are weight gain, headache, prolonged bleeding time, and alopecia. Hepatitis and thrombocytopenia occur rarely.

Drug Interactions

CNS depressants may potentiate the sedative effects of valproic acid when given concurrently. Valproic acid has antiplatelet effects that may be potentiated by the anticoagulant effects of warfarin and aspirin if either is used concurrently with valproic acid.

Therapy Considerations

Valproic acid is available in oral dosage forms, including an extended-release form of divalproex (Depakote ER). Daily dosage can be gradually increased to obtain the desired blood concentration as a means to decrease the GI adverse effects. Typical dosage range is shown in Table 13-7

TABLE 13-8			
POTENTIAL DRUG INTERACTIONS WITH CARBAMAZEPINE			
EFFECT	**DRUG CATEGORY**	**GENERIC NAME**	**TRADE NAME**
↓The drug's effect	Anticoagulant	warfarin	Coumadin
	Asthma therapy	theophylline	Theo-Dur
	Anticonvulsant	valproic acid	Depakene
	Oral contraceptives	estrogen/progestin	many
	Benzodiazepine	diazepam	Valium
	Antidepressant	bupropion	Wellbutrin
↑ Carbamazepine effect	Azole antifungal	ketoconazole	Nizoral
	H$_2$-blocker	cimetidine	Tagamet
	Ca channel blocker	diltiazem	Cardizem
	SSRI	fluoxetine	Prozac
	Macrolide antibiotic	erythromycin	E-Mycin
SSRI = selective serotonin reuptake inhibitor.			

for the maintenance therapy, but the dosage for treatment of acute mania may be higher.

Carbamazepine (Equetro)

Carbamazepine is another antiepileptic drug that has a mood-stabilizing effect in the treatment of bipolar disorder. It is effective in treating acute mania and preventing manic and depressive episodes of bipolar disorder. The mechanism of action for efficacy in bipolar disorder is unknown.

Adverse Effects

GI effects (eg, nausea, vomiting, diarrhea, anorexia, constipation) occur with carbamazepine therapy, but taking the drug with food can minimize these adverse effects. The most frequent adverse effects have a CNS origin and include drowsiness, confusion, headache, dizziness, vertigo, blurred vision, and slurred speech. These CNS effects diminish after a few weeks of therapy, but beginning therapy with a lower dose and gradually increasing the dose can help reduce them. Some blood diseases (eg, aplastic anemia, leukopenia) occur rarely, but monitoring of blood cell counts is necessary.

Drug Interactions

Use of carbamazepine with other drugs that also cause sedation should be avoided. Also, carbamazepine is metabolized by the liver and causes the induction of liver P450 enzymes (see Chapter 3), which increases the metabolism rate of many other drugs as well as its own. Examples of drugs that are metabolized by these same P450 enzymes are shown in Table 13-8. Dosage adjustment of these drugs

may be necessary to retain their effectiveness if they are used concurrently with carbamazepine. Note that women taking oral contraceptives cannot rely on their efficacy while carbamazepine is also being used. Drugs that inhibit these P450 enzymes (see Table 13-8) will cause an increase in blood concentration of carbamazepine and may cause toxicity if the dosage of carbamazepine is not decreased. Grapefruit juice should be avoided with carbamazepine because it can increase the amount of carbamazepine absorbed, resulting in a higher blood concentration.

Recall from Chapter 2 that liver enzymes metabolize drugs and typically inactivate the drug. An induction of P450 liver enzymes increases the number of enzyme molecules present, causing a faster rate of metabolism and faster inactivation of the drug; a faster inactivation results in a diminished effect from the drug.

Therapy Considerations

The usual maintenance therapy dosage range for carbamazepine is shown in Table 13-7. The initial therapy for an acute manic episode should be lower than the target dose and taken in divided doses with meals. The rate of dosage increase should be gradual and conducted over days to weeks, depending on the adverse effects and the therapeutic response obtained. Because carbamazepine induces its own metabolism, the dosage may also have to be readjusted during the first month of therapy until the metabolism rate has stabilized.

Table 13-9

Dosage Range of Benzodiazepines for Anxiety

GENERIC NAME	TRADE NAME	DOSAGE RANGE[a] (MG/DAY)
alprazolam	Xanax	0.5 to 4
chlordiazepoxide	Librium	15 to 100
clorazepate	Tranxene	15 to 60
diazepam	Valium	4 to 40
lorazepam	Ativan	2 to 6
oxazepam	Serax	30 to 120

[a]Usual adult oral dosage range for maintenance therapy.

Antipsychotic Drugs

Some patients with bipolar disorder have symptoms of psychosis (eg, hallucinations, delusions, disordered flow of thought, and diminished ability to recognize reality) during acute episodes of bipolar disorder. Antipsychotic drugs (see Table 13-3) are effective treatment of psychotic symptoms. The antipsychotic drugs are used alone or in combination with a mood stabilizer for the treatment of acute manic episodes. Antipsychotic drugs can also be used as maintenance therapy in the treatment of bipolar disorder because they can also stabilize the mood. They are typically used in combination with a mood stabilizer when used for maintenance therapy. As discussed earlier in this chapter, selection of an atypical antipsychotic drug is preferred due to the more favorable adverse effect profile.

Section Summary

Bipolar disorder requires drug therapy to treat acute manic and depressive episodes as well as to prevent these episodes. Duration of therapy varies from long-term to lifetime depending on the number of episodes, the nature of the episodes, and the patient's family history.

Mood stabilizers (lithium, valproic acid, and carbamazepine) are effective to treat acute manic episodes and as maintenance therapy to prevent episodes. The major disadvantage of lithium is the low TI, but it also has other significant adverse effects, ranging from headache, polyuria, and fine hand tremor to renal toxicity and hypothyroidism. Because lithium is excreted by the kidney and has a low TI, drugs that affect kidney function have the potential to initiate toxic symptoms from lithium. Valproic acid and carbamazepine are antiepileptic drugs that are also mood stabilizers for bipolar disorder. They are less toxic than lithium, and the incidence of significantly disconcerting adverse effects is lower, making them more favorable mood stabilizers for bipolar disorder than lithium. Antipsychotic drugs are used to treat psychotic symptoms

that sometimes occur in bipolar disorder and for maintenance therapy as a mood stabilizer; atypical antipsychotic drugs are preferred.

Drugs for Treating Anxiety Disorders

The SSRIs and SNRIs are considered the drugs of choice for anxiety disorders. The pharmacology of the antidepressants is discussed earlier in this chapter. The benzodiazepines and buspirone (BuSpar) are also medications used in the treatment of anxiety disorders and are discussed in this section. All of the drugs used to treat anxiety disorders have an array of adverse effects. Dosage regimens are increased gradually during initial therapy so that the patient can be monitored for therapeutic response as well as onset of adverse effects. It should be noted that nondrug therapy (eg, psychotherapy, behavioral therapy) is indicated for all anxiety disorders, and patients usually respond best to a combination of drug and nondrug therapy.

Drugs for Treating Generalized Anxiety Disorder

The drugs of choice for initial treatment of acute symptoms of GAD are the benzodiazepines, diazepam (Valium) being a notable example (Table 13-9). The major advantage of using benzodiazepines in the management of acute anxiety symptoms is that the onset of action is rapid (minutes to hours). Buspirone (BuSpar) is an alternative option for relief of anxiety symptoms; however, it has a slower onset of action compared with the benzodiazepines and therefore should not be used when immediate treatment is required. The SSRIs and SNRIs are the primary medications used in the management of GAD. Similar to their activity in major depression, the onset of action of these antidepressants is slow (weeks). Depending on the severity of the anxiety, the duration of treatment varies from months to years. Patients should avoid caffeine and other stimulant drugs, which could exacerbate feelings of anxiety.

Benzodiazepines

There are over a dozen benzodiazepines, and these drugs have several therapeutic uses in addition to GAD, including sedation to treat insomnia, management of alcohol withdrawal symptoms, treatment of certain seizure disorders, treatment of muscle spasms, and use as a preoperative medication. Among the benzodiazepines, some are used preferentially for one or more of these clinical purposes because of the drug's onset of action, duration of action, or extent of metabolism by the liver (for patients with impaired liver function).

The benzodiazepines are lipid-soluble drugs and thus readily enter the CNS, the site of virtually all of their therapeutic and adverse effects. The mechanism of action of benzodiazepines is that they bind to a receptor in the CNS (the benzodiazepine receptor), which potentiates the effect of GABA, an inhibitory neurotransmitter in the CNS. The enhanced activity of GABA reduces the feeling of anxiety.

Adverse Effects

Benzodiazepines are controlled substances but have a relatively low potential for abuse and thus are Schedule IV drugs (see Table 1-7). There is a degree of physical dependence associated with the benzodiazepines, especially following long-term use. Withdrawal symptoms range from anxiety, insomnia, and tremors following short-term use and with lower doses to panic, paranoia, hypertension, delirium, and convulsions with abrupt discontinuation following long-term use (months) and with higher doses. To reduce the severity of the withdrawal symptoms following long-term therapy, the dosage should be tapered over several weeks.

The most common adverse effect is CNS depression causing drowsiness, which usually occurs for the first few days and then diminishes. Benzodiazepines with a longer t½ can be administered at bedtime. Some patients experience amnesia for the time following the drug administration and thus may require a change in drug therapy; some benzodiazepines cause a higher incidence of amnesia than others. Because of their lipid solubility, benzodiazepines cross the placental barrier readily and should be avoided during pregnancy; they are in pregnancy risk categories D and X (see Table 3-6). They also enter breast milk and should not be used by women who are breastfeeding their infants.

Drug Interactions

The most serious drug interaction is the combination of benzodiazepines with any other CNS depressant; the sedative effects of benzodiazepines will be enhanced with these combinations. Benzodiazepines have a weak respiratory depression effect, and thus an overdose of any benzodiazepine used alone would rarely be life threatening. However, the combination of benzodiazepines with any other CNS depressant (see Table 8-2), including alcohol, causes a potentiation of the respiratory depression effect, and the combination can be fatal.

Therapy Considerations

Benzodiazepines begin relieving symptoms of GAD quickly. The dose of benzodiazepine should be initially low and gradually increased until the desired level of anxiety relief is achieved, the maximum dosage is reached, or the adverse effects become limiting. The advantage of using benzodiazepines beyond 4 to 6 months must be weighed against the problems associated with physical dependence. When benzodiazepines are discontinued, the dose should be tapered gradually. Patients should be cautioned regarding drowsiness and the dangers of using any other CNS depressant while on benzodiazepine therapy.

Buspirone (BuSpar)

Buspirone is effective in the treatment of GAD and is an alternative to the benzodiazepines, but it takes 4 to 6 weeks of therapy for the maximum effect. Advantages of buspirone compared with benzodiazepines are that it does not have an abuse potential, it causes minimal sedation, and it does not potentiate CNS-depressant effects of other drugs. The mechanism of action of buspirone is not known, but it does not bind to the benzodiazepine or GABA receptors.

Adverse Effects

The most frequent adverse effects are nausea, headache, dizziness, nervousness, and dysphoria.

Drug Interactions

Buspirone is metabolized by P450 enzymes, so drugs that inhibit these same selected enzymes may increase the blood level of buspirone if used concurrently. Examples of these P450 inhibitors are erythromycin (E-Mycin) and azole antifungals such as ketoconazole (Nizoral). Grapefruit juice also increases buspirone levels. These interactions can enhance the likelihood and intensity of adverse effects.

Therapy Considerations

Buspirone is an option for the treatment of persistent anxiety but not for patients who need immediate relief of anxiety symptoms. It is useful for treatment of patients who cannot tolerate any of the adverse effects from the benzodiazepines and in patients who have a history of alcohol or other drug abuse. The initial dose of buspirone is low and is gradually increased. The usual maintenance dose is 20 to 30 mg/day, with a maximum dose of 60 mg/day. Some benefit may be observed after several days of therapy, but 4 to 6 weeks are necessary for maximal effect.

Antidepressants

Antidepressants are effective in the treatment of GAD and offer a benefit to patients with depressive symptoms and GAD. Paroxetine (Paxil), escitalopram (Lexapro), the extended-release form of venlafaxine (Effexor XR), and duloxetine (Cymbalta) have been approved for treatment of GAD. The pharmacological characteristics of these antidepressants were discussed earlier in this chapter. Like buspirone, it takes weeks for the antidepressants to demonstrate maximal response.

Drugs for Treating Panic Disorder

Benzodiazepines and antidepressants (SSRIs, venlafaxine, TCAs) are used to treat panic disorder. The adverse effects and drug interactions for these drugs were discussed earlier, and these drugs have their advantages relative to these effects. Generally, the antidepressants are preferred to the benzodiazepines for treatment of panic disorder because of the physical dependence potential with the benzodiazepines. In addition, if depression accompanies panic disorder, the antidepressants offer another benefit. A therapeutic response occurs faster with the benzodiazepines (1 to 2 weeks) compared with the antidepressants (3 to 5 weeks), as does the maximum response (4 to 6 vs 8 to 10 weeks). As with the treatment of major depression, the SSRIs have a more favorable adverse effect profile and are the preferred antidepressants for panic disorder. Commonly used SSRIs are paroxetine (Paxil) and sertraline (Zoloft).

The treatment objectives are to alleviate the acute phase of panic disorder, which includes panic attacks and the anticipatory anxiety, and then to maintain the patient on drug therapy. Maintenance antidepressant therapy is typically continued for 1 to 2 years. A low initial dose is used to begin therapy and gradually increased to obtain the optimal relief of symptoms with minimal adverse effects. When drug therapy is discontinued, the dosage should be tapered over months and the patient monitored for signs of relapse.

Drugs for Treating Social Anxiety Disorder

The objective of therapy is to alleviate symptoms of anxiety (tachycardia, sweating, flushing, tremor) and to reduce the anxiety and fear that cause the patient to avoid specific social or public situations. The drugs of choice are the SSRIs, such as paroxetine (Paxil) and sertraline (Zoloft). Venlafaxine (Effexor XR) is efficacious in the treatment of SAD and has been effective in patients who did not respond to SSRIs. MAOIs, particularly phenelzine (Nardil) and tranylcypromine (Parnate), are also effective as alternatives to the SSRIs to treat SAD. When switching from an SSRI to an MAOI (or vice versa), at least 2 weeks should elapse after discontinuing one and beginning the other (except

5 weeks when going from the long-duration fluoxetine to an MAOI). Therapeutic effects take about 4 to 6 weeks and maximal effects about 12 weeks.

Benzodiazepines such as alprazolam (Xanax) and clonazepam (Klonopin) are alternatives to the SSRIs. The therapeutic response from benzodiazepines is rapid (1 to 2 weeks) compared with the SSRIs. The most lipid-soluble benzodiazepines, diazepam (Valium) and clorazepate (Tranxene), are useful for acute anxiety treatment because they begin relieving anxiety within 1 hour of administration, but they have a shorter duration of action. Benzodiazepines should be avoided in patients who have risk of alcohol or other drug dependency. The use of β-blockers (see Chapter 12) such as propranolol (Inderal) or atenolol (Tenormin) have been of benefit to alleviate the autonomic-based symptoms (tachycardia, sweating, blushing, tremor) associated with performance anxiety when administered within a couple hours of the performance.

> *In Chapter 16, you will learn that β-blockers are considered performance-enhancing drugs in some sports and thus are banned for use in these sports by the International Olympic Committee and National Collegiate Athletic Association.*

Drugs for Treating Obsessive-Compulsive Disorder

The objective of therapy is to alleviate symptoms of OCD so that the patient is able to function in social, work, and athletic environments at an optimum level but at the same time minimize the adverse effects of drug therapy. Even with drug and behavioral therapy combined, rarely are all symptoms alleviated. Lack of sufficient response from serotonin in the CNS is considered to play at least a partial role in OCD symptoms.

The SSRIs are the drugs of choice for OCD. If one SSRI is not effective, another should be used instead. The average dose of SSRIs to treat OCD is generally higher than the average dose to treat depression or other anxiety disorders. Dosages would typically be in the higher half of the ranges shown in Table 13-6. Response to SSRIs also takes longer, with initial response occurring after 6 to 8 weeks, compared with 4 to 6 weeks for maximum response in the treatment of depression. If several weeks of trials with a higher dosage of 2 or 3 SSRIs fail to attain sufficient benefit, clomipramine (Anafranil), a TCA, is an alternative. Clomipramine has somewhat better efficacy in the treatment of OCD, but the adverse effects are less desirable (eg, sedation, anticholinergic, and seizures at higher doses). After maintaining the same effective dose for 1 to 2 years, the dosage of SSRI can be tapered over months. If relapse occurs, therapy should be resumed; if relapse occurs repeatedly after additional courses of therapy, lifelong treatment may be necessary.

Drugs for Treating Posttraumatic Stress Disorder

Objectives of therapy are to alleviate the disabling effect that is caused by the patient reexperiencing the event, to stabilize the patient emotionally, and to minimize drug adverse effects. The drugs of choice for treatment of PTSD are SSRIs such as paroxetine (Paxil) and sertraline (Zoloft); the SNRI venlafaxine is also used in the treatment of PTSD. Dosage of the antidepressant should be gradually increased during initial therapy. Maintenance therapy should be continued for 1 to 2 years. Drug therapy should be decreased slowly and the patient monitored for symptoms of relapse. Some patients require drug therapy indefinitely. The TCAs such as amitriptyline and MAOIs such as phenelzine (Nardil) have shown benefit as alternatives in patients who do not respond to SSRI or SNRI therapy. In addition to the antidepressants, the atypical antipsychotics may be used in patients with persistent symptoms. The α_1-receptor antagonist prazosin (see Chapter 12) has been investigated as an agent to decrease nightmares associated with PTSD.

Section Summary

There are several types of anxiety disorders: general anxiety, panic, social anxiety, obsessive-compulsive, and posttraumatic stress. All of these can be treated with SSRIs, although the benzodiazepines are the drugs of choice for relief of acute symptoms because they produce a rapid response in patients. The benzodiazepines, such as diazepam (Valium), have CNS effects that include sedation, an abuse potential (Class IV drugs), and physical dependence with withdrawal syndrome. Another drug that is used to treat GAD and offers an alternative to the use of benzodiazepines is buspirone (BuSpar). This drug does not have the CNS depression effects or abuse potential of benzodiazepines, but there are other drug interactions that may be problematic in some patients. In general, drug therapy for anxiety disorders is gradually increased to obtain the target dose for long-term maintenance therapy. When the drugs are discontinued, they are tapered over weeks to months to minimize the risk of relapse and to monitor the patient for symptoms. Therapy for anxiety disorders typically continues for 1 or more years and in some cases indefinitely as a result of repeated relapse.

DRUGS FOR TREATING ATTENTION DEFICIT/HYPERACTIVITY DISORDER

The intent of therapy for ADHD is to improve the patient's ability to focus and reduce the hyperactivity and impulsive behavior so that the patient can perform better in the school or work environment and socially. Accomplishing these outcomes with acceptable adverse effects requires monitoring the patient and making appropriate dosage regimen adjustments. The most frequently used drugs for treatment of ADHD are CNS stimulants, such as amphetamines and methylphenidate. A few other drugs that are not stimulants are used as alternatives when the stimulants are ineffective or inappropriate.

Stimulant Drugs

The stimulant drugs, methylphenidate and the amphetamines, will be discussed together because their use, effects, and therapy considerations are similar. These drugs have been on the market for many years, and consequently the therapeutic outcomes are well documented and the short-term effects have been well studied; some of the ramifications of long-term use are still uncertain.

The amphetamines are a group of drugs that include dextroamphetamine (Dexedrine), methamphetamine (Desoxyn), and amphetamine, which is a mixture of dextroamphetamine (dextro form) and levamfetamine (levo form). A mixture of amphetamine and dextroamphetamine is also available (Adderall). Like amphetamine, methylphenidate (Ritalin) is a 50:50 mixture of 2 isomers (dextro and levo). The dextro isomer alone is available as dexmethylphenidate (Focalin). Since most of the efficacy to treat ADHD is in the dextro isomer of methylphenidate, the dose for dexmethylphenidate is one-half the dose of methylphenidate. Another stimulant is lisdexamfetamine (Vyvanse), a prodrug that is metabolized to dextroamphetamine and thus has essentially the same effects as dextroamphetamine.

> *Recall from Chapter 2 that a prodrug is given in an inactive form but is converted to the active drug, typically by enzymes in the GI tract or liver.*

Amphetamines and methylphenidate increase the effects of norepinephrine and dopamine in the CNS and peripheral nervous system. The level of these neurotransmitters in the CNS is thought to affect symptoms of ADHD. It is unclear whether these drugs are affecting ADHD by other mechanisms as well.

Adverse Effects

Characteristics of amphetamines, including adverse reactions, are discussed in Chapter 16 as the example of CNS stimulant drugs of this type, all of which are performance-enhancing drugs. In summary, potential adverse effects include decreased appetite, insomnia, abdominal cramps, headache, anxiety, sweating, irritable mood, talkativeness, rapid speech, dilated pupils, and dizziness. Some cardiovascular effects, including increased blood pressure, dysrhythmias, and anginal pain, can occur with use of stimulant medications. More severe psychiatric reactions can be associated with simulant use; some of the reported reactions include severe anxiety, violent or aggressive behavior, mania, and psychosis. Of the adverse effects, the ones of most concern at doses used to treat ADHD are appetite suppression and insomnia.

Another adverse effect for which there is still some debate is whether stimulant ADHD medications affect final patient height. These drugs slow the growth of children early in therapy. It is possible that the anorexic adverse effect contributes to the slower growth rate, which is approximately 1 cm per year during the first 1 to 3 years of therapy. There is some conflicting evidence as to whether the growth delay is temporary and whether the children eventually reach a normal or reduced final height.

Because amphetamines and methylphenidate stimulate the CNS at therapeutic doses, they increase alertness, reduce fatigue, and increase mood. Euphoria can occur, especially as the dose is increased. The elevated mood and euphoria are the basis for the abuse potential associated with these drugs; consequently, they are controlled substances (Class II) (see Table 1-7). With continued use, tolerance develops to the elevated mood, appetite suppression, and cardiovascular effects. However, physical dependence can also occur with continued use, resulting in withdrawal symptoms (eg, depression, increased appetite, fatigue) if the drug is abruptly discontinued. The tendency for abuse seems to be lower (due to less euphoria) for long-acting CNS stimulants that have been developed for once-per-day dosing, including lisdexamfetamine (Vyvanse).

Drug Interactions

The major concern regarding drug interactions is to avoid other CNS stimulants such as caffeine and nasal decongestants, which can enhance the adverse effects of the amphetamines and methylphenidate. MAOIs should not be used in combination with amphetamines or methylphenidate due to the potential for hypertensive crisis.

Therapy Considerations

The therapeutic effect is observed within 1 hour of the first dose, and the duration of action is up to 6 hours. However, observation of the patient's behavior over days is necessary to evaluate the efficacy of the dosage regimen. Dosage is usually increased gradually until behavioral target outcomes are reached or adverse effects are too undesirable. If the desired therapeutic outcome cannot be reached after a sufficient trial with either amphetamine or methylphenidate, a trial with the other drug (amphetamine or methylphenidate) can be attempted.

Typical dosage is 5 to 10 mg 2 or 3 times per day for the short-acting amphetamines or methylphenidate, with the last dose by late afternoon. Maximum daily dosage for children aged 6 years or older is 60 mg and 40 mg for methylphenidate

and dextroamphetamine, respectively. A significant disadvantage of these dosage forms is that multiple dosing per day decreases adherence. To provide once-per-day dosing, delayed-delivery products have been developed for dextroamphetamine (Dexedrine Spansules), amphetamine mixture (Adderall-XR), and methylphenidate (Ritalin LA, Concerta, and Metadate CD). The delayed-delivery products release some of the dose immediately and some later in the day; products are taken in the morning to minimize insomnia. Some caution is needed when administering Concerta tablets to be sure that they are not chewed, which could release the extended-release portion of the drug sooner than desired. Metadate CD and Ritalin LA are capsules that can be separated so that the drug can be sprinkled on a small amount of applesauce and swallowed (not chewed). The immediate-acting methylphenidate is available in tablets, chewable tablets, and an oral solution. An intermediate-acting dosage form of methylphenidate is also available that requires 1 to 2 doses per day (Ritalin SR, Metadate ER, Methylin ER).

Another relatively new dosage form for methylphenidate that has been approved for children and adolescents (6 to 17 years old) is the transdermal patch (Daytrana). The patch is applied to the hip and worn for 9-hour intervals during the day. It takes an average of about 3 hours for methylphenidate to be detected in the blood, with peak levels at 7 to 9 hours. The transdermal patch offers the advantage of once-per-day application, is useful for children who do not swallow medication readily, and can be applied before the child wakes up in the morning. In long-term studies, transdermal therapy was discontinued in some patients because of application-site reaction, anorexia, and insomnia. The concern with growth suppression also exists with this dosage form.

Although stimulant drugs have been used for many years to treat ADHD and their benefits during short-term use have been documented, some controversy remains regarding their use in children. Already mentioned is the potential for growth suppression. In addition, some critics feel that a combination of behavioral intervention and drug therapy is the best treatment, but most parents fail to try behavioral interventions once drug therapy is implemented. The benefit of stimulant therapy used for more than 2 years is also controversial; critics indicate that some data show that the initial advantages are no longer evident beyond 2 years of treatment. Additional studies and data analysis are needed to resolve these issues.

Nonstimulant Drugs

The nonstimulant drugs pose an option for use if the stimulant drugs are not effective, if the adverse effects are not well tolerated, or if there is evidence of current drug abuse problems with the patient.

Atomoxetine (Strattera)

Atomoxetine is a selective norepinephrine reuptake inhibitor that is approved for maintenance treatment of

ADHD in children, adolescents, and adults. Studies have not demonstrated efficacy equal to methylphenidate, making the drug a second-line agent in those that have not responded to or tolerated stimulants. It is not a controlled substance and has no abuse potential, which is an advantage over the stimulant medications. However, the drug is not without some potential problems, having a suicide rate slightly higher than placebo and reports of rare cases of liver damage. Patients taking atomoxetine should be advised regarding the signs of liver damage (eg, dark urine, jaundice, upper-quadrant pain, unexplained flu-like symptoms). There is a potential for weight loss and growth suppression with atomoxetine, although the risk appears to be lower than with the stimulant medications.

Centrally Acting α_2 Receptor Agonists

Extended-release guanfacine (Intuniv) and extended-release clonidine (Kapvay) are both nonstimulant medications approved for ADHD treatment in children and adolescents. Both of the medications bind to α_2 receptor in the CNS; however, the mechanism of action of these medications in treatment of ADHD symptoms is not known. Similar to other nonstimulant medications, their efficacy in ADHD is less than that of the stimulants, but they have advantages in that they are not controlled substances and do not have abuse potential. Guanfacine and clonidine were originally approved as antihypertensives, so low blood pressure is an adverse effect of both. Additional adverse effects include drowsiness and fatigue.

Antidepressants

The antidepressants bupropion (Wellbutrin) and the TCAs are alternate options to the therapy with stimulants. These drugs may not be as efficacious as the CNS stimulants for treatment of ADHD, but they offer the advantage of no abuse potential, lower incidence of sleep problems, and less appetite suppression. The antidepressants are slower to produce the maximum therapeutic effect (about 3 weeks).

Section Summary

ADHD affects children and can continue into adulthood. Methylphenidate is the most commonly used drug, but amphetamines are equally effective; if treatment goals are not achieved with one, a trial with the other can be attempted. These drugs allow the patient to remain focused longer on any given task and reduce the hyperactivity and impulsivity symptoms. Methylphenidate and amphetamines are categorized as CNS stimulants but also have adverse effects due to action in the peripheral nervous system. The major adverse effects of concern are suppressed appetite and insomnia. Historically, the CNS stimulants have been administered 2 to 3 times per day because of their relatively short duration of action. However, newer oral dosage forms, including a transdermal patch, have provided once-per-day dosing.

Nonstimulant drugs are available as alternatives to methylphenidate and amphetamines. These are useful for patients who do not respond to the CNS stimulants or for whom adverse effects, including the potential for drug abuse, preclude the use of stimulants. Among these are atomoxetine (Strattera), guanfacine (Intuniv), clonidine (Kapvay), bupropion (Wellbutrin), and the TCAs.

Some controversies remain regarding drug therapy for ADHD, particularly long-term therapy with stimulants. Effects on growth rate, reduced motivation to use behavioral strategies, and diminished effectiveness beyond 2 years of therapy remain controversial issues.

DRUGS FOR TREATING INSOMNIA

Prescription drugs for insomnia are called *hypnotics* because at therapeutic doses they can induce sleep. All drugs used to treat insomnia cause sedation and thus allow the patient to fall asleep and/or stay asleep. Whether insomnia is intermittent, short term, or chronic, the basic treatment principles are the same: determine the cause, employ nondrug measures as much as possible (Box 13-2), and use drug therapy at the lowest effective dose for the shortest time possible. Pinpointing and treating the cause of the insomnia may eliminate the need for additional therapy for insomnia. For example, if insomnia is caused by depression or anxiety disorders, treatment of those conditions may resolve the insomnia.

Benzodiazepines

Benzodiazepines and benzodiazepine-like drugs (Table 13-10) are the preferred hypnotic drugs for treatment of insomnia. The benzodiazepines that are used to treat anxiety (see Table 13-9) also have hypnotic (sleep-inducing) effects at higher doses but are not typically used to treat insomnia. The benzodiazepine-like drugs chemically do not look like benzodiazepines, but they combine with the same receptor as benzodiazepines and thus are discussed together. These 2 groups of drugs have the advantage of low abuse potential, low potential for suicide (unless taken with alcohol), and few drug interactions. The benzodiazepines with longer duration of action, such as flurazepam (Dalmane) or quazepam (Doral), have residual drowsiness in the morning and thus may impair coordination and performance. Some patients experience memory impairment after using benzodiazepine or benzodiazepine-like drugs. Tolerance to the hypnotic effect (thus diminished efficacy) occurs with these drugs, but the amount of time for tolerance to develop varies from 2 weeks for triazolam (Halcion) to 6 months for eszopiclone (Lunesta). Discontinuing the hypnotic drug for a short period can restore the effectiveness.

Box 13-2

NONDRUG MEASURES TO TREAT INSOMNIA

- Avoid caffeine beverages and nicotine later in the day, especially in the evening.
- Avoid stimulant-causing medications later in the day, especially in the evening, including caffeine-containing OTC products and nasal decongestants.
- Do not take dose of diuretics in the evening.
- Establish a routine wake-sleep schedule.
- Make the bedroom environment conducive for sleep (room-darkening blinds, carpeting to muffle noises, comfortable mattress, moderate room temperature).
- Do not take naps during the day.
- Exercise several times per week during the day, but not prior to bedtime.
- Relax before bedtime; avoid engaging in physically, mentally, or emotionally stressful activities.
- Sleep long enough to feel rested but do not lie around in bed.
- Avoid unnecessary trips to the bathroom by minimizing fluid intake prior to bedtime.
- Avoid alcohol prior to bedtime; it may facilitate sleep onset but may disrupt sleep quality.
- Do not remain in bed if you cannot fall asleep within 20 to 30 minutes. Get up and do something relaxing until you feel drowsy.
- Do not use the bed as the place to read, eat, or watch television.

Table 13-10

BENZODIAZEPINE RECEPTOR AGONISTS USED TO TREAT INSOMNIA

GENERIC NAME	TRADE NAME	DURATION OF ACTION
estazolam	ProSom	Intermediate
eszopiclone[a]	Lunesta	Intermediate
flurazepam	Dalmane	Long
quazepam	Doral	Long
temazepam	Restoril	Intermediate
triazolam	Halcion	Short
zaleplon[a]	Sonata	Ultrashort
zolpidem[a]	Ambien	Short[b]

[a]Benzodiazepine-like drugs.

[b]There is a controlled-release formulation of zolpidem (Ambien CR) that has an intermediate duration of action.

Hypnotic drugs with a shorter onset of action provide a quicker onset of sleep; drugs with a longer duration of action help the patient stay asleep. Thus, a patient who has difficulty falling asleep would benefit most from a quick-onset, shorter-duration drug such as zaleplon (Sonata), whereas a patient who awakens frequently in the middle of the night or too early in the morning would benefit from a drug with a longer duration of action such as eszopiclone (Lunesta). In all situations, periodically assessing the effectiveness of therapy, the onset of tolerance, and the occurrence of adverse effects is expected.

Other Drugs

Trazodone (Desyrel) has already been discussed as treatment for depression. Because of the significant sedative properties, trazodone is used to counter the CNS stimulant properties of SSRIs that are also antidepressants. It has the advantage of not causing tolerance. Because trazodone is not a controlled substance, it can also be used in patients with a history of drug dependency. Doxepin (Silenor) is a tricyclic antidepressant with antihistamine properties that is approved for treatment of insomnia. This particular agent is used for patients with sleep maintenance insomnia (difficulty staying asleep). Other tricyclic antidepressants such as amitriptyline are also used to treat insomnia.

As discussed in Chapters 8 and 10, first-generation antihistamines have prominent sedative properties. Diphenhydramine (Nytol, Sominex) and doxylamine (Unisom) are OTC antihistamines approved to promote sleep. They have the disadvantages of anticholinergic adverse effects, quicker onset of tolerance than benzodiazepines, and long duration of action, which may cause impaired daytime function, including athletic activity.

Melatonin is a naturally occurring hormone synthesized from serotonin that plays a role in regulating the sleep-wake cycle. Melatonin is available as an OTC supplement; it has sedative properties and has been used as self-therapy to treat jet lag and insomnia. Low doses (0.3 to 2 mg) before bedtime have been effective in treating intermittent insomnia without sedation lingering in the morning. Results for use to treat jet lag (typically 5 to 8 mg/dose) when crossing several time zones have been mixed. Adverse effects from melatonin have been minimal, but no long-term studies have established its safety or efficacy for treating insomnia.

Ramelteon (Rozerem) is a melatonin agonist that has been approved to treat sleep-onset insomnia. Adverse effects have not been prominent, it is not a controlled substance, and it does not cause tolerance.

Valerian is an herbal supplement that is used to promote onset of sleep (see Chapter 15), but it is not useful to help maintain sleep throughout the night. It takes several days of use before a sleep-promoting response occurs from valerian.

Section Summary

Treatment for insomnia should include identifying the cause of the insomnia and using nondrug measures to facilitate sleep. Treatment should be for as short a time as possible using the lowest dosage possible. Benzodiazepines and benzodiazepine-like drugs are the most frequently used prescription therapy to treat insomnia. These are relatively safe but have the disadvantages of having an abuse potential and allowing patients to develop tolerance to the hypnotic effect after continued use. Drugs with a shorter duration of action are useful to treat patients who have difficulty falling asleep, whereas drugs with longer duration of action assist patients who awaken throughout the night, but the longer-duration drugs may also have residual drowsiness in the morning.

Trazodone (Desyrel) is useful to treat insomnia caused by SSRIs and to treat insomnia in patients with a history of drug dependency. Other antidepressants such as amitriptyline and doxepin are also used for insomnia. First-generation antihistamines are available as OTC sleep aids (Nytol, Sominex, Unisom) but have anticholinergic adverse effects, a higher incidence of residual morning drowsiness, and tolerance that occurs relatively quickly. Melatonin and valerian are supplements that are used to promote sleep and may be useful for intermittent insomnia in some patients. Ramelteon (Rozerem) is a melatonin agonist and is useful to initiate sleep, can be used for long-term therapy, and can be used in patients with a history of drug dependency.

Drugs for Treating Eating Disorders

The primary treatment for AN and BN is psychotherapy and nutritional counseling. Getting the patient to admit the existence of a problem and the need for help can be the initial hurdle. Not surprisingly, patients with milder symptoms tend to have better outcomes. Even with treatment, symptoms tend to linger, and relapses occur.

Drug Therapy for Anorexia Nervosa

There are no drugs specifically FDA approved for treatment of AN. Antidepressants are used to treat comorbid conditions (eg, depression, anxiety, OCD) as discussed previously in this chapter.

Drug Therapy for Bulimia Nervosa

Antidepressants have demonstrated beneficial outcomes in the treatment of BN. The SSRIs (discussed previously in this chapter) are the agents of choice, and fluoxetine (Prozac) is the one FDA-approved drug for this use. It may take 4 to 8 weeks for the maximum beneficial effect to be evident. Dosage is often at the higher end (60 mg/day) of the antidepressant dosage range. The goal of therapy is to reduce the incidence of binge-and-purge behavior; the results are best when combined with psychotherapy. Comorbid conditions are treated as needed with conventional therapy.

Section Summary

Psychotherapy and nutritional counseling are the primary therapy for AN and BN. Effective drug therapy is sparse for the treatment of eating disorders. Antidepressants, particularly SSRIs, are used for management of coexisting psychiatric conditions in patients with AN. Fluoxetine (Prozac) is approved by the FDA for treatment of BN because it can reduce the incidence of binge-and-purge behavior.

ROLE OF THE ATHLETIC TRAINER

Treatment of psychiatric disorders poses an array of health care concerns, such as obtaining the appropriate diagnosis, selecting the appropriate drug therapy and the best dosage, incorporating psychotherapy as part of the treatment plan, monitoring the patient for adverse effects, encouraging the patient to comply with therapy, and being sensitive to the stigma sometimes associated with the diagnosis of these disorders.

It is important for athletic trainers to be aware of the characteristics of these disorders and the drugs used to treat them so that the athletic trainer can assist in the referral of undiagnosed patients and can be of assistance to the patient in the following ways:

- Reinforcing the necessity for the patient to adhere to the prescribed dosage regimen

- Being adamant that the patient should not abruptly discontinue medications or begin OTC medications or herbal remedies without the physician's approval

- Identifying some symptoms of adverse drug reactions that may require a change in dosage regimen

- Encouraging the patient to continue with the dosage regimen while waiting for the onset of therapeutic benefit, knowing that many of these drugs require weeks of therapy before significant changes in behavior are observed

- Preventing the patient from participating in some events that may be hazardous during a time when adverse drug effects, such as CNS sedation, are having a negative impact on balance, coordination, or other skills

- Assisting the athlete in applying for therapeutic use exemptions when the drug therapy includes drugs banned from competition

- Being aware that although drug therapy may restore the patient's desire and enthusiasm for athletic participation, some of the adverse effects may be a hindrance to achieving the intended level of performance

CASE STUDY

As the athletic trainer for the basketball team, Nate travels over the Thanksgiving break with the team to the annual Las Vegas Men's Invitational Basketball Tournament. It is a week-long event, and he notices rather quickly that the freshman center is being ignored by many of the other team members. Upon closer observation, Nate realizes why. The freshman seems to talk incessantly, even when the coach is talking. Nate notices that this player also interrupts other team players when they are contributing to a conversation. He doesn't seem to think before he speaks and frequently gets into trouble because of it. Nate thinks the freshman has ADHD and approaches him about it. The freshman admits that he has had a problem interacting with others for a long time and indicates that school is hard for him because he can't seem to concentrate enough to learn the information. He tells Nate that when he was in elementary school, his mother took him to a doctor but the physician said, "Boys will be boys" and dismissed his problems in school to his high energy level. Nate tells the freshman that when they return home he will refer him to a physician. Nate knows that if this player does have ADHD, he will likely be placed on medication, either a stimulant or a nonstimulant drug. Nate intends to identify the side effects of these drugs so he is prepared if the freshman center complains of any of them. What adverse effects should the athlete expect from these medications? How do the stimulant medications differ from the nonstimulant medications?

REFERENCE

1. American Psychiatric Association. *Diagnostic and Statistical Manual of Mental Disorders*, Fifth Edition. Arlington, VA: American Psychiatric Association; 2013.

BIBLIOGRAPHY

Alderman CP, McCarthy LC, Marwood AC. Pharmacotherapy for post-traumatic stress disorder. *Expert Rev Clin Pharmacol.* 2009;2(1):77-86.

Bucci KK, Possidente CJ, Talbot KA. Strategies to improve medication adherence in patients with depression. *Am J Health Syst Pharm.* 2003;60:2601-2605.

Kaplan G, Newcorn JH. Pharmacology for child and adolescent attention-deficit hyperactivity disorder. *Pediatr Clin North Am.* 2011;58:99-120.

Manos MJ, Tom-Revzon C, Bukstein OG, Crismon ML. Changes and challenges: managing ADHD in a fast-paced world. *J Manag Care Pharm.* 2007;13(9,S-b):S1-S13.

Schultz SH, North SW, Shields CG. Schizophrenia: a review. *Am Fam Physician.* 2007;75(12):1821-1829.

Willer B, Leddy JJ. Management of concussion and post-concussion syndrome. *Curr Treat Options Neurol.* 2006;8:415-426.

CHAPTER 14: ADVANCE ORGANIZER

Foundational Concepts

- Disease Process
  - Type 1 Diabetes Mellitus
  - Type 2 Diabetes Mellitus
  - Long-Term Complications
- Diagnosis and Monitoring
- Nondrug Measures
- Patient Adherence
- Section Summary

Drug Therapy for Type 1 Diabetes Mellitus

- Insulin Preparations
  - Insulin Administration
  - Adverse Effects
    - Hypoglycemia
    - Weight Gain
    - Immune Responses
    - Lipohypertrophy
  - Drug Interactions
- Amylin-Like Compounds
- Section Summary

Drug Therapy for Type 2 Diabetes Mellitus

- Oral Antidiabetic Drugs
  - Sulfonylureas
  - Glinides (Meglitinides)
  - Biguanides
  - Glitazones (Thiazolidinediones)
  - α-Glucosidase Inhibitors
  - DPP-4 Inhibitors (Gliptins)
  - SGLT Inhibitors
- Other Oral Antidiabetic Agents
- Incretin-Like Compounds (Incretin Mimetics, GLP-1 Analogs)
- Pramlintide
- Insulin
- Section Summary

Role of the Athletic Trainer

14

Drugs for Treating Diabetes Mellitus

CHAPTER OBJECTIVES

At the end of this chapter, the reader will be able to:
- Describe the disease process for the development of type 1 and type 2 diabetes mellitus
- Differentiate between type 1 and type 2 diabetes mellitus
- Recall the signs and symptoms of hypoglycemia and its treatment
- Explain how blood glucose levels are monitored and maintained
- Explain nondrug and drug-related interventions to control type 1 and type 2 diabetes mellitus
- List how insulin can be administered
- Summarize the role of the athletic trainer in the monitoring of blood glucose levels as well as nondrug and drug therapies for patients with diabetes mellitus

ABBREVIATIONS USED IN THIS CHAPTER	
A1C. glycosylated hemoglobin	**LDL.** low-density lipoprotein
ADA. American Diabetes Association	**NPH.** neutral protamine Hagedorn
CNS. central nervous system	**OTC.** over-the-counter
DPP-4. dipeptidyl peptidase 4	**rDNA.** recombinant deoxyribonucleic acid
FDA. Food and Drug Administration	**SGLT.** sodium-glucose–linked transporter
GERD. gastroesophageal reflux disease	**SMBG.** self-monitoring of blood glucose
GI. gastrointestinal	**t½.** half-life

In this chapter, the term *diabetes* refers to diabetes mellitus. This disease is very prevalent in the United States; it is estimated that there are over 29 million Americans who have diabetes and that nearly one-third of cases have not been diagnosed. The incidence of type 2 diabetes is increasing due to the rising prevalence of obesity and sedentary lifestyles. Consequently, it is important for the athletic trainer to understand not only the treatment principles for

diabetes, which typically includes regular exercise, but also the symptoms in undiagnosed athletes. Part of the challenge for the patient regarding diabetes therapy is to properly adjust insulin dosage, adhere to diet and exercise regimens, monitor blood glucose, and obtain early treatment of diabetes complications. The purpose of this chapter is to provide information for the athletic trainer for improving diabetes care through a better understanding of the therapeutic

Houglum JE, Harrelson GL, Seefeldt TM.
Principles of Pharmacology for Athletic Trainers, Third Edition (pp 269-288).
© 2016 Taylor & Francis Group.

Figure 14-1. Insulin production and function.

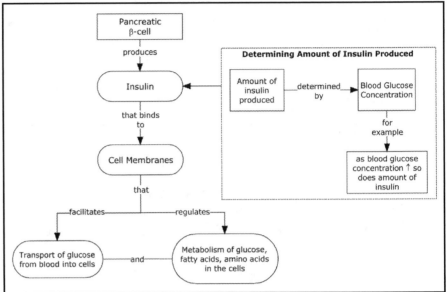

<table>
<tr><td align="center">Box 14-1</td></tr>
</table>

SYMPTOMS OF UNCONTROLLED DIABETES[a]

- Polyuria (increased urine output)
- Polyphagia (increased appetite)
- Polydipsia (increased thirst)
- Unexplained weight loss
- Fatigue
- Blurred vision
- Irritability

[a]Ketosis (ketone bodies in blood) is another symptom of uncontrolled type 1 diabetes.

---

goals of treatment, an ability to recognize the signs and symptoms of potential problems, and a desire to provide encouragement to the patient with diabetes.

FOUNDATIONAL CONCEPTS

There are 2 major types of diabetes: type 1 and type 2. Among diabetic patients, 10% or fewer have type 1, and although onset occurs prior to age 20 years in most patients, some cases are diagnosed later. At least 90% of people with diabetes have type 2. Onset of type 2 diabetes occurs most often after age 40 but can occur at any age. Type 1 diabetes requires daily insulin, and some cases of type 2 diabetes are also managed best with insulin. The disease process differentiates these 2 types of diabetes and dictates the treatment options.

Disease Process

The β-cells of the pancreas produce insulin in response to the blood glucose concentration; more is released as the blood glucose level increases. The insulin binds to cell membranes such as liver, muscle, and adipose; facilitates the transport of glucose from the blood into the cells; and regulates the metabolism of glucose, fatty acids, and amino acids in the cells (Figure 14-1). Through these processes, insulin maintains the fasting blood glucose at < 100 mg/dL and quickly reduces spikes in glucose concentration after carbohydrate ingestion, keeping the 2-hour postprandial glucose at ≤ 120 mg/dL.

Type 1 Diabetes Mellitus

Patients with type 1 diabetes do not and cannot produce insulin because the β-cell function is destroyed. This is an autoimmune disease because the β-cells are destroyed by the person's own antibodies. Some people may be genetically predisposed to produce these antibodies but never do so unless they also encounter an environmental trigger (eg, virus, chemical, dietary substance) that initiates the production of these antibodies. As the antibodies slowly destroy the β-cells, hyperglycemia eventually appears because the insulin is not present to facilitate the movement of glucose out of the blood and into the cells. As hyperglycemia is sustained and worsens, the blood glucose level exceeds the threshold of glucose the kidney can reabsorb (180 mg/dL) through the active uptake mechanism (see Figure 2-8) and glucose is spilled into the urine, initiating the onset of acute symptoms (Box 14-1). Glucose in the urine acts as a diuretic causing polyuria, one of the major acute symptoms of uncontrolled diabetes. Other symptoms are increased thirst (polydipsia), which occurs because of the polyuria, and polyphagia (increased appetite), which occurs because

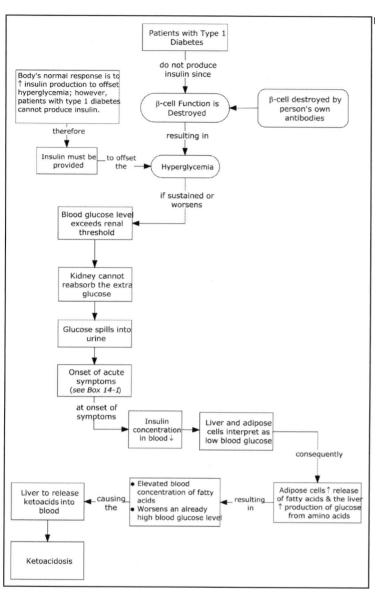

Figure 14-2. Onset of symptoms in type 1 diabetes.

so many calories are being excreted in the urine. Weight loss also occurs because of the excreted calories.

Insulin functions by combining with a receptor on the surface of the cell and initiating a sequence of events within the cell similar to the receptor theory of drug action discussed in Chapter 3. The specific sequence of events within the cell differs depending on the type of cell affected. For example, insulin facilitates the transport of glucose from the blood into the muscle and adipose cells for use as an energy source. In the liver, insulin causes a decrease in glucose production and an increase in glycogen production, whereas in the fat cell, insulin suppresses fatty acid release and causes an increase in fatty acid and triglyceride synthesis.

Besides regulating glucose metabolism, insulin also plays a role in regulating fatty acid and amino acid metabolism (see Figure 14-1). As the symptoms of diabetes unfold and the insulin concentration in the blood diminishes, the liver and adipose cells begin functioning as if the blood glucose level is low (that is the tissue's interpretation of the hormone signal [ie, no insulin]). Consequently, the adipose cells increase the release of fatty acids in the blood and the liver increases the production of glucose from amino acids (gluconeogenesis) and releases it into the blood because these tissues are responding to the hormone signal of low insulin. Unfortunately, these responses by adipose and liver cells not only elevate blood concentration of fatty acids but also exacerbate the already high blood glucose level (Figure 14-2).

In people without diabetes, these same effects on fatty acid, amino acid, and glucose metabolism occur as a means

---

Box 14-2

CRITERIA FOR DIAGNOSIS OF DIABETES

1. A1C ≥6.5% (using method that is certified and standardized)

   or

2. Fasting plasma glucose ≥126 mg/dL (Fasting is defined as no caloric intake for at least 8 hours.)

   or

3. Two-hour plasma glucose ≥200 mg/dL during an oral glucose tolerance test[a] (The test should be performed as described by World Health Organization, using a glucose load containing the equivalent of 75 g anhydrous glucose dissolved in water.)

   or

4. Symptoms of hyperglycemia plus a casual plasma glucose ≥200 mg/dL (Casual is defined as any time of day without regard to time since last meal. The classic symptoms of hyperglycemia include polyuria, polydipsia, and unexplained weight loss.)

---

[a]In the absence of unequivocal symptoms of hyperglycemia, criteria 1 to 3 should be confirmed by repeat testing.

Adapted from Standards of Medical Care in Diabetes–2014. *Diabetes Care.* 2014;37(suppl 1):S14-S80.

Box 14-3

POTENTIAL LONG-TERM COMPLICATIONS OF DIABETES

- Hypertension
- Heart disease and stroke
- Retinopathy
- Kidney disease
- Diminished sensation in hands and feet
- Foot problems including infections
- Amputations of lower limb
- Sexual dysfunction
- Periodontal disease

---

of providing energy sources when insulin levels diminish because blood glucose levels are low. In people without diabetes, as a means to conserve glucose, the liver also makes ketoacids (also called *ketones* or *ketone bodies*) from the fatty acids and releases them into the blood (ketosis). The ketoacids provide an alternative energy source, especially for the central nervous system and muscle, which will use them in place of glucose. Therefore, in people without diabetes, the ketoacids are an advantage because they are used as an alternate energy source, thus conserving the low level of glucose. However, in people with diabetes, the low insulin level sends the wrong signal to the liver (because the blood glucose level is not low) and the liver produces ketoacids although the blood glucose level is high. These ketoacids continue to be made beyond any need for them, and thus they accumulate in the blood. Because these are acids, their accumulation in the blood eventually leads to ketoacidosis (a drop in the blood pH) that eventually leads to death if the situation is not corrected with insulin. Acetone is another ketone body (but not an acid) that has no metabolic function. Acetone is a volatile compound that is excreted by the lungs and gives the breath a fruity or sweet odor, which is a sign of a ketosis.

Type 2 Diabetes Mellitus

Unlike people with type 1 diabetes, type 2 diabetic patients continue to produce insulin. The major underlying defect is the existence of insulin resistance; that is, for one or more reasons, the response of the cell (liver, muscle, adipose) to insulin is diminished. In response to insulin resistance, the pancreas increases the production of insulin to compensate for the reduced effectiveness of the insulin, but the release may not be synchronized with the glucose-based need. The blood glucose level increases higher than normal after meals (postprandial hyperglycemia), and the fasting blood glucose may also be higher than normal but not quite high enough to be categorized as diabetes. As this process continues for years, the patient may go undiagnosed because there are often no symptoms. Even when the fasting blood glucose level becomes high enough to be diagnostic for diabetes (Box 14-2), the patient often goes undiagnosed for 4 to 7 years unless hyperglycemia is revealed through diabetic screening or other blood tests. Unfortunately, by the time of diagnosis, many patients have already lost some β-cell function and the underlying causes of the long-term complications (Box 14-3) have already begun. A major concern, besides the long-term complications, is that as the diabetes progresses throughout the years, the insulin resistance increases and the insulin production decreases as β-cell function continues to diminish, making it more difficult to control the blood glucose. The progressive nature of the disease process necessitates routine glycemic monitoring (ie, glycosylated hemoglobin [A1C], fasting blood glucose, postprandial blood glucose) and aggressive adjustment in therapy when the glycemic goals are not being reached.

However, the complexity of diabetes goes beyond the secretion of insulin and cellular insulin resistance. Other hormones also affect glucose levels and the amount of insulin secreted by the pancreas in type 2 diabetes. Incretins, for example, are peptide hormones released by the gastrointestinal (GI) tract in response to absorption of food. These hormones have 4 major effects that are of interest regarding the treatment of diabetes. Incretins cause the pancreas to increase the release of insulin when blood glucose is rising. Probably most importantly, the incretins have demonstrated in vitro that they may preserve the insulin-producing capacity of β-cells, a significant factor in the progression of type 2 diabetes. The incretins decrease the appetite, which is of particular benefit because most patients with type 2 diabetes are overweight. A fourth effect of the incretins is that they reduce the secretion of glucagon from the β-cells of the pancreas. Glucagon is a hormone with metabolic effects much the opposite of insulin. One effect in particular is that glucagon increases the blood glucose level by enhancing glucose synthesis from amino acids (gluconeogenesis) and the breakdown of glycogen (glycogenolysis). Patients with type 2 diabetes have a diminished incretin response, which may be a contributing factor to postprandial hyperglycemia. The incretin hormones have a half-life (t½) of 2 to 7 minutes, being inactivated by the enzyme dipeptidyl peptidase 4 (DPP-4), which is present in and around certain blood vessels.

Another process that does not function properly in diabetic patients is the regulatory effects of amylin. This is also a peptide hormone and is cosecreted with insulin by the pancreatic β-cells. Amylin decreases GI motility, thereby slowing the rate of glucose absorption. It reduces the release of glucagon, thus decreasing the glycemic-enhancing effects that glucagon has on the liver. These effects on GI motility and glucagon release provide a means of reducing the rapid rise and magnitude of postprandial hyperglycemia. Through an action in the central nervous system, amylin also decreases appetite. Insufficient regulatory effects from amylin contribute to the diabetes disease process.

The primary risk factors for type 2 diabetes are obesity (especially around the abdomen), a sedentary lifestyle, and age. Although age is a risk factor, obesity and sedentary lifestyle in the United States is resulting in an increasing prevalence of type 2 diabetes among children and adolescents aged 6 to 19 years. Evidence indicates that lifestyle changes (eg, diet and exercise) can prevent the onset of type 2 diabetes in some patients. There is also evidence for a genetic link that may contribute to the etiology; the incidence of type 2 diabetes is higher in African Americans, Native Americans, Hispanic/Latino Americans, Asian Americans, and Pacific Islanders.

As mentioned, people with type 2 diabetes may be hyperglycemic yet asymptomatic for years. When symptoms occur, they are usually similar to those of type 1 diabetes (see Box 14-1) but may be milder. Other symptoms may include complications from coronary heart disease and hypertension. Because patients with type 2 diabetes produce some insulin, cellular metabolism is maintained in sufficient balance so that ketoacidosis is not an outcome of type 2 diabetes. The exception may be during significant physiological stress, such as caused by pregnancy or infection, or during psychological stress.

Long-Term Complications

Long-term complications are of major concern for both type 1 and type 2 diabetes (see Box 14-3). The major goals of diabetes management are to prevent occurrence of acute hypoglycemic episodes and to prevent these long-term complications. Heart disease and stroke are the leading cause of death among patients with diabetes. The occurrence of long-term complications is directly related to the extent and duration of hyperglycemia and to the abnormal lipid metabolism, hence the need for treatment of type 2 diabetes regardless of symptoms. Although the progression of some long-term complications has already begun by the time type 2 diabetes is diagnosed, the incidence and severity of these complications can be minimized in patients who have tightly controlled hyperglycemia through close monitoring of blood glucose levels, appropriate adjustments in insulin or other drug therapy, and proper diet and exercise.

Diagnosis and Monitoring

Hyperglycemia is determined by measuring the blood glucose concentration using any of 4 tests (see Box 14-2): fasting plasma glucose, casual plasma glucose, oral glucose tolerance test, and A1C. For the fasting plasma glucose test, the patient fasts for at least 8 hours prior to the blood being drawn. In contrast, casual plasma glucose concentration means the concentration is determined at any time with no special instructions regarding eating (or fasting) prior to the test. The oral glucose tolerance test requires an oral administration of 75 g of glucose 2 hours prior to the blood sample. The A1C level gives an indication of what the average glucose control has been during the previous 2 to 3 months; a high glucose level yields a higher A1C. Diagnostic for diabetes is a fasting glucose level of ≥ 126 mg/dL, a casual plasma glucose of ≥ 200 mg/dL with symptoms of hyperglycemia, an oral glucose tolerance test of ≥ 200 mg/dL at 2 hours, or A1C ≥ 6.5%. A second test result should be obtained to confirm the diagnosis. Preferably, the same test is repeated, but alternatively one of the other tests may be used for confirmation. The patient's symptoms are also used as a diagnostic indicator.

Monitoring blood glucose level is an important part of diabetes care for type 1 and 2 diabetes. The goal is to minimize hyperglycemia but also to prevent hypoglycemia (< 70 mg/dL) because of too much insulin. Self-monitoring of blood glucose (SMBG) is the norm and allows the patient to check the level several times throughout the day (≥ 3 times/day for patients using multiple insulin injections or insulin pump) and to make adjustments in insulin, exercise, and diet accordingly. The involvement of the patient in this self-care decision making is a necessary component of the diabetes management plan. Hand-held devices and reagent strips containing the appropriate chemicals and

TABLE 14-1

GLYCEMIC RECOMMENDATIONS BY AGE[a]

AGE GROUP (YR)	PLASMA BLOOD GLUCOSE (MG/DL)			
	Preprandial	*Postprandial*	*Bedtime*	*A1C*
6 to 12[b]	90 to 180	nr	100 to 180	< 8%
13 to 19[b]	90 to 130	nr	90 to 150	< 7.5%
Adult	70 to 130	< 180	nr	< 7%

[a]Should be individualized based on duration of diabetes, pregnancy status, age, comorbid conditions, hypoglycemia unawareness, and individual patient considerations.

[b]For type 1 diabetes.

nr = no recommendation.

Adapted from Standards of Medical Care in Diabetes–2014. *Diabetes Care.* 2014;37(suppl 1):S14-S80.

enzymes for self-monitoring are readily available and relatively easy to use. Several continuous glucose-monitoring devices are also available, most of which use an electrode sensor inserted into the subcutaneous tissue of the abdomen. These continuous monitoring devices provide a digital display of the patient's blood glucose and provide warning if the glucose level is too high or too low. Educating the patient regarding SMBG and the strategy of making appropriate adjustments is necessarily an ongoing process to ensure that the patient can make the best decisions. For adults with diabetes, the recommendations of the American Diabetes Association (ADA) are for the blood glucose level to be at 70 to 130 mg/dL before meals (preprandial) and < 180 mg/dL at peak postprandial (1 to 2 hours after starting the meal). Table 14-1 lists ADA recommendations for SMBG for different age groups. These glycemic goals should be individualized (eg, in infants, children, and elderly; during pregnancy; during acute illness; in poorly motivated patients) if necessary to avoid hypoglycemic episodes and to achieve the A1C goal.

Measuring A1C is another means of monitoring glycemic control as well as diagnosing diabetes. Hemoglobin in red blood cells reacts spontaneously with glucose to form glycosylated hemoglobin. Because this reaction is spontaneous, it cannot be regulated by the cell, and thus the concentration of A1C directly depends on the concentration of glucose in the blood. Normal A1C for people without diabetes is < 6%. The general goal recommended by the ADA for nonpregnant adult patients with diabetes is < 7%, if it can be achieved without significant hypoglycemia. However, goals should be individualized for patients such as for children (see Table 14-1), patients with history of severe or frequent hypoglycemia, or patients with long-standing diabetes (≥ 30 years) with minimal or stable microvascular complications. Values ≥ 7% are indicative of inadequate control and the need for some adjustments in therapy.

Measuring A1C does not replace SMBG but provides another piece of information to assess the effectiveness of the overall therapy and should be performed 2 to 4 times per year, depending on whether the patient is meeting the treatment goals and/or has had a change in therapy.

The A1C is usually the prime indicator of glycemic control (ie, the success of the drug therapy, diet, and exercise program). Tight glycemic control is generally advocated (A1C < 7%) because research has demonstrated the connection between tight glycemic control and lower incidence of the microvascular complications (eg, nephropathy, retinopathy, neuropathy). The evidence is less convincing regarding tight glycemic control and lower incidence of the other long-term complications, called *macrovascular complications* (eg, hypertension, stroke, coronary artery disease, peripheral vascular disease). It is generally assumed that some level of glycemic control is beneficial to reduce the risk of macrovascular complications. Studies have found conflicting data on the impact of tight glycemic control (A1C < 7%) on cardiovascular outcomes. The differences in impact of tight glycemic control on macrovascular outcomes have been associated with how long the patient has had diabetes and whether cardiovascular disease was present at the time of initiation of diabetes treatment. In addition, there is some evidence that too aggressive of an approach may increase the death rate among individuals who are at high risk for heart disease. It is clear that intensive glycemic control may need to be tempered for some patients who are at high risk for certain complications. Additionally, for the best therapeutic outcomes, glycemic control must be coupled with appropriate monitoring and treatment of conditions such as hypertension, elevated blood cholesterol, eye disease, reduced kidney function, and foot problems to curb the incidence of more serious consequences.

BOX 14-4

SOME NUTRITIONAL RECOMMENDATIONS FOR DIABETES[a]

- Saturated fat intake should be < 10% of total calories.

- Substitute mono- and polyunsaturated fats for saturated fats.

- Cholesterol consumption should be < 300 mg/day.

- Monitor carbohydrate intake as a component of glycemic control.

- Vitamin or mineral supplementation provide no benefit without underlying deficiencies to people with diabetes compared with the general population.

- Avoid routine supplementation with antioxidants (eg, vitamins E and C and carotene).

- Eat ≥ 2 servings of fish/week (not commercially fried) for n-3 polyunsaturated fatty acids.

- Minimize trans fat intake.

- Use a variety of sources for carbohydrate (eg, fruits, vegetables, whole grains, low-fat milk).

- Foods with sucrose (table sugar) can substitute for other carbohydrates in the meal plan. However, this substitution should be kept to a minimum to avoid replacing more nutrient-rich carbohydrates with table sugar.

- Limit alcohol consumption to ≤ 1 drink/day for women and ≤ 2 drinks/day for men.

- If using insulin or insulin secretagogues, alcohol consumption increases risk for hypoglycemia.

[a]Individuals with diabetes and are pregnant or have comorbid disease may need other special dietary considerations.

Adapted and selected from Nutrition Therapy Recommendations for the Management of Adults with Diabetes. *Diabetes Care.* 2014;37(suppl 1):S120-S143.

Foot ulcers are a common complication of neuropathy and vascular disease among diabetic patients. Nerve damage diminishes sensation in the feet; thus, any damage to the feet such as cuts, bruises, or blisters may go unnoticed until significant damage has occurred. Poor circulation to the feet can diminish the rate of healing and exacerbate the problem. The majority of diabetes-related amputations of the lower extremities have foot ulcers as a precipitating complication. Consequently, patients with diabetes should undergo an annual comprehensive foot examination, examine their feet daily, wear shoes that fit properly, and immediately attend to any problems.

Nondrug Measures

Diet and exercise are the foundation of the nondrug measures to treat diabetes. Each of these factors can improve glycemic control as demonstrated by lower A1C, fasting glucose, and postprandial glucose, particularly in individuals with type 2 diabetes. Patients with type 2 diabetes are typically overweight or obese, but even modest weight loss can reduce insulin resistance in these patients. Appropriate diet

and exercise have also demonstrated improved cholesterol and blood pressure, which are factors linked to long-term complications. The ADA recommends that all individuals with diabetes should receive individualized medical nutrition therapy. Some nutritional recommendations for patients with diabetes are shown in Box 14-4.

Routine exercise is important for patients with either type 1 or type 2 diabetes, the goal being to reduce the risk for long-term complications, particularly macrovascular disease. Considering the disease process of type 2 diabetes, with long-term complications often beginning prior to diagnosis, the need for exercise as part of the diabetes management plan is very important. In addition, evidence demonstrates some benefits of exercise for type 2 diabetes regarding improved glycemic control (Box 14-5). For example, exercise improves the utilization of glucose by muscle, which contributes to glucose control. Prior to exercise, the existence of conditions such as hypertension, autonomic neuropathy, retinopathy, or peripheral neuropathy should be determined because they may pose some problems to be considered when planning the exercise regimen. Barring the existence of these problems, the level of exercise recommended by the ADA for people with diabetes is at least 150 minutes/week of moderate-intensity aerobic activity (50% to 70% of maximum heart rate). Resistance

---

Box 14-5

EFFECTS OF EXERCISE FOR TYPE 2 DIABETES

- Hypoglycemia during exercise rarely occurs to individuals who are taking metformin, glitazones, or β-glucosidase inhibitors, but may occur to individuals taking insulin or insulin secretagogues.

- Exercise reduces A1C and is independent of weight loss.

- Higher-intensity exercise has a greater effect on A1C.

- Weight loss success is greater with the combination of exercise and diet management.

- Exercise improves glucose utilization by muscles.

- Exercise has a synergistic effect with insulin on glucose utilization.

- The effect of exercise on insulin/glucose utilization lasts 24 to 72 hours after exercise, depending on the duration and intensity of exercise.

- Exercise has demonstrated improvement in cardiovascular parameters that are important components for reducing risk for cardiovascular disease.

Box 14-6

RECOMMENDATIONS FOR THE ATHLETE REGARDING EXERCISE

- Be sure the intended exercise is suitable for your health status.

- Wear or carry medical identification to identify that you have diabetes.

- If just beginning an exercise program, gradually increase the intensity and duration.

- Learn how duration and intensity of exercise affect your blood glucose.

- Stay hydrated during exercise.

- Do not exercise if blood glucose is > 250 mg/dL and test for ketones is positive.

- Ingest carbohydrate prior to exercise if blood glucose is below predetermined level.

- Have carbohydrate available during exercise.

- Ingest carbohydrate as soon as you feel symptoms of hypoglycemia.

- Follow diet, insulin dosage, and exercise as planned with diabetes health care professional.

- Vary some aspect of exercise to avoid boredom.

- Exercise with someone to provide support.

- Set exercise goals and write them down.

- Do not neglect proper foot care as needed for your exercise.

---

exercise also provides improved glycemic control, and some patients may gain an additional advantage by combining aerobic and resistance exercise. The ADA recommends that individuals with type 2 diabetes do resistance training twice a week. Box 14-6 lists suggestions for the patient with diabetes regarding exercise.

Maintaining the effective balance of carbohydrate intake, exercise, and insulin dosage is very important. Hypoglycemia is a significant concern during, or even hours following, exercise in patients using insulin or insu-lin secretagogues (ie, drugs that increase the secretion of insulin, such as sulfonylureas and glinides). If the glucose level prior to exercise is < 100 mg/dL in these patients, they should ingest carbohydrate prior to exercise. For patients who are experiencing frequent episodes of hypoglycemia, the patient's diabetes management professional may recommend a change of diet or drug therapy to accommodate for planned exercise. Hypoglycemia, from planned or unplanned exercise, should be treated with 15 to 20 g of glucose-containing carbohydrate. Individuals with type 2

TABLE 14-2

SYMPTOMS OF HYPOGLYCEMIA

MILD	MODERATE	SEVERE	NOCTURNAL
Sweating	Mood changes	Poor responsiveness	Morning headache
Intense hunger	Headache	Unconscious	Nightmares
Inability to concentrate	Irritability	Coma	Lips/tongue tingling
Palpitations, tachycardia	Confusion		Profuse sweating
Tremor	Blurred vision		Restless sleep
Anxiety	Drowsiness		

diabetes and not taking insulin or insulin secretagogues rarely experience hypoglycemia, even during exercise.

Individuals with type 1 or type 2 diabetes can participate in athletic activities at all levels, from leisure activities to professional sport, as long as they have good glycemic control and do not have complications that preclude the activity. For patients who are taking insulin or an insulin secretagogue, monitoring for hypoglycemia must be a concern and is a part of the glycemic control plan. The knowledge, education, and experience of patients to provide self-care (SMBG, insulin adjustment, dietary adjustment, and awareness of hypoglycemia symptoms) will in part determine the extent of their athletic/exercise participation.

Patient Adherence

Adherence to the diabetes management program by patients is a major obstacle in reaching the glycemic goal, as well as other goals relative to the long-term complications of diabetes. Although tight glycemic control reduces both short- and long-term complications (and cost) of diabetes, and the advent of new antidiabetic drugs in the past several years has provided additional options for patients to reach their glycemic goals (A1C target, decreased postprandial hyperglycemia, fewer hypoglycemic episodes), more than half of patients fail to reach A1C <7%. Even fewer patients meet all of the other therapeutic goals. Lack of sufficiently aggressive prescribed therapy sometimes contributes to goals not being reached, but patient adherence with the pharmacotherapy, blood glucose monitoring, diet, and exercise regimens are major contributors. Patients must be educated regarding the connection between diabetic complications and maintaining their glycemic goals, the importance of each component of the diabetes management program in reaching the goals, and the proper procedures to appropriately monitoring blood glucose and adjust insulin. Consider the complexity of disease management for the patient who has to inject insulin a few times a day (and/or take oral antidiabetic drugs), monitor blood glucose

≥3 times a day, monitor carbohydrate and calorie intake with each meal, make adjustment in insulin dosage based on changes in diet or exercise, and be aware of signs and symptoms of hypoglycemia (Table 14-2). With this extent of complexity as part of the overall therapy for diabetes, it is not surprising that patient adherence with the diabetes management program is a challenge. Table 14-3 lists some common factors that are hindrances to patient adherence and some suggestions that may be helpful to support adherence. Athletic trainers can assist patients in achieving their goals by being cognizant of these factors and providing the needed encouragement to the patient.

Section Summary

Diabetes is a common chronic illness, type 2 being more common and occurring in over 90% of the patients with diabetes. The pancreas does not produce insulin in patients with type 1 diabetes, whereas in type 2 diabetes, insulin is produced but resistance to its effects at the target cells (liver, muscle, fat) and diminished production of insulin are major problems. Type 1 diabetes has an acute onset of an array of symptoms, including polyuria, polydipsia, polyphagia, and unexplained weight loss. A primary goal of treatment is to keep glycemic control as close to normal as possible to avoid the development of the long-term complications of the disease (eg, cardiovascular disease, retinopathy, neuropathy, amputations). For type 2 diabetes, hyperglycemia often begins years prior to diagnosis because there are no symptoms of the initial hyperglycemia. Consequently, some progression of the long-term complications may have begun prior to diagnosis. For both type 1 and type 2 diabetes, tight control of blood glucose, proper diet, and appropriate exercise can curb the progression of long-term complications. Hence, pharmacological treatment regimens, with monitoring of blood glucose and A1C, are aimed at accomplishing tight glycemic control.

TABLE 14-3
DIABETIC THERAPY ADHERENCE

HINDERING FACTORS	HELPFUL SUGGESTIONS
• Fear of requiring insulin injections may delay use of appropriate therapy • Lack of personal support system • Financial cost • Does not understand the disease, including need for glycemic control • Frequent doses of antidiabetic drugs • Too many different medications • Adverse effects from medications • Poor communication with diabetes management professional	• Encourage patient to ask questions • Reenforce the long-term advantage of good glycemic control • Suggest patient write down daily medication schedule to remember • Recommend patient keep written record of problems with therapy for discussion with diabetes management professional • Suggest exercise with team or friend as support mechanism

DRUG THERAPY FOR TYPE 1 DIABETES MELLITUS

Because people with type 1 diabetes do not make insulin, treatment must include insulin, although diet, exercise, and SMBG are also necessary components to good glycemic control. The pancreas of cows and pigs was the source of insulin until 1982, when the US Food and Drug Administration (FDA) approved human insulin made by recombinant DNA (rDNA) technology. This technology uses bacteria, yeast, or mammalian cells to synthesize human insulin and modifications of it; consequently, the production and use of pork and beef insulin has been phased out. The focus of this section is the use of insulin to obtain appropriate glycemic control in patients with type 1 diabetes.

Insulin Preparations

The most important clinical differences among insulin products are their onset and duration of action. Insulin preparations can be grouped into 4 categories: rapid acting, short acting, intermediate acting, and long acting. Rapid-acting has the fastest onset and shortest duration of action; long-acting has the slowest onset and longest duration of action (Table 14-4).

Regular insulin is unmodified insulin. This is a clear and colorless aqueous solution that can be used intravenously. Regular insulin forms aggregates of insulin molecules after subcutaneous injection, slowing the onset of action somewhat (0.5 to 1 hour) and providing a duration of 5 to 8 hours (short acting).

Rapid-acting preparations include insulin glulisine, insulin lispro, and insulin aspart (see Table 14-4). These have a slightly different structure than regular human insulin (ie, modified human insulin), which is often reflected in the generic name. For example, lispro insulin has 2 amino acids switched around (lysine and proline), whereas aspart insulin has aspartic acid in place of one proline. These forms of modified human insulin decrease the ability of the insulin molecules to form aggregates and thus increase their solubility after subcutaneous injection, making them rapid acting (15-minute onset). Like regular insulin, these are all clear, colorless solutions and are the only other (besides regular) insulin that can be used intravenously.

NPH (neutral protamine Hagedorn) insulin is intermediate acting and is prepared by forming a complex between a protein (protamine) and regular insulin. The protein bound to insulin decreases the solubility of the molecule so the insulin has a slower onset and longer duration than regular insulin of 1 to 2 and 18 to 24 hours, respectively.

Recall from Chapter 2 that increased rate of solubility and blood flow will increase the rate of absorption from subcutaneous injection sites.

Insulin glargine and detemir are long-acting insulins. Insulin glargine is a chemical modification of human insulin involving glycine and arginine components (amino acids). These structural changes increase the ability of insulin molecules to form aggregates, thus prolonging the time to be absorbed. For detemir, a fatty acid is added to one of the amino acids in the insulin structure, allowing it to bind to protein at the injection site, thus delaying absorption.

TABLE 14-4					
EXAMPLES OF INSULIN PREPARATIONS[a]					
GENERIC NAME	TRADE NAME	TYPE	ONSET[b] (HR)	PEAK[b] (HR)	DURATION[b] (HR)
lispro	Humalog	Rapid acting	0.25 to 0.5	0.5 to 1.5	3 to 5
aspart	NovoLog	Rapid acting	0.25	1 to 2	3 to 5
glulisine	Apidra	Rapid acting	0.25	0.5 to 1.5	4 to 6
regular	Humulin R	Short acting	0.5 to 1	2 to 4	5 to 8
	Novolin R	Short acting	0.5 to 1	2 to 4	5 to 8
NPH	Humulin N	Intermediate acting	1 to 2	6 to 14	18 to 24
	Novolin N	Intermediate acting	1 to 2	6 to 14	18 to 24
glargine	Lantus	Long acting	1 to 2	None	18 to 24
detemir	Levemir	Long acting	1 to 2	Relatively flat	12 to 24
[a]All are human insulin or modified human insulin derived from rDNA technology.					
[b]Site of injection, blood flow to the site, and dose of insulin will affect values.					

Absorption rate after subcutaneous injection of insulin glargine or detemir is fairly constant, and thus they do not have the same peak effect of other insulin preparations. The relatively flat absorption profile poses an advantage in that both insulin glargine and detemir have demonstrated fewer hypoglycemic episodes compared with NPH insulin.

In general, the rapid-acting and short-acting insulins are used at mealtime to handle the postprandial increase in blood glucose concentration. Injecting a dose of insulin aspart 10 minutes prior to breakfast is the bolus component of insulin therapy. Using 1 or 2 injections of intermediate- or long-acting insulin is considered the basal component. Balancing the right combination of bolus and basal insulin injections, along with the individual patient's diet and exercise routines, to achieve tight glycemic control with minimal hypoglycemic episodes is a significant challenge for the patient and the patient's diabetes management professionals.

> *A bolus therapy of insulin is given as one dose and is intended to provide the impact of the dose as soon as possible to reduce the spike in blood glucose that would otherwise occur soon after a meal. Basal therapy is one or more dosage units that are intended to keep the blood glucose within the desired level for the longer time between meals. The purpose of the basal-bolus therapy is to more closely mimic the normal pattern of insulin release by the pancreas.*

Caution is necessary when mixing different insulin preparations in the same syringe because some combinations are incompatible with each other due to differences in pH or various other components (eg, protamine). The procedure for mixing also requires a specific order and process by which insulin is properly drawn into the syringe. The objective in mixing insulins is to reduce the number of daily injections needed to obtain the desired basal-bolus insulin therapy. There are stable mixtures of several insulin combinations commercially available, such as NPH:regular at 50:50, lispro protamine:lispro at 75:25, and aspart protamine:aspart at 70:30.

Insulin Administration

Because insulin is a polypeptide, it cannot be given orally because the digestive system would break it into the amino acid components. Insulin lispro, aspart, and glulisine (rapid acting), regular (short acting), and insulin detemir and glargine (long acting) are clear solutions. NPH insulin is a suspension. The solutions are clear and colorless, whereas the suspensions are cloudy and have particles (Figure 14-3). If there are any particles or color associated with the solutions, they should be discarded. The most common concentration available is 100 units of insulin per mL, designated 100 U. Also available is 500 U for patients requiring high doses of insulin. Syringes are marked in units and are produced in sizes that will hold up to 30, 50, and 100 units (0.3, 0.5, 1.0 mL). Box 14-7 lists a few points to remember regarding insulin.

Insulin is stable at room temperature for about 1 month. Consequently, insulin vials that are in current use can remain at room temperature; others should be refrigerated. Suspensions must be evenly dispersed prior to each use to ensure a more consistent dose, but because insulin is a protein, foaming will result if the suspension is shaken. To evenly disperse the particles in the suspension, the vial

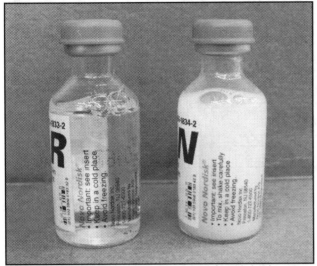

Figure 14-3. Clear solution of regular insulin (left) and cloudy suspension of NPH insulin (right).

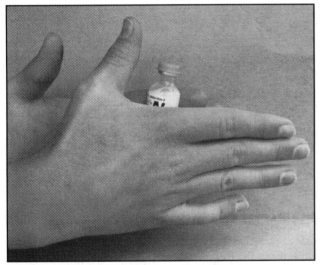

Figure 14-4. Dispersing insulin evenly in the vial by gently rolling it between the hands.

should be gently rolled between the palms of the hands (Figure 14-4).

Rotating the injection site is important for both comfort and consistent absorption. The arms, thighs, abdomen, and buttocks are the typical sites of injection. Rate of absorption varies among these sites and thus patients are advised to use the same general anatomic site but placing the injections about 1 inch apart. The abdomen provides the most consistent absorption, least affected by exercise, and thus it is the recommended site for all injections. Alternatively, diabetic patients who must give themselves multiple injections per day may be advised to consistently use the same anatomic site for each time of the day but to rotate anatomic sites throughout the day, so that, for example, the first injection of the day is always in the abdomen and the second injection of the day is always in the thigh.

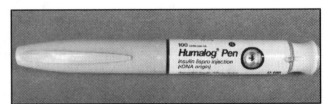

Figure 14-5. An example of an insulin pen; the insulin and needle are self-contained.

Insulin pens (Figure 14-5) are available as an alternative to a vial of insulin and syringe. The insulin pen is a device that has a pen-like shape and size but contains a cartridge of insulin. Various types of insulin and insulin combinations are available as insulin pens. There are disposable (one-time use) pens as well as reusable pens that can be refilled with new cartridges and fresh needles. Prior to administering the insulin, the patient can adjust the amount of insulin through a dial on the pen. Insulin pens provide a more convenient means of carrying and administering insulin.

The technology for insulin pumps has improved to make them increasingly popular (Figure 14-6). These contain a battery-operated pump controlled by computer technology to deliver the insulin from a reservoir of insulin. External pumps require thin tubing that connects the pump to the subcutaneous administration site (Figure 14-7). The pump reservoir is filled every few days with the appropriate insulin (Figure 14-8). Internal pumps are also available and are implanted just under the skin and contain a reservoir of insulin that lasts for months. Insulin pumps deliver a small basal rate of insulin throughout the day to maintain a more constant level of blood glucose, but the patient can give a bolus dose of insulin as needed, just prior to a meal, for example. The pump can be reprogrammed to change the delivery of insulin as needed. There are also blood glucose-monitoring devices that have been developed

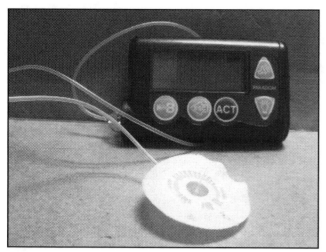

Figure 14-6. Insulin pump with tubing and adhesive patch to secure cannula.

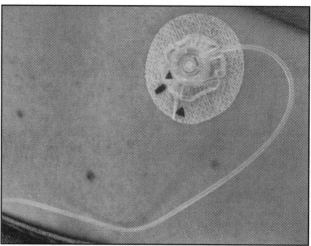

Figure 14-7. Infusion set held in place with adhesive patch.

to communicate with the insulin pump for more closely controlled release of insulin.

Adverse Effects

Although insulin is a protein that has normal physiologic functions, administration of insulin as a medication does have adverse effects. These adverse effects include hypoglycemia, weight gain, immune responses, and lipohypertrophy, which are addressed here.

Hypoglycemia

Hypoglycemia (blood glucose < 70 mg/dL) is of major concern because it limits the patient's activity during that time, and, if severe enough, it can cause coma and death. Hypoglycemia occurs when there is too much insulin relative to the amount of glucose in the blood. The cause of hypoglycemia may be a calculation error regarding the amount of insulin needed, a measurement error of the desired insulin, or a significant unplanned change in diet or exercise. Other reasons for a change in the insulin required are pregnancy, illness such as infection, or surgery. If occurrences of hypoglycemia are too frequent, adjustments in insulin therapy or diet/exercise are necessary.

Symptoms of hypoglycemia are shown in Table 14-2. These symptoms may begin as the blood glucose concentration drops below 60 mg/dL; the number of symptoms and severity increases as the glucose continues to drop. There are automatic counterregulatory mechanisms to prevent the hypoglycemia from continuing, such as the release of glucagon and epinephrine, which signal the liver to add glucose to the blood. Another effect of epinephrine is to cause some of the early symptoms of hypoglycemia (particularly the tremor, palpitations, and tachycardia). However, the longer the person has diabetes, the greater the likelihood that the release of glucagon diminishes, and subsequently in some patients also a reduced epi-

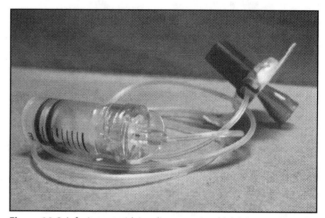

Figure 14-8. Infusion set with insulin reservoir, which is inserted into the pump, tubing, adhesive patch, and cannula (the protective material is removed from the cannula prior to insertion under the skin).

nephrine response. These patients may have hypoglycemia unawareness (ie, no symptoms). Loss of the early warning signs of hypoglycemia makes it even more imperative that patients with hypoglycemia unawareness measure blood glucose routinely and whenever hypoglycemia is suspected. Some patients experience nocturnal hypoglycemia and may awake with some of the symptoms. Repeated hypoglycemic episodes require reevaluation of the diabetes management program.

Steps to treat hypoglycemia should be taken as soon as symptoms appear. Oral administration of 15 to 20 g of any glucose-containing carbohydrate is the recommended treatment. Patients with moderate hypoglycemia may require assistance; severe hypoglycemia is a medical emergency. For mild to moderate hypoglycemia, the treatment with carbohydrate should be repeated if the effect of treatment is not apparent in 10 to 20 minutes or if SMBG is not > 60 mg/dL in 15 minutes. The use of 10 g of glucose will increase blood glucose by approximately 40 mg/dL over

	TABLE 14-5		
DRUGS THAT MAY ALTER BLOOD GLUCOSE			
CATEGORY	**GENERIC NAME**	**BRAND NAME**	**EFFECT ON GLUCOSE**
β-blockers[a]	propranolol	Inderal	Hypoglycemia; ↓ glucose release from liver
Corticosteroids	prednisone	generic	Hyperglycemia; ↑ glucose release from liver
β-agonists	albuterol	Proventil	Hyperglycemia; ↑ glucose release from liver
Nasal decongestants	pseudoephedrine	many OTC	Hyperglycemia; ↑ glucose release from liver
Thiazide diuretics	hydrochlorothiazide	Hydrodiuril	Hyperglycemia; ↓ insulin effect and release from pancreas
Alcohol	alcohol	Many	Hypoglycemia; ↓ glucose release from liver
[a]Also masks some symptoms of hypoglycemia and may delay recovery from hypoglycemia.			

30 minutes. Examples of carbohydrate containing 10 g of carbohydrate include 2 teaspoons of sugar, one-half cup of orange juice, one-third of a can of soda (nondiet), or 6 Life Savers (Wm. Wrigley Jr. Company). Patients using insulin or insulin secretagogues should consider having a source of carbohydrate always readily available. Patients who are unconscious will require parenteral glucose or glucagon.

Weight Gain

The use of insulin typically is accompanied by weight gain. This can be minimized through the diet and exercise components of therapy.

Immune Responses

Allergic reactions to insulin are rare now that pork and beef sources of insulin are not being used. Symptoms of allergic reactions range from skin rashes to difficulty breathing.

Lipoatrophy is a depression in the skin at the site of injection due to loss of fat at that site and is likely an immune-based response caused by impurities in the insulin preparation. With the highly purified insulins now used, lipoatrophy is not very common.

Lipohypertrophy

Repeatedly injecting insulin at the same site (ie, not rotating injection sites) can cause lipohypertrophy. This is a lumpy area under the skin due to increased fat deposits from the fat synthesis characteristic of insulin. Insulin absorption from an area of lipohypertrophy is unpredictable so those sites should not be used for insulin injections. Lipohypertrophy can be remedied by rotating injection sites.

Drug Interactions

Drugs that can affect the release of glucose (either increase or decrease) should be used with caution in patients with either type 1 or type 2 diabetes. The change in blood glucose caused by these drugs (Table 14-5) may be significant enough to warrant a change in the diabetes management program, especially if the tightly controlled glycemia is disrupted enough by the drug interaction to cause hypoglycemia.

Nonselective β-blockers pose a special potential problem for people with diabetes. As discussed in Chapter 12, these drugs block the effects of epinephrine. Among the effects of nonselective β-blockers (see Box 12-5) is that they inhibit the production and release of glucose into the blood from the liver (ie, inhibit gluconeogenesis and glycogenolysis). This is one of the automatic counterregulatory measures that help curb hypoglycemia. Additionally, some of the early symptoms of hypoglycemia (eg, tremor, palpitations, and tachycardia) are initiated by the autonomic nervous system effects of epinephrine. The consequences for some diabetic patients is that β-blockers may increase the occurrence of hypoglycemic episodes, delay the recovery from these episodes, and require the patient to be more cognizant of the symptoms of hypoglycemia that are not mediated through β-adrenergic receptors (eg, sweating, inability to concentrate). Consequently, β-blockers should be used with caution in diabetic patients. Alcohol used in moderate to high doses also can disrupt glycemic control by inhibiting gluconeogenesis, again posing a threat of hypoglycemia.

Corticosteroids such as hydrocortisone to treat inflammation (see Chapter 6) and prednisone to treat asthma (see Chapter 9) increase gluconeogenesis and thus may cause hyperglycemia in diabetic patients (see Boxes 6-1 and 6-2). Drugs that enhance the sympathetic nervous system responses also have the potential to increase blood glucose through their β-adrenergic agonist activity. Albuterol, used to treat asthma (see Chapter 9), has β-adrenergic activity, and pseudoephedrine, a nasal decongestant (see Chapter 10) used for its α-adrenergic activity, has some β-adrenergic activity. Thiazide diuretics (see Chapter 12) have the potential to cause hyperglycemia by inhibiting the effect of insulin and reducing insulin secretion. All of these drugs have the potential to disrupt glycemic control, and thus adjustments in insulin may be necessary if they are added or removed from therapy.

Amylin-Like Compounds

Pramlintide (Symlin) is a synthetic peptide that is similar in chemical structure to the hormone amylin, which is secreted by the β-cells of the pancreas. Pramlintide (also called an *amylin receptor agonist*) combines with the amylin receptor to mimic the effects of amylin: reduce appetite, slow the absorption of food, and inhibit the release of glucagon from the β-cells of the pancreas. Postprandial blood glucose is thereby reduced by 2 mechanisms: delaying absorption of carbohydrate and reducing the glycemic effects of glucagon on the liver. The approved indication for pramlintide is to accompany the mealtime use of insulin, thus curbing the postprandial glucose elevation in either type 1 or type 2 diabetes. It is injected subcutaneously prior to meals. To prevent hypoglycemia when used with insulin, the manufacturer recommends that the bolus dose of the rapid- or short-acting insulin prior to the meal be reduced by 50% and blood glucose levels be monitored closely. The most common adverse effect is nausea, ranging from mild to severe, although this can be minimized by starting at a lower dose and gradually increasing to the desired dose. Because pramlintide decreases GI motility, it may have a significant impact on the effectiveness of some other drugs (eg, analgesics, antibiotics) if they are administered within 1 hour before or 2 hours after pramlintide.

Section Summary

Treatment of type 1 diabetes with insulin is a requirement for these patients. Insulin is most commonly administered subcutaneously. Multiple injections are often needed to maintain tight glycemic control, although insulin pumps also provide an option for some patients. The advent of rDNA technology has generated several insulin alternatives in addition to regular human insulin and has replaced the use of insulin extracted from cow and pig pancreas. The new insulin products are more highly purified and result in fewer allergic reactions and adverse effects at the site of injection. Insulin preparations are grouped into categories based on their onset and duration of action: rapid, short, intermediate, and long. A combination of types of insulin is useful to achieve optimum glycemic control: rapid and short acting to achieve control at mealtime and intermediate and long acting for basal-level control. Hypoglycemia is of major concern when treating with insulin. It is important for diabetic patients to be cognizant of the symptoms of hypoglycemia, such as tremor, sweating, and tachycardia, and to have a source of carbohydrate readily available at the onset of these symptoms. Some drugs may also pose a problem to the person with type 1 diabetes to maintain the desired glycemic control; these include corticosteroids,

β-blockers, β-agonists, and alcohol. It is noteworthy that β-blockers also mask the early symptoms of hypoglycemia besides inhibiting the counterregulatory effects of epinephrine that may otherwise aid in the recovery from hypoglycemia.

DRUG THERAPY FOR TYPE 2 DIABETES MELLITUS

The foundation of treatment for type 2 diabetes is diet and exercise, with appropriate drug therapy added as soon as necessary to achieve the glycemic goals. Initial treatment may be limited to diet and exercise if it is reasonable that the glycemic goals can be achieved. In other cases, aggressive drug therapy is warranted at the outset. Considering that most patients have had hyperglycemia for years prior to diagnosis, it is important that initial treatment be sufficiently aggressive with antidiabetic drug therapy to achieve A1C <7% as quickly as possible. As the disease progresses, insulin resistance and β-cell failure become worse, necessitating the increase in dosage of the drug therapy or adding another drug to the therapy that acts by a different mechanism. There are several categories of antidiabetic drugs used to treat type 2 diabetes that act by different mechanisms (Table 14-6). Use of any other drug that affects glucose metabolism (see Table 14-5) can disrupt glycemic control being achieved from the oral antidiabetic agents.

Oral Antidiabetic Drugs

Oral antidiabetic agents are only used to treat type 2 diabetes, not type 1. This group of drugs used to be called *oral hypoglycemic drugs*, but with the introduction of several new drugs, not all of the orally effective drugs cause hypoglycemia. Typically, if one drug in a category is not effective for a patient, the other drugs in that category will not be either. Selection of the appropriate drug will be dependent upon the level of glycemic control, other medications the patient is taking, and existence of other conditions (eg, heart, kidney, and liver function). Compared with insulin therapy for patients with type 1 diabetes, the risk for hypoglycemia is less with oral antidiabetic drugs, principally those that increase insulin release (eg, sulfonylureas, glinides). Hypoglycemia unawareness rarely exists. Nonetheless, changes in daily routine, such as the addition of strenuous exercise or missing a meal, may precipitate hypoglycemia.

Sulfonylureas

The sulfonylureas, such as tolbutamide (Orinase) and glipizide (Glucotrol), exert their effect by increasing the release of insulin from the pancreas and thus are among the drugs referred to as *insulin secretagogues*. These are the

	TABLE 14-6		
DRUGS FOR TREATING TYPE 2 DIABETES			
CATEGORY	**GENERIC NAME**	**BRAND NAME**	**CHARACTERISTICS OF CATEGORY**
Sulfonylureas	tolbutamide tolazamide chlorpropamide glyburide glipizide glimepiride	Orinase Tolinase Diabenese DiaBeta Glucotrol Amaryl	Oral; ↑ release of insulin; potential hypoglycemia; weight gain
Glinides	repaglinide nateglinide	Prandin Starlix	Oral; ↑ release of insulin; potential hypoglycemia; control postprandial hyperglycemia
Biguanides	metformin	Glucophage	Oral; ↓ release of glucose from liver; may ↑ glucose use by muscles; GI adverse effects; weight loss; lactic acidosis caution
Glitazones	rosiglitazone pioglitazone	Avandia Actos	Oral; reduces insulin resistance (insulin sensitizer); edema, weight gain; liver function and heart failure caution; increased risk of myocardial infarction and sudden cardiac death with rosiglitazone
α-glucosidase inhibitors	acarbose miglitol	Prelose Glyset	Oral; ↓ absorption of glucose from small intestine; controls postprandial hyperglycemia; abdominal adverse effects
DPP-4 inhibitors	sitagliptin saxagliptin linagliptin alogliptin	Januvia Onglyza Tradjenta Nesina	Oral; ↑ effect of incretins to ↑ insulin and ↓ glucagon; may preserve β-cell function; controls postprandial hyperglycemia
SGLT inhibitors	canagliflozin dapagliflozin empagliflozin	Invokana Farxiga Jardiance	Oral; ↓ reabsorption of glucose by the kidneys; may increase risk of certain infections
Incretin-like drugs	exenatide liraglutide albiglutide	Byetta Victoza Tanzeum	Injected sc; ↑ effect of incretins to ↑ insulin and ↓ glucagon; may preserve β-cell function; controls postprandial hyperglycemia; weight loss; GI adverse effects
Amylin-like drugs	pramlintide	Symlin	Injected sc; mimics amylin effects to ↓ glucagon, slow glucose absorption, and reduce appetite; controls postprandial hyperglycemia; weight loss; nausea
Insulin	Many	See Table 14-1	Injected sc; hypoglycemia potential; weight gain
sc = subcutaneously.			

oldest group of oral drugs to treat type 2 diabetes, but some are newer than others and are sometimes subcategorized as first- and second-generation sulfonylureas to differentiate the newer from older drugs. The major pharmacological differences between the first- and second-generation sulfonylureas are the potency (and thus dose) and duration of action. Therapeutically, the potency is of little consequence because they are all equally effective at equipotent doses. Because of their longer duration of action, the second-generation sulfonylureas can be used with once-daily dosing, whereas the dosing of first-generation drugs is 1 to 3 doses per day. The exception is chlorpropamide (Diabenese), which is a first-generation drug but has the longest duration and is used once per day. The liver and kidney are the tissues for metabolism and excretion of these drugs. Dosage adjustments may be necessary in patients with compromised liver or kidney function, which is common among elderly patients. Chlorpropamide is of particular concern because it has the longest duration of action and thus has the greatest potential for accumulation in patients with compromised kidney function.

In addition to the drugs listed in Table 14-5, disruption of glycemic control can occur due to drug interactions with sulfonylureas if they are used concurrently with aspirin, phenylbutazone (nonsteroidal anti-inflammatory drug), fluconazole (antifungal drugs), sulfonamide antibiotics (antibacterial drugs), and cimetidine (inhibits production of acid in the stomach). These drugs alter the pharmacokinetic or pharmacodynamic properties of sulfonylureas or affect insulin release from the pancreas directly. Use of alcohol with sulfonylureas has produced upper body flushing for up to several hours after alcohol consumption in some people, chlorpropamide having the highest incidence. Hypoglycemia is the adverse effect of major concern, and therefore close monitoring should occur in patients who are taking other drugs that can increase the hypoglycemic effects or who have coexisting conditions that affect liver or kidney function. Weight gain is also a common adverse effect with sulfonylureas.

Glinides (Meglitinides)

Repaglinide (Prandin) and nateglinide (Starlix) are glinides that, like sulfonylureas, stimulate the pancreas to release insulin but by binding to a different receptor in the pancreas. Because they stimulate insulin release, the glinides are also grouped with sulfonylureas as secretagogues or sometimes differentiated as short-acting secretagogues. Because insulin release is increased, weight gain can occur with the use of these drugs. In contrast to sulfonylureas, the glinides have a much shorter onset and duration of action, with the t½ being approximately 1 hour. These drugs are given immediately prior to meals to control postprandial blood glucose levels. Hypoglycemia is a concern, although the incidence is minimized if the patient eats within 30 minutes of taking the dose.

Biguanides

Metformin (Glucophage) is the only biguanide currently available in the United States and is considered the drug of choice for most type 2 diabetic patients. The primary antidiabetic mechanism of this drug is to reduce the release of glucose by the liver, likely by inhibiting gluconeogenesis, and, to a lesser extent, it increases glucose utilization by muscles. It is excreted unchanged in the urine. Compared with the sulfonylureas, metformin is much less likely to cause hypoglycemia. Adverse effects are nausea, diarrhea, vomiting, metallic taste, and anorexia; the latter may result in weight loss. A rare but potentially fatal adverse effect is lactic acidosis arising from the ability of metformin to inhibit the use of lactic acid for gluconeogenesis. Part of this concern regarding

lactic acidosis exists because another drug in this category (phenformin) was removed from the market because of the high incidence of lactic acidosis. Consequently, patients with impaired liver or kidney function or conditions that may contribute to lactic acid production (eg, chronic hypoxic respiratory disease, heart failure) should not take metformin. Besides the effects of alcohol on glucose metabolism (see Table 14-5), heavy alcohol consumption will potentiate the effect of metformin on lactic acid metabolism. Cimetidine (Tagamet), used to treat heartburn, gastroesophageal reflux disease, and peptic ulcer disease (see Table 11-2), can increase metformin blood levels by inhibiting the renal excretion, which may necessitate a reduction in the metformin dose.

Glitazones (Thiazolidinediones)

This group of drugs is also called the *thiazolidinediones* and includes rosiglitazone (Avandia) and pioglitazone (Actos). The glitazones cause fat and muscle to be more responsive to insulin (reduces insulin resistance) and are therefore sometimes called *insulin sensitizers*. When administered with insulin, the dose of insulin is reduced. Because insulin must be present for the glitazones to be effective, there is no risk for hypoglycemia directly from the glitazones. One disadvantage of the glitazones is that they take 2 to 3 months for their maximum activity to be realized, whereas other antidiabetic drugs can be evaluated and adjusted (titrated) within a couple weeks or less. Glitazones can be used alone or in combination with insulin or other antidiabetic drugs. Fixed-dose combinations are available such as pioglitazone with metformin (Actoplus).

Liver function should be monitored when glitazones are used, primarily because another drug in this category (troglitazone) was removed from the market due to liver toxicity. The most concerning adverse effects associated with the glitazones involve the cardiovascular system. Edema and weight gain can occur as adverse effects. Glitazones can cause or exacerbate congestive heart failure in some patients, so patients should be monitored closely for symptoms of heart failure, such as edema and weight gain. These drugs are contraindicated in patients with New York Heart Association Functional Classification III or IV heart failure (see Table 12-5). Rosiglitazone can increase the risk of myocardial infarction, angina, and sudden cardiac death. Consequently, patients must be assessed for known risk factors of myocardial ischemia. There is also an increased risk for fractures, particularly in women, with use of glitazones. Considering the potential for these significant adverse effects, the glitazones have become less favorable options for treatment of type 2 diabetes.

α-Glucosidase Inhibitors

The mechanism of action for the α-glucosidase inhibitors, acarbose (Precose) and miglitol (Glyset), is that they prevent the conversion of carbohydrates (sucrose and starches) in the small intestine. Because carbohydrates need to be converted to their monomer units (primarily glucose, galactose, and fructose) for absorption, the α-glucosidase inhibitors decrease the amount of glucose absorbed. These drugs are used to control postprandial hyperglycemia and are taken immediately at the beginning of the meal. Systemic adverse effects are minimal because the majority of the drug is not absorbed. The unabsorbed carbohydrate proceeds to the large intestine and provides nutrient for the resident bacteria. Consequently, the most common adverse effects of the α-glucosidase inhibitors are flatulence, diarrhea, and abdominal cramps. Hypoglycemia and weight gain are not adverse effects from the α-glucosidase inhibitors. If hypoglycemia occurs because of insulin or other antidiabetic therapy while using α-glucosidase inhibitors, products containing specifically glucose or lactose (milk) can be used to remedy the hypoglycemia, but not sucrose (table sugar) or other carbohydrates.

DPP-4 Inhibitors (Gliptins)

The DPP-4 inhibitors are incretin based in their mechanism of action. DPP-4 is the enzyme that inactivates the incretin hormones. Inhibitors of DPP-4 (also called *gliptins* or *incretin enhancers*) increase the t½ of the incretins and prolong their activity. Currently, there are 4 FDA-approved DPP-4 inhibitors: sitagliptin (Januvia), saxagliptin (Onglyza), linagliptin (Tradjenta), and alogliptin (Nesina). Not surprisingly, the DPP-4 inhibitors have effects similar to the incretin hormones: they stimulate insulin secretion, inhibit glucagon release, reduce postprandial glucose, and possibly preserve β-cell function. These effects translate therapeutically into lower postprandial hyperglycemia and A1C values. Body weight is not affected, but DPP-4 inhibitors help to stabilize weight when used in combination with other antidiabetic drugs that cause weight gain (eg, sulfonylureas) or weight loss (eg, metformin). A significant advantage over the incretin-like compounds is that the DPP-4 inhibitors are orally effective and have fewer significant adverse effects; GI adverse effects are not common. The incidence of hypoglycemia is very low.

Sodium-Glucose–Linked Transporter Inhibitors

The sodium-glucose–linked transporter (SGLT) inhibitors are a new class of oral antidiabetic agents, and 3 of these agents have been approved: canagliflozin (Invokana), dapagliflozin (Farxiga), and empagliflozin (Jardiance). SGLT is a protein that transports sodium and glucose and is responsible for the reabsorption of glucose in the urine that has been filtered by the kidneys. By inhibiting this transport, the amount of glucose in the urine increases and the plasma glucose decreases. Because these drugs rely in the urinary excretion of glucose, they should not be used in patients with poor renal function. Hypoglycemia is a possible adverse effect, especially when combined with insulin or other agents that cause hypoglycemia. An interesting adverse effect of the SGLT inhibitors is that they increase the risk of certain infections, particularly urinary tract infections and vaginal fungal infections. There have also been concerns about cardiovascular-related adverse effects, including increased low-density lipoprotein cholesterol and low blood pressure.

Other Oral Antidiabetic Agents

Two medications that have traditionally been used in the treatment of other conditions have also received approval for treatment of type 2 diabetes. Bromocriptine (Cycloset) has traditionally been used in the treatment of Parkinson disease and related conditions. It has recently been approved for type 2 diabetes. The mechanism of action of the antidiabetic effect is unknown. Colesevelam (Welchol) has been used to treat high cholesterol and is now approved for type 2 diabetes. The mechanism of the antidiabetic action of this agent is also unclear.

Incretin-Like Compounds (Incretin Mimetics, GLP-1 Analogs)

These compounds, like the DPP-4 inhibitors, are incretin-based in their mechanism. The incretin-like compounds (also called *incretin mimetics*) mimic the effects of the incretins, which are a group of GI hormones produced by the intestinal cells and released into the blood in response to food absorption. One specific incretin compound is glucagon-like peptide-1 (GLP-1); drugs that are a slight modification of GLP-1 are GLP-1 analogs. The incretins have a short t½ (approximately 2 to 7 minutes) and therefore are not used therapeutically; the incretin-like compounds have a longer t½.

Exenatide (Byetta) was the first incretin-like compound (GLP-1 analog) approved for therapeutic use, but 2 others have since been approved. Exenatide reduces postprandial hyperglycemia and A1C and may cause weight loss. Like DPP-4 inhibitors, exenatide may preserve β-cell function. Exenatide is a peptide and thus is not effective orally; it is injected subcutaneously twice per day using a pen injector. Liraglutide (Victoza) is administered once daily by subcutaneous injection, whereas albiglutide (Tanzeum) only has to be administered once a week.

Hypoglycemia is an adverse effect associated with the incretin mimetics, especially if used with another antidiabetic drug that causes hypoglycemia (eg, sulfonylureas). These agents reduce gastric emptying and therefore may slow the absorption of other medications, causing drug interactions. The most common adverse effects are nausea, vomiting, and diarrhea. Pancreatitis has been reported in a small percentage of patients. Among these patients with pancreatitis, most had at least one other risk factor for acute pancreatitis (eg, gallstones, alcohol use). All patients using incretin mimetics should be advised to seek medical care if they experience abdominal pain.

Pramlintide

Pramlintide (Symlin) is an amylin-like drug that is used to treat either type 1 or type 2 diabetes and was discussed previously. Pramlintide is injected before meals to control postprandial hyperglycemia. Nausea is the most common adverse effect.

Insulin

Insulin is also used to treat type 1 diabetes, and specific examples of available formulations were discussed previously. When insulin is used for treatment of type 2 diabetes, it can be used alone or added to oral antidiabetic drug therapy when oral therapy alone is not sufficiently effective to achieve glycemic goals. Short- or rapid-acting insulin is frequently used as bolus therapy prior to meals to control postprandial hyperglycemia and as an oral antidiabetic drug for basal therapy. As β-cell function diminishes with disease progression, the use of insulin becomes necessary. In addition, it may be in the best interest for some individuals with type 2 diabetes to be managed with insulin earlier rather than later in the disease progression, both for optimal glycemic control and to allay the progression of long-term complications.

Section Summary

Type 2 diabetes is treated with diet, exercise, and one or more of an array of drug treatment options. Most patients have already been hyperglycemic for years prior to diagnosis, so it is important to get the hyperglycemia under control quickly. An A1C < 7% is a typical target goal, but the level of postprandial glycemia, the number of hypoglycemic episodes, and fasting blood glucose are also useful indicators of glycemic control. Also important are the proper monitoring and treatment of the long-term complications. As type 2 diabetes progresses, β-cell function typically diminishes as insulin resistance increases, necessitating an increase in the dosage of the antidiabetic drug(s) and/or addition of one or more other antidiabetic drugs with a different mechanism of action. Failure to reach glycemic goals is a common problem in the treatment of type 2 diabetes, and nonadherence with therapy is a major cause. Adequate patient education related to the disease and good communication between patient and health care professionals, including the athletic trainer, can improve adherence.

There are several drugs used to treat type 2 diabetes:

- The sulfonylureas and glinides increase insulin secretion and may cause weight gain and hypoglycemia.
- Metformin reduces glucose production by the liver but does not cause hypoglycemia or weight gain.
- Glitazones are insulin sensitizers that improve the cellular effectiveness of insulin and do not cause hypoglycemia or weight changes when given alone.
- The α-glucosidase inhibitors act in the small intestine to inhibit absorption of glucose and are useful to minimize postprandial hyperglycemia.
- DPP-4 inhibitors cause a decrease of glucagon release and increase of insulin release, stabilize weight, and may preserve β-cell function.
- The SGLT inhibitors increase glucose excretion in the urine and lower plasma glucose.
- The incretin mimetics have an incretin-based mechanism so their activity and uses are similar to the DPP-4 inhibitors, but they must be injected subcutaneously.
- Pramlintide is an amylin receptor agonist that reduces glucagon release, GI motility, and appetite but must be injected subcutaneously.
- Insulin is available as many preparations of short, intermediate, and long durations of action and is an important option for treatment of type 2 diabetes.

ROLE OF THE ATHLETIC TRAINER

Appropriate treatment of diabetes is complex, and, in addition to proper drug selection and administration, treatment requires routine monitoring of blood glucose, diet, and exercise. Several factors regarding diabetes and management of the disease offer opportunities for the athletic trainer to play a significant role in improving diabetes care. Nearly one-third of people with diabetes have not been diagnosed, most people with diabetes do not reach their treatment goals, many diabetic patients do not properly monitor or treat their diabetes as prescribed, and exercise is a component of therapy for nearly all patients. For the athletic trainer to take advantage of opportunities to improve diabetes care, he or she should do the following:

- Know and be able to recognize the symptoms of uncontrolled diabetes
- Understand and be able to explain to a diabetic patient the important connection between tight glycemic control and the short- and long-term complications of diabetes
- Be willing to be supportive and be a source of encouragement to a diabetic patient who may be struggling with the daily complexity of achieving and maintaining glycemic control
- Know which athletes have diabetes and recommend that they have a medical alert identification (Figure 14-9)
- Be able to recognize the symptoms of hypoglycemia and have a source of carbohydrate available for athletes who become hypoglycemic

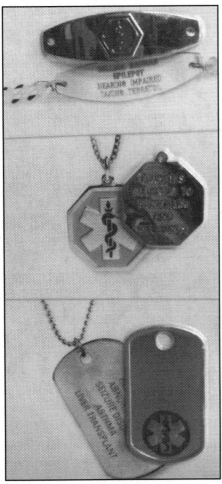

Figure 14-9. Examples of medial alert identification (front and back view of each style).

- Promote diabetes education by encouraging communication with patients by being willing to answer or find the answers to questions that patients have regarding diabetes
- Encourage diabetic patients to have regular medical exams to monitor for early signs of long-term complications
- Provide education and assistance regarding appropriate foot care and encourage the patient to have a comprehensive foot exam at least once per year

CASE STUDY

The girls' lacrosse team you are covering is into its third overtime. You know that Cate, the team's center, has played the entire game and continues as the game is about to go into its fourth overtime. You also know that she has had type 1 diabetes since she was 4 years old. She takes very good care of herself (eg, controls her diabetes with her insulin pump, eats a healthy diet, uses regular glucose testing), so she is usually not a concern for you. However, you notice that Cate has not been attentive to the game during the past several minutes, missing several passes. She is also stumbling and is not her normally coordinated self. During the break between the third and fourth overtimes, you have Cate test her blood glucose level and find that she has a reading of 58 mg/dL. As you observe her testing her glucose level, you notice other signs that tell you she is having a hypoglycemic episode. You inform the coach that Cate will not be able to play in the next overtime period. What are the hypoglycemic signs you are likely to see in Cate? What are your options to manage her hypoglycemia?

BIBLIOGRAPHY

American Diabetes Association. http://www.diabetes.org.

American Diabetes Association. Standards of medical care in diabetes–2014. *Diabetes Care.* 2014;37(suppl 1):S14-S80.

American Diabetes Association. Diagnosis and classification of diabetes mellitus. *Diabetes Care.* 2014;37(suppl 1):S81-S90.

Colberg SR, Sigal RJ, Fernhall B, et al. Exercise and type 2 diabetes. The American College of Sports Medicine and the American Diabetes Association: joint position statement. *Diabetes Care.* 2010;33(12):e147-e167.

Evert AB, Boucher JL, Cypress M, et al. Nutrition therapy recommendations for the management of adults with diabetes. *Diabetes Care.* 2014;37(suppl 1):S120-S143.

Jimenez CC, Corcoran MH, Crawley JT, Hornsby WG, Peer KS, Philbin RD, Riddell MC. National Athletic Trainers' Association position statement: management of the athlete with type 1 diabetes mellitus. *J Athl Train.* 2007;42(4):536-545.

Simon JL, Timaeus S, Misita C. SGLT2 inhibitors: a new treatment option for type 2 diabetes. *Pharmacy Times.* http://www.pharmacytimes.com/publications/health-system-edition/2014/September2014/SGLT2-Inhibitors-A-New-Treatment-Option-for-Type-2-Diabetes. Accessed July 26, 2015.

Stein SA, Lamos EM, Davis SN. A review of the efficacy and safety of oral antidiabetic drugs. *Expert Opin Drug Saf.* 2013;12(2):153-175.

Terry T, Raravikar K, Chokrungvaranon N, Reaven PD. Does aggressive glycemic control benefit macrovascular and microvascular disease in type 2 diabetes? Insights from ACCORD, ADVANCE, and VADT. *Curr Cardiol Rep.* 2012;14(1):79-88.

Wallia A, Molitch ME. Insulin therapy for type 2 diabetes mellitus. *JAMA.* 2014;311(22):2315-2325.

CHAPTER 15: ADVANCE ORGANIZER

Foundational Concepts

- Federal Regulations
- Safety, Efficacy, and Quality
- Adverse Effects and Drug Interactions
- Section Summary

Selected Herbal and Fitness Supplements

- St. John's Wort
  - Uses
  - Effects
  - Adverse Effects and Drug Interactions
- Ginkgo
  - Uses
  - Effects
  - Adverse Effects and Drug Interactions
- Saw Palmetto
  - Uses
  - Effects
  - Adverse Effects and Drug Interactions
- Echinacea
  - Uses
  - Effects
  - Adverse Effects and Drug Interactions
- Black Cohosh
  - Uses
  - Effects
  - Adverse Effects and Drug Interactions
- Feverfew
  - Uses
  - Effects
  - Adverse Effects and Drug Interactions
- Garlic
  - Uses
  - Effects
  - Adverse Effects and Drug Interactions
- Valerian
  - Uses
  - Effects
  - Adverse Effects and Drug Interactions
- Ginseng
  - Uses
  - Effects
  - Adverse Effects and Drug Interactions
- Creatine
  - Uses
  - Effects
  - Adverse Effects and Drug Interactions
- β-Hydroxy-β-Methylbutyrate
  - Uses
  - Effects
  - Adverse Effects and Drug Interactions
- Energy Drinks
- Section Summary

Role of the Athletic Trainer

15

Herbal and Fitness Supplements

CHAPTER OBJECTIVES

At the end of this chapter, the reader will be able to:

- Discuss the difference between a dietary supplement and an herbal supplement
- Explain the federal regulations that govern herbal supplements
- Explain the safety, efficacy, and quality components of herbal supplements
- Recall the uses, effects, adverse effects, and drug interactions of commonly used herbal and fitness supplements as well as energy drinks
- Summarize the role of the athletic trainer regarding herbal and fitness supplements

The use of herbal supplements has become extremely popular in the United States. Estimates of the number of people who use herbal supplements range from 30 to 60 million, many of whom do not report their herbal use to health care professionals. It is now a multi-billion-dollar business annually.

A number of people use herbal supplements to maintain good health, and others use them to treat existing diseases. Some people view herbal supplements as a substitute for conventional prescription or over-the-counter (OTC) therapy, and others view them as an adjunct to such therapy. Regardless of

ABBREVIATIONS USED IN THIS CHAPTER	
A1C. glycosylated hemoglobin	**HDL.** high-density lipoprotein
ADP. adenosine diphosphate	**HMB.** β-hydroxy-β-methylbutyrate
ATP. adenosine triphosphate	**LDL.** low-density lipoprotein
BPH. benign prostatic hyperplasia	**MAO.** monoamine oxidase
CGMP. current good manufacturing practice	**NSAID.** nonsteroidal anti-inflammatory drug
COX. cyclooxygenase	**OTC.** over-the-counter
DSHEA. Dietary Supplement Health and Education Act	**PAF.** platelet-activating factor
	PG. prostaglandin
FDA. Food and Drug Administration	**SSRI.** selective serotonin reuptake inhibitor
GABA. gamma-aminobutyric acid	**TCA.** tricyclic antidepressant
GI. gastrointestinal	**TX.** thromboxane

Houglum JE, Harrelson GL, Seefeldt TM.
Principles of Pharmacology for Athletic Trainers, Third Edition (pp 291-306).
© 2016 Taylor & Francis Group.

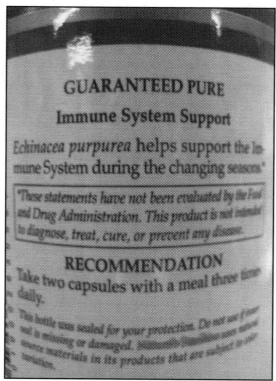

Figure 15-1. Label for echinacea product with statement for use and federally mandated disclaimer statement.

the reason that people use them, very often they do not view herbals as "drugs" and thus do not realize there are many of the same concerns of adverse effects, toxicity, and drug interactions that accompany the use of conventional drugs. The purpose of this chapter is to give the athletic trainer an awareness of the uses, effects, and potential problems associated with herbal and fitness remedies. This information may be of benefit to reduce athletes' inappropriate use of herbal supplements and subsequent suboptimum participation in athletics. In addition, an overview of the adverse effects associated with the use of energy drinks is provided.

FOUNDATIONAL CONCEPTS

Dietary supplements is a broad term that includes herbs, vitamins, minerals, amino acids, enzymes, fish oils, and extracts. Herbal medicines are obtained from plant sources and are used for health-related purposes. Many conventional drugs are also derived from plants but have been purified such that a single ingredient is isolated from the plant and identified as the active ingredient. Besides the usual oral dosage forms of tablets and capsules, some herbal supplements are marketed as teas, bulk powder extracts, oils, and nutrition bars. Some herbs are used topically as creams, ointments, and tinctures, but these topical products are not "supplements."

Federal Regulations

The Dietary Supplement Health and Education Act (DSHEA) of 1994 defined dietary supplements as a subcategory of foods. Therefore, from a legal standpoint, herbal supplements are not considered drugs, and some people oppose calling them drugs. Nonetheless, as mentioned in Chapter 1, legal, ethical, and therapeutic issues should all be considered in the discussion of whether a substance is a drug. If it looks like a drug, acts like a drug, and is used like a drug, it should be considered a drug for the patient's benefit, regardless of the legal classification.

According to DSHEA, all ingredients of dietary supplements that were in use prior to October 15, 1994, can be marketed without prior approval from the US Food and Drug Administration (FDA). That means that companies are not required to demonstrate efficacy or safety to the FDA prior to marketing the product. However, they have the responsibility to be able to substantiate the safety of the dietary ingredients and to have adequate evidence to demonstrate that the label claims are not false or misleading. If the FDA has evidence that the product is not safe (ie, presents a significant or unreasonable risk) after it has been on the market or that the product information is false or misleading, the FDA is authorized to take enforcement actions. The FDA has taken some enforcement actions regarding dietary supplements, the most notable being the removal of ephedra found in the ma huang plant, which was banned from the US market in 2004 due to deaths caused by its use. Examples of other actions have included warnings to companies because certain dietary supplements contained prescription drugs, heavy metals, or pesticide residues or because the product was subpotent compared with the label claim. Manufacturers do not have to register their dietary supplements or their company with the FDA, so there is no comprehensive list of dietary supplements. Ingredients that were introduced as dietary supplements after 1994 must be approved by the FDA based on adequate safety data provided by the manufacturer.

Other aspects of DSHEA restrict or otherwise regulate the labeling of dietary supplements. Labels cannot be compared with OTC or prescription drugs, for example related to their strength, quality, or effect. The labels cannot claim effectiveness in the treatment of disease, disease symptoms, or conditions that lead to disease, but labels can make truthful claims regarding health and a nutritional role of the ingredients. Therefore, claims can include statements regarding the effect of the ingredients on the structure and function of the body but not on the prevention or treatment of a specific disease. For example, a label cannot claim that a dietary supplement is effective to treat depression but can claim a benefit for emotional stability; it cannot claim to treat osteoporosis but it can claim to promote healthy bones (Figure 15-1). Because athletic performance is a "normal"

Box 15-1

REQUIREMENTS OF MANUFACTURERS UNDER THE CGMP RULE

- Employ qualified employees and supervisors.

- Design and construct physical plant in a manner to protect dietary ingredients and dietary supplements from becoming adulterated during manufacturing, packaging, labeling, and holding.

- Use equipment and utensils that are of appropriate design, construction, and workmanship for the intended use.

- Establish and use master manufacturing and batch production records.

- Establish procedures for quality control operations.

- Hold and distribute dietary supplements and materials used to manufacture dietary supplements under appropriate conditions of temperature, humidity, light, and sanitation so that the quality of the dietary supplement is not affected.

- Keep a written record of each product complaint related to the CGMP rule.

- Retain records for 1 year past the shelf life date, if shelf life dating is used; or 2 years beyond the date of distribution of the last batch of dietary supplements associated with those records.

Adapted from US Food and Drug Administration. Fact sheet: Dietary supplement current good manufacturing practices (CGMPs) and interim final rule (IFR) facts. http://www.fda.gov/Food/GuidanceRegulation/CGMP/ucm079496.htm. Accessed September 8, 2014.

condition in contrast to a disease or "abnormal" condition, claims supported by evidence for ergogenic aids have been acceptable. Products that contain a structure/function claim must include the following disclaimer on the label: "This statement has not been evaluated by the FDA. This product is not intended to diagnose, treat, cure, or prevent any disease" (see Figure 15-1).

Other label requirements for dietary supplements mandate that the product must be labeled as a supplement and the label must include several elements:

- The name and location of the manufacturer, packer, or distributor

- The name of the dietary supplement

- A complete list of ingredients

- The quantity of the product

- Nutritional labeling

Nondietary ingredients must also be listed, such as coloring agents, stabilizers, flavoring, and preservatives. Dietary supplements must be intended for ingestion and not for use by topical, sublingual, or other routes of administration.

The DSHEA included a provision for the FDA to develop and implement regulations for Current Good Manufacturing Practices (CGMP) for dietary supplements. The CGMP rule was issued in 2007 and is aimed at directly addressing the problematic areas of dietary supplements related to identity, purity, strength, and composition of the products and applies to all dietary supplements manufactured or distributed in the United States. Some of the requirements of manufacturers under the CGMP rule are

shown in Box 15-1. For the consumer, this rule helps to ensure that products meet certain quality standards, are not contaminated, and are accurately labeled. The CGMP rule does not regulate the use of dietary supplements nor ensure the safety of the labeled ingredient, much less the efficacy of the product to affect the health as anticipated by the consumer.

Safety, Efficacy, and Quality

As previously mentioned, ingredients of dietary supplements that were marketed prior to DSHEA do not have to demonstrate safety. New ingredients since that time must demonstrate safety, but if no specific claims are made on the label, proof of efficacy is not required. Even for claims of efficacy that are within the confines of DSHEA, the data required are not the extensive requirements of new OTC or prescription drugs. Because herbs have been available for generations, the reports of therapeutic benefit in the nonscience literature, coupled with selected results from small clinical studies, provide the impetus for consumers to use herbal supplements for specific health benefits. Because no claims of efficacy are on the label, there are no regulations that require proof of such efficacy.

Safety and efficacy are also related to quality; poor quality can result in poor safety and efficacy. Some aspects of product quality have been addressed through the new CGMP rule. However, the amount of active ingredients in herbal products will vary depending upon how and where the herb was grown as well as how it was processed. Therefore, the amount of active ingredient can change

Box 15-2

SELECTED HERBS WITH ANTICOAGULANT AND/OR ANTIPLATELET PROPERTIES

- Alfalfa
- Anise
- Bilberry
- Bladderwrack
- Bromelain
- Cat's claw
- Celery
- Coleus
- Cordyceps
- Dong quai
- Evening primrose oil
- Fenugreek
- Feverfew
- Garlic
- Ginger

- Ginkgo biloba
- Ginseng
- Grape seed
- Green tea
- Guggul
- Horse chestnut seed
- Horseradish
- Licorice
- Prickly ash
- Red clover
- Reishi
- Sweet clover
- Saw palmetto
- Turmeric
- White willow

from one manufacturer to another and from batch to batch. Up until the CGMP rule, no standards were established or regulations in place to guarantee that the specified amount of active ingredient was actually in the herbal product. In some cases, the active ingredient has not been identified, and only the weight of dried plant material can be specified. Additionally, no aspect of DSHEA, including the CGMP rule, requires dietary supplements to contain a minimum therapeutic dose, only that the product contains the dose claimed on the label. Studies have demonstrated the presence of potentially toxic contaminants or prescription drugs in some herbal products that were manufactured without regard to good manufacturing practices.

Adverse Effects and Drug Interactions

Because herbal supplements are processed plant products, there are many ingredients in each herb, and oftentimes multiple herbs are combined in the same tablet or capsule. Consequently, there can be many active ingredients in any one tablet or capsule. For example, St. John's wort is a mixture of at least 10 compounds that may contribute to its biological activity. With so many compounds being added to the bloodstream, it seems reasonable to expect some adverse reactions and drug interactions. Most of these may be relatively minor or occur at a low incidence in the general population, but as more people continue to take more

herbal supplements along with their OTC and prescription regimens, it becomes more likely that the athletic trainer will encounter athletes with these herbal-related problems. As an example of the potential for drug interactions with herbal supplements, consider Box 15-2, which lists selected herbs that reportedly have some anticoagulant and/or antiplatelet properties and thus may enhance that effect in patients who are also on therapy with aspirin, nonsteroidal anti-inflammatory drugs (NSAIDs), or warfarin.

The adverse effects for selected herbal supplements are discussed later in this chapter and range from gastrointestinal (GI) upset to liver toxicity. Among the drug interactions that are the easiest to predict are the combinations of an herbal supplement with another drug (either OTC or prescription) that has similar pharmacological effects; one will accentuate the effects of the other. For example, ginkgo enhances the anticoagulant effect of aspirin and other NSAIDs and may increase bleeding time. As with the addition of any drug to a therapeutic regimen that includes a drug with a narrow therapeutic window (see Chapter 3), extra caution is necessary with the addition of herbal supplement to such therapy, and consultation with a physician or pharmacist should be done prior to adding an herbal supplement to these drugs. Athletes should be instructed to inform their physician and pharmacist of all herbal and fitness supplements they are taking.

Section Summary

Although herbal supplements cannot claim efficacy in the treatment of disease or symptoms, they have become a mainstay of daily self-therapy for millions of people. Herbal supplements are also promoted as useful adjuncts to maintain good health and normal body functions. Proof of safety and efficacy are not requirements for the marketing of the herbal supplements. The CGMP rules are aimed at improving the quality control of dietary supplements. Although herbal supplements are not promoted as drugs, they contain a mixture of chemicals that can have adverse effects and may interact with prescription and OTC drugs.

SELECTED HERBAL AND FITNESS SUPPLEMENTS

There are hundreds of herbs and herbal products available. Some of the most commonly used herbal and fitness supplements are mentioned in this section.

St. John's Wort

St. John's wort (*Hypericum perforatum*) is one of the most commonly used herbal supplements. It grows wild in Asia, Europe, and North America and has been available in Europe for many years as a prescription medication for treatment of depression. The name originated from the Old English term *wort*, meaning "plant," and from the fact that *H perforatum* flowers near the feast of St. John in June. This herb contains many compounds, and no single entity has been identified as being responsible for the effects. Among these compounds is hypericin. Although it is not likely that hypericin is responsible for all of the effects of St. John's wort, extracts of St. John's wort are often standardized to contain 0.3% hypericin with a typical dose of 300 mg 3 times per day. Sometimes the content of another compound, hyperforin, at 3% to 5% is used instead of hypericin to standardize the product.

Uses

St. John's wort has been used for several conditions, but the one for which there are the most data is treating mild to moderate depression. Many clinical studies have been conducted to compare the effect of St. John's wort with placebo or with prescription antidepressants (see Chapter 13) such as selective serotonin reuptake inhibitors (SSRIs) and tricyclic antidepressants (TCAs). Most of these studies, along with meta-analyses of these studies, have demonstrated effectiveness greater than placebo and equivalent to the antidepressant efficacy of SSRIs and TCAs for treatment of mild to moderate depression. Although as a whole these studies indicate that St. John's wort is effective, most of these clinical studies had design flaws, such as using low doses of antidepressant medication as a comparison and use of a small number of patients. Additionally, none of the clinical studies determined effects after long-term use, and clinical studies do not support the use of St. John's wort for moderate to severe depression. Clinical data are minimal and show negative results for other uses, such as treatment of obsessive-compulsive disorder, insomnia, attention deficit disorder, anxiety, premenstrual syndrome, menopausal symptoms, or HIV.

Effects

Although St. John's wort is among the most studied herbal supplements, the mechanism by which it elicits the antidepressant effects is uncertain. The most commonly accepted mechanism is that it blocks the reuptake of serotonin, norepinephrine, and dopamine at the nerve terminal, thus enhancing the response of these compounds in the central nervous system (CNS). Some components of St. John's wort also appear to inhibit monoamine oxidase, an enzyme that inactivates these neurotransmitters. These are the same mechanisms by which conventional antidepressant drugs work (see Chapter 13). Other effects of St. John's wort are the basis for the array of potential drug interactions discussed next.

Adverse Effects and Drug Interactions

The advantages that proponents mention for the use of St. John's wort for treatment of depression are fewer adverse effects from St. John's wort that occur at a lower incidence than reported for the use of SSRIs, TCAs, or monoamine oxidase inhibitors to treat depression. Adverse effects from St. John's wort have been few, of low incidence, and generally not serious, the most common of which has been GI upset. Photosensitivity has also been reported in a few patients; consequently, caution is advised with the use of St. John's wort in fair-skinned patients or together with other photosensitizing drugs (eg, tetracyclines and sulfonamide antibiotics; see Chapter 5). Avoiding overexposure to the sun or any ultraviolet treatment would be prudent while using St. John's wort.

A significant disadvantage of St. John's wort is the many potential drug interactions (Table 15-1). These interactions can pose some significant problems, such as diminished control of blood cholesterol, increased risk for blood clots, and increased adverse effects from TCA therapy. St. John's wort induces P450 enzymes (see Chapter 2) and consequently reduces the effectiveness of all other drugs metabolized by the same enzyme (see Chapter 3). St. John's wort also increases the synthesis of a certain transport protein (p-glycoprotein) in the small intestine and kidney that is responsible for facilitating the excretion of drugs. By affecting the transport proteins in this way, St. John's wort increases the excretion and decreases the effectiveness of drugs that are handled by this mechanism. For example, these mechanisms are thought to be the cause of a reduced blood level of oral contraceptive and subsequent unexpected pregnancy that has occurred in women taking St. John's wort with oral contraceptives.

Other potential drug interactions can occur if St. John's wort is used along with traditional antidepressant drugs or other drugs that increase neurotransmitter levels. Use of SSRIs, TCAs, or monoamine oxidase inhibitors with St. John's wort can increase the intensity of the serotonin response to cause serotonin syndrome. The risk for serotonin syndrome increases when 2 or more drugs that enhance serotonin are used together. This syndrome can potentially be fatal and has an array of symptoms, including headache, sweating, dizziness, confusion, ataxia, tremor, agitation, tachycardia, and coma. Adrenergic agonists such as nasal decongestants (see Chapter 10) and higher doses of caffeine, as well as foods with high tyramine content (see Box 13-1), may enhance neurotransmitter responses and should also be avoided with St. John's wort to prevent undesirable intensified responses such as increased blood pressure and heart rate.

Ginkgo

Ginkgo, also known as ginkgo biloba, is prepared from an extract of the leaves from the *Ginkgo biloba* tree. The extract is a complex mixture of many chemicals, and evidence indicates that the therapeutic benefits are derived from multiple components within this complex mix rather

TABLE 15-1			
POTENTIAL DRUG INTERACTIONS WITH ST. JOHN'S WORT			
DRUG	**TRADE NAME**	**THERAPEUTIC USE**	**EFFECT DUE TO ST. JOHN'S WORT**
alprazolam	Xanax	Treat anxiety	↓
digoxin	Lanoxin	Treat heart failure	↓
phenelzine[a]	Nardil	Treat depression	↑
oral contraceptives	Many	Prevent pregnancy	↓
phenytoin	Dilantin	Anticonvulsant	↓
omeprazole	Prilosec	Treat heartburn/ulcers	↓
fluoxetine[b]	Prozac	Treat depression	↑
simvastatin	Zocor	Reduce cholesterol	↓
amitriptyline[c]	Elavil	Treat depression	↑
warfarin	Coumadin	Prevent blood clots	↓
[a]Monoamine oxidase inhibitor. [b]Selective serotonin reuptake inhibitor. [c]Tricyclic antidepressant.			

than from one entity. Flavonoids (flavone glycosides), terpenoids (ginkgolides, bilobalide), and ginkgolic acid are components of the chemical mixture. Some ginkgo products are standardized to contain 24% flavone glycosides and 6% terpenoids. The extraction procedure is intended to exclude as much ginkgolic acid as possible because it is potentially toxic. Ginkgo is available OTC and by prescription in Europe and is one of the most popular drugs. Typical daily dosage range is 120 to 240 mg.

Uses

A well-studied effect of ginkgo is its ability to improve blood flow to various tissues. Most of the uses of ginkgo presume a benefit, at least in part, from this improved blood flow. Ginkgo has been used to improve memory and concentration, treat senile dementia and Alzheimer's dementia, and treat intermittent claudication (ie, impaired circulation in the legs). Other uses are to treat symptoms of premenstrual syndrome, anxiety, macular degeneration, glaucoma, sexual dysfunction due to antidepressant drugs, and tinnitus.

Several studies have evaluated the effectiveness of ginkgo in treating Alzheimer's dementia and senile dementia, and the results in some studies have shown improved cognitive function in some patients compared with placebo, but these clinical studies have used a relatively small number of patients. In one large study of 3069 volunteers, use of ginkgo was not effective in reducing the incidence or rate of development of dementia or the occurrence of Alzheimer's disease.[1] The value of improving short-term memory in

normal adults or in the elderly with mildly impaired memory has shown positive results in some, but not all, studies.

Double-blind, placebo-controlled clinical studies have demonstrated the benefit of ginkgo to treat intermittent claudication, allowing the treated patients to walk a longer distance pain free compared with the placebo group, but again these have been small studies of short duration. A recent review analyzed data from several studies of ginkgo biloba in intermittent claudication and found that a small, but not statistically significant, increase in walking distance was observed with ginkgo compared with placebo.[2] Fewer studies have been conducted regarding all other uses for ginkgo, although some benefit has been demonstrated.

Effects

Primary effects of ginkgo are that it relaxes vascular smooth muscle, inhibits platelet-activating factor (PAF), and decreases prostaglandin production by inhibiting COX (see Chapter 6). All of these effects may play some role in facilitating blood flow. These same effects on smooth muscle, PAF, and COX may be suspected as contributing to other therapeutic responses attributed to ginkgo, such as prevention of blood clots, reduced inflammation, and treatment of asthma, but the impact of ginkgo by itself in these treatment areas appears to provide insignificant therapeutic benefit.

Adverse Effects and Drug Interactions

Adverse effects are relatively few but include a low incidence of mild GI upset and headache. Spontaneous bleeding has been reported, likely due to the effect of ginkgo on prostaglandins and PAF. Consequently, ginkgo should be used with caution in patients with bleeding problems or if using aspirin or other anticoagulants. The safety of ginkgo has not been established for use during pregnancy. Seizures have been reported in patients with epilepsy; thus, use of ginkgo is not recommended in patients being treated for seizures.

Saw Palmetto

The lipid extract of berries of the American dwarf palm (*Serenoa repens* or *Sabal serrulata*) is known as saw palmetto. This extract is a mixture of many compounds, including several fatty acids, polysaccharides, and sterols. Although it is sold only as a dietary supplement in the United States, it holds the status of a drug in several countries as an accepted medicinal treatment for benign prostatic hyperplasia (BPH). It is available as berries, tablets, capsules, liquid extract, and teas. Typical dosage is 320 mg per day of the extract standardized to contain 85% to 95% sterols and fatty acids.

Uses

Although historically saw palmetto has been used as a urinary antiseptic and to increase libido, breast size, and sperm production, only its use to treat BPH has been the most extensively studied. BPH is characterized by proliferation of prostate cells and symptoms of urinary hesitancy, decrease in urinary stream, and increased daytime and nighttime urinary frequency. Results of clinical trials examining the effects of saw palmetto in treatment of BPH have been mixed. Many placebo-controlled clinical studies have demonstrated effectiveness of saw palmetto compared with placebo, and some have even shown symptomatic improvement approximately equal to finasteride (Propecia), a drug used to treat BPH. However, more recent well-designed clinical trials failed to show a difference between saw palmetto and placebo in relief of BPH symptoms.[3,4]

Effects

The mechanism for the purported benefit in BPH is not clear, and several theories have been proposed. Saw palmetto may inhibit enzymes in the prostate that impact testosterone metabolism. It may also block receptors that are important the development of BPH symptoms, including androgen receptors and α_1 receptors. Saw palmetto does not seem to affect the serum levels of prostate-specific antigen, an enzyme used in the diagnosis of prostate cancer, and therefore does not cause misleading prostate-specific antigen values.

Adverse Effects and Drug Interactions

The incidence of adverse effects is quite low with saw palmetto but, as expected, increases with larger doses. Adverse effects include headache, decreased libido, diarrhea, and mild GI upset, which can be minimized by taking saw palmetto with meals. Because of the potential effects on androgen and estrogen receptors, saw palmetto should be avoided during pregnancy, in women who may become pregnant, or while breastfeeding. Patients should not self-medicate with saw palmetto as a substitute for appropriate diagnosis when symptoms of BPH occur; existence of prostate cancer must be ruled out through appropriate tests. Saw palmetto has been reported to have effects on platelet function; because of this, patients taking aspirin, warfarin, or other anticoagulants should not use saw palmetto.

Echinacea

Commercial products of echinacea are extracted from any one of 3 species of the purple coneflower native to North America: *E angustifolia*, *E pallida*, and *E purpurea*. Various parts of these plants, including the roots and leaves, are used to make the herbal products. Echinacea products are available in variety of forms for topical and oral use (eg, tinctures, syrups, juices, creams, ointments, capsules, tablets). The specific active compounds have not been identified but could be among any of the chemical groups present, such as glycoproteins, glycosides, polysaccharides, and essential oils. Echinacea products that are standardized have typically used a component of the extract called *phenolic compounds* as the ingredients with a standard percentage.

Uses

North American Indians not only applied echinacea to wounds to expedite healing and to prevent infections but also used it internally to treat sore throat, toothache, colds, and cough. The major uses for echinacea continue to include wound healing, but it is also used to treat topical infections, psoriasis, eczema, and viral infections such as the flu and common cold. In general, the mechanism of action that warrants these uses is not by directly affecting the microbes but by enhancing various aspects of the immune system and by inhibiting the inflammatory response.

Effects

There have been many in vitro and animal studies that confirm the ability of echinacea to initiate various immunological responses. These in vitro responses include enhanced macrophage phagocytosis, increased production of tumor necrosis factor, and increased levels of interleukin-1 and interferon beta-2 in selected cells. Animal studies have demonstrated a reduction of inflammation and edema. Regarding systemic use in humans, several placebo-controlled, double-blind clinical studies have focused on assessing the benefit of echinacea in the prevention and treatment of upper respiratory infections. It has been proposed that the timing of echinacea administration may be critical for use against the common cold, having the greatest effect if taken prior to infection. There have been some positive results upon analysis of the few studies of echinacea to prevent clinical symptoms in volunteers inoculated with the cold virus. The results of most other studies have not been encouraging, usually failing to demonstrate a statistically significant difference in the occurrence or duration of cold symptoms compared with placebo. Nonetheless, echinacea remains one of the most popular herbal supplements. Reports from people who claim personal benefits from using echinacea to prevent and treat various infections, including the common cold, provide the basis for its popularity. At this point, no definitive conclusion can be reached regarding the extent of therapeutic effectiveness of echinacea to treat the common cold.

Adverse Effects and Drug Interactions

Nausea, vomiting, and diarrhea have been reported. Allergic reactions, including anaphylaxis, are the most significant adverse effects and occur more frequently in people who have asthma, allergic rhinitis and other atopic disorders, or allergies to the daisy family of plants (eg, daisies, ragweed, chrysanthemums, marigolds). Patients who have autoimmune diseases should avoid using echinacea. Safety has not been established in women who are pregnant or breastfeeding.

Black Cohosh

Black cohosh is prepared as an extract of the rhizomes and roots of *Cimicifuga racemosa* (also known as *Actaea racemosa*), which is indigenous to the eastern North America. It was used by North American Indians to treat various gynecological conditions, which continues to be the major use of the herbal product. The primary active ingredients have been identified, and thus the potency of this herbal product can be specified based on the milligrams (1 to 2 mg/day) of 27-deoxyactein, one of the active triterpene compounds in the extract. However, not all products are standardized, and the extraction process varies among products; hence, the amount of active ingredients and the existence of additional components vary. These differences likely contribute to some of the discrepancies in the literature regarding the effectiveness of black cohosh. The standardized product that has been used in Germany for over 50 years and in more clinical research studies than any other is Remifemin (distributed by Enzymatic Therapy Inc).

Uses

The main use of black cohosh is to treat menopausal symptoms, but long-term studies are lacking, and thus it should not be used for longer than 6 months. It is also used to relieve symptoms of premenstrual syndrome and menstrual cramps, and although the use of black cohosh has not been studied as extensively for these conditions, it is generally considered to be safe and effective.

Effects

Black cohosh reduces hot flashes, mood swings, depression, night sweats, sleep disturbances, and headaches associated with menopause. Although clinical studies comparing black cohosh with menopause hormone therapy have been conducted with small numbers of patients, most results have shown the effectiveness to be comparable. The effects observed with black cohosh may be due to multiple mechanisms, including inhibition of luteinizing hormone release from the pituitary gland and activity at the serotonin receptors. Black cohosh also causes relaxation of uterine smooth muscle to relieve menstrual cramps. There is no clinical evidence that black cohosh prevents osteoporosis associated with menopause.

There remains some uncertainty as to whether black cohosh can be used in women with a history of estrogen-sensitive cancers. The issue is whether it stimulates these cancer cells, such as through binding to their estrogen receptor. Use of different black cohosh products may be the reason for some discrepancy in the research. Several studies using Remifemin have shown no stimulation of estrogen-sensitive breast cancer cells in vitro, no increased risk for breast cancer in an animal model, and no adverse ramifications in women with a history of breast cancer. Until this issue is definitively settled, use of black cohosh should be avoided in patients with a history of estrogen-dependent cancer.

Adverse Effects and Drug Interactions

The adverse effects from black cohosh are minimal; mild GI upset is the most common complaint at usual doses. Higher doses may cause dizziness, vomiting, and headaches. Black cohosh should not be used during pregnancy and lactation. Drug interactions have not been confirmed with clinical studies. Nonetheless, it seems prudent to seek medical advice before using in combination with hormone products such as estrogen replacement therapy, oral contraceptives, and anti-estrogen therapy.

Feverfew

The leaves and flowers from *Tanacetum parthenium* are the source of feverfew herbal preparations. The extract from the plant yields over 30 compounds that have been identified, of which parthenolide exists in the highest concentration. Because this specific active ingredient has been identified, products containing feverfew can be standardized based on the parthenolide content. Although parthenolide is not the only active ingredient, the content of parthenolide provides a benchmark to compare various products. A typical dosage is 125 mg of feverfew contains at least 0.2% parthenolide. Different methods of preparing feverfew products will yield various levels of parthenolide. Drying the leaves and using them to form a powder for tablets or capsules is common. Using liquid carbon dioxide to extract the active ingredients produces a more potent product with a typical dose of 6.25 mg. Chewing the whole leaf has been another method of administration.

Uses

The major use for feverfew is to prevent migraine headaches. Several small clinical studies have demonstrated efficacy in patients who have frequent migraine headaches. A few placebo-controlled clinical studies have shown that daily use of feverfew can reduce the incidence and intensity of acute attacks but not necessarily the duration of each attack. The nausea and vomiting associated with the migraine headaches was also reduced. One clinical study that did not demonstrate a difference from the placebo group used an alcoholic extract; the other studies used dried leaves or a carbon dioxide extract. Another study showed a difference in patients with 4 or more headaches per month but not in patients with less frequent migraines. Many differences exist in the research designs among these studies, including duration of treatment (2 months vs 2.5 years), dosage, and product (6.25 mg carbon dioxide extract vs 82 mg powdered leaves) and number of patients (17 vs 170). There is less evidence to support effectiveness to treat acute migraine attacks.

Feverfew has also been used to treat fever, dysmenorrhea, psoriasis, rheumatoid arthritis, and osteoarthritis, but evidence of effectiveness for these uses is minimal.

Effects

Feverfew has many physiologic effects, which is not surprising considering the abundance of compounds in the plant. The mechanism for its use to treat migraine headaches is not clear but may result from synergistic effects from multiple compounds acting by different mechanisms. It has been proposed that parthenolide alone does not reduce migraine headaches but may be contributing along with other compounds to produce the overall effect. Among the diverse effects that have been studied in vitro or in animals are inhibition of prostaglandin synthesis and inhibition of platelet aggregation but by some mechanism different from that of aspirin and NSAIDs. Besides prostaglandins, other mediators of inflammation are also inhibited. Feverfew inhibits serotonin release from platelets, which may be contributory to the prevention of migraine headaches although other mechanisms appear to be significant, including a direct effect on vascular smooth muscle. There is also evidence of thrombolytic activity, antimicrobial activity, and antitumor activity in vitro.

Adverse Effects and Drug Interactions

Adverse effects are relatively few, although studies regarding long-term use have not been conducted. Ulceration of the mouth and swelling of the lips, tongue, and mouth may occur in some patients who chew the leaves or drink tea prepared from feverfew. With any of the oral products, abdominal discomfort occurs in some people, although usually minor, but can include indigestion, nausea, vomiting, and diarrhea. Abrupt withdrawal of feverfew can cause post-feverfew syndrome, which includes nervousness, muscle stiffness, joint pain, tension, headaches, and insomnia. Individuals who plan to discontinue taking feverfew should do so gradually to avoid post-feverfew syndrome. Feverfew should not be used during pregnancy or while breastfeeding. People who are allergic to the *Asteraceae* family of plants (eg, chamomile, ragweed, sunflower, chrysanthemum, yarrow) may also be allergic to feverfew.

Theoretically, because feverfew inhibits platelet aggregation, there could be a drug interaction with any other drug that affects blood coagulation. Consequently, caution should be used if combining feverfew with aspirin, NSAIDs, or warfarin. Potential additive effects could also occur if feverfew is combined with other herbs that have anticoagulant effects (see Box 15-2).

Garlic

There has been a lot of research conducted regarding the potential therapeutic uses of garlic (*Allium sativum*). It is an herb that is cultivated nearly everywhere in the world. It is commercially available as cloves, garlic oil (garlic extracted with oil), tablets, freeze-dried powder, and minced bulbs. The components of garlic include alliin, several enzymes, amino acids, lipids, minerals, and vitamins. Allicin gives garlic the characteristic odor and is produced from alliin by the enzymatic action of alliinase, an enzyme that is activated when the garlic clove is crushed or ground. Heat destroys this enzyme and thus prevents the further production of allicin, considered one of the therapeutically active ingredients in garlic. Typical dosage of garlic varies because of the various forms that are available and the unstable nature of allicin, which breaks down into other compounds. Some clinical studies have used 600 to 900 mg of garlic powder standardized to 1.3% alliin as a means of obtaining dosing consistency.

Part of the problem in conducting clinical studies of the effects of garlic is that the odor of garlic makes it difficult to conduct double-blind placebo studies. In addition, as with so many herbs, the dose of active ingredient may vary among products. For example, products that are ground have activated alliinase to produce allicin, but allicin is not very stable, so the amount begins to diminish soon after it is produced. Studies may need to be conducted for at least 6 months because data indicate that the results may vary at ≤3 months compared with ≥6 months in the same patient.

Uses

Garlic has been used for its antiviral, antibacterial, and anticancer effects in the past, but recently the most common use for it has been to obtain various cardiovascular benefits. Many people now use garlic to reduce blood pressure, improve blood lipid levels, inhibit plaque formation from atherosclerosis, and prevent platelet aggregation. Regarding blood lipids, garlic has been used to increase high-density lipoprotein cholesterol and decrease low-density lipoprotein cholesterol as well as total cholesterol and triglycerides.

Effects

It is well established that garlic has antiseptic activity when applied topically to kill bacteria, fungi, and viruses. However, it is irritating to the skin when applied topically and can cause blistering. Garlic is not effective orally as an antimicrobial agent and therefore is not used to treat systemic infections. One exception might be to prevent the common cold. Some evidence, although not proof, indicates that daily use of garlic may reduce the number and duration of colds, but there is no evidence that garlic is effective if used after the onset of a cold. There is suggestive clinical evidence that people who use garlic as a routine part of their diet may have a lower incidence of stomach and colon cancer.

Garlic inhibits platelet aggregation by inhibiting thromboxane synthesis (see Figure 6-3). Other cardiovascular effects are less conclusive. Although some studies have shown a decrease in blood pressure with use of garlic, the effects have been small, and in some cases there were aspects of the research design that were criticized. An analysis of clinical trials studying the impact of garlic on blood pressure concluded that garlic was superior to placebo in lowering blood pressure; this effect was larger in hypertensive patients.[5] Because of studies completed by the mid-1990s, garlic was suspected to have cholesterol-lowering benefits. Many studies have been conducted since then that have failed to show such a benefit, particularly of garlic to sustain a cholesterol-lowering effect at 6 months or more. An analysis of several clinical trials of garlic found that a modest decrease in total cholesterol and triglycerides was observed with garlic treatment; however, no significant changes in low-density lipoprotein or high-density lipoprotein cholesterol were observed.[6] Animal studies have shown a benefit of garlic in slowing the atherosclerotic process, and clinical studies have demonstrated an indirect, but inconclusive, benefit.

Adverse Effects and Drug Interactions

Garlic is generally recognized as safe by the FDA. Large doses have not demonstrated toxicity in laboratory animals. The most common adverse effect is the odor. Other potential adverse effects are upset stomach, heartburn, nausea, vomiting, and flatulence. Although studies have not proven the safety of garlic during pregnancy or while breastfeeding, it is generally assumed that garlic is safe, considering it is a commonly used food.

The only notable potential drug interaction is if garlic is combined with any drug or other herb that also inhibits blood clotting or platelet aggregation, including aspirin, warfarin, and herbs listed in Box 15-2.

Valerian

The rhizomes and roots from *Valeriana officinalis* are used to obtain valerian. The active ingredient has not been identified, although one component, valerenic acid, is used to standardize dosage forms at 0.8% valerenic acid. Other components of valerian include amino acids, valepotriates, fatty acids, alkaloids, and flavonoids. The typical daily dosage varies depending on whether the product is dried root (2 to 3 g), alcohol extract (400 to 900 mg), or aqueous extract (250 to 500 mg).

Uses

The major use of valerian is to improve sleep. However, the clinical studies are conflicting, with some demonstrating a quicker onset of sleep with valerian and others showing no difference compared with placebo. It has been suggested that daily use of valerian for some weeks may be necessary for it to be effective as a sleep aid. Valerian is also used to relieve general anxiety and stress, but there are fewer studies to document this benefit.

Effects

Valerian appears to increase the availability of GABA, an inhibitory neurotransmitter in the brain that causes sedation. The effect on GABA is also the basis for the antianxiety response. The increased availability of GABA is similar to the mechanism of benzodiazepines, a group of conventional drugs used to treat both insomnia and anxiety. Valerian does not appear to produce a morning hangover effect as typically observed with conventional drugs for insomnia.

Adverse Effects and Drug Interactions

Mild GI upset in some patients and potential for drowsiness are the primary adverse effects. The potential for drowsiness warrants caution when driving a vehicle after taking valerian. Studies in animals and case reports in humans indicate additional sedation when combined with alcohol. It seems prudent to avoid valerian if other CNS depressants are to be used.

Ginseng

The 2 most common varieties of ginseng available are American (*Panax quinquefolius*) and Asian (*Panax ginseng*). These are also called Western and Korean ginseng, respectively. The Asian variety is considered more potent. Ginseng products may be prepared from the unprocessed root or from an extract of the root, which is available as capsules, powder, or tea. The pharmacologic activity is usually attributed to the many compounds called ginsenosides (or panaxosides) found in ginseng. Some ginsenosides appear to have opposite pharmacologic effects. The components vary among the ginseng products, including the ginsenoside content, and therefore the effects observed may vary. Many other compounds, including oils, vitamins, and peptides, are in ginseng products. Dosage is usually 200 to 600 mg daily of extract standardized to contain 4% to 7% ginsenosides, or up to 2 g of the dry root.

Uses

A popular use of ginseng is to improve overall health and to help the body accommodate physical and emotional stresses. More specifically, ginseng is used to prevent colds and flu, prevent cancer, improve concentration and stamina, improve the feeling of well-being in the elderly, enhance appetite, increase physical performance and endurance, relieve menopausal symptoms, improve sleep, treat depression, improve emotional stability, reduce blood glucose in people with type 2 diabetes, treat impotence, and lower blood pressure. Although the data are not convincing to recommend use for these conditions, the herb is used nonetheless.

Effects

A considerable variety of pharmacologic effects have been noted with in vitro and animal studies, and some have a degree of confirmation with clinical studies, but typically with a small number of patients. Examples of effects that have been reported include stimulating DNA, protein, and lipid synthesis; diminishing pain and inflammation; causing hypertension and hypotension; reducing blood glucose; lowering glycosylated hemoglobin blood levels; improving some immune parameters and psychomotor and cognitive ability; and an aspirin-like effect of inhibiting platelet aggregation. Although some effects may be relatively minor in magnitude, they may be significant for patients with pre-existing conditions (eg, diabetes mellitus or hypertension) or on selected drug therapy (anticoagulants).

As with some other herbal supplements, seemingly most reported uses for ginseng have at least one or more clinical studies to support the claim but also conflicting or inconclusive data from other reports. With that in mind, some general statements can be made regarding the effectiveness of ginseng based on clinical studies. Ginseng may improve the menopausal symptoms of mood, sleep disturbances, and well-being, but there is little evidence that it alleviates vasomotor symptoms (eg, hot flashes). Several double-blind, placebo-controlled studies have shown a significant reduction in the number of colds and flu-like symptoms when ginseng was taken for several months. Results concerning blood glucose have been contradictory; in some cases, American ginseng decreased blood glucose, whereas results with Asian ginseng have been mixed. Studies indicate that ginseng has the ability to enhance mood and increase feelings of well-being, although these effects may be more prominent in older adults. When improvement in cognitive function has been demonstrated, the quantitative

measure has generally been small. Data are insufficient regarding cancer prevention activity. Other effects from ginseng that have some data to suggest efficacy are to treat male impotence and to improve appetite and sleep.

The impact of ginseng on athletic performance has been studied based on the potential for this herb to improve cognitive and psychomotor skills. Asian ginseng has been studied most extensively as an ergogenic aid, but the results have been inconsistent. Some of the ergogenic claims associated with ginseng include increased energy, longer duration of exercise, increased red blood cell production, and improved pulmonary function. Many of the clinical studies have suffered from design flaws, including small sample size and short duration, which complicates drawing conclusions from the data. Also some of the claims related to athletic performance have been extrapolated from findings in animal studies or clinical trials that did not include healthy athletes; caution is needed in this type of extrapolation because data from animal studies or clinical trials in older patients, patients with compromised health, or patients who are not physically active does not necessarily correlate to enhanced athletic performance. Because of these problems with the research, there are not sufficient data to support the use of ginseng as an athletic performance enhancer. Further research is needed to definitively confirm or disprove the purported effects of ginseng.

Adverse Effects and Drug Interactions

Because ginseng causes a wide range of effects, there are many potential adverse effects; hypertension, insomnia, nervousness, irritability, headache, euphoria, and vomiting are among the most common. Consequently, ginseng should be avoided in patients with insomnia, hypertension, headaches, or psychological imbalance. Pregnant patients should avoid ginseng. Ginseng may provide an additional drop in blood glucose when used with other blood glucose-lowering agents (see Chapter 14) and thus must be used with caution in individuals with diabetes mellitus. It is not recommended that ginseng be used with anticoagulant drugs such as aspirin, NSAIDs, or warfarin.

Creatine

Creatine is the most well studied and most commonly used dietary supplement for ergogenic purposes. As a fitness supplement, creatine is available alone and in combination with other potential ergogenic aids such as beta-alanine. There are several forms of creatine available, but creatine monohydrate is the most commonly used.

Uses

The primary use of creatine is to enhance athletic performance. Creatine has been used to increase muscle mass and strength and to increase the number of repetitions of an activity that can be performed. The effects of creatine supplementation in various neurological and musculoskeletal conditions, including Parkinson's disease, muscular dystrophy, and polymyositis, have been studied; however, the current evidence is insufficient to support use of creatine in these conditions.

Effects

Creatine is naturally found in the body, primarily in skeletal muscle. There are 2 forms of creatine in the body: free creatine and phosphocreatine. Phosphocreatine serves as an energy source in the skeletal muscle. The phosphate group of phosphocreatine can be transferred to adenosine diphosphate to produce adenosine triphosphate (ATP). The ATP provides the energy for skeletal muscle contraction. The body has other pathways for the production of ATP; however, during intense exercise, the body cannot generate new ATP at a high enough rate to sustain the necessary muscle contraction. In these situations, the phosphocreatine is used to supply the needed ATP. The administration of supplemental creatine leads to increased creatine accumulation in muscle and therefore increases the amount of phosphocreatine available to generate ATP.

Several studies have examined the effects of creatine on athletic performance. Although there have been mixed results from these studies, most have supported the ergogenic effects of creatine. The effects of creatine are most apparent in short-duration but high-intensity activity. A position statement from the International Society of Sports Nutrition determined that creatine is effective in improving high-intensity exercise capacity and in increasing lean body mass.[7] The form of creatine may be important in the effects observed. Creatine monohydrate is the form that is most commonly used. Creatine ethyl ester is likely ineffective because it is converted to creatinine instead of creatine in the body.

Adverse Effects and Drug Interactions

Weight gain, muscle cramps, and nausea are adverse effects that have been reported with creatine. There is some controversy regarding the potential for kidney injury and liver dysfunction with creatine supplementation. Case reports have been published for both of these toxicities. In many of these reports, the patient was using doses of creatine that were higher than recommended, so it is possible that these effects occur with overdose. The findings are also complicated by the use of multiple supplements by the patients described in some of the case studies; in these cases, it is not possible to confirm what product actually caused the adverse effect. Other studies of creatine supplementation have not found these adverse effects. In an overall healthy athlete, creatine appears to be safe. However, patients with baseline kidney or liver disease should not use creatine. Also because of the potential effects on the kidney, creatine should not be used in com-

bination with other medications that can negatively affect kidney function.

β-Hydroxy-β-Methylbutyrate

β-hydroxy-β-methylbutyrate (HMB) is a metabolite of leucine, a branched-chain amino acid.

Uses

Leucine supplementation has been reported to increase lean body mass, improve muscle strength, and inhibit muscle breakdown after intense exercise. It has been proposed that the ergogenic effects observed with leucine are actually produced, at least in part, by a metabolite. HMB supplementation produces similar effects as leucine, and therefore, it is possible that HMB is mediating leucine's ergogenic activity. In addition to their use as fitness supplements, they have been studied for their benefit in muscle wasting in patients with chronic illnesses such as cancer and acquired immunodeficiency syndrome (AIDS).

Effects

Several clinical trials have examined the athletic performance enhancement effect of HMB. Results of clinical trials have been mixed. Some studies have shown increased muscle strength and reduced signs of muscle injury following exercise. Other studies have failed to show a beneficial effect of HMB supplementation. There has been considerable variation in the design of the studies, particularly related to the dose of HMB and the timing of administration relative to exercise; this variation is likely a contributor to the conflicting results. An analysis of the clinical studies of HMB concluded that the effects of the supplement are highest when it is taken 30 to 60 minutes before high-intensity exercise. There are also chronic effects of HMB administration; these effects are maximized when the supplement is taken for 2 weeks before the high-intensity activity.[9] The mechanism of action of HMB is not fully understood; however, it likely involves increased protein synthesis and inhibition of protein degradation.

Adverse Effects and Drug Interactions

HMB appears to be well tolerated. Recent animal studies have found that HMB supplementation produced insulin resistance. Insulin resistance is a feature of type 2 diabetes mellitus. This adverse effect has not been observed in human HMB trials. Further study is required to determine the potential effects of HMB on insulin sensitivity, blood glucose, and risk for diabetes mellitus.

Energy Drinks

The use of energy drinks and energy shots is very common, particularly among athletes. These products have been promoted as a mechanism to improve athletic performance, which has increased their popularity among athletes. The primary ingredient in energy drinks is caffeine (see Table 16-3). Many energy drinks also contain guarana extract, which also contains caffeine. Caffeine acts as a CNS stimulant, and the ergogenic effects of caffeine are discussed in Chapter 16. The athletic trainer should note that energy drinks contain a variety of other ingredients besides caffeine. These additional ingredients can include sugars, B vitamins, amino acids (such as taurine), and herbal extracts (such as guarana, ginseng, and ginkgo biloba) and may contribute to the effects and toxicity potential from energy drinks. One of the challenges in understanding the effects of these additional ingredients is that the specific amounts of them are not always included on the energy drink label.

Many concerns regarding the safety of energy drinks have been raised in recent years. Several deaths have been linked to energy drink consumption, and there has been a significant increase in emergency department visits related to energy drinks. Much of the information on energy drink toxicity comes from case reports of individuals who experienced toxicity after consumption of an energy drink or from research done on the individual ingredients in energy drinks. Potential toxicity associated with energy drinks includes cardiovascular risk, seizures, liver dysfunction, and kidney dysfunction. Additional concerns arise if energy drinks are combined with alcohol.

The caffeine component of energy drinks is the most well understood in terms of toxicity. It should be noted that because energy drinks can contain multiple ingredients that contain caffeine as well as other stimulants, a combined stimulant effect can result from energy drink consumption. Adverse effects associated with caffeine include increased heart rate, increased blood pressure, nervousness, difficulty sleeping, and GI upset. Overdoses of caffeine are associated with more serious complications, including cardiac dysrhythmias; fatal overdoses of caffeine are possible. Other components of energy drinks can also contribute to cardiovascular toxicity. Some energy drinks contain bitter orange (*Citrus aurantium*), which has an active ingredient called synephrine; synephrine has similar effects as epinephrine in the autonomic nervous system (see Chapter 12) and can cause increased blood pressure and cardiac dysrhythmias.

If energy drinks are consumed, moderation is essential to avoid toxicity associated with overdose. Users should also be aware of caffeine and other stimulants that they may consume in other beverages, foods, medications, or supplements to avoid accidental overdose or toxicity from combined stimulant effects. Energy drinks should never be mixed with alcohol. Because of toxicity concerns, the American Academy of Pediatrics has recommended against consumption of energy drinks by children and adolescents.[8] Other patient groups should also be advised to not consume energy drinks. This includes patients with preexisting cardiovascular conditions and neurologic disorders. Patients with diabetes mellitus should also not consume energy drinks due to the cardiovascular risks and the exacerbation of hyperglycemia from the sugar content.

Section Summary

Conducting clinical studies with herbal supplements poses some significant problems that are not encountered in most studies with conventional drugs. Herbal supplements are a mixture of many compounds, each of which may have some pharmacological effect, and usually the compound of primary interest has not been identified and is not supplied in standardized dosages for use by all studies. Among studies there is inconsistency of dosage, duration of treatment, product contents, and study design. One common aspect of the herbal clinical studies is that they almost all use a small number of participants (tens or hundreds rather than thousands). These inconsistencies and small sample sizes often yield variable results that are difficult to interpret. Based on the popularity of the herbal supplements, it is obvious that the general population has greater confidence in the efficacy of these products than is warranted by the clinical data. Table 15-2 summarizes the effects and cautions for the herbal supplements discussed in this chapter.

ROLE OF THE ATHLETIC TRAINER

The role of the athletic trainer regarding herbal supplements is not much different from that regarding OTC or prescription drugs: understand the basic uses, effects, and potential drug interactions and be cognizant of their potential for changes in the patient. However, with herbals it is also important to consider that standardization of active ingredients and the quality controls that regulate their production are relatively new approaches to regulating the herbal industry. Consequently, the pharmacologic response from any herbal product may be significantly greater or less than expected. In addition, patients may not report the use of herbal supplements as they would OTC or prescription medications because patients may not view herbals as drugs or their use of them as a potential problem. If a patient complains of a new symptom and the existence of a conventional drug is not the cause, inquiry should be made regarding the use of herbal supplements. Similarly, if the patient experiences a change in the therapeutic response or adverse effects from current drug therapy, the addition of an herbal supplement should be questioned as a possible cause. Although herbal supplements do not fall under the legal classification of drugs, the athletic trainer should consider the potential for significant effects on the athlete just as with OTC and prescription drugs. Box 15-3 lists some additional general advice that may be useful for athletes who are considering the use of herbal supplements.

TABLE 15-2

SUMMARY OF EFFECTS AND CAUTIONS WITH SELECTED HERBAL SUPPLEMENTS

HERBAL SUPPLEMENT	USE SUPPORTED BY SOME CLINICAL DATA	CAUTIONS[a]
St. John's wort	Treat mild to moderate depression	Decreased effectiveness of oral contraceptives; do not use with other antidepressants (see Table 15-1)
Ginkgo	Treat senile dementia and Alzheimer's dementia; treat intermittent claudication; improve memory	Caution if taking anticoagulants or aspirin, or if history of seizures
Ginseng	Improve mood, reduce fatigue, increase stamina; antidepressant; prevent colds; improve menopausal symptoms; ergogenic potential	Caution in patients taking anticoagulants or aspirin or being treated for diabetes mellitus or hypertension
Saw palmetto	Treat benign prostatic hyperplasia	GI discomfort
Echinacea	Improve wound healing; boost immune system	Caution in patients with autoimmune diseases
Black cohosh	Treat symptoms of menopause, premenstrual syndrome, and menstrual cramps	GI discomfort
Feverfew	Prevent migraine headache	GI discomfort; post-feverfew syndrome; caution with anticoagulants or aspirin
Garlic	Cardiovascular benefits; prevent colds	Bad breath; GI discomfort; caution with anticoagulants or aspirin
Valerian	Sleep aid; anxiety	Drowsiness; caution while driving; avoid other CNS depressants, including alcohol
Creatine	Improved athletic performance	May cause weight gain; should not be used by patients with kidney or liver disease
HMB	Improved athletic performance	Possible association with insulin resistance

CNS = central nervous system; GI = gastrointestinal; HMB = β-hydroxy-β-methylbutyrate.

[a]All herbal supplements should be used with caution in women who are pregnant or breastfeeding. Studies have not been conducted to demonstrate safety during these conditions or the herbal is contraindicated on basis of the theoretical mechanism of action of herbal components.

There are hundreds of herbal supplements about which the athletic trainer may need to obtain current information regarding uses, effects, adverse effects, or drug interactions. Listed in Box 15-4 are some Internet sites that may provide an easily accessible source for needed information.

CASE STUDY

You are on a road trip with the university's women's track and field team. You notice that Pam, the team's 21-year-old sprinter who competes in the 100-m and 4 × 100-m relay, has a number of tablets she is taking with her meal. You are surprised because you recall from Pam's history form that the only medication she listed was her "rescue inhaler" and her long-acting medication for her asthma, a contraceptive, and occasional acetaminophen for headache. After the meal, you speak with her to ask her what she is taking so you can update her history form. Pam indicates that she is just taking herbal supplements that she has taken since high school when her parents suggested she use them, like they do, to maintain good health. She states that she is taking the same ones her parents started her on: St. John's wort, ginseng, gingko biloba, and echinacea. You realize that the side effects of some of these herbal supplements are deleterious for Pam and explain to her that these supplements may be interacting with her current prescription medications as well as contributing to her complaints of headaches. Which

---

Box 15-3

RECOMMENDATIONS TO ATHLETES REGARDING USE OF HERBAL SUPPLEMENTS

- Do not use herbals as a substitute for needed medical treatment.
- Look for a verification of standardization on the label.
- Only use products that show the quantity of herb on the label.
- Keep using the same manufacturer's brand that has been working for you.
- Do not use if you are pregnant or breastfeeding.
- Regard herbals as you would drugs by reporting your use to your doctor and pharmacist and by being aware that drug interaction and adverse effects are possible.
- Use products that contain only one herb per product.
- Be skeptical of claims that sound too good to be true. The therapeutic effects from herbal supplements are generally modest at best.
- Avoid herbals if you are younger than 18 years because most herbal research has been in adults.
- Consult your doctor or pharmacist before taking herbals if you are taking medication that must be closely monitored (eg, blood thinners) or if modest changes in effectiveness could have significant consequences (eg, drugs for heart conditions, diabetes, asthma, seizures).

Box 15-4

INTERNET SITES THAT PROVIDE INFORMATION REGARDING HERBAL SUPPLEMENTS

- http://nccam.nih.gov

  National Center for Complementary and Alternative Medicine. Provides search capability to obtain printable information regarding many herbal supplements.

- http://ods.od.nih.gov

  Office of Dietary Supplements, NIH. Provides information and search capability for dietary supplements including herbs. Information includes fact sheets, PowerPoint presentations, or other written reports.

- www.supplementquality.com/index.html

  Dietary Supplement Quality Initiative. Provides news, information, and summary of research regarding dietary supplements, including herbal supplements. Contains search capabilities.

- http://healthlibrary.epnet.com/GetContent.aspx?token=e0498803-7f62-4563-8d47-5fe33da65dd4&chunkiid=33802

  Sponsored by iHerb.com. Provides a summary of scientific evidence with references regarding uses for hundreds of herbs and other dietary supplements.

- www.pdrhealth.com/home/home.aspx

  From the publishers of *Physicians' Desk Reference*. Provides information such as uses, dosages, effects, warnings, and references regarding prescription, OTC, and herbals and supplements as an alphabetical listing.

- www.consumerlab.com

  Consumer Lab. Conducts quality tests on dietary supplements and reports findings on website. A subscription is required for full access to the quality reports.

of these herbal supplements should she not be taking and why? What are the potential side effects of each of the supplements she is taking?

REFERENCES

1. DeKosky ST, Williamson JD, Fitzpatrick AL, et al. Ginkgo biloba for prevention of dementia: a randomized controlled trial. *JAMA.* 2008;300(19):2253-2262.

2. Nicolaï SPA, Kruidenier LM, Bendermacher BLW, et al. Ginkgo biloba for intermittent claudication (review). *Cochrane Database Syst Rev.* 2013;6:CD006888.

3. Bent S, Kane C, Shinohara K, et al. Saw palmetto for benign prostatic hyperplasia. *N Engl J Med.* 2006;354(6):557-566.

4. Barry MJ, Meleth S, Lee JY, et al. Effect of increasing doses of saw palmetto extract on lower urinary tract symptoms: a randomized trial. *JAMA.* 2011;306(12):1344-1351.

5. Ried K, Frank OR, Stocks NP, Fakler P, Sullivan T. Effect of garlic on blood pressure: a systematic review and meta-analysis. *BMC Cardiovasc Disord.* 2008;8:13.

6. Reinhart KM, Talati R, White CM, Coleman CI. The impact of garlic on lipid parameters: a systematic review and meta-analysis. *Nutr Res Rev.* 2009;22:39-48.

7. Buford TW, Kreider RB, Stout JR, et al. International Society of Sports Nutrition position stand: creatine supplementation and exercise. *J Int Soc Sports Nutr.* 2007;4:6.

8. Committee on Nutrition and the Council on Sports Medicine and Fitness. Sports drinks and energy drinks for children and adolescents: are they appropriate? *Pediatrics.* 2011;127:1182-1189.

9. Wilson JM, Fitschen PJ, Campbell B, et al. International Society of Sports Nutrition position stand: beta-hydroxy-beta-methylbutyrate (HMB). *J Int Soc Sports Nutr.* 2013;10:6.

BIBLIOGRAPHY

Bahrke MS, Morgan WP, Stegner A. Is ginseng an ergogenic aid? *Int J Sport Nutr Exerc Metab.* 2009;19(3):298-322.

Bent S. Herbal medicine in the United States: review of efficacy, safety, and regulation. *J Gen Intern Med.* 2008;23(6):854-859.

Borrelli F, Izzo AA. Herb-drug interactions with St. John's wort (*Hypericum perforatum*): an update on clinical observations. *AAPS J.* 2009;11(4):710-727.

Bucci LR. Selected herbals and human exercise performance. *Am J Clin Nutr.* 2000;72(suppl):624S-636S.

Buell JL, Franks R, Ransone J, Powers ME, Laquale KM, Carlson-Phillips A. National Athletic Trainers' Association position statement: evaluation of dietary supplements for performance nutrition. *J Athl Train.* 2013;48(1):124-136.

Campbell B, Wilborn C, La Bounty P, et al. International Society of Sports Nutrition position stand: energy drinks. *J Int Soc Sports Nutr.* 2013;10:1.

Chen CK, Muhamad AS, Ooi FK. Herbs in exercise and sport. *J Physiol Anthropol.* 2012;31:4.

Clauson KA, Shields KM, McQueen CE, Persad N. Safety issues associated with commercially available energy drinks. *J Am Pharm Assoc.* 2005;48:e55-e67.

Diener HC, Pfaffenrath V, Schnitker J, Friede M, Henneicke-von Zepelin H-H. Efficacy and safety of 6.25 mg t.i.d. feverfew CO_2 extract (MIG-99) in migraine prevention-a randomized, double-blind, multicenter-placebo-controlled study. *Cephalagia.* 2005;25(11):1031-1041.

Evans RW, Taylor FR. "Natural" or alternative medications for migraine prevention. *Headache.* 2006;46(6):1012-1018.

Gerlinger-Romero F, Guimaraes-Ferreira L, Giannocco G, Nunes MT. Chronic supplementation of beta-hydroxy-beta methylbutyrate (HMB) increases the activity of the GH/IFG-1 axis and induces hyperinsulinemia in rats. *Growth Horm IGF Res.* 2011;21(2):57-62.

Gualano B, Roschel H, Lancha AH, Brightbill CE, Rawson ES. In sickness and in health: the widespread application of creatine supplementation. *Amino Acids.* 2012;43:519-529.

Hall M, Trojian TH. Creatine supplementation. *Curr Sports Med Rep.* 2013;12(4):240-244.

Higgins JP, Tuttle TD, Higgins CL. Energy beverages: content and safety. *Mayo Clin Proc* 2010;85(11):1033-1041.

Kreider RB, Wilborn CD, Taylor L, et al. ISSN exercise and sport nutrition review: research and recommendations. *J Int Soc Sports Nutr.* 2010;7:7.

Liddle DG, Connor DJ. Nutritional supplements and ergogenic aids. *Prim Care Clin Office Pract.* 2013;40:487-505.

Luberto CM, White C, Sears RW, Cotton S. Integrative medicine for treating depression: an update on the latest evidence. *Curr Psychiatry Rep.* 2013;15(9):391.

McHughes M, Timmermann BN. A review of the use of CAM therapy and the sources of accurate and reliable information. *J Manag Care Pharm.* 2005;11(8):695-703.

Sarris J. St. John's wort for the treatment of psychiatric disorders. *Psychiatr Clin North Am* 2013;36(1):65-72.

Schoop R, Klein P, Suter A, Johnston SL. Echinacea in the prevention of induced rhinovirus colds. A meta-analysis. *Clin Therap.* 2006;28(2):174-183.

Shergis JL, Zhang AL, Zhou W, Xue CC. Panax ginseng in randomised controlled trials: a systematic review. *Phytother Res.* 2013;27:949-965.

Shi S, Klotz U. Drug interactions with herbal medicines. *Clin Pharmacokinet.* 2012;51(2):77-104.

Tacklind J, Macdonald R, Rutks I, Stanke JU, Wilt TJ. Serenoa repens for benign prostatic hyperplasia. *Cochrane Database Syst Rev.* 2012;12:CD001423.

US Food and Drug Administration. Fact sheet: Dietary supplement current good manufacturing practices (CGMPs) and interim final rule (IFR) facts. http://www.fda.gov/Food/GuidanceRegulation/CGMP/ucm079496.htm. Accessed September 8, 2014.

Williams M. Dietary supplements and sports performance. *J Int Soc Sports Nutr.* 2006;3(1):1-6.

Winterstein AP, Storrs CM. Herbal supplements: considerations for the athletic trainer. *J Athl Train.* 2001;36(4):425-432.

Wolk BJ, Ganetsky M, Babu KM. Toxicity of energy drinks. *Curr Opin Pediatr.* 2012;24(2):243-251.

Yonamine CY, Teixeira SS, Campello RS, et al. Beta hydroxyl beta methylbutyrate supplementation impairs peripheral insulin sensitivity in healthy sedentary Wistar rats. *Acta Physiol.* 2014;212(1):62-74.

CHAPTER 16: ADVANCE ORGANIZER

Stimulants

- Amphetamines
  - Pharmacodynamics
  - Possible Ergogenic Effects
  - Adverse Effects
- Caffeine
  - Pharmacodynamics
  - Possible Ergogenic Effects
  - Adverse Effects
- Ephedrine
  - Pharmacodynamics
  - Possible Ergogenic Effects
  - Adverse Effects
- Section Summary

Anabolic Agents

- Anabolic Steroids
  - Pharmacodynamics
  - Possible Ergogenic Effects
  - Adverse Effects
- Human Growth Hormone
  - Pharmacodynamics
  - Possible Ergogenic Effects
  - Adverse Effects
- β-Agonists
  - Pharmacodynamics
  - Possible Ergogenic Effects
  - Adverse Effects
- Section Summary

Diuretics

- Pharmacodynamics
- Possible Ergogenic Effects
- Adverse Effects
- Section Summary

Anti-Inflammatory Drugs

- Corticosteroids
  - Pharmacodynamics
  - Possible Ergogenic Effects
  - Adverse Effects
  - Section Summary

β-Blockers

- Pharmacodynamics
- Possible Ergogenic Effects
- Adverse Effects
- Section Summary

Oxygen Delivery Enhancers

- Erythropoietin
  - Pharmacodynamics
  - Possible Ergogenic Effects
  - Adverse Effects
- Section Summary

Role of the Athletic Trainer

16

Performance-Enhancing Drugs

Michael Powers, PhD, ATC, CSCS, EMT

Chapter Objectives

At the end of this chapter, the reader will be able to:

- Identify the general classifications of ergogenic drugs and the specific drugs within each classification

- Explain the pharmacodynamics of each drug and specific physiological and psychological effects each has on the human body

- Discuss the efficacy of each drug as it relates to athletic performance

- Identify the adverse effects associated with each drug

- Identify the drugs that are available over-the-counter (OTC) and those available by prescription only

- Discuss the ethical and legal issues associated with ergogenic drug use

Ergogenic drug use, or *doping*, as it is often referred to, was previously defined by the International Olympic Committee (IOC) as the administration of or use by a competing athlete of any substance foreign to the body or of any physiological substance taken in abnormal quantity or taken by an abnormal route of entry into the body with the sole intention of increasing in an artificial manner his or her performance in competition. More recently, the World Anti-Doping Agency (WADA) simply defined doping as the possession, administration, or attempted

administration of a prohibited substance or the presence of a prohibited substance or its metabolites or markers in an athlete's sample. The modern-day competitiveness of both professional and amateur athletics has resulted in ergogenic drug use by many athletes in hopes of achieving an edge over the competition. However, doping in athletics is not new. Ancient Greek Olympic athletes consumed herbs and mushrooms to improve performance, and the use of drugs by American athletes dates back to the 1800s. The use of stimulants, anabolic steroids, and other drugs became popularized in the 1950s and 1960s, forcing the IOC to begin drug testing at the 1968 Olympic Games in Mexico City. It was during these games that the first drug disqualification occurred when a Swedish entrant in the modern pentathlon tested positive for excessive alcohol.

Today, numerous drugs are ingested or otherwise administered for a performance-enhancing effect. Many drugs can be purchased OTC, whereas others require a prescription from a licensed practitioner. When the US Food and Drug Administration (FDA) passed the Dietary Supplement Health and Education Act of 1994, it allowed numerous compounds to be classified as nutritional supplements instead of drugs. Although many athletes turned to these products because of their availability and implied safety, drug use in professional and amateur athletics is still widespread. In 1998, a large number of prohibited drugs were found by police in a raid during the Tour de France. The scandal led to a major reappraisal of the role of public

Houglum JE, Harrelson GL, Seefeldt TM.
Principles of Pharmacology for Athletic Trainers, Third Edition (pp 309-345).
© 2016 Taylor & Francis Group.

ABBREVIATIONS USED IN THIS CHAPTER

AAS. anabolic-androgenic steriod	**IOC.** International Olympic Committee
ADHD. attention deficit/hyperactivity disorder	**LDL.** low-density lipoprotein
AIDS. acquired immuno-deficiency syndrome	**MI.** myocardial infarction
cAMP. cyclic adenosine monophosphate	**MLB.** Major League Baseball
CBA. collective bargaining agreement	**NCAA.** National Collegiate Athletic Association
CNS. central nervous system	**NHL.** National Hockey League
DNA. deoxyribonucleic acid	**NFL.** National Football League
EPO. erythropoietin	**NSAID.** nonsteroidal anti-inflammatory drug
FDA. Food and Drug Administration	**OTC.** over-the-counter
FFA. fatty free acid	**PGA.** Professional Golfers' Association
GI. gastrointestinal	**RBCs.** red blood cells
Hb. hemoglobin	**rEPO.** recombinant erythropoietin
HDL. high-density lipoprotein	**RNA.** ribonucleic acid
hGH. human growth hormone	**t½.** half-life
IBA. inhaled β_2-agonist	**VO$_2$.** oxygen consumption
IGF-1. insulin-like growth factor-1	**WADA.** World Anti-Doping Agency

authorities in anti-doping affairs. It also highlighted the need for an independent international agency, which would set unified standards for drug testing and coordinate the efforts of sports organizations. The IOC took the initiative and convened the World Conference on Doping in Sport in February 1999. Following the proposal of the Conference, the WADA was established in November 1999. Four years later, at the 2003 World Conference on Doping in Sport, all major sports federations and nearly 80 governments gave their approval to the WADA by backing a resolution that accepts the WADA Code as the basis for the fight against doping in sports. The World Code was put into effect prior to the 2004 Olympic Games in Athens, Greece, with the mission of promoting, coordinating, and monitoring on an international basis, the fight against doping in sport.

Substances are included on the prohibited list if they meet 2 of 3 criteria:

1. Medical or scientific evidence that the substance has the potential to enhance or enhances sport performance;

2. The substance represents an actual or potential risk to the health of the athlete; and

3. The substance violates the "spirit of sport" as identified in the WADA code.

Some of the primary classifications of drugs used in the athletic setting and prohibited by WADA include stimulants, anabolic agents, diuretics, anti-inflammatory agents, β-blockers, and oxygen delivery enhancers (Table 16-1).

STIMULANTS

Stimulant is a name given to several groups of drugs that tend to increase arousal and alertness via central nervous system (CNS) stimulation. The US Anti-Doping Agency defines a *stimulant* as an agent, especially a chemical agent, such as caffeine, that temporarily arouses or accelerates physiological or organic activity. These agents include street drugs commonly called uppers (or speed) and Ecstasy (or Molly). Stimulants are commonly prescribed for a number of medical conditions including obesity, narcolepsy, and depression. It is not uncommon for an athletic trainer to care for patients taking stimulants such as methylphenidate (Ritalin and Concerta) or amphetamines (Adderall) because these drugs are also commonly prescribed for attention deficit hyperactivity disorder (ADHD) (Table 16-2). Likewise, stimulants such as levmetamfetamine (Vicks Inhaler), pseudoephedrine (Sudafed), and phenylephrine (Sudafed PE) are commonly used as nasal decongestants. This class of drugs has also found its way into the athletic arena and, in one form or another, they have been used to enhance performance for almost 2 centuries. In fact, one of the earliest reported drug-related deaths in sport was a British cyclist who died in 1968 after he was administered strychnine by his coach. Although there are conflicting reports regarding his death, the coach was later banned from cycling for his part in doping. Thus, it is not surprising that stimulants were some of the first drugs used and studied as ergogenic aids and were the first class of drugs to be banned by the IOC (see Table 16-1). Those more commonly found in the athletic setting include amphetamines, ephedrine, and caffeine.

Amphetamines

Amphetamine was first synthesized in 1887 by a German chemist named Edeleano who named it *phenylisopropylamine*. In the 1930s, ephedrine was the only effective drug being used in the treatment of asthma, and at that time

TABLE 16-1

THE WORLD ANTI-DOPING CODE PROHIBITED SUBSTANCE LIST (2015 LIST)

SUBSTANCES PROHIBITED AT ALL TIMES (IN- AND OUT-OF-COMPETITION)

S0. NON-APPROVED SUBSTANCES

Any pharmacological substance which is not addressed by any of the subsequent sections of the List and with no current approval by any governmental regulatory health authority for human therapeutic use (eg, drugs under pre-clinical or clinical development or discontinued, designer drugs, substances approved only for veterinary use) is prohibited at all times.

S1. ANABOLIC AGENTS

Anabolic agents are prohibited.

1. ANABOLIC ANDROGENIC STEROIDS (AAS)

a. Exogenous AAS including:

1-androstendiol	gestrinone	norclostebol
1-androstanedione	4-hydroxytestosterone	norethandrolone
bolandiol	mestanolone	oxabolone
bolasterone	mesterolone	oxandrolone
boldenone	metandienone	oxymesterone
boldione	metenolone	oxymetholone
calusterone	methandriol	prostanozol
clostebol	methasterone	quinbolone
danazol	methyldienolone	stanozolol
dehydrochlormethyl-testosterone	methyl-1-testosterone	stenbolone
desoxymethyltestosterone	methylnortestosterone	1-testosterone
drostanolone	methyltestosterone	tetrahydrogestrinone
ethylestrenol	metrebolone	trenbolone
fluoxymesterone	mibolerone	and other substances with similar chemical structure or similar biological effect(s)
formebolone	nandrolone	
furazabol	19-norandrostenedione norboletone	

b. Endogenous AAS when administered exogenously:

androstenediol

androstenedione

dihydrotestosterone

prasterone

testosterone

and their metabolites and isomers

2. OTHER ANABOLIC AGENTS, INCLUDING BUT NOT LIMITED TO

clenbuterol

selective androgen receptor modulators (SARMs)

tibolone

zeranol

zilpaterol

(continued)

TABLE 16-1 (CONTINUED)

THE WORLD ANTI-DOPING CODE PROHIBITED SUBSTANCE LIST (2015 LIST)

S2. PEPTIDE HORMONES, GROWTH FACTORS AND RELATED SUBSTANCES

The following substances, and other substances with similar chemical structure or similar biological effect(s), are prohibited:

1. Erythropoiesis-Stimulating Agents [e.g. darbepoietin (dEPO), erythropoietin (EPO), EPO-mimetic peptides (EMP), and methoxy polyethylene glycol-epoetin beta (CERA)

2. Hypoxia-inducible factor (HIF) stabilizers and HIF activators

3. Chorionic Gonadotrophin (CG) and Luteinizing Hormone (LH) and their releasing factors, in males;

4. Corticotrophins and their releasing factors;

5. Growth Hormone (GH) and its releasing factors including Growth Hormone Releasing Hormone (GHRH) and its analogues, Growth Hormone Secretagogues (GHS) and GH-Releasing Peptides (GHRPs)

In addition, the following growth factors are prohibited

Fibroblast Growth Factors (FGFs); Hepatocyte Growth Factor (HGF); Insulin-like Growth Factor-1 (IGF-1) and its analogues; Mechano Growth Factors (MGFs); Platelet-Derived Growth Factor (PDGF); Vascular-Endothelial Growth Factor (VEGF) and any other growth factor affecting muscle, tendon or ligament protein synthesis/degradation, vascularisation, energy utilization, regenerative capacity or fibre type switching.

S3. BETA-2 AGONISTS

All beta-2 agonists, including all optical isomers, eg, d- and l- where relevant, are prohibited.

Except:

- Inhaled salbutamol (maximum 1600 micrograms over 24 hours);

- Inhaled formoterol (maximum delivered dose 54 micrograms over 24 hours); and

- Inhaled salmeterol in accordance with the manufacturers' recommended therapeutic regimen.

The presence in urine of salbutamol in excess of 1000 ng/mL or formoterol in excess of 40 ng/mL is presumed not to be an intended therapeutic use of the substance and will be considered as an Adverse Analytical Finding (AAF) unless the Athlete proves, through a controlled pharmacokinetic study, that the abnormal result was the consequence of the use of the therapeutic inhaled dose up to the maximum indicated above.

S4. HORMONE AND METABOLIC MODULATORS

The following are prohibited:

1. Aromatase inhibitors including, but not limited to: aminoglutethimide; anastrozole; androsta-1,4,6-triene-3,17-dione (androstatrienedione); 4-androstene-3,6,17 trione (6-oxo); exemestane; formestane; letrozole and testolactone.

2. Selective estrogen receptor modulators (SERMs) including, but not limited to: raloxifene, tamoxifen, toremifene.

3. Other anti-estrogenic substances including, but not limited to: clomiphene, cyclofenil, fulvestrant.

4. Agents modifying myostatin function(s) including, but not limited to: myostatin inhibitors.

5. Metabolic modulators:

Activators of the AMP-activated protein kinase (AMPK) and Peroxisome Proliferator Activated Receptor δ (PPARδ) agonists, Insulins and Trimetazidine.

S5. DIURETICS AND OTHER MASKING AGENTS

The following diuretics and masking agents are prohibited, as are other substances with a similar chemical structure or similar biological effect(s).

(continued)

TABLE 16-1 (CONTINUED)

THE WORLD ANTI-DOPING CODE PROHIBITED SUBSTANCE LIST (2015 LIST)

Including, but not limited to:

- Desmopressin; probenecid; plasma expanders, eg, glycerol and intravenous administration of albumin, dextran, hydroxyethyl starch and mannitol.

- Acetazolamide; amiloride; bumetanide; canrenone; chlortalidone; etacrynic acid; furosemide; indapamide; metolazone; spironolactone; thiazides, eg, bendroflumethiazide, chlorothiazide and hydrochlorothiazide; triamterene and vaptans, eg, tolvaptan.

Except:

- Drospirenone; pamabrom; and topical dorzolamide and brinzolamide.

- Local administration of felypressin in dental anaesthesia.

The detection in an Athlete's Sample at all times or In-Competition, as applicable, of any quantity of the following substances subject to threshold limits: formoterol, salbutamol, cathine, ephedrine, methylephedrine and pseudoephedrine, in conjunction with a diuretic or masking agent, will be considered as an Adverse Analytical Finding unless the Athlete has an approved therapeutic use exemption for that substance in addition to the one granted for the diuretic or masking agent.

SUBSTANCES PROHIBITED IN COMPETITION

In addition to the categories S0 to S5 defined above, the following categories are prohibited In-Competition:

S6. STIMULANTS

All stimulants, including all optical isomers (eg, d- and l-) where relevant, are prohibited.

a: Non Specified Stimulants:

adrafinil	cropropamide	mesocarb
amfepramone	crotetamide	metamfetamine(d-)p-methylam-
amphetamine	fencamine	phetamine
amfetaminil	fenetylline	modafinil
amiphenazole	fenfluramine	norfenfluramine
benfluorex	fenproporex	phendimetrazine
benzylpiperazine	fonturacetam	phentermine
bromantan	furfenorex	prenylamine
clobenzorex	mefenorex	prolintane
cocaine	mephentermine	

A stimulant not expressly listed in this section is a Specified Substance.

b: Specified Stimulants:

benzfetamine	famprofazone	methylhexaneamine
cathine**	fenbutrazate	methylphenidate
cathinone and its analogues	fencamfamin heptaminol	nikethamide
dimethylamphetamine	hydroxyamfetamine	norfenefrine
ephedrine***	isometheptene	octopamine
epinephrine****	levmetamfetamine	oxilofrine
etamivan	meclofenoxate	pemoline
etilamfetamine	methylenedioxymeth-amphetamine	pentetrazol
etilefrine	methylephedrine***	phenethylamine

(continued)

TABLE 16-1 (CONTINUED)

THE WORLD ANTI-DOPING CODE PROHIBITED SUBSTANCE LIST (2015 LIST)

phenmetrazine	pseudoephedrine*****	strychnine
phenpromethamine	selegiline	tenamfetamine
propylhexedrine	sibutramine	tuaminoheptane

and other substances with a similar chemical structure or similar biological effect(s).

Except:

Imidazole derivatives for topical/ophthalmic use and those stimulants included in the 2015 Monitoring Program*.

* Bupropion, caffeine, nicotine, phenylephrine, phenylpropanolamine, pipradrol, and synephrine: These substances are included in the 2015 Monitoring Program, and are not considered Prohibited Substances.

** Cathine: Prohibited when its concentration in urine is greater than 5 micrograms per milliliter.

*** Ephedrine and methylephedrine: Prohibited when the concentration of either in urine is greater than 10 micrograms per milliliter.

**** Epinephrine (adrenaline): Not prohibited in local administration, e.g. nasal, ophthalmologic, or co-administration with local anaesthetic agents.

***** Pseudoephedrine: Prohibited when its concentration in urine is greater than 150 micrograms per milliliter.

S7. NARCOTICS

The following narcotics are prohibited:

buprenorphine	hydromorphone	oxymorphone
dextromoramide	methadone	pentazocine
diamorphine (heroin)	morphine	pethidine
fentanyl (and its derivatives)	oxycodone	

S8. CANNABINOIDS

- Natural, e.g. cannabis, hashish and marijuana, or synthetic 9-tetrahydrocannabinol (THC).

- Cannabimimetics, eg, "Spice", JWH-018, JWH-073, HU-210.

S9. GLUCOCORTICOSTEROIDS

All glucocorticosteroids are prohibited when administered by oral, intravenous, intramuscular or rectal routes.

SUBSTANCES PROHIBITED IN PARTICULAR SPORTS

P.1 ALCOHOL

Alcohol (ethanol) is prohibited In-Competition only, in the following sports. Detection will be conducted by analysis of breath and/or blood. The doping violation threshold is equivalent to a blood alcohol concentration of 0.10 g/L.

- Air Sports
- Archery
- Automobile
- Motorcycling
- Powerboating

P.2 BETA-BLOCKERS

Beta-blockers are prohibited In-Competition only, in the following sports, and also prohibited Out-of-Competition where indicated.

(continued)

Table 16-1 (continued)

The World Anti-Doping Code Prohibited Substance List (2015 list)

- Archery (also prohibited out-of-competition)
- Automobile
- Billiards (all disciplines)
- Darts
- Golf
- Shooting (also prohibited out-of-competition)
- Skiing/Snowboarding (FIS) in ski jumping, freestyle aerials/halfpipe and snowboard halfpipe/big air
- Underwater sports (CMAS) in constant-weight apnoea with or without fins, dynamic apnoea with and without fins, free immersion apnoea, Jump Blue apnoea, spearfishing, static apnoea, target shooting and variable weight apnoea.

Beta-blockers include, but are not limited to, the following:

acebutolol	carvedilol	nadolol
alprenolol	celiprolol	oxprenolol
atenolol	esmolol	pindolol
betaxolol	labetalol	propranolol
bisoprolol	levobunolol	sotalol
bunolol	metipranolol	timolol
carteolol	metoprolol	

For a current list of banned substances visit the WADA web site at http://www.wada-ama.org/.

Adapted from The World Anti-Doping Code 2015 Prohibited List. World Anti-Doping Agency. https://www.wada-ama.org/en/resources/science-medicine/prohibited-list Published September 20, 2014. Accessed May 15, 2015.

it was obtained naturally from the ephedra plant. Fear that the demand for the ephedrine could not be met by its natural supply led to numerous attempts at producing synthetic ephedrine. In an attempt to do this, a University of California Los Angeles graduate student named Gordon Alles produced the d isomer of phenylisopropylamine, later named *dextroamphetamine* (Dexedrine). A mixture of the d and l isomers was then developed and marketed as a nasal decongestant under the brand name Benzedrine. Before that time, a Japanese chemist accidentally produced methamphetamine while also attempting to produce synthetic ephedrine. This was later marketed under the brand name Methedrine. These drugs became collectively referred to as *amphetamines* and in the late 1930s became available by prescription (in tablet form) for the treatment of narcolepsy and ADHD. It was not long after the medical use that their psychomotor stimulant effects were realized, and during World War II amphetamines were widely distributed to soldiers on both sides to help them keep fighting.

Although it is unclear when amphetamine use by athletes began, the American Medical Association and the National Collegiate Athletic Association (NCAA) alleged in 1957 that there was widespread use in athletics to improve performance. Concern for safety began when a Danish

cyclist collapsed and died during the 1960 Olympic Games in Rome, Italy. Originally diagnosed as excessive heat, the cyclist's death was later revealed as a result of amphetamine overdose. This concern only heightened when one of Great Britain's most successful cyclists died while using amphetamines during the 1967 Tour de France. The ergogenic use of amphetamines became more than a question of ethics and safety with the passage of the Controlled Substance Act (Title II of the United States Comprehensive Drug Abuse Prevention and Control Act of 1970). Under this act, amphetamines are classified as controlled substances, making it a felony to possess them without a prescription from a licensed practitioner. However, this does not appear to be a deterrent because amphetamine use continues to be one of the most common causes of positive drug tests in athletics. Athletes with a documented medical condition (such as ADHD) requiring the use of a prohibited substance are usually required to obtain a therapeutic use exemption. In 2011, a total of 105 Major League Baseball (MLB) players were granted exemptions for Adderall. That calculates to about one in every 10 players, which is a much higher rate than the general population and suggests illicit use. Thus, it is not surprising that the number of positive drug tests

	TABLE 16-2	
	BRANDS OF STIMULANT MEDICATIONa	
MEDICATION	**DURATION (HR)**	**ACTIVE DRUG**
Adderall	4	Amphetamine aspartate Amphetamine sulfate Dextroamphetamine saccharate Dextroamphetamine sulfate
Adderall XR	8 to 10	Amphetamine aspartate Amphetamine sulfate Dextroamphetamine saccharate Dextroamphetamine sulfate
Concerta	12	Methylphenidate
Dexedrine	4 to 5	Dextroamphetamine sulfate
Dexedrine Spansule	8	Dextroamphetamine sulfate
Methylin	4	Methylphenidate
ProCentra	4 to 6	Dextroamphetamine sulfate
Ritalin	4	Methylphenidate
Ritalin SR	8	Methylphenidate
Vyvanse	12	Lisdexamfetamine dimesylate
Zenzedi	4 to 6	Dextroamphetamine sulfate
All of the above are classified as a Schedule II controlled substance and are listed as banned substances. aTypically used in the treatment of ADHD.		

for Adderall has increased in both the National Football League (NFL) and MLB in recent years.

Pharmacodynamics

Amphetamines are stimulants of both the CNS and the sympathetic division of the peripheral nervous system. The effects are similar to those of cocaine; however, they last much longer. These sympathomimetic amines (see Chapter 12) increase synaptic dopamine and norepinephrine primarily by stimulating presynaptic release rather than by blockade of reuptake (see Figure 13-1), as in the case with cocaine. As a result, their concentrations increase dramatically in a dose-dependent manner, resulting in greater amounts in the synaptic cleft where they can act on receptors. Dopamine is also a neurotransmitter that, in certain parts of the brain, activates the pleasure center. Amphetamines are structurally related to the catecholamines epinephrine and norepinephrine and act directly on some of the same adrenergic receptors, thus acting as α- and β-agonists. As discussed in Chapter 12, α- and β-sympathetic receptors are cell membrane receptors sensitive to epinephrine and norepinephrine and are found on most cells throughout the body, including the cells of the heart, lungs, and surrounding blood vessels. Consequently, amphetamines exert effects such as increased blood pressure, heart rate, respiratory rate, metabolic rate, and increased plasma free fatty acid levels. Unlike the true catecholamines, amphetamines are able to readily cross the blood-brain barrier, which allows them to act as some of the most potent CNS stimulants.

Possible Ergogenic Effects

It is possible that the CNS stimulant effect of amphetamines would enhance strength, power, speed, reaction time, and agility. Because of their direct and indirect adrenergic stimulation, increases in cardiac output, minute ventilation, and metabolic rate occur, as well as enhanced arousal and alertness. This can also result in an increase in plasma free fatty acid levels that may provide a glycogen-sparing effect and enhance endurance. An oral dose of amphetamine has been shown to induce wakefulness, alertness, energy, motivation, and a decreased sense of fatigue and need for sleep. Additionally, an elevation of mood and an increased self-confidence and ability to concentrate have been observed. The release of dopamine typically induces a sense of elation and aroused euphoria, which may last several hours.

Although improvements in cognitive performance are common, reports have been mixed regarding the effects of amphetamines on athletic performance. Studies conducted over 40 years ago on trained runners, swimmers, and track and field athletes showed positive results, whereas other studies on untrained athletes failed to demonstrate a performance benefit. Many of the earlier studies came under a great deal of criticism, mainly due to small subject number, methodological flaws, and lack of appropriate statistical analyses. Studies conducted 10 to 20 years later demonstrated improvement in anaerobic endurance when amphetamines were administered. However, because there was no increase in oxygen consumption (VO_2) and lactic acid levels increased, it was concluded that amphetamines did not provide any true physiological improvement but only provided a masking of the fatigue due to their CNS stimulant effects. Overall, the amount of change induced by the amphetamines appears to be small, on the order of a few percent. However, in many events, a percent improvement can make the difference between winning and losing. Thus, many athletes still think that the margin of improvement provided by these drugs is beneficial.

Adverse Effects

Some of the possible signs of amphetamine use can be found in Box 16-1. The minor adverse effects associated with amphetamine use include decreased appetite, fever, sweating, headache, restlessness, anxiety, blurred vision, sleeplessness, confusion, and dizziness. Although amphetamines may initially stimulate libido, chronic amphetamine use often leads to decreased sex drive. The serious adverse effects associated with amphetamine abuse are essentially the same as for cocaine and include arrhythmias, sudden cardiac death, stroke, and psychosis. Amphetamines can increase body temperature. As a result, there have been a number of heat stroke fatalities associated with amphetamine use.

All amphetamines can cause catecholamine-mediated cardiotoxicity. Other cardiovascular adverse effects include palpitations, hypertension, myocardial hypertrophy, aneurysm, and coronary artery disease. Amphetamine use is associated with both hemorrhagic and ischemic stroke. Although the mechanism for this is unclear, hypertension has been suggested as the cause. Users of large amount of amphetamines over a long time can develop an amphetamine psychosis, a mental disorder similar to paranoid schizophrenia. Although amphetamine users may feel a temporary boost in self-confidence and power, abuse of the drug can lead to delusions, hallucinations, and a feeling of paranoia. Auditory, tactile, and visual hallucinations are also common. These feelings can cause a person to act in a bizarre, and even violent, fashion. In most people, these effects disappear when they stop using the drug.

Amphetamines cause both physical and psychological dependence. Users can become dependent on the drug to

---

BOX 16-1

SIGNS OF AMPHETAMINE USE

- Dilated pupils
- Dry mouth
- Frequent lip licking
- Restlessness, difficulty sitting still
- Reduced appetite
- Abdominal cramps
- Weight loss
- Irritable, moody
- Tremors
- Argumentative
- Talkative, rapid speech
- Anxiety
- Hallucinations

---

avoid the down feeling they often experience when the drug's effect wears off and those who abruptly stop using amphetamines often experience withdrawal symptoms, such as fatigue, long periods of sleep, irritability, and depression. The length and severity of the depression is often related to the dose and frequency of amphetamine use. Amphetamines also have the potential to produce tolerance (see Chapter 3), which means that when the drug is used on a regular basis, an increased amount of the drug is needed to achieve the desired effects.

Caffeine

Caffeine, known chemically as trimethylxanthine, is a methylxanthine derivative related to theophylline and theobromine. It is probably the most popular drug in the world, and it is found in coffee, tea, cocoa, chocolate, some soft drinks, energy drinks, and numerous medications (Table 16-3). It is also widely used by athletes in their daily lives and during training and competition. However, caffeine is banned by the NCAA (Table 16-4). A test is considered positive if the concentration in the urine exceeds 15 µg/mL. This would be the equivalent of ingesting about 6 cups of coffee before testing. Although the IOC had also banned caffeine at one time, the WADA did not include it on its original list of banned substances that took effect in January 2004 (see Table 16-1). Thus, it is no longer banned by the IOC. However, the WADA continues to monitor the use of caffeine during competition, and, if trends are observed, it is possible that it will once again be banned.

TABLE 16-3

CAFFEINE CONTENT OF SOME COMMON FOODS AND BEVERAGES

ITEM	SIZE (OZ)	CAFFEINE CONTENT (MG)
7-Up or Diet 7-Up	12	0
Mug Root Beer	12	0
Sprite	12	0
Hot cocoa	8	1 to 8
Coffee, decaf	8	2 to 5
5-Hour Energy (decaf)	1.9	6
Tea	8	15 to 80
RC Cola	12	18
Barq's Root Beer	12	22
Coca-Cola	12	35
Pepsi Cola	12	38
Mr. Pibb	12	40
Dr. Pepper	12	42
Sunkist Orange Soda	12	42
Diet Coca-Cola	12	46
Surge	12	52
Mountain Dew	12	55
Josta	12	58
Coffee	8	60 to 180
Vault[a]	12	70
Jolt Cola	12	71
Amp[a]	8	71
Rock Star[a]	8	80
Red Bull[a]	8.4	83
Monster Energy[a]	8	92
Arizona Energy[a]	8	129
Stacker 2 6-Hour Power[a]	2	149
Starbucks Doubleshot	15	162
Jolt Endurance Shot[a]	2	200
5-Hour Energy[a]	1.9	215
Extreme Energy 6 Hour[a]	2	220
NOS Energy Drink[a]	16	224
Rockstar Energy Shot[a]	2.5	229
5-Hour Energy Extra Strength[a]	1.9	242
Anacin	tablet	32
Excedrin	tablet	65
NoDoz	tablet	100
Vivarin and Dexatrim	tablet	200

[a]Marketed as an energy drink.

TABLE 16-4

THE NATIONAL COLLEGIATE ATHLETIC ASSOCIATION LIST OF BANNED DRUG CLASSES

THE NCAA BANS THE FOLLOWING CLASSES OF DRUGS:

- Stimulants

Amphetamine (Adderall); caffeine (guarana); cocaine; ephedrine; fenfluramine (Fen); methamphetamine; methylphenidate (Ritalin); phentermine (Phen); synephrine (bitter orange); methylhexaneamine, "bath salts" (mephedrone); etc.

exceptions: phenylephrine and pseudoephedrine are not banned.

- Anabolic Agents

(sometimes listed as a chemical formula, such as 3,6,17-androstenetrione)

Androstenedione; boldenone; clenbuterol; DHEA (7-Keto); epi-trenbolone; etiocholanolone; methasterone; methandienone; nandrolone; norandrostenedione; stanozolol; stenbolone; testosterone; trenbolone; etc.

- Alcohol and Beta Blockers (banned for rifle only)

Alcohol; atenolol; metoprolol; nadolol; pindolol; propranolol; timolol; etc.

- Diuretics and Other Masking Agents

Bumetanide; chlorothiazide; furosemide; hydrochlorothiazide; probenecid; spironolactone (canrenone); triameterene; trichlormethiazide; etc.

- Street Drugs

Heroin; marijuana; tetrahydrocannabinol (THC); synthetic cannabinoids (eg, spice, K2, JWH-018, JWH-073)

- Peptide Hormones and Analogues

Growth hormone(hGH); human chorionic gonadotropin (hCG); erythropoietin (EPO); etc.

Drugs Subject to Restrictions

- Local anesthetics (under some conditions)
- Beta-2 agonists permitted only by prescription and inhalation
- Caffeine if concentrations in urine exceed 15 micrograms/mL

(continued)

TABLE 16-4 (CONTINUED)
THE NATIONAL COLLEGIATE ATHLETIC ASSOCIATION LIST OF BANNED DRUG CLASSES
The institution and the student-athlete shall be held accountable for all drugs within the banned drug class regardless of whether they have been specifically identified.
Additional examples of banned drugs can be found at www.ncaa.org/drugtesting.
National Collegiate Athletic Association Banned Drugs. National Collegiate Athletic Association. http://www.ncaa.org/health-and-safety/policy/2014-15-ncaa-banned-drugs Published June 2014. Updated November 7, 2014. Accessed May 15, 2015.

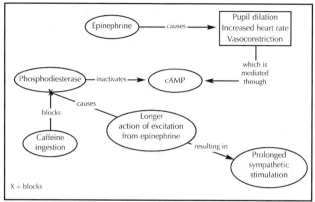

Figure 16-1. How caffeine affects physiological function.

Pharmacodynamics

Caffeine, like amphetamines and cocaine, is a CNS stimulant; however, the effects are milder than those of amphetamines and cocaine. It crosses the membranes of all tissues in the body, including the blood-brain barrier. Because of this, it can exert its effects on both the CNS and the peripheral tissues, resulting in a number of physiological effects. Caffeine interferes with adenosine at multiple sites in the brain. Adenosine is another xanthine that occurs naturally in the human body and acts as a neurotransmitter. As adenosine is created in the brain, it binds to adenosine receptors, causing drowsiness by depressing nerve cell activity. In the brain, adenosine binding also causes vasodilation (presumably to let more oxygen in during sleep). Caffeine is an adenosine receptor antagonist and thus has the opposite effect as adenosine. Therefore, instead of slowing down nerve cell activity, caffeine increases the cell's activity. Because it also blocks adenosine's ability to cause vasodilation, caffeine causes cerebral vasoconstriction. This effect is one reason for the use of caffeine in some headache medicines such as Anacin; caffeine will constrict the blood vessels to help relieve some types of headaches. As discussed in Chapter 7, caffeine may enhance the general analgesic effect when used in combination with other pain relievers, although the mechanism is unclear and caffeine has no analgesic properties when used alone. As mentioned previously, epinephrine is the fight-or-flight hormone, and it has a number of effects on the body such as pupil dilation, increased heart rate, and vasoconstriction. Some of this activity of epinephrine is mediated through the second messenger cyclic adenosine monophosphate (cAMP). Caffeine blocks phosphodiesterase, an enzyme that inactivates cAMP, so the excitatory signals from epinephrine, through cAMP, persist longer. Thus, the effect of caffeine is

to disable braking systems in the brain (adenosine) and the body (phosphodiesterase), resulting in a prolonged sense of wakefulness and alertness (Figure 16-1).

Possible Ergogenic Effects

There appear to be 3 primary mechanisms by which caffeine might provide an ergogenic effect. First, the metabolic theory suggests that caffeine will provide improved endurance due to an increase in fat availability and muscle lipid oxidation with a consequent glycogen sparing effect. The binding of caffeine to adenosine receptors might also block muscle glucose uptake and further reduce carbohydrate use. Second, caffeine may also provide a performance effect via changes in skeletal muscle ion handling. It has been proposed that caffeine can stimulate Na^+-K^+ ATPase activity and Ca^{2+} kinetics. An increased skeletal muscle Ca^{2+} presumably could enhance the strength of muscle contraction. Finally, caffeine has direct effects on the CNS as a stimulant, which can alter the perception of fatigue, increase alertness, and increase motor unit recruitment. The first mechanism would make this a drug of choice for the endurance athlete, whereas the latter 2 would play a greater role in strength and power competitions and events requiring arousal and alertness.

In the 1970s, a number of studies provided support for the ergogenic use of caffeine because improvements in time to exhaustion, work rate, and other measures of endurance were observed. Increased plasma free fatty acid levels and decreased respiratory exchange ratios (indicating increased fat oxidation) were commonly observed, providing support for the metabolic theory. However, during the 1980s, there was a great amount of variability in published findings and conclusions. One factor making caffeine research difficult is the fact that individuals ingest varying levels of caffeine in their habitual diet. Thus, it is difficult to establish groups of subjects with similar tolerance levels to the drug. Several well-controlled studies were published in the 1990s reexamining the performance effects of caffeine. Overall, varying doses of caffeine (ranging from 3 to 13 mg/kg) were shown to improve endurance performance by approximately

20% to 50%. The improvements in performance were associated with increases in plasma epinephrine and free fatty acids and an associated glycogen-sparing effect. However, improvements did not always occur at lower doses. Furthermore, not all studies have reported hormonal and metabolic changes along with improvements in performance. These observations support the central fatigue theory and the ergogenic role of caffeine as a CNS stimulant. Thus, it appears unlikely that increased fat oxidation and glycogen sparing is the prime ergogenic mechanism. More recently, a number of systematic reviews have been performed and have concluded that caffeine is effective for enhancing sport performance in trained athletes when consumed in low-to-moderate dosages (~3 to 6 mg/kg).[1-3] The improvements observed in endurance have been highly variable between studies (Table 16-5). It is suggested that the high degree of variability may be dependent on a number of factors, including ingestion timing, ingestion mode, and subject habituation. It is recommended that the caffeine is ingested no more than 60 minutes before exercise. Evidence also suggests that habitual caffeine use may dampen the degree of performance improvement observed when caffeine naive.

Investigations of high-intensity anaerobic exercise are not as positive as the endurance studies (Table 16-6). In a recent meta-analysis, Brown[2] concluded that caffeine failed to provide an ergogenic effect during repeat sprint performance in team sport athletes. Of the 8 studies included in the analysis, 4 of them independently reported significant benefits on sprint performance; however, these findings were not supported when the data were pooled. In contrast, Astorino[1] found that 11 (65%) of 17 studies revealed significant improvements in performance ranging from 1.0% to 20.0%. Ergogenic doses as small as 100 mg were demonstrated in college athletes; however, the most widely administered dose predominantly shown to be ergogenic was 6 mg/kg. Improvements were uncommon in performance of laboratory-based tests, such as the Wingate test, whereas studies in which exercise bouts completed by athletes simulating the demands of sport, such as swimming, sprint cycling, and repeated sprinting, tended to reveal enhanced performance with caffeine ingestion. Trained athletes appear to be more apt to experience the ergogenic effects of caffeine for high-intensity exercise such as resistance training, tests of peak power, or swimming compared with less active individuals. Data further suggest that the improvements in strength and power are most likely due to caffeine's effect on the CNS, as opposed to a direct effect on muscle. It is interesting to note that in one study, performance improved following ingestion of 6 and 9 mg/kg body mass, whereas urinary levels remained within acceptable limits for NCAA drug testing (see Table 16-4).[4] Only a 13-mg/kg dose or higher would have produced a positive urine test. However, in a separate study, ingesting 9 and 13 mg/kg body mass would have resulted in a positive urine test.[5]

Adverse Effects

The adverse effects associated with caffeine ingestion have been well established. The more minor ones include anxiety, jitters, dizziness, headache, inability to focus, irritability, insomnia, diuresis, and gastrointestinal distress. In the performance studies mentioned previously, these adverse effects were rare at dosages at or below 6 mg/kg but were prevalent at higher doses. One of the more common problems is the effect that caffeine has on sleep. Adenosine receptor activity is important to sleep, and especially to deep sleep. Under the influence of caffeine, one might still be able to fall asleep, but the benefits of deep sleep would probably be missed.

Caffeine can also have a mild diuretic effect. This is of concern for the athlete because dehydration could not only impair performance but also lead to heat illness. However, the majority of the research does not support caffeine-induced diuresis during exercise because core temperature, sweat loss, plasma volume, and urine volume are usually normal when exercising following caffeine ingestion.[6] Because of this, it is now widely accepted that habitual use of caffeine does not influence hydration status negatively. As with most drugs, ingesting higher doses worsens the adverse effects. Adverse effects associated with higher doses also include cardiac arrhythmias and hallucinations. In massive doses, caffeine is lethal. A fatal dose of caffeine can range from 3 to 10 g (about 170 mg/kg body mass), resulting in seizures, tachycardia, or ventricular dysrhythmias. Like the performance effects, the adverse effects associated with caffeine ingestion vary considerably across individuals.

There is also concern that ingesting caffeine on a regular basis (habitual use) might predispose an athlete to increased risk for a number of diseases, such as cardiovascular disease and cancer. However, due to conflicting reports, claims of both acute and chronic adverse effects on the cardiovascular system are inconclusive at this time. The majority of studies examining cardiovascular health have concluded that caffeine consumption does not increase the risk of coronary heart disease or stroke. Habitual caffeine use can lead to a number of other disorders, including anxiety, sleep disorders, dependence, and withdrawal (hence, a degree of physical dependence). Typical withdrawal symptoms associated with caffeine are headache, fatigue, and muscle pain. These symptoms can occur within 24 hours after the last dose of caffeine. Although caffeine is a mild CNS stimulant and may increase dopamine in the CNS, it is generally not considered addicting. This is because most caffeine users, unlike amphetamine users, do not lose control of their caffeine intake.

Ephedrine

The plant species *Ephedra sinica*, *Ephedra equisetina*, and *Ephedra intermedia*, collectively known by their

TABLE 16-5

THE EFFECTS OF CAFFEINE SUPPLEMENTATION ON ENDURANCE PERFORMANCE

REFERENCE	RESEARCH PROTOCOL	RESULTS
Ivy, 1979 *Med Sci Sports Exerc*	Endurance-trained subjects 2 x 250 mg caffeine 120-min cycling at 80 rpm	Increased work production and VO_2 Increased fat oxidation
Casal, 1985 *Med Sci Sports Exerc*	Endurance-trained subjects 400 mg caffeine 45-min run at 75% VO_2 max	Serum FFAs increased No change in VO_2, VCO_2, or RER
Fisher, 1986 *Int J Sports Med*	Habitual caffeine users 5 mg/kg caffeine 60-min run at 75% VO_2 max	Increased exercise VO_2 RER decreased FFA levels increased
Falk, 1989 *Eur J Appl Physiol*	Endurance-trained subjects 5 mg/kg caffeine TTE at 90% VO_2 max	No change in TTE No change in FFA levels
Berry, 1991 *Med Sci Sports Exerc*	Aerobically trained subjects 7 mg/kg caffeine Incremental treadmill test	No change in VO_2, VCO_2, or RER
Dodd, 1991 *Eur J Appl Physiol*	Moderately trained subjects 3 and 5 mg/kg caffeine Graded VO_2 test to exhaustion	Increased resting heart rate Increased resting and exercise FFAs No change in VO_2 or anaerobic threshold
Graham, 1991 *J Appl Physiol*	Endurance-trained subjects 9 mg/kg caffeine TTE at 85% VO_2 max (running and cycling)	44% increase in running TTE 51% increase in cycling TTE Increased plasma epinephrine No change in FFAs or RER
Spriet, 1992 *Am J Physiol*	Recreational cyclists 9 mg/kg caffeine Cycling TTE at 80% VO_2 max	27% increase in TTE 55% decrease in muscle glycogenolysis
Graham, 1995 *J Appl Physiol*	Endurance-trained subjects 3, 6, or 9 mg/kg caffeine TTE at 85% VO_2 max	3 mg/kg: 22% increase in TTE 6 mg/kg: 22% increase in TTE 9 mg/kg: No change in endurance. Increased epinephrine, glycerol, and FFAs
Pasman, 1995 *Int J Sports Med*	Endurance-trained subjects 5, 9, or 13 mg/kg caffeine TTE at 80% maximal power	5, 9, and 13 mg/kg increased TTE 24% to 25%, serum FFAs and glycerol increased
Anderson, 2000 *Int J Sport Nutr Exerc Metab*	Trained female rowers 6 and 9 mg/kg caffeine 2000-m rowing	Both dosages improved 2000-m rowing time
Bruce, 2000 *Med Sci Sports Exerc*	Trained rowers 6 and 9 mg/kg caffeine 2000-m rowing	Both dosages improved 2000-m rowing time and power

(continued)

TABLE 16-5 (CONTINUED)

THE EFFECTS OF CAFFEINE SUPPLEMENTATION ON ENDURANCE PERFORMANCE

REFERENCE	RESEARCH PROTOCOL	RESULTS
Bell, 2002 *J Appl Physiol*	Caffeine users vs nonusers 5 mg/kg caffeine TTE at 80% VO$_2$ max	Nonusers experienced greater increases in TTE than users and the effect lasted longer in the nonusers
Hunter, 2002 *Int J Sport Nutr Exerc Metab*	Trained cyclists 6 mg/kg caffeine 100-km time trials	No change in performance Mean heart rate higher with caffeine No change in peripheral fatigue
Bell, 2003 *Med Sci Sports Exerc*	Recreational cyclists 2.5 and 5 mg/kg caffeine TTE at 80% VO$_2$ max	Improved TTE
Bridge, 2006 *J Sports Sci*	Endurance-trained males 3 mg/kg caffeine 8-km run performance	1.2% improvement in performance time
Wiles, 2006 *J Sports Sci*	Trained cyclists 5 mg/kg caffeine 1-km cycling time trial	Improved performance time, mean speed, mean power, and peak power
Beck, 2008 *J Strength Cond Res*	Untrained men 201 mg caffeine TTE at 85% VO$_2$ max	No change in TTE
Hogervorst, 2008 *Med Sci Sports Exerc*	Trained cyclists 100 mg caffeine TTE at 75% VO$_2$ max following 2.5-h exercise	27% increase in TTE compared with carbohydrate ingestion 84% increase in TTE compared with control Cognitive performance improved
Jenkins, 2008 *Int J Sport Nutr Exerc Metab*	Trained cyclists 1, 2, and 3 mg/kg caffeine Cycling performance	2 mg/kg increased performance by 4% 3 mg/kg increased performance by 3%
Bortolotti, 2014 *J Int Soc Sports Nutr*	Trained cyclists 6 mg/kg caffeine 20-km cycling time trial	No change in speed, power, or RPE
FFA=free fatty acid; RER=respiratory exchange ratio; RPE=rating of perceived exertion; TTE=time to exhaustion.		

Chinese name *ma-huang*, are indigenous to northwestern India, Pakistan, and China. For centuries, the dried stem of these plants has been used as a remedy for numerous medical conditions. In 1923, scientists discovered that the ma-huang plant has 2 primary active ingredients, ephedrine and pseudoephedrine, and in the 1930s ephedrine was the only effective drug being used in the treatment of asthma. At that time, ephedrine was sold OTC and remained available without a prescription until 1954. Like amphetamine, ephedrine and certain ephedrine alkaloids are banned by both the WADA and the NCAA (see Tables 16-1 and 16-4). Pseudoephedrine was on the IOC banned substances list until 2004, when it was replaced by the WADA list. Although the WADA initially only monitored pseudoephedrine, it began prohibiting large doses (>150 µg/mL) in 2010 and continues to do so today. Pseudoephedrine is not included on the NCAA banned substance list. The NFL decided to ban ephedrine before the start of the 2002 season, during which time a number of players tested positive and were suspended. However, the use of ephedrine appears to have declined recently, as the illicit use of ADHD drugs like Ritalin and Adderall has gained popularity.

TABLE 16-6
THE EFFECTS OF CAFFEINE SUPPLEMENTATION ON STRENGTH AND ANAEROBIC PERFORMANCE

REFERENCE	RESEARCH PROTOCOL	RESULTS
Bond, 1986 *Br J Sports Med*	Intercollegiate sprinters 5 mg/kg caffeine Muscle strength	No change in knee extension strength No change in knee flexion strength No change in muscle power
Williams, 1987 *Am J Phys Med*	Physically active subjects 7 mg/kg caffeine Muscle strength and endurance	No change in hand grip strength No change in endurance No change in EMG characteristics
Williams, 1988 *Br J Sports Med*	Caffeine-naïve males 7 mg/kg caffeine Maximal cycling	No change in PP, TTPP, total work, and fatigue
Collomp, 1991 *Int J Sports Med*	Recreationally active subjects 5 mg/kg caffeine Wingate anaerobic test	No change in PP, mean power, or fatigue Increased catecholamines and lactate
Jacobson, 1991 *J Sports Med Phys Fitness*	Recreationally active subjects 300 and 600 mg caffeine Muscle strength and endurance	No change in maximal strength No change in muscle endurance
Anselme, 1992 *Eur J Appl Physiol*	Healthy men and women 250 mg caffeine 6-s sprints on a cycle ergometer	Increased anaerobic power
Collomp, 1992 *Eur J Appl Physiol*	Trained and untrained swimmers 250 mg caffeine 2 x 100-m swim sprints	Trained subjects increased swim velocity Blood lactate increased in both groups
Jacobson, 1992 *Br J Sports Med*	Trained athletes 7 mg/kg caffeine Muscle strength and power	Improvements were observed in some strength, work, and power parameters
Jackman, 1996 *J Appl Physiol*	Endurance-trained subjects 6 mg/kg caffeine TTE at 100% VO_2 max	20% increase in TTE Increased plasma epinephrine No change in glycogen at fatigue
Greer, 1998 *J Appl Physiol*	Healthy men 6 mg/kg caffeine Wingate tests	No improvement in performance
Kalmar, 1999 *J Appl Physiol*	Healthy males 6 mg/kg caffeine Knee extensor strength	Improved muscle activation and isometric TTE
Paton, 2001 *Med Sci Sports Exerc*	Male team sport athletes 6 mg/kg caffeine Ten 20-m sprints	No improvement in performance

(continued)

TABLE 16-6 (CONTINUED)

THE EFFECTS OF CAFFEINE SUPPLEMENTATION ON STRENGTH AND ANAEROBIC PERFORMANCE

REFERENCE	RESEARCH PROTOCOL	RESULTS
Plaskett, 2001 *J Appl Physiol*	Caffeine-naïve males 6 mg/kg caffeine Time to maintain 50% MVC	Knee extensors
Jacobs, 2003 *Med Sci Sports Exerc*	Strength-trained men 4 mg/kg caffeine Leg/bench press and Wingate test	No improvement in performance
Meyers, 2005 *J Appl Physiol*	Caffeine-naïve males 6 mg/kg caffeine Time to maintain 50% MVC	Increases TTE during submaximal isometric contractions
Stuart, 1995 *Med Sci Sports Exerc*	Male rugby players 6 mg/kg caffeine Tests of speed, power, and passing accuracy	Improved speed, power, and passing accuracy
Beck, 2006 *J Strength Cond Res*	Resistance-trained men 201 mg caffeine Muscle strength and endurance Wingate test	Increased bench press 1-RM No change in PP, mean power, or fatigue
Crowe, 2006 *Int J Sport Nutr Exerc Metab*	Recreationally active subjects 6 mg/kg caffeine Two 60-s bouts of max cycling	No improvement in PP or work output No change in cognitive performance
Greer, 2006 *Appl Phys Nutr Metab*	Recreationally active males 5 mg/kg caffeine Wingate test with EMG	No change in PP, mean power, or fatigue No change in EMG variables
Kalmar, 2006 *J Appl Physiol*	Healthy males 6 mg/kg caffeine Knee extension strength	No change in muscle activation or knee extensor strength
Kalmar, 2006 *Exp Brain Res*	Healthy males 6 mg/kg caffeine Plantar flexion strength	No change in muscle activation or plantar flexion strength
Lorino, 2006 *J Strength Cond Res*	Physically active males 6 mg/kg caffeine Agility and Wingate tests	No change in agility No change in PP, mean power, or fatigue
Schneiker, 2006 *Med Sci Sports Exerc*	Male team sport athletes 6 mg/kg caffeine 18 4-s cycle ergometer sprints	Increased total work and mean power

(continued)

TABLE 16-6 (CONTINUED)

THE EFFECTS OF CAFFEINE SUPPLEMENTATION ON STRENGTH AND ANAEROBIC PERFORMANCE

REFERENCE	RESEARCH PROTOCOL	RESULTS
Wiles, 2006 *J Sports Sci*	Trained cyclists 5 mg/kg caffeine 1-km time trial	Improved performance and power output
Forbes, 2007 *Int J Sports Nut Exerc Metab*	Healthy young men and women 2 mg/kg caffeine Bench press at 70% 1RM and Wingate tests	Increased bench press repetitions, no change in Wingate performance
Green, 2007 *Int J Sports Physiol Perform*	Trained males and females 6 mg/kg caffeine Repetitions to failure	Increased leg press repetitions on third (final) set, no change in bench press
Astorino, 2008 *Eur J Appl Physiol*	Strength-trained men 6 mg/kg caffeine Bench/leg press 1RM and reps	No change in 1RM or muscle endurance
Beck, 2008 *J Strength Cond Res*	Untrained men 201 mg caffeine 1RM bench press	No change in bench press strength
Beaven, 2008 *Int J Sports Nutr Exerc Metlab*	Male rugby players 200/400/800 mg caffeine 10-m sprints/resistance exercise	Improved sprint performance
Bliss, 2008 *Med Sci Sports Exerc*	Colligate shot putters 100 mg caffeine Shot put distance	Increased distance thrown
Carr, 2008 *J Sports Med Phys Fitness*	Team sports athletes 6 mg/kg caffeine 5 sets of 6 x 20-m sprints	Improved sprint performance
Del Coso, 2008 *Med Sci Sports Exerc*	Endurance-trained males 5 mg/kg caffeine Maximal cycling power Knee extension MVIC	Increased cycling power Improved maximum voluntary isometric contraction following fatigue
Glaister, 2008 *Med Sci Sports Exerc*	Physically active males 5 mg/kg caffeine Multiple 30-m sprint trials	Improved fastest sprint times
Hoffman, 2008 *J Strength Cond Res*	Strength-trained men 110 mg (in a supplement) Barbell squats at 75% 1RM	Increased number of repetitions on fifth set (6 sets total)

(continued)

TABLE 16-6 (CONTINUED)

THE EFFECTS OF CAFFEINE SUPPLEMENTATION ON STRENGTH AND ANAEROBIC PERFORMANCE

REFERENCE	RESEARCH PROTOCOL	RESULTS
Hudson, 2008 *J Strength Cond Res*	Strength-trained men 6 mg/kg caffeine 4 sets of arm curls and leg extensions to fatigue	Increased leg extension repetitions on set 1 only, no change in curl performance
Park, 2008 *Int J Sport Nutr Exerc Metab*	Healthy college students 6 mg/kg caffeine Knee extension strength	Improved uninjured isometric knee extension strength and muscle activation
Pruscino, 2008 *Int J Sports Nutr Exerc Metlab*	Elite male swimmers 6.2 mg/kg caffeine Two 200-m freestyle time trials	No change in performance
Williams, 2008 *J Strength Cond Res*	Strength-trained men 300 mg caffeine 1RM bench press/pulldown and Wingate test	No change in performance
Woolf, 2008 *Int J Sport Nutr Exerc Metab*	Recreationally active males 5 mg/kg caffeine Wingate anaerobic test Chest and leg press strength	No change in leg press strength Increased chest press strength Increased peak power during Wingate test
Woolf, 2009 *J Strength Cond Res*	Caffeine-naïve football players 5 mg/kg caffeine 40-yd sprint, 20-yd shuttle, bench press	No improvement in speed, anaerobic capacity, or bench press strength
Astorino, 2012 *Amino Acids*	Female soccer athletes 1.3 mg/kg (255 mL Red Bull) Modified T test	No change in repeated sprint performance or RPE

EMG = electromyography; PP = peak power; RPE = rating of perceived exertion; TTE = time to exhaustion; TTPP = time to peak power.

Pharmacodynamics

Like amphetamine, ephedrine and pseudoephedrine are classified as sympathomimetic alkaloids because they directly stimulate the sympathetic or fight-or-flight nervous system. They are structurally similar to amphetamine and have direct α- and β-agonistic properties, as well as catecholamine-releasing actions. Thus, they augment the availability and action of the natural neurotransmitter norepinephrine in the brain and in the heart. Ephedrine is easily absorbed following oral administration, with peak plasma levels occurring within 1 hour of ingestion. Its plasma half-life (t½) is approximately 3 to 6 hours and varies depending on urine pH. Unlike pseudoephedrine, ephedrine also mediates its effects by causing the release of circulating epinephrine.

The increased catecholamine release following ephedrine ingestion is subjected to negative feedback systems, which then tend to inhibit catecholamine release and actions (Figure 16-2). These negative feedback systems include adenosine and prostaglandin release in the synaptic junction and elevated phosphodiesterase enzyme activity, which results in degradation of cAMP. Caffeine interferes with this negative feedback mechanism by inhibiting both adenosine and phosphodiesterase activity and preventing degradation of cAMP. Aspirin also interferes with the negative feedback mechanism via its inhibition of prostaglandin

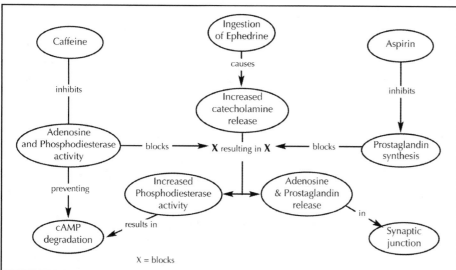

Figure 16-2. How caffeine and aspirin can potentiate the effects of ephedrine.

synthesis. Thus, it is conceivable that either of these mechanisms would potentiate the effects of ephedrine. Because of this, it is common to find athletes ingesting the combination of ephedrine, caffeine, and aspirin.

Possible Ergogenic Effects

Because ephedrine is a sympathomimetic and a CNS stimulant, it is commonly used as an energy enhancer. Thermogenic and lipolytic effects have also led to the claim that ephedrine can improve endurance via increased fat utilization and glycogen sparing during exercise, similar to caffeine. It has been suggested that the thermogenic effects of combining ephedrine and caffeine are synergistic. Like ephedrine, caffeine has a stimulating effect on the CNS and energy metabolism. However, the primary reason for combining the 2 drugs is to potentiate the effects of the ephedrine. Many of the ergogenic claims associated with ephedrine originated from earlier studies investigating its antiobesity and anorectic effects. For some time now, ephedrine and the combination of ephedrine and caffeine have been considered effective weight loss agents, although not all studies support this. Originally, the observed weight loss was attributed solely to the appetite suppressing effects of ephedrine. More recently, increases in metabolism and, more specifically, fat metabolism have been suggested as the mechanism. For example, increases in resting VO_2, fat oxidation, and fat loss were commonly observed during clinical trials investigating the effects of ephedrine and the combination of ephedrine and caffeine. However, it must be noted that only clinically obese individuals were used as subjects in these investigations. Thus, it is likely that the subjects may have been deficient in metabolic rate and/or fat metabolism.

Although the research concerning ephedrine and performance in an athletic population is limited, most of the investigations do not support ergogenic claims. Although ephedrine ingestion has been observed to increase resting VO_2 and fat oxidation in healthy individuals, these changes have not been observed during exercise. Similar observations have been made following pseudoephedrine ingestion. Like VO_2 and fat oxidation, a number of other performance measures have also been unaffected by supplementation. Sidney and Lefcoe[7] administered 24 mg of ephedrine and found no improvements in muscle strength, endurance, power, lung function, reaction time, hand-eye coordination, anaerobic capacity, speed, cardiorespiratory endurance, ratings of perceived exertion, or recovery. Similarly, a single 120-mg dose of pseudoephedrine had no effect on 40-km cycling time, maximal muscle force, or muscle endurance during repeated isometric contractions.[8] More recently, Swain et al[9] administered pseudoephedrine (1 and 2 mg/kg) to trained cyclists and found no changes in ratings of perceived exertion or time to exhaustion.

Performance improvements have been observed when higher doses of ephedrine and caffeine have been combined. Bell et al[10] observed that the combination of caffeine and ephedrine significantly increased cycling time to exhaustion by 38% over a placebo condition, whereas caffeine and ephedrine on their own failed to provide such an effect. In a separate study, the combination of caffeine and ephedrine improved cycling time to exhaustion by 64% over a placebo condition.[11] In both of these studies, ratings of perceived exertion were significantly lower following supplementation, but heart rate was significantly elevated as well. The authors attributed the improvement to CNS stimulation because no changes were observed for VO_2, carbon dioxide production, or fat oxidation. More recently, Bell and Jacobs[12] administered 75 mg of ephedrine with 375 mg of caffeine and observed a slight (5%) but significant improvement running time during a Canadian Forces Warrior Test (3.2-km run while wearing field gear).

Adverse Effects

The spectrum of adverse health events associated with the use of ephedrine cannot be overlooked. Adverse effects were commonly observed in many performance studies. Although it is likely that the occurrence of adverse effects in many cases was the result of misuse, they have also been regularly observed in subjects involved in clinical trials with controlled doses. Some of the minor adverse effects associated with ephedrine include tremors, palpitations, headache, restlessness, anxiety, and insomnia. Because of its direct sympathomimetic effects, ephedrine can cause increases in heart rate, contractility, cardiac output, and peripheral resistance. Thus, increases in both heart rate and blood pressure are common observations following ephedrine ingestion. Although these effects are not serious in most users, the consequences can be severe in those with underlying heart disease, hypertension, diabetes, and those sensitive to ephedrine. A number of investigators have warned against possible interactions between ephedrine and nonsteroidal anti-inflammatory drugs. It is possible that the effects of ephedrine combined with the inhibited production of prostaglandins (vasodilators) might cause a greater than expected rise in blood pressure. The more serious adverse effects of ephedrine use include seizures, severe hypertension, arrhythmias, psychosis, hepatitis, stroke, myocardial injury, and intracranial hemorrhage. It is important to note that the adverse effects do not always depend on the dose consumed because serious problems can occur in susceptible persons with use of low dosages. Furthermore, the toxicity of sympathomimetic agents is exacerbated by physical exercise, dehydration, and increases in body temperature, which are all commonly experienced by athletes during training and competition. Although they are not common, cases of fatal intoxication following ephedrine ingestion have been reported. In instances of ephedrine overdose, cardiovascular and CNS stimulant effects predominate, with myocardial infarction and cerebrovascular accident causing death most often.

Section Summary

Although their efficacy as ergogenic aids can be debated, stimulants continue to be some of the most popular drugs used to enhance performance. In a 2004 survey[13] of collegiate hockey teams, 52% of the players reported stimulant use, which included ephedrine (48%), pseudoephedrine (44%), and amphetamines (4%). The stimulant users had good knowledge about the potential side effects of ephedrine, including sudden death, hypertension, and insomnia, and the majority of the athletes (80%) were aware of the current NCAA ban of ephedrine. Over 40% stated they would use a banned substance if it would help them get to the National Hockey League (NHL). At the time of the study, the NHL did not have a policy for formal testing and penalties with regards to stimulant use; however, they were added to the prohibited substance list as part of the Collective Bargaining Agreement signed in 2013.

The performance gains achieved through amphetamine use appear to be minimal and primarily via CNS stimulation and a masking of fatigue. Greater improvements have been observed from caffeine and the combination of caffeine and ephedrine. Although CNS stimulation is most likely the cause of this, physiological effects such as enhanced fat utilization and glycogen sparing may contribute as well. All stimulants are associated with adverse effects, which worsen with increasing dosages. At this time caffeine and pseudoephedrine can be sold OTC. Caffeine is found in coffee, tea, cocoa, chocolate, some soft drinks, and numerous nutritional supplements marketed as energy boosters and fat burners, whereas pseudoephedrine is an active ingredient in many sinus and allergy medications. Ephedrine and amphetamines are only available with a prescription from a licensed physician for the treatment of medical conditions; thus their use as performance enhancers would be considered illegal. All of the stimulants discussed in this chapter are banned by various sport organizations.

ANABOLIC AGENTS

Anabolic agents are those substances that promote tissue growth. This can occur through a number of pathways; however, the most notable is through enhancing protein synthesis or inhibiting protein degradation. Many athletes turn to drugs developed to enhance tissue growth in the hopes of increasing muscle size and strength. The most common drugs used for this purpose include anabolic-androgenic steroids, human growth hormone (hGH), and *β-agonists*.

Anabolic Steroids

Testosterone is the natural steroid hormone primarily produced by the testes that is responsible for the androgenic and anabolic effects observed during male adolescence and adulthood. The natural and synthetic derivatives of this hormone are known as anabolic-androgenic steroids (AAS). These steroids were first developed as treatments for medical conditions such as delayed puberty, micropenis, aplastic anemia, and hypogonadism in children and for reproductive dysfunction, anemia, hereditary angioedema, metastatic breast cancer, and protein deficiency in adults. They are also commonly used in the management of infection, surgery, burns, acquired immunodeficiency syndrome (AIDS), and trauma. It was not long after the medical use began that their possible influence on performance was recognized, dating as far back as World War II when they were used to improve performance and increase aggressiveness in German troops. In the 1960s, the apparent use of these drugs by Olympic athletes was severe enough to warrant testing for them. However, it was not until the 1976 Olympic Games in Montreal, Canada, that suitable methods were available to enforce a ban. A list of banned anabolic agents can be found in Tables 16-1 and 16-4. Probably the most notorious violation of the IOC's drug policy came in 1988, when Canadian sprinter Ben Johnson was stripped of his gold medal in the 100 meter after testing positive for the use of AAS. In the 1980s, widespread use was also reported in professional football, while use at the collegiate level was realized following the first drug test administered by the NCAA in 1986. Since that time, a number of studies have reported use at the collegiate level. Even more alarming is the fact that a number of studies also report use of AAS by high school students, many of them not even involved in athletics. Recent studies have consistently shown that AAS users typically ingest a wide variety of additional drugs. These include other performance-enhancing drugs as well as classic drugs of abuse.

Once considered drugs for strength and power sports only, AAS use has spread into many other areas, including swimming, boxing, track and field, and winter sports such as snowboarding and bobsledding. Before 2002, MLB had no official policy on steroid use among players. As part of a collective bargaining agreement, players and owners agreed to hold survey testing in 2003 and to put formal testing and penalties into place if more than 5% of the results were positive. It was later announced that 5% to 7% of the test results were positive, resulting in a policy for formal testing and penalties in 2004. Even the Professional Golfers' Association Tour included AAS on its list of prohibited substances as part of the first-ever antidoping program that began in 2008. The development of drugs referred to as *designer steroids* (norboletone and tetrahydrogestrinone) created a challenge to drug testing. These were simple chemical modifications of known banned AAS that could not be detected in existing testing protocols.

It is important to note that the controversy surrounding AAS use is more than a question of ethics and moral judgment. The Anabolic Steroid Control Act of 1992 classified AAS as Schedule III controlled substances. Because of this, it is a felony to possess AAS without a prescription from a licensed physician. Likewise, the illicit distribution of these drugs is also a felony. The use of testosterone precursors such as androstenedione and androstenediol (also steroid hormones) was popularized in the late 1990s as they were classified as nutritional supplements and were available for sale OTC. However, an amendment to the Controlled Substances Act (cited as the Anabolic Steroid Control Act of 2004) classified these hormones as AAS and included them as Schedule III controlled substances. Thus, they are now available as prescription drugs for medical use only. Dehydroepiandrosterone, the immediate precursor to androstenedione, was not included in the amendment and is still available OTC as a supplement.

Pharmacodynamics

Steroid hormones are lipid soluble and passively diffuse across the cell membrane. Once inside the cell, they bind to receptors and interact with the cell's genetic material (DNA). The stimulation of messenger RNA results in the production of new proteins that mediate the hormone's function. Virtually every cell in the body has receptors for AAS. However, physiologically, the anabolic and androgenic effects of AAS are inseparable. When the steroid molecule binds with receptor molecules in various tissues, the same type of receptor produces the anabolic and the androgenic effects. Thus, the effect the steroid has on the cell depends on several factors:

- The location of the cell
- The type of cell
- The type of steroid-metabolizing enzymes contained within the cell

Some of the anabolic effects from the endogenous hormone include increased muscle mass, accelerated bone growth; increased bone density; increased heart, liver, and kidney size; enhanced erythropoiesis; and an enlarged larynx. These are seen in both men and women. The androgenic effects include spermatogenesis; changes in genital size and function; and axillary, facial, and pubic hair growth. Multiple preparations of AAS have been developed, and new forms are made to avoid detection by screening and provide different means of administration. Many attempts have been made in the production of synthetic steroids to eliminate the androgenic effects and enhance the anabolic effects. However, this is most likely physiologically impossible.

Anabolic steroids are often classified as either testosterone based, dihydrotestosterone based or 19-nortestosterone based (Nandrolone). These drugs can be administered orally or parenterally (by intramuscular injection or transdermal application). Those taken orally usually have a short t½, generally on the order of several hours, whereas those injected tend to have a longer t½, usually around 1 to 3 days. Orally ingested compounds are absorbed from the gastrointestinal tract and must first pass through the liver before entering the blood to be distributed throughout the body. To prevent rapid breakdown by the liver, many oral AAS are chemically modified by the manufacturer by a process called alkylation (C-17 alkylated steroids). Injected steroids are slowly absorbed into the bloodstream without a first pass through the liver (see Chapter 2). Consequently, the liver experiences a much lower concentration than with orally administered AAS. Most injected steroid compounds are not alkylated but are chemically modified to form esters. Esters increase the half-lives of injectable AAS because they have a slower rate of breakdown. The ester also makes the steroid compound less water soluble and more fat soluble. This makes it more difficult for the blood to pick it up and carry it into circulation, and likewise slows the rate the drug can leave the injection site. When a steroid has an ester attached, the steroid is rendered inactive because the ester prevents it from binding to a receptor. As a result, an inactive deposit of steroid can sit at the site of injection, releasing slowly for days into the bloodstream. Once free in the blood, the ester is removed by enzymes, and the steroid is rendered active.

Possible Ergogenic Effects

Regardless of administration, AAS are believed to increase muscle mass and strength by 3 mechanisms. First, AAS increase protein synthesis. As mentioned above, the binding of the steroid hormone to specific steroid receptors located in cells of target tissues stimulates an increased production of messenger and ribosomal RNA.[14] The increased amount of RNA is then used by the muscle cells to produce more protein, leading to increases in muscle mass and strength. Second, AAS inhibit protein degradation. Glucocorticoids are hormones that have a catabolic effect on the body via protein degradation. They are released during times of stress, which would include intense exercise or training. Anabolic steroids compete with glucocorticoids for receptor sites, thus inhibiting protein degradation. It has been suggested that it is through this mechanism that AAS provide the greatest increases in muscle size and strength. Through an improved use of protein, AAS can convert a negative nitrogen balance to a positive one, increasing nitrogen retention. Finally, it has been suggested that the use of AAS provides a psychological effect. Individuals taking AAS frequently exhibit aggressive behavior, a state of euphoria, and a diminished sense of fatigue, allowing them to train at higher intensities and longer durations. The possibility of a placebo effect associated with this psychological result cannot be ruled out.

A number of studies have shown that increased levels of testosterone can increase protein synthesis, muscle strength, and lean body mass. However, other studies investigating the efficacy of AAS use for enhanced strength provide inconsistent results. Results of studies evaluating AAS are difficult to evaluate because of methodological and dosing differences. For example, in an analysis of studies investigating AAS and muscle strength, Haupt and Rovere[15] concluded that an athlete must have been intensively trained in resistance training prior to AAS use and that the intense training must continue during this use. They also concluded that improvements in muscle strength can only occur if the athlete maintains a high-protein, high-caloric diet when using AAS. Likewise, Elashoff et al[16] attempted to analyze 30 studies investigating the effects of AAS on muscle strength. Twenty-one of those studies were eliminated from the analysis, primarily due to methodological flaws. From the remaining 9 studies, they concluded that AAS may slightly enhance muscle strength in previously trained athletes. However, no firm conclusion could be made regarding the effects of AAS on overall athletic performance. They also pointed out that the stud-

ies they reviewed used low dosages and that it is difficult to generalize the results of clinical investigations to the actual athletic setting. Individuals who use AAS often use 10 to 100 times the therapeutic dose and often stack (taking more than one AAS simultaneously) a number of different steroids. In one study of weight-training athletes taking AAS, the lowest dosage reported was equivalent to 350% of the usual therapeutic dose.[17]

The majority of strength-training studies in which body weight was assessed report greater increases in weight under steroid treatment than under placebo treatment. In studies using higher dosing over longer periods, the effects seem to be more pronounced. Although it has been suggested that the increase is due to greater lean body mass, the extent to which increased water and electrolyte retention accounts for body mass changes remains to be resolved. However, the American College of Sports Medicine acknowledges that AAS, in the presence of adequate diet, can contribute to increases in body weight, often in the lean mass compartment, and that the gains in muscular strength achieved through high-intensity exercise and proper diet can be increased by the use of AAS in some individuals. It is generally accepted that adequate protein intake and high-intensity training in previously trained individuals are required for these gains to occur.

Adverse Effects

The immediate and long-term adverse effects associated with AAS use are well established and typically involve the hepatic, reproductive, cardiovascular, musculoskeletal, immune, and psychological systems (for review see Kersey[18]). Hepatic abnormalities are probably the most serious adverse effects of AAS use currently documented. Changes in liver enzyme levels are generally used to monitor liver function. Elevations in these enzymes have been reported during AAS use but return to normal when use is discontinued. Cholestatic jaundice and peliosis hepatis (blood-filled cysts of unknown etiology) are relatively common and typically occur when alkylated agents, such as methyltestosterone, methandrostenolone, oxymetholone, oxandrolone, and stanozolol, are used. As mentioned previously, the alkylated agents are those primarily administered orally. However, a few alkylated steroids that are usually administered orally are also available as injectable compounds (methandrostenolone and stanozolol), and these have similar effects on the liver as the oral AAS. Nonalkylated agents, such as testosterone and nortestosterone, are less likely to produce liver damage.

Hypogonadism has also been associated with AAS use. This results in a decline in sperm count, abnormal sperm morphology, and testicular atrophy. The mechanism for this involves a negative loop of the pituitary and gonads, causing a dose-dependent depression of luteinizing hormone and follicle-stimulating hormone. This is also associated with significant decreases in plasma testosterone. Androgenic hormones can also be converted to the female sex hormones estradiol and estrone in the extragonadal tissues. This results in feminizing effects such as increased voice pitch and gynecomastia in males.

The use of AAS can lead to detrimental changes in serum lipid profiles. These changes, which include decreases in high-density lipoprotein cholesterol and increases in low-density lipoprotein cholesterol, have been associated with the development of cardiovascular disease. The more serious cardiovascular effects include hypertension, myocardial ischemia, and sudden cardiac death. As an example, electrocardiographic changes reflecting altered myocardium in the hypertrophied heart were observed in power athletes taking large doses of AAS. However, the true relationship between AAS use and serious cardiovascular effects is not fully understood at this time.

Another area of concern with AAS use is the potential psychological effects. Cooper et al[19] found that AAS use directly caused significant disturbances in personality profile as assessed by the Diagnostic and Statistical Manual of Mental Disorders. Aggressive behavior, mood changes, and psychiatric events, including acute paranoia, delirium, mania or hypomania, and homicidal rage, have been reported with AAS use. Episodes of depression, anxiety, and hostility have also been reported. Anabolic steroid users have reported higher rates of aggressive feelings, verbal aggression, and aggression toward objects while on the agents as compared with off of them. The general conclusion is that these episodes are not frequent when lower dosages are used but are more prevalent at higher dosages. It has also been suggested that AAS are addictive and that body type dissatisfaction and an obsession with increases in size and strength obtained with AAS contribute to patterns of dependent use and abuse.[20]

Although the effects of AAS use by females are not as well documented as those of males, adverse effects include hirsutism (changes in hair growth patterns, including facial hair), acne, deepening of the voice, clitoral hypertrophy, kidney and liver dysfunction, decreased breast mass, increased abdominal fat accumulation, male pattern baldness, and general virilization. The nonmedical use of AAS can also have serious consequences for adolescents, such as severe facial and body acne, premature skeletal maturation (premature closing of the growth plates), and decreased spermatogenesis.

Although clinical testing is the most reliable method of detecting illicit AAS use, there are numerous physical signs that may cause suspicion (Box 16-2). These include muscular hypertrophy, oily skin and acne, jaundice in the skin or eyes, gynecomastia, hepatomegaly, testicular atrophy and edema, and mood changes or aggression.

Human Growth Hormone

hGH, otherwise known as *somatotropin*, is a polypeptide hormone that mediates numerous metabolic and growth

---

Box 16-2

SIGNS OF ANABOLIC STEROID USE

- Dramatic increase in body bulk
- Wide and erratic mood swings
- Increased aggressiveness ("steroid rage") and irritability
- Irrational behavior and depression
- Increased presence of acne (oily skin and hair)
- Jaundice, usually only with the use of oral anabolic steroids
- Hypertension, increased low-density lipoprotein cholesterol, and decreased high-density lipoprotein cholesterol
- In males, premature balding, gynecomastia (increased breast size), testicular atrophy, and decreased sperm production
- In females, male pattern balding, enlarged clitoris, growth of coarse facial hair, deepened voice, reduction in breast size, and change in or cessation of menstruation

---

processes in the human body. Although a number of growth hormone peptides exist in the body, the most common is a single-strand polypeptide composed of 191 amino acids (about 21% of all circulating hGH). This hormone is used clinically to treat children's growth disorders and adult growth hormone deficiency. In recent years, replacement therapies with hGH have become extremely popular in the battle against aging. Touted as the fountain of youth, reported effects of hGH therapy include decreased body fat, increased lean mass, increased bone density, increased energy levels, improved skin tone and texture, improved immune system function, and an enhanced sense of well-being. However, the research involving hGH has not been limited to the aging because its role as an anabolic agent in a young, healthy population has also been investigated. At this time, hGH is still considered to be a very complex hormone and many of its functions are still unknown.

hGH has been used by competitors in a variety of sports since the 1970s. Although it has been banned by the NCAA and IOC for quite some time (see Tables 16-1 and 16-4), traditional urine analyses were not able to distinguish between its natural and synthetic forms. Thus, the ban could not be enforced. However, in the early 2000s, blood tests were developed that could detect doping with hGH. Because of this, the WADA collected approximately 3000 blood samples at the 2004 Olympic Games in Athens, Greece, with hGH being the primary target. This testing continued at the 2008 Olympic Games in Beijing, China. The use of hGH continues to be controversial because a wide range of both amateur and professional athletes have been implicated in or confessed to illicit hGH use. As a result, hGH has been banned by other sport organizations such as the NHL and MLB. The NFL began testing for hGH during the 2014 season. Although hGH is not classified as a controlled substance, its prescription and distribution for athletic enhancement is considered illegal.

Pharmacodynamics

hGH is synthesized in and secreted from the anterior pituitary gland in a pulsatile manner throughout the day. Under basal conditions, hGH levels in a normal adult are relatively low. Surges of secretion occur at 3- to 5-hour intervals, with the greatest surge occurring 60 to 90 minutes after the onset of deep sleep. The secretion of hGH is regulated by 2 hypothalamic hormones: GH-releasing hormone, which stimulates its release, and somatostatin, which inhibits it. A number of factors are known to affect these hormones and hGH secretion, such as age, sex, diet, exercise, stress, and other hormones. Secretion can be suppressed by a negative feedback on the hypothalamus and pituitary. This occurs when blood levels of hGH increase.

The effects of hGH on tissues are exerted directly and through the mediation of insulin-like growth factors. Because polypeptide hormones are not fat soluble, they cannot penetrate the sarcolemma. Thus, hGH exerts its effects directly by binding to receptors on target cells, such as muscle and fat cells. The binding to a receptor activates a secondary messenger, which then directs its actions to specific areas in the cell. Through this mechanism, hGH is a potent anabolic agent because it promotes muscle, bone, and cartilage growth via enhanced cellular amino acid uptake and protein synthesis. However, hGH also exerts its anabolic effect indirectly via another potent anabolic hormone: insulin-like growth factor-1 (IGF-1).

hGH mediates numerous metabolic processes, such as promotion of glucose and amino acid transport into muscle and fat, diversion of amino acids from oxidation to protein synthesis, retention of intracellular electrolytes, and stimulation of lipolysis in fat and muscle. Thus, it has the ability to alter the source of fuel from carbohydrate to fat.[21] However, because more than one form of it exists in the human body, the overall physiological effects of hGH are not completely understood at this time.

Possible Ergogenic Effects

Exogenous hGH administration requires intramuscular or subcutaneous injection of recombinant hGH. Recombinant hGH is primarily used to increase muscle size and strength. However, the possible anabolic effects combined with the lipolytic effects make it an appealing drug for bodybuilders and those concerned with cosmetic appearance. Increases in lean body mass have been observed in hGH- or IGF-1-deficient adult patients and in an elderly population (who have typically low hGH concentrations) after receiving hGH treatment. In addition to increases in muscle mass, improvements in muscle strength and exercise capacity have also been observed in the hGH-deficient population. When groups of young healthy subjects are administered hGH, the results are not as consistent. In an examination of power-trained athletes, Deyssig et al[22] observed significant increases in serum hGH, IGF-1, and IGF-1 binding protein following 6 weeks of hGH treatment. However, these increases were not associated with any changes in lean body mass or strength. Likewise, in 2 separate studies, hGH administration failed to increase muscle protein synthesis and muscle strength in both trained[23] and untrained[24] young men. Whole-body protein synthesis rates increased but were attributed to decreased amino acid oxidation. They concluded that the increases in fat-free mass commonly observed during hGH treatment were probably from lean tissue other than skeletal muscle. In contrast, Crist et al[25] observed a significant increase in fat-free weight, a significant decrease in percent body fat, and an improved ratio of fat-free weight to fat weight in highly conditioned subjects following 6 weeks of hGH treatment. The primary cause of these changes appeared to be lipolysis. Elevations in circulating levels of IGF-1 were also observed in that study. Some of these studies were included in a recent analysis of hGH and its effects on performance. Liu et al[26] analyzed 27 studies investigating the effects of hGH on a young healthy population. Studies that included patients with a medical condition or administered hGH as a treatment for a specific illness were excluded from the analysis. They concluded that although hGH might increase lean body mass in the short term, it does not appear to improve strength or athletic performance. They also pointed out that the studies they reviewed likely used dosages lower than those used by athletes. It is important to note that when exogenous hGH is administered, it is only in one form. As mentioned previously, numerous forms of hGH are found in the body and these may be the true source of the anabolic potential.

Adverse Effects

Although the use of exogenous hGH is fairly common among athletes and bodybuilders, the data from this population are limited. Thus, the majority of what is known regarding the adverse effects of excess hGH has been obtained through the clinical evaluation of acromegaly (Box 16-3). Acromegaly is the clinical condition in which the pituitary gland naturally oversecretes hGH. It is characterized by bony overgrowth, which is particularly noticeable in the mandible, the supraorbital ridges, and the enlargement of the hands and feet. Other clinical symptoms can include facial and aural soft tissue swelling; profuse sweating; deepening of the voice; gigantism; accelerated osteoarthritis; and visceral growth of cardiac, hepatic, renal, pulmonary, and thyroidal tissue. Growth hormone administration may have profound adverse effects on other hormonal systems and metabolic processes. Prolonged exposure to excessive amounts of hGH can also cause a suppression of endogenous hGH release and insulin resistance. In one of the few studies involving an athletic population, diminished hGH response to natural stimuli was observed following 6 weeks of exogenous hGH treatment.[25] In the previously mentioned analysis, Liu[26] also concluded that hGH use by healthy young subjects is frequently associated with adverse events. However, a complete understanding of the adverse effects experienced by a healthy athletic population injecting hGH is not possible at this time.

β-Agonists

As discussed in Chapter 12, a β-agonist is defined as any compound that stimulates β-adrenergic receptors. Oral or inhaled forms of these drugs are traditionally used for the treatment of bronchial ailments. For example, short-acting inhaled β_2-agonists are commonly used prophylactically before exercise by those diagnosed with asthma or exercise-induced asthma (see Table 9-6). However, because of their sympathomimetic properties, concerns have been raised regarding the potential unfair competitive advantage they provide. They have gained even greater popularity as performance enhancers as their potential anabolic effects have been realized. Common β-agonists include albuterol (also known as *salbutamol* in other countries), bambuterol and clenbuterol (neither approved for therapeutic use in the United States), and terbutaline. At this time, clenbuterol, which at one time was the most popular β-agonist used to enhance performance, is not approved by the FDA for human use and has been banned by the NCAA and the WADA (it was banned by the IOC in 1992 as a stimulant but is now classified as an anabolic agent). Its anabolic properties have seen it used in food-producing animals to increase lean meat yield. However, concerns about toxicity to humans from contaminated meat led to its use for this purpose being banned in the United States in 1991. Despite this, at the 1992 Olympic Games in Barcelona, Spain, 2 American athletes tested positive for clenbuterol and were disqualified from competition. However, because β_2-agonists are commonly used in the management of asthma, the NCAA and the WADA allow for the use of some inhaled β_2-agonists (IBAs), but only with prior written notification (Table 16-7). The WADA recently dropped the requirement of a therapeutic use exemption for the use of salbutamol and salmeterol and now only requires a simplified declaration of use. Sports with the highest percentage of athletes approved for inhaled IBA use during international competition include cycling, triathlon, swimming, cross-country skiing, and some ice sports.

Pharmacodynamics

As mentioned previously, β-adrenergic receptors are characterized by their interaction with epinephrine and

Box 16-3
Adverse Effects Associated With Excessive Growth Hormone

METABOLIC CHANGES

Diabetes mellitus

Hypercalciuria

Impaired glucose tolerance

Insulin resistance

NEUROMUSCULAR MANIFESTATIONS

Headache

Hypertrophic neuropathy

Myopathy

Nerve impingement (carpal tunnel syndrome)

Sleep apnea

Visual field loss

SKIN AND CONNECTIVE TISSUE GROWTH

Excessive sweating

Facial and acral (fingers, feet ,etc) soft tissue swelling

Hirsutism

Laryngeal thickening (causing deep voice)

SKELETAL AND ARTICULAR CHANGES

Articular cartilage growth (accelerated osteoarthritis)

Cranial growth

Costal growth (barrel chest)

Gigantism

Mandibular growth (lantern jaw)

Nasal cartilage growth

Phalangeal bony overgrowth

Vertebral bony overgrowth

VISCERAL GROWTH

Cardiac (ventricular and septal thickening)

Hepatic

Pulmonary

Renal

Thyroid

norepinephrine. The β-receptors can be classified as either β_1 or β_2 based on their affinity for certain compounds (see Chapter 12). Stimulation of β_1-receptors is associated with increased heart rate and cardiac contractility. Simulation of β_2-receptors is generally associated with bronchial and vascular smooth muscle relaxation and a stabilizing effect on

TABLE 16-7

β-AGONISTS PERMITTED BY WADA IN INHALANT FORM WITH A THERAPEUTIC USE EXEMPTION

GENERIC NAME	TRADE NAME
formoterol[a]	Foradil
salbutamol	Proventil
	Ventolin
salmeterol[b]	Serevent
terbutaline	Brethaire

[a]The presence in urine of salbutamol in excess of 1000 ng/mL or formoterol in excess of 40 ng/mL is presumed not to be an intended therapeutic use of the substance and will be considered as an adverse analytical finding unless the athlete proves, through a controlled pharmacokinetic study, that the abnormal result was the consequence of the use of the therapeutic inhaled dose up to the maximum indicated above.

[b]Use of salbutamol and salmeterol by inhalation no longer requires a therapeutic use exemption but rather a simplified declaration of use.

mast cells, thus preventing the release of histamine and other inflammatory mediators. β-agonists bind to β-receptors on cardiac and smooth muscle tissues. They also have important actions in other tissues, especially bronchial smooth muscle and the liver. In general, β-agonists can be classified as sympathomimetic amines (eg, amphetamine and ephedrine). Thus, they mimic the actions of sympathetic adrenergic stimulation acting through β-adrenergic receptors.

Possible Ergogenic Effects

Interest in β-agonists as performance enhancers began with studies involving veterinary applications. In animal models, β-agonists have been shown to prevent protein breakdown, increase skeletal muscle hypertrophy, and decrease fat deposition. The primary mechanism behind the anabolic effects appears to be a reduction of protein degradation. The dosages used to achieve the anabolic and lipolytic effects were much greater than those used for bronchodilation (up to 100 times). Similar anabolic effects have not been observed in human studies (Table 16-8). More recently, a number of systematic reviews have been performed and have concluded that oral β-agonist administration can improve muscle strength, anaerobic power and endurance performance in trained nonasthmatic subjects and that these improvements are commonly associated with hormonal and metabolic changes.[27-29] As seen in the animal studies, the dose needed to obtain an ergogenic effect is higher than that used for therapeutic purposes in asthma. There is also minimal support for increases in strength in nonathletic populations; however, these were also not associated with an anabolic effect (the proposed ergogenic mechanism).

In contrast to oral administration, inhaled $β_2$-agonists seem to be without relevant effect on performance in trained nonasthmatic athletes (Table 16-9). While the majority of studies have demonstrated improved pulmonary function, this should not be regarded as ergogenic. A review by 9 international experts looked at 26 separate studies involving over 400 participants and concluded that there was no evidence that inhaled $β_2$-agonists improve aerobic or anaerobic capacity.[29] For example, Meeuwisse et al[30] failed to observe improvements in anaerobic power in highly trained athletes following administration of albuterol in aerosol form. In a similar study, Lemmer et al[31] administered twice the normal dosage (360 μg) of albuterol and still found no improvement. Additionally, McKenzie et al[32] administered therapeutic doses of albuterol in aerosol form to healthy track and field athletes and found no change in pulmonary function, VO$_2$ max, heart rate, and anaerobic threshold. It is interesting to note that a paper published in the *Clinical Journal of Sports Medicine* reported that asthmatic athletes have consistently outperformed healthy athletes in every Olympic Games since 2000.[33] Unpublished data from the IOC Independent Asthma Panel show that 19.1% of swimmers were approved to use IBAs at the Beijing Olympics and won 32.9% of the individual medals awarded. In addition, 17.3% of cyclists were permitted to use IBAs and won 28.9% of individual medals. At this time, the efficacy of β-agonist use for performance enhancement remains unclear. Despite the lack of solid evidence from human trials, these drugs have become very popular at all levels of competition. Like hGH, the lipolytic potential of β-agonists makes them desirable for bodybuilders as well as strength and power athletes.

Adverse Effects

The majority of what is known regarding adverse effects associated with β-agonists has been obtained from patients being treated with these drugs and from people who have eaten meat from animals treated with the drugs. Common adverse effects can be found in Figure 16-3. Adverse effects of β-agonists are considered minimal if they are inhaled using recommended doses. These include skeletal muscle tremor, nervousness, and palpitations. Some of the other adverse effects include headaches and insomnia. However, the fact that little is known about β-agonists, particularly at dosages used for the anabolic effects, makes it a very dangerous drug. A recent animal study[34] using albuterol injections at doping doses reported bone loss because of the treatment. The bone loss occurred independently of an anabolic effect on muscle mass and was equally severe in sedentary and exercising rats. At higher doses, more serious adverse effects

Table 16-8

Effects of Oral β_2-Agonists on Performance in Nonasthmatic Subjects

REFERENCE	DRUG AND SUBJECTS	RESULTS
Martineau, 1992 *Clin Sci (Lond)*	Salbutamol, 16 mg/day (3 wk) Healthy subjects	Inconsistent improvements in muscle strength
Caruso, 1995 *Med Sci Sports Exerc*	Albuterol, 16 mg/day (6 wk) Strength-trained subjects	Improved isokinetic strength, power, and work
Collomp, 2000 *Int J Sports Med*	Salbutamol, 6 mg Healthy, moderately trained	Improved cycling TTE and substrate availability
Collomp, 2000 *J Appl Physiol*	Salbutamol, 12 mg/day (3 wk) Healthy, recreational athletes	Improved cycling TTE and substrate availability
Van Baak, 2000 *Med Sci Sports Exerc*	Salbutamol, 4 mg Healthy, active males	Improved isokinetic strength and cycling TTE
Collomp, 2002 *Int J Sports Med*	Salbutamol, 12 mg/day (3 wk) Healthy, moderately trained	No change in mean power during 10 min of max cycling
Caruso, 2005 *J Strength Cond Res*	Albuterol, 16 mg/day (3 wk) Healthy men	Improved isokinetic knee flexion and extension strength
Collomp, 2005 *Int J Sports Med*	Salbutamol, 4 mg Healthy, recreational athletes	Improved PP and AP during a Wingate test
Le Panse, 2005 *Int J Sports Med*	Salbutamol 12 mg/day (3 wk) Strength trained and sedentary	Improved PP and TTPP during a Wingate test
Arlettaz, 2006 *Int J Sports Med*	Salbutamol, 4 mg Healthy, moderately trained	No change in cycling TTE or lactate
Le Panse, 2006 *Br J Sports Med*	Salbutamol, 12 mg/day (4 wk) Trained and sedentary females	Improved Wingate PP and TTPP, no change in lean body mass
Le Panse, 2007 *Br J Sports Med*	Salbutamol, 4 mg Healthy, moderately trained	Improved PP, mean power, and TTPP
Andersen, 2009 *J Exerc Physiol*	Salbutamol, 4 mg Highly endurance trained	Improved running TTE
Crivelli, 2011 *Acta Physiol*	Salbutamol, 6 mg Recreational male athletes	No change in maximal isometric strength or fatigue
Decorte, 2014 *Scand J Med Sci Sports*	Salbutamol Healthy, strength trained	Improved muscle power, total work, and muscle endurance

AP = average power; PP = peak power; TTE = time to exhaustion; TTPP = time to peak power.

could include cardiac arrhythmias. Myocardial hypertrophy has been reported as an adverse effect of clenbuterol and other β-agonists in animal studies. This is a known factor in sudden cardiac death in athletes. Reports of adverse effects by illegal users of clenbuterol in the United States are understandably minimal. However, it has been anecdotally reported that the deaths of 2 professional bodybuilders from Europe were the result of clenbuterol use.

It is important to recognize that regular use of IBAs leads quickly to tolerance and their bronchoprotective effect is rapidly diminished. For this reason, the minimum dose and frequency of IBAs to protect against bronchospasm and to

TABLE 16-9

EFFECTS OF INHALED β_2-AGONISTS ON PERFORMANCE IN NONASTHMATIC SUBJECTS

REFERENCE	DRUG AND SUBJECTS	RESULTS
McKenzie, 1983 *Med Sci Sports Exerc*	Salbutamol, 800 µg/day (1 wk) Endurance trained	No change in VO$_2$ max or anaerobic threshold
Bedi, 1988 *Can J Sport Sci*	Albuterol, 180 µg Cyclists and triathletes	Endurance performance unchanged, final sprint improved
Booth, 1988 *NZ J Physiother*	Salbutamol, 100 µg Cyclists	No change in maximum workload during max incremental cycling
Gong, 1988 *Arch Environ Health*	Albuterol, 180 µg Cyclists	No change in VO$_2$ max or sprint TTE in 0.21 ppm ozone
Meeuwisse, 1992 *Med Sci Sports Exerc*	Salbutamol, 200 µg Cyclists	No change in VO$_2$ max or final sprint performance
Morton, 1992 *Clin J Sport Med*	Salbutamol, 200 µg Endurance-trained runners	No change in VO$_2$ max, running TTE, or Wingate test performance
Signorile, 1992 *Int J Sports Med*	Albuterol, 360 µg Recreational athletes	Increased peak power during 15-s Wingate test
Fleck, 1993 *Int J Sports Med*	Albuterol, 360 µg Highly trained cyclists	No change in VO$_2$ max, RPE, or workload
Morton, 1993 *Clin J Sport Med*	Salbutamol, 200 µg Power athletes	No change in isokinetic strength or anaerobic performance
Unnithan, 1994 *Pediatr Pulmonol*	Terbutaline, 500 µg Healthy adolescent boys	No change in VO$_2$ max or running time to VO$_2$ max, submax RER elevated
Heir, 1995 *Scand J Med Sci Sports*	Salbutamol, 50 µg/kg Cross-country skiers, marathon runners	No change in VO$_2$ max, running TTE decreased
Lemmer, 1995 *Int J Sports Med*	Albuterol, 360 µg Highly trained cyclists	No change in Wingate test performance or lactate
Morton, 1996 *Clin J Sport Med*	Salmeterol, 50 µg Cyclists and triathletes	No change in isokinetic strength, anaerobic performance, reaction time, or motor control
Norris, 1996 *Eur J Appl Physiol Occup Physiol*	Salbutamol, 400 µg Cyclists	No change in VO$_2$ max, 20-km cycling time, or anaerobic performance
Carlsen, 1997 *Scand J Med Sci Sports*	Salbutamol, 800 µg/salmeterol, 50 µg Cross-country skiers, biathletes, distance runners	No change in VO$_2$ or anaerobic threshold, running TTE decreased
McDowell, 1997 *J Allergy Clin Immunol*	Salmeterol, 42 µg Cyclists	No change in anaerobic performance or lactate
Larsson, 1997 *Med Sci Sports Exerc*	Terbutaline, 3 mg Cross-country skiers, distance runners, cyclists	No change in VO$_2$, ventilation, or running TTE in cold air

(continued)

TABLE 16-9 (CONTINUED)

EFFECTS OF INHALED β_2-AGONISTS ON PERFORMANCE IN NONASTHMATIC SUBJECTS

REFERENCE	DRUG AND SUBJECTS	RESULTS
Sandsund, 1998 *Eur J Appl Physiol Occup Physiol*	Salbutamol, 400 µg Cross-country skiers	No change in VO_2 max, running TTE, or lactate
Sue-Chu, 1999 *Scand J Med Sci Sports*	Salmeterol, 50 µg Cross-country skiers	No change in VO_2, running TTE, or lactate in cold air
Carlsen, 2001 *Respir Med*	Formoterol, 9 µg Cross-country skiers, others	No change in VO_2 max, maximum ventilation, or running TTE
Goubault, 2001 *Thorax*	Salbutamol, 200/800 µg Triathletes	No change in cycling TTE, lactate, or psychomotor performance
Stewart, 2002 *Med Sci Sports Exerc*	Salbutamol, 400 µg/formoterol, 12 µg Highly trained athletes	No change in VO_2 max or anaerobic performance
van Baak, 2004 *Int J Sports Med*	Salbutamol, 800 µg Cyclists and triathletes	Time trial performance increased (1.9%), no change in lactate
Riiser, 2006 *Med Sci Sports Exerc*	Formoterol, 18 µg Cross-country skiers	No change in VO_2 max, maximum ventilation, or running TTE in hypobaric conditions
Tjorhom, 2007 *Scand J Med Sci Sports*	Formoterol, 18 µg Cross-country skiers	No change in VO_2, ventilation, or running TTE in cold air
Decorte, 2008 *Med Sci Sports Exerc*	Salbutamol, 200/800 µg Healthy, physically active	No change in maximal cycling power or leg extension force
Sporer, 2008 *Med Sci Sports Exerc*	Salbutamol, 200/400/800 µg Cyclists and triathletes	No change in VO_2 max, peak power, or 20-km running time
Dickinson, 2011 *Br J Sports Med*	Salbutamol, 800/1600 µg Trained soccer athletes	No change in VO_2 or RER, increased lactate, and heart rate
Decorte, 2014 *Med Sci Sports Exerc*	Salbutamol, 200/800 µg Highly endurance trained	Improved muscle endurance
Dickinson, 2014 *Clin J Sport Med*	Salbutamol, 1600 µg/day (6 wk) Trained athletes	No change in VO_2, 3-km run time, or bench/leg press strength
Dickinson, 2014 *J Sports Sci Med*	Salbutamol, 1600 µg Trained runners	No change in VO_2, RPE, lactate, or 5-km run time
RER = respiratory exchange ratio; RPE = rating of perceived exertion; TTE = time to exhaustion.		

manage symptoms are recommended to minimize this loss of therapeutic effect. Thus, the chronic ergogenic use of these drugs by an asthmatic athlete could have detrimental effects during an actual asthma episode.

Section Summary

Increased protein synthesis, decreased protein degradation, or a combination is the primary mechanism by which anabolic agents promote muscle growth. There are conflicting reports regarding the efficacy of these drugs for increasing muscle size and strength. A number of studies report increases in strength and lean body mass when AAS are administered. However, not all studies are in agreement with this. hGH appears to be effective when treating hGH- or IGF-1-deficient patients, whereas its effects on a healthy population remain unclear, and, at this time, the scientific literature is lacking in evidence to support the ergogenic use

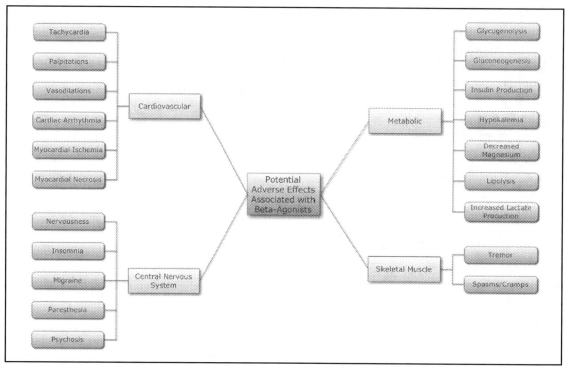

Figure 16-3. Potential effects associated with β-agonists. (Adapted from Sears MR. Adverse effects of beta-agonists. *J Allergy Clin Immunol.* 2002;110[6 suppl]:S322-S328; and Lulich KM. Adverse reactions to beta 2-agonist bronchodilators. *Med Toxicol.* 1986;1[4]:286-299.)

of β$_2$-agonists. All of the anabolic agents discussed in this chapter have been associated with adverse effects, some serious in nature. These drugs are not available OTC, and each one has been banned by various sport organizations.

DIURETICS

Any drug that promotes the formation of urine by the kidney is considered to be a diuretic. Clinically, diuretics are used to treat hypertension (see Chapter 12) and edema associated with conditions such as heart failure and hepatic and renal disease. The majority of the drugs classified as diuretics are available by prescription only. However, xanthines such as caffeine and pamabrom have a weak diuretic effect on the body and are commonly included in OTC medications to relieve fluid retention associated with menstruation. Theophylline, another xanthine with mild diuretic effects, is a prescription drug that is also naturally present in tea. Although the FDA has not approved a diuretic for the treatment of obesity or weight loss, they are commonly used by athletes for that purpose as well. In fact, rapid weight loss (water loss) can be achieved when using these drugs. Thus, diuretics are prohibited by the WADA, NCAA, and other sport governing bodies. In 1992, the IOC reported that diuretics were the fourth most commonly abused drug, behind AAS, stimulants, and narcotics. A survey of female collegiate athletes[35] found that 10% of them used diuretics to lose weight. Use was greatest among volleyball players (24%). This may be even greater in sports that have weight classes such as boxing, weightlifting, and wrestling or those that emphasize appearance and a leaner body type like gymnastics and cheerleading. For example, 2 Bulgarian weight lifters were stripped of their gold medals after testing positive for a diuretic at the 1988 Olympic Games in Seoul, Korea. Twelve years later, the entire team was expelled from the Olympic Games in Sydney, Australia, after 3 of the athletes tested positive for diuretics. Although it is likely that these athletes were trying to make weight, it is possible that the drugs were administered to dilute their urine and mask the use of other banned drugs during testing.

Pharmacodynamics

Diuretics increase water excretion by increasing the excretion of solutes in the renal tubular system. The more commonly used are loop, thiazide, and potassium sparing diuretics. Loop diuretics, such as bumetanide (Bumex) and furosemide (Lasix), act on the loop of Henle and have a very strong diuretic effect (see Figure 12-3). They do so by greatly increasing the excretion of sodium and chloride. Thiazide diuretics such as hydrochlorothiazide and potassium-sparing diuretics such as amiloride act on the distal tubule and collecting duct and have a weaker effect than loop diuretics. Like loop diuretics, they increase the excretion of sodium and chloride. Unlike the others, potassium-sparing diuretics increase this excretion through a mechanism that decreases excretion of potassium. Regardless of which drug is used, diuresis occurs through osmotic changes and decreased water reabsorption in the tubular system.

Possible Ergogenic Effects

Although not very common, athletic trainers do encounter athletes prescribed diuretics to control hypertension. However, this would be considered medical use as opposed to ergogenic use. Most athletes who use diuretics for ergogenic benefit do so to lose weight, although the benefit of weight loss in the form of water could easily be debated. However, an improvement in vertical jump performance has been reported following rapid diuretic-induced weight loss. This was most likely due to the lighter load during the jump. Other improvements in performance have been noted in individuals suffering from cardiac or pulmonary disease. In contrast, studies examining running and cycling performance, VO$_2$ max, and strength in healthy individuals report either no change or a decline in performance. Thus, any true ergogenic benefit is unlikely. Diuretics are also commonly used by athletes to mask the use of other drugs. They are used to dilute the urine so that the presence of other ergogenic drugs or their metabolites cannot be detected. Although they had their own classification at one time, diuretics are now classified as masking agents by the WADA and the NCAA (see Tables 16-1 and 16-4). It is the opinion of these and other governing bodies that the use of diuretics is more for the masking of other drugs than for weight loss or any direct ergogenic benefit.

Adverse Effects

Common side effects associated with diuretic use are listed in Box 16-4; additionally, hypokalemia, hyponatremia, and other electrolyte imbalances are also possible complications. Thiazide diuretics can cause photosensitivity. This would be a concern for an outdoor athlete because even brief exposure to sun can cause severe sunburn, itching, rash, and redness. The most obvious concern with diuretic use in an athletic population is dehydration. Exercise and diuretic use can each independently cause fluid and electrolyte loss. When they are combined, this loss is even greater. It is well accepted that dehydration can lead to muscle cramping. Most diuretics stimulate diuresis via increased sodium excretion. Thus, it is likely that this sodium loss would increase the occurrence of cramping more so than water and electrolyte loss through sweating alone. Even without cramping, dehydration can impair performance because it can lead to a decrease in plasma volume and cardiac output. The magnitude of plasma volume decrease is greater following diuretic dehydration than with other forms of dehydration such as exercise and can result in hypotension. Decreases in resting plasma volume have been observed in athletes and healthy individuals follow-

---

Box 16-4

COMMON SIDE EFFECTS ASSOCIATED WITH DIURETIC USE

- Thirst
- Dryness of mouth
- Fatigue
- Muscle weakness and soreness

- Numbness
- Paresthesia
- Nausea
- Vomiting
- Diarrhea

---

ing acute diuretic administration. This hypovolemia can compromise venous return to the heart. When this occurs, heart rate increases and peripheral blood vessels constrict to maintain cardiac output and blood pressure. If cardiac output cannot be maintained during exertion, heat exhaustion can occur. These cardiovascular adaptations to hypovolemia occur at the expense of thermoregulation as blood flow to the skin decreases. If severe enough, this can cause impaired thermoregulation, leading to heat stroke. It is important to note that the adverse effects of diuretic use can be exacerbated with ingestion of either alcohol, caffeine, or other xanthines. As mentioned previously, these drugs also have a diuretic effect on the body.

Section Summary

Diuretics are commonly used for weight loss both in and out of the athletic setting. Although the ergogenic effects of fluid loss are easily debated, many athletes such as wrestlers and football players attempting to cut weight may find benefit in this practice. However, it is important to note that only limited support exists for a performance improvement associated with diuretic-induced weight loss. Thus, an ergogenic effect beyond a particular weight loss goal is unlikely. The most obvious concern with diuretic use in an athletic population is dehydration and the complications associated with it, such as cramping, hypovolemia, impaired thermoregulation, and electrolyte loss. Although recent research shows that diuretics are still being used for weight loss, it is more likely that they are used to mask the presence of other performance-enhancing drugs or their metabolites in the urine. The WADA, NCAA, and other sport-governing bodies have banned their use during competition and now classify them as masking agents or urine manipulators.

ANTI-INFLAMMATORY DRUGS

Musculoskeletal breakdown is almost inevitable during athletic competition and intense training. This type of breakdown is generally accompanied by pain and inflammation. Because of this, the use of nonprescription and prescription anti-inflammatory drugs is one of the most common pharmaceutical interventions in athletics. Anti-inflammatory drugs are generally separated into 2 classifications: nonsteroidal anti-inflammatory drugs and corticosteroids (see also Chapter 6).

Corticosteroids

Corticosteroids, which consist of glucocorticoids and mineralocorticoids, are a class of steroid hormones synthesized from cholesterol within the adrenal cortex. Levels of glucocorticoids are elevated in stressful situations, such as intense training, and are thought to be the primary endocrine response to starvation, as amino acids are converted to carbohydrate to maintain essential glucose levels in the brain. Exogenous corticosteroids are drugs with a sterol structure similar to that of cortisol, which is the primary circulating glucocorticoid found in the human body. They are commonly used as glucocorticoid replacement therapies in Addison's disease or other forms of adrenal insufficiency. Other therapeutic effects of glucocorticoids were first realized when it was unexpectedly reported that cortisone had powerful anti-inflammatory activity that dramatically improved the condition of patients with rheumatoid arthritis. Thus, these hormones are mainly used as anti-inflammatory drugs, which also provide an analgesic effect as inflammation is relieved. Some examples used in the treatment of musculoskeletal injury include dexamethasone, hydrocortisone, cortisone, prednisolone, and prednisone. At this time, the systemic use of glucocorticoids is prohibited by the WADA when administered orally, rectally, or by intravenous or intramuscular injection. The use of adrenocorticotropic hormone, which stimulates the secretion of glucocorticoids, is also prohibited (see Tables 16-1 and 16-4). However, local and intra-articular injections of glucocorticoids are permitted if the governing body receives medical notification.

Pharmacodynamics

Glucocorticoids are produced in the adrenal gland and are generally regarded as protein catabolic hormones. The secretion of these hormones is stimulated by adrenocorticotropic hormone. Glucocorticoids stimulate gluconeogenesis from amino acids derived from protein catabolism, decrease glucose use, and can cause insulin resistance. The direct effect on skeletal muscle is known from the marked muscle wasting and weakness in Cushing's syndrome (increased glucocorticoid production). Likewise, loss of muscle protein due to increased protein breakdown and decreased protein synthesis has been observed in response to glucocorticoid treatment. Like many other hormones, glucocorticoids exert their effect by binding to specific receptors.

As endogenous anti-inflammatory compounds, glucocorticoids protect tissue from damage caused by its own defense reactions and the products of these reactions during stress. They inhibit the synthesis of almost all known cytokines and other molecules required for immune function. Thus, they inhibit the function of key cells that comprise the inflammatory response. They also prevent the breakdown of phospholipids and their conversion to inflammatory mediators. One of the most important anti-inflammatory effects is their ability to inhibit the recruitment of leukocytes to the inflammatory site and to modify the capillary and membrane permeability that occurs during the tissue injury response. By doing so, glucocorticoids inhibit a critical step in the initiation of the inflammatory process.

Possible Ergogenic Effects

Theoretically, the reduced glucose use and increased use of fatty acids associated with corticosteroids would provide a glycogen-sparing effect and improve performance. However, the research involving corticosteroid use and performance is limited, and the studies that exist do not support the claims of enhanced performance. The catabolic properties of these drugs would suggest that their use would only impair performance. Thus, their use in athletics appears to be restricted to the treatment of chronic and painful musculoskeletal injury. Local injection is the method of choice in this situation. However, it is possible that a reduction in pain could allow an athlete to continue training and competing at a more intense level, providing an ergogenic effect. The same would be true for the use of narcotic analgesic medications that are also banned by the WADA, NCAA, and most other sport governing bodies (see Tables 16-1 and 16-4). Once again, clinical studies supporting the ergogenic benefits of corticosteroids do not exist.

Adverse Effects

There are numerous ways in which corticosteroids can be administered. When taken orally, these drugs act systemically and can have profound effects on the body. Cushing's syndrome provides a primary example of adverse effects associated with elevated glucocorticoid levels. Some of these adverse effects include hypertension, acne, glaucoma, avascular necrosis, obesity, psychiatric problems, and poor wound healing. It is common for patients to experience weight gain during corticosteroid therapy. This can progress to a more extreme cushingoid appearance (swollen effect), with moon face, buffalo neck, and hirsutism. The development of diabetes mellitus is possible with long-term corticosteroid use, and existing diabetes can be exacerbated.

Although local injection reduces the risks of systemic effects, there are still complications. The anti-inflammatory and catabolic properties can adversely affect the healing process. Because the pain feedback mechanism is lost, the potential for further injury exists. The possibility of tendon and ligament weakening justifies concern for joint injury and tendon rupture. It is actually recommended that athletes be kept out of training for several weeks following corticosteroid injection. One of the primary concerns in an athletic population would be the long-term complication of corticosteroid-induced osteoporosis.

Section Summary

At this time, evidence supporting the ergogenic use of corticosteroids in healthy individuals does not exist. When used by an injured athlete, the decreased inflammation and resultant reduction in pain may allow training and competition to continue. However, this may also increase the risk for reinjury. Although the adverse effects appear to be minor, continued use and increasing doses can increase the risk for more serious adverse effects. Although the use of glucocorticoids is prohibited by a number of organizations when administered orally, rectally, or by intravenous or intramuscular injection, local and intra-articular injections are generally permitted.

β-BLOCKERS

Beta-adrenergic antagonists, also known as *beta-blockers* (β-blockers), are drugs primarily used for conditions that affect the cardiovascular system (see Chapter 12). In an athletic population, these drugs are more commonly prescribed to control hypertension. As performance enhancers, β-blockers are used to counteract the effects of anxiety associated with athletic competition, which include increases in heart rate, nervousness, and skeletal muscle tremor. Although the physiological response to beta blockade may not be desirable for many types of sports or athletic events, it may provide benefit for activities requiring precision and accuracy. Unofficial tests at the 1984 Olympic Games in Los Angeles, California, indicated that a majority of the athletes competing in the pentathlon used β-blockers. As a result, the IOC banned β-blockers in 1985. This ban was subsequently altered and now affects only precision sports such as archery, shooting, modern pentathlon, bobsled, skiing, bowling, and golf (see Table 16-1). However, the extent of β-blocker use in athletic competition is not fully understood. Anecdotal reports of use during golf competition lead the Professional Golfers' Association to include β-blockers on their list of prohibited substances when it began drug testing for the first time in 2008. Players may apply for an exemption if it is substantiated that there is a medical need, which is particularly important because the antidoping program includes players on the seniors' Champions Tour. Although the NCAA has banned the use of β-blockers during rifle competition, they have not been banned from golf competition (see Table 16-4).

Pharmacodynamics

β-blockers are drugs that were developed to bind to sympathetic cell membrane receptors sensitive to the catecholamines, epinephrine and norepinephrine. As mentioned previously (see amphetamines), these receptors are found on most cells throughout the body, including the cells of the heart, lungs, and surrounding blood vessels. β-blockers work by decreasing heart rate, stroke volume (overall cardiac output), and mean arterial blood pressure and are used to lower blood pressure and decrease the work of the heart in ischemic heart conditions and heart failure. They are commonly used to treat hypertension, angina, arrhythmias, migraine headache, and anxiety and are frequently given after myocardial infarction. Their central anxiolytic effect (reduction in anxiety) occurs in direct proportion to their lipophilic binding and their ability to cross the blood-brain barrier.

Possible Ergogenic Effects

β-blockers are commonly used to reduce performance anxiety in musicians, teachers, and business executives. Although reports are mostly anecdotal, short-acting, low-dose preparations, such as propranolol, are generally recommended. Improvements have been observed in these populations; however, it is difficult to generalize these improvements to sport competition. Sport competition creates anxiety, which is associated with an increase in sympathetic nervous system activity and increased levels of catecholamines. Even before competition begins, an athlete will experience anxiety symptoms such as elevations in heart rate and blood pressure and skeletal muscle tremor. β-blockers are used to decrease this type of anxiety during athletic competition. Although decreases in cardiac output would not be beneficial for an endurance athlete, β-blocker use could improve performance in sports requiring precision and accuracy. For example, experienced shooters fire during diastole. Thus, a slower heart rate would increase time during diastole and possibly improve shooting performance. At this time, investigation into the efficacy of β-blocker use during sport competition is very limited. Metoprolol use has been associated with a 13% improvement in pistol shooting, with the greatest effect being observed in the more skilled shooters.[36] It was suggested that the improvement was more due to the drug's effect on hand tremor rather than on heart rate. Similar observations have been made when oxprenolol is administered. However, not all studies have shown improvement. For example, although cardiovascular changes have been observed, β-blockade has not been shown to improve bowling performance. It appears that their effects on performance and physiological changes, such as lipid and lactic acid levels, depend on the intensity of the activity and whether a cardioselective or nonselective drug is used. β-blockers have no effect on strength or power, and their negative inotropic and chronotropic effects are undesirable for endurance athletes.

Adverse Effects

The most common adverse effects associated with beta blockade are bradycardia and hypotension. Other adverse effects include bronchospasm, heart failure, arrhythmias, fatigue, impaired glucose control in diabetes mellitus, and aggravation of peripheral vascular disease. It is important to note that these reactions can be accentuated with alcohol, which is also used to enhance performance in similar sports or events. Endurance athletes should avoid using β-blockers because of their negative effect on cardiac output, oxygen consumption, and overall exercise capacity. Other possible adverse effects during exercise include increased perceived exertion levels, earlier lactate threshold and fatigue, and possible exacerbation of exercise-induced bronchospasm or asthma. Because these drugs can inhibit lipolysis and glycogenolysis, hypoglycemia may occur after intense exercise. β-blocker use should also be avoided by athletes with first- or second-degree heart block and by those with asthma.

Section Summary

Although the benefit of beta blockade in the treatment of various medical conditions is well accepted, their use as performance enhancers is not. Any possible benefit would only apply to sports requiring precision such as shooting and archery. However, at this time support for their ability to improve this type of performance is very limited. Furthermore, any sport requiring strength, power, speed, or endurance would only be impaired by β-blockade. There are also numerous adverse effects associated with these drugs. Thus, caution is warranted with their use.

OXYGEN DELIVERY ENHANCERS

In endurance sports such as running, cycling, and cross-country skiing, the ability to deliver oxygen to the working muscles over long periods of time is a critical component to performance. This is evident as VO_2 during exercise and maximal VO_2 are generally higher in trained compared with untrained athletes. Oxygen consumption by the working muscles is dependent on the cardiovascular system's ability to deliver the oxygen from the lungs. Erythrocytes, or red blood cells (RBCs), are responsible for this delivery. RBCs contain hemoglobin, which binds to oxygen to form an unstable compound called oxyhemoglobin. In tissues where the oxygen concentration is low, hemoglobin releases its oxygen. Thus, changes in the hemoglobin concentration (Hb) or its oxygen saturation can have an impact on physical performance. Because of this, numerous attempts have been made to alter these variables. In blood doping, units of whole blood are collected from an athlete. The RBCs are then separated from the plasma, frozen, and stored in glycerol. This is usually done 2 to 3 months before competition to allow for erythropoiesis (the production of RBCs) and restoration of normal Hb. Three to 5 days before competition, the RBCs are infused resulting in an increased Hb. It is well accepted that this procedure can improve oxygen delivery and endurance performance. However, this is an invasive procedure and is associated with certain risks. Because of this, attempts have been made to find alternative pharmaceutical methods for increasing Hb and oxygen delivery. One of the more popular drugs used for this purpose is erythropoietin (EPO).

Erythropoietin

EPO is a glycoprotein hormone made of 165 amino acids that plays a primary role in erythropoiesis. It is secreted by the kidneys in response to low oxygen levels in the blood, resulting in an increased bone marrow production of RBCs. The gene encoding EPO was cloned in 1985, which led to its synthetic production. Recombinant EPO (r-EPO) is produced by inserting the gene into a cell and stimulating the cell to produce it. It was originally developed for treating patients suffering from bone marrow failure and those with certain types of anemia, such as anemia due to chronic renal failure, anemia associated with cancer and chemotherapy, and anemia secondary to zidovudine treatment of AIDS. The r-EPO assists these patients in raising their hematocrit (index of RBC level) and oxygen-carrying capacity, relieving the symptoms of their chronic disease. However, it was not long after its development that the ergogenic potential of r-EPO was also realized. Although the prevalence of r-EPO use in sport is unknown, anecdotal reports suggest that it is widespread among endurance athletes. Because r-EPO potentially gives an unfair advantage in competition, it has been banned by various sport governing bodies (see Tables 16-1 and 16-4). Probably the greatest controversy surrounding the use of r-EPO has occurred during the Tour de France. Before the start of the 1998 Tour, a team masseur named Willy Voet was stopped at the Franco-Belgium border where his car was found to contain more than 400 doping products, including r-EPO. This led to an investigation of teams and individual riders by authorities, resulting in numerous disqualifications. Since that time, numerous high-profile athletes have either admitted to taking or tested positive for r-EPO and have been penalized. However, despite improvements in doping control, penalties, and possible risks, r-EPO continues to be very popular among athletes.

Pharmacodynamics

Normal levels of EPO are approximately 0 to 19 mU/mL; however, large individual and interindividual variations exist during the day and in response to different physiological situations. The kidney cells that make EPO are specialized and are sensitive to low oxygen levels in the blood. Thus, oxygen availability in the kidneys is the primary regulator of EPO production. Hypoxia due to anemia or low plasma oxygen pressure leads to an increase in EPO secretion. Following secretion, EPO binds to receptors in the bone marrow, which stimulate the differentiation and proliferation of erythroid precursors. This also stimulates the release of reticulocytes into the circulation and the synthesis of cellular hemoglobin. The end result of this process is an increased RBC production and Hb. Exogenous r-EPO is administered intravenously or subcutaneously and has a plasma t½ of approximately 6 to 8 hours (the t½ is longer following subcutaneous injection). It binds to the same receptors and has the same physiological effect as endogenous EPO. Early clinical trials showed that r-EPO was capable of increasing the hematocrit by 3% to 4% in as little as 3 to 4 weeks. This treatment has also resulted in a restoration of Hb and physical performance levels and an overall improvement in quality of life in patients with certain diseases. In patients with chronic heart failure, r-EPO has been shown to increase oxygen delivery and Hb and enhance exercise capacity. It is important to note that these patients can be considered a deficient population. The question is whether the same changes would occur in healthy individuals.

Possible Ergogenic Effects

Like a diseased population, improved physical performance in healthy individuals would depend on an increased Hb and enhanced maximal VO_2. Although large variations have been observed across subjects, the general conclusion is that r-EPO will increase the Hb and hematocrit in trained subjects. Other variables such as blood volume, resting heart rate, and VO_2 during submaximal exercise do not appear to change. However, the increases in Hb and hematocrit have been associated with increases in maximal VO_2. These observations have been consistent across most individuals. In fact, the increases observed are similar to those observed following blood doping. Even in well-trained athletes, it appears that r-EPO will increase erythropoiesis and enhance physical performance. Increases in maximal VO_2 following r-EPO administration have been associated with improvements in time to exhaustion, which is a standard measure of endurance performance. For example, an increased hematocrit (43% to 51%) has been observed in endurance trained athletes following 4 weeks of r-EPO administration. This was associated with a 7% increase in VO_2 max and a 9% increase in time to exhaustion. Interestingly, the ergogenic effect lasted for 3 weeks after r-EPO administration had stopped. Thus, it has become well accepted that the use of r-EPO can provide an ergogenic effect during both maximal and submaximal exercise. However, many have suggested that the use of r-EPO as a performance-enhancing agent is a dangerous practice.

Adverse Effects

The medical risks associated with blood doping have been estimated from carefully controlled research studies, and the unsupervised use of blood doping will increase these risks. It is the position of the American College of Sports Medicine that the use of blood doping in an attempt to improve athletic performance is unethical, unfair, and exposes the athlete to unwarranted and potentially serious health risks. The use of r-EPO can cause a reduction in endogenous EPO production. Although the effects of long-term use are not fully understood, endogenous levels return to normal when short-term use is discontinued. The use of r-EPO also has the potential for increased blood viscosity and thrombosis with potentially fatal results. Exercise training can stimulate RBC production and increase Hb, but this is usually associated with an increase in plasma volume as well. In contrast, the increase in RBC mass during r-EPO therapy generally occurs without an increase in the total blood volume. When used to gradually elevate the hematocrit in anemic patients, r-EPO therapy usually is uneventful. The same cannot be said for healthy subjects. When r-EPO is administered to healthy individuals and the normal hematocrit level is exceeded, blood viscosity increases. Thus, the increased RBC density caused by r-EPO can increase the viscosity of the blood and increase the risk for thrombotic events. The increased viscosity can also overload the heart, increasing the chances of myocardial infarction and stroke. Because of this, it has been suggested that r-EPO use contributed to the unexpected deaths of several well-trained endurance athletes during the 1990s. This may be of even greater concern with athletes during training or competition due to the interaction between dehydration and environmental stress.

Other adverse effects associated with r-EPO include headaches, hypertension, and seizures. Hypertension develops in 25% to 35% of renal patients treated with r-EPO, whereas elevations in systolic blood pressure have been observed in trained athletes during submaximal exercise. Those with a history of thrombosis, heart disease, or hypertension may have increased chances of adverse effects. The chance of seizures may be increased in those with history of seizures. Rare side effects include flu-like symptoms and bone and muscle pain. There are also rare reports of antibody formation toward r-EPO in humans.

Section Summary

Very few would debate the ergogenic value of r-EPO. However, very few would also debate the dangers associated with this prescription drug. For this reason, r-EPO has been banned by numerous sport-governing organizations since the early 1990s. However, in the absence of a valid procedure to detect r-EPO doping, in-competition health checks were introduced by organizations such as the International Ski Federation and the International Cycling Union. These health checks excluded athletes from competition when their Hb or hematocrit values exceeded an predetermined limit. This reduced the danger to athletes but did nothing to eliminate the use of r-EPO. Through the past decade, both direct and indirect methods for detecting r-EPO were investigated. No single indirect marker was found that satisfactorily demonstrated r-EPO use. Because of this, a combination of blood and urine tests together formed the procedure and strategy approved by the IOC for detecting r-EPO use at the 2000 Olympic Games in Sydney, Australia, and the 2002 Olympic Games in Salt Lake City, Utah. In June 2003, the WADA's Executive Committee accepted the results of an independent report stating that urine tests alone can be used to detect the presence of r-EPO and concluded that urinary testing is the only scientifically validated method for direct detection of r-EPO. Thus, the urine test alone is now used. A new long-acting EPO (3-times-longer t½) called *darbepoetin* is also banned.

ROLE OF THE ATHLETIC TRAINER

Ergogenic drug use continues to create controversy at all levels of athletic competition. Little evidence is available to evaluate the efficacy and safety of these drugs at the doses and regimens that are actually used by athletes, and few studies provide long-term data on their use. At this time, there is support in the scientific literature for the use of some drugs (eg, caffeine, AAS), whereas it does not exist for others (eg, β-agonists, glucocorticoids). The potential for adverse effects, sometimes serious in nature, exists with the use of any drug. Because of the health risks associated with ergogenic drug use, it is important that athletic trainers and other health care professionals provide intervention in the form of education, information, medical care, and referral when necessary. In addition, the athletic trainer's role in ergogenic drug use includes many facets, such as the following:

- Athletic trainers are in a unique position to assess and assist ergogenic drug abusers and those who may become ergogenic drug abusers.

- It is imperative that athletic trainers and other health care professionals become educated regarding the efficacy, safety, and legalities of ergogenic drug use.

- Athletic trainers should maintain an open, honest, and evidence-based dialogue with athletes, coaches, administrators, and parents regarding ergogenic drug use.

- Because many athletes may not be open about their drug use, it is also important that the athletic trainer recognizes the adverse effects and general signs and symptoms of this type of drug use.

- The athletic trainer must also accept the role of liaison and refer the athlete to counseling when it is believed that this type of intervention is necessary.

- The athletic trainer must understand that many athletes may use potentially ergogenic drugs for nonergogenic reasons, such as symptomatic relief during illness (eg, decongestants) or control of certain conditions (eg, ADHD). Regardless of the reason, many of these drugs are banned, and their use could result in penalties. The athletic trainer must provide guidance and possible referral for the athlete in these situations.

CASE STUDY 1

A high school baseball athlete reports to his athletic trainer complaining of a rapid and strong heart beat, which the athletic trainer determines to be palpitations. The athlete's medical history is unremarkable and he denies any drug use; however, the athletic trainer notes that his pupils appear dilated and he seems to be very restless. The athletic trainer also notes that the athlete has lost weight since the beginning of the season. Which drug classification might the athletic trainer suspect the athlete is using? Given his setting and recent trends in performance enhancing drug use, which drug is he most likely using?

CASE STUDY 2

A collegiate distance runner has asked her athletic trainer for advice regarding caffeine use. She states that she rarely ingests coffee, tea, or soda but is considering using energy drinks prior to her races and wants her athletic trainer's opinion. What should his response be?

REFERENCES

1. Astorino TA, Roberson DW. Efficacy of acute caffeine ingestion for short-term high-intensity exercise performance: a systematic review. *J Strength Condition Res.* 2010;24(1):257-265.
2. Brown SJ, Brown J, Foskett A. The effects of caffeine on repeated sprint performance in team sport athletes—a meta-analysis. *Sport Sci Rev.* 2013;22(1-2):25-32.
3. Ganio MS, Klau JF, Casa DJ, Armstrong LE, Maresh CM. Effect of caffeine on sport specific endurance performance: a systematic review. *J Strength Condition Res.* 2009;23(1):315-324.
4. Graham TE, Spriet LL. Metabolic, catecholamine and exercise performance responses to varying doses of caffeine. *J Appl Physiol.* 1995;78:867-874.
5. Pasman WJ, VanBaak MA, Jeukendrum AE, DeHann A. The effect of different dosages of caffeine on endurance performance time. *Int J Sports Med.* 1995;16:225-230.
6. Armstrong LE, Casa DJ, Maresh CM, Ganio MS. Caffeine, fluid-electrolyte balance, temperature regulation, and exercise-heat tolerance. *Exerc Sport Sci Rev.* 2007;35(3):135-140.
7. Sidney KH, Lefcoe NM. The effects of ephedrine on the physiological and psychological responses to submaximal and maximal exercise in man. *Med Sci Sports Exerc.* 1977;9:95-99.

8. Gillies H, Derman W, Noakes T, Smith P, Evans A, Gabriels G. Pseudoephedrine is without ergogenic effects during exercise. *J Appl Physiol.* 1996;81:2611-2617.

9. Swain RA, Harsha DM, Baenziger J, Saywell RM. Do pseudo-ephedrine or phenylpropanolamine improve maximum oxygen uptake and time to exhaustion? *Clin J Sports Med.* 1997;7:168-173.

10. Bell DG, Jacobs I, McLellan TM, Zamecnik J. Reducing the does of combined caffeine and ephedrine preserved the ergogenic effect. *Aviat Space Environ Med.* 2000;71:415-419.

11. Bell DG, Jacobs I, Zamecnik J. Effects of caffeine, ephedrine, and their combination on time to exhaustion during high intensity exercise. *Eur J Appl Physiol.* 1998;77:427-433.

12. Bell DG, Jacobs I. Combined caffeine and ephedrine ingestion improves run times of Canadian Forces Warrior Test. *Aviat Space Environ Med.* 1999;70:325-329.

13. Brents RT, Marsh E. Patterns of ephedra and other stimulant use in collegiate hockey athletes. *Int J Sport Nut and Exer Metab.* 2006;16(6):636-643.

14. Rogozkin V. Metabolic effects of anabolic steroid on skeletal muscle. *Med Sci Sports Exerc.* 1999;11:160-163.

15. Haupt HA, Rovere GD. Anabolic steroids: a review of the literature. *Am J Sports Med.* 1984;12:469-484.

16. Elashoff JD, Jacknow AD, Shain SG, Braunstein GD. Effects of anabolic androgenic steroids on muscular strength. *Ann Intern Med.* 1991;115:387-393.

17. Burkett LN, Falduto MT. Steroid use by athletes in a metropolitan area. *Phys Sports Med.* 1984;12:69-74.

18. Kersey RD, Elliot DL, Goldberg L, et al. National Athletic Trainers' Association Position Statement: Anabolic-Androgenic Steroids. *J Athl Train.* 2012;47(5):567–588.

19. Cooper CJ, Noakes TD, Dunne T, Lambert MI, Rochford K. A high prevalence of abnormal personality traits in chronic users of anabolic-androgenic steroids. *Br J Sports Med.* 1996;30:246-250.

20. Copeland J, Peters R, Dillon P. Anabolic-androgenic steroid use disorder among a sample of Australian competitive and recreational users. *Drug Alcohol Depend.* 2000;60:91-96.

21. Goodman HM, Grichting G. Growth hormone and lipolysis: a reevaluation. *Endocrinology.* 1983;113:1697-1702.

22. Deyssig R, Frisch H, Blum WF, Waldhor T. Effect of growth hormone treatment, hormonal parameters, body composition and strength in athletes. *Acta Endocrinol.* 1993;128:313-318.

23. Yarasheski KE, Campbell JA, Smith K, Rennie MJ, Holloszy JO, Bier DM. Effects of growth hormone and resistance exercise on muscle growth in young men. *Am J Physiol.* 1992;262:E261-E267.

24. Yarasheski KE, Zachwieja JJ, Angelopoulos TJ, Bier DM. Short-term growth hormone treatment does not increase muscle protein synthesis in experienced weight lifters. *J Appl Physiol.* 1993;74:3073-3076.

25. Crist DM, Peake GT, Egan PA, Waters DL. Body composition response to exogenous GH during training in highly conditioned adults. *J Appl Physiol.* 1988;65:579-584.

26. Liu H, Bravata DM, Olkin I, et al. Systematic review: the effects of growth hormone on athletic performance. *Ann Intern Med.* 2008;148(10):747-758.

27. Kindermann W, Meyer T. Inhaled β2 agonists and performance in competitive athletes. *Br J Sports Med.* 2006;40(Suppl I):i43–i47.

28. Pluim BM, de Hon O, Staal JB, et al. β2-agonists and physical performance: a systematic review and meta-analysis of randomized controlled trials. *Sports Med.* 2011;41(1):39-57.

29. Wolfarth B, Wuestenfeld JC, Kindermann W. Ergogenic effects of inhaled β2-agonists in non-asthmatic athletes. *Endocrinol Metab Clin N Am.* 2010;39:75-87.

30. Meeuwisse WH, McKenzie DC, Hopkins SR, Road JD. The effect of salbutamol on performance in elite nonasthmatic athletes. *Med Sci Sports Exerc.* 1992;24:1161-1166.

31. Lemmer JT, Fleck SJ, Wallach JM, et al. The effects of albuterol on power output in non-asthmatic athletes. *Int J Sports Med.* 1995;16:243-249.

32. McKenzie DC, Rhodes EC, Stirling DR, et al. Salbutamol and treadmill performance in non-atopic athletes. *Med Sci Sports Exerc.* 1983;15:520-522.

33. McKenzie DC, Fitch KD. The asthmatic athlete: inhaled Beta-2 agonists, sport performance, and doping. *Clin J Sport Med.* 2011;21:46-50.

34. Bonnet N, Benhamou CL, Beaupied H, et al. Doping dose of salbutamol and exercise: deleterious effect on cancellous and cortical bones in adult rats. *J Applied Phys.* 2007;102(4):1502-1509.

35. Martin M, Schlabach G, Shibinski K. The use of nonprescription weight loss products among female basketball, softball, and volleyball athletes from NCAA Division I institutions: issues and concerns. *J Athl Train.* 1998;33(1):41-44.

36. Kruse P, Ladefoged J, Nielsen U, Paulev P, Sorensen J. Beta-blockade used in precision sports: effect on pistol shooting performance. *J Appl Physiol.* 1986;61:417-420.

CHAPTER 17: ADVANCE ORGANIZER

History

Sports Organizations and Drug Testing

Legal Considerations

Components of a Drug-Testing Program

- Policy
  - Purpose
  - Banned Substances
  - Testing Types and Methods
  - Consequences
  - Appeal
  - Treatment
- Participants
  - Donor (Athlete)
  - Drug-Testing Administrator
  - Third-Party Administrators
  - Collectors
  - Laboratories
  - Medical Review Officer (Results Recipient)
- Methodology
  - Specimen Types
    - Urine
    - Blood
    - Oral Fluid
    - Hair
    - Sweat
  - Banned Drugs
    - Stimulants
    - Narcotic Analgesics
    - Diuretics
    - Anabolic Agents
    - Peptide Hormones
    - β-Blockers
    - Other Prohibited Substances and Manipulators
  - Sample Collection and Chain of Custody
  - Specimen Adulteration
  - Specimen Analysis
    - Laboratory Analysis
    - On-Site Screening Devices
  - Results Verification and Applying Sanctions

Development of a Drug-Testing Program

Current and Future Challenges in Drug Testing in Sports

Role of the Athletic Trainer

17

Drug Testing in Sports

Cindy Thomas, MS, AT-R and Nathan Burns, MS, ATC

CHAPTER OBJECTIVES

After the end of this chapter, the reader will be able to:

- Discuss the historical progression of performance-enhancing drug use in sport from the ancient Olympic Games to current day

- Identify and compare the various sports organizations that administer drug-testing programs

- Explain relevant case law pertaining to drug testing in sport, including an understanding of the protections guaranteed by the Constitution of the United States

- Identify and describe the necessary components of a sports drug-testing policy

- Explain the responsibilities of the drug-testing administrator, collector, and laboratory

- Compare the applicability, methodology, advantages, and disadvantages of the various types of biological specimens used in drug testing

- Identify and locate sports organizations' banned drug lists and explain why specific drug classes are prohibited

- Explain why the specimen collection process is an integral part of the drug-testing process and include a discussion on specimen adulteration

- Describe the difference between laboratory specimen screening and confirmation procedures and provide examples of each method

- Identify the steps necessary in the development and implementation of a sports drug-testing program.

Sport has a responsibility to maintain a level playing field. Competitors are expected to abide by the rules of fair play. Some athletes use chemical and pharmacologic substances in pursuit of competitive superiority.[1] The sports world has responded to this unethical and risky behavior of manipulating performance to dominate the opponent by developing drug-testing programs. Unfortunately, these programs are not accepted as the total solution to the doping woes tarnishing sport today. To the contrary, drug testing in sport is often considered a necessary evil. It is necessary to deter the use of performance-enhancing substances and other dangerous drugs by athletes, yet the very process has been challenged as an invasion of privacy and regarded as inconvenient, time consuming, humiliating, and ineffective. Heralded as the cure for athlete doping practices, drug testing has become commonplace in sport. Today's elite athlete has reached a conundrum of sorts: compete clean as an underdog, give up competing instead of doping, or give in and dope to compete.[2] Athletes of all ages can sometimes let the drive for success be so compelling that they can lose sight of what is fair and right, and often this drive outweighs the risk of serious medical

Houglum JE, Harrelson GL, Seefeldt TM.
Principles of Pharmacology for Athletic Trainers, Third Edition (pp 347-379).
© 2016 Taylor & Francis Group.

ABBREVIATIONS USED IN THIS CHAPTER

CAS. Court of Arbitration for Sport	**IOC.** International Olympic Committee
CCF. Custody and Control Form	**LC.** liquid chromatography
CSMAS. Committee on Competitive Safeguards and Medical Aspects of Sports	**MRO.** medical review officer
DEA. Drug Enforcement Administration	**MS.** mass spectrometry
DHEA. dehydroepiandrosterone	**NCAA.** National Collegiate Athletic Association
EPO. erythropoietin	**NFL.** National Football League
FBS. Football Bowl Subdivision	**NOC.** National Olympic Committee
FDA. Food and Drug Administration	**USADA.** United States Anti-Doping Agency
GC. gas chromatography	**USOC.** United States Olympic Committee
GC/MS. gas chromatography with mass spectrometry	**WADA.** World Anti-Doping Agency
hGH. human growth hormone	**SAMSHA.** Substance Abuse and Mental Health Services Administration
IAAF. International Association of Athletics Federations	**THC.** tetrahydrocannabinol
IAF. International Athletics Foundation	**TLC.** thin-layer chromatography
IGF-1. insulin-like growth factor-1	**TPAs.** third-party administrators
	TUEs. therapeutic use exceptions

complications from the use of performance-enhancing substances.[3] As long as athletes choose an unethical path of improving performance and endangering their lives, drug-testing programs will continue as an attempt to promote integrity in athletics.

The purpose of this chapter is to provide the athletic trainer with a detailed understanding of sports drug testing. A chronological history is presented demonstrating how performance-enhancing substances have been used since the earliest recorded competitive setting. Conversely, numerous sports organizations have developed antidoping initiatives in response to drug use in sport, and these programs are described along with the legal battles that

have been fought in an effort to eliminate these unethical and risky behaviors. The various components necessary to implement drug testing are explained, along with details on policy content and methodology. Finally, a perspective of doping issues facing the future of sport is examined.

Drug use or doping in sport has become a complex, multidimensional problem. The term *doping* is believed to be derived from the Dutch word *doop*, which is a viscous opium juice, the drug of choice of the ancient Greeks. *Doping control* has been adopted as a common international term for drug testing in sports.[4,5] The International Olympic Committee (IOC) defines doping as "the administration of or use by a competing athlete of any substance foreign to the body or any physiological substance taken in abnormal quantity or taken by an abnormal route of entry into the body with the sole intention of increasing in an artificial or unfair manner his or her performance in competition."[6] Although anabolic steroids and other performance-enhancing agents and processes are most widely used by athletes, many routinely use and abuse alcohol, tobacco, marijuana, cocaine, and a variety of other licit and illicit drugs. Like performance-enhancing substances, these drugs also pose serious health-related problems, and their use must be addressed. It is well documented that athletes use a variety of drugs for a multitude of reasons.[7] It is important to recognize that abuse of drugs in sport is not just an individual problem limited to athletes; it is a burgeoning problem threatening our youth and public health.[8] Adolescents seem particularly vulnerable to the lure of performance-enhancing substances. Many engage in risk-taking behavior and experimentation when coping with puberty. Adolescents, by nature, feel invincible and shun the health risks associated with substance use. Adolescents are also intensely preoccupied with body image.[3] Drug testing has been shown to be extremely effective at reducing drug use in schools and businesses nationwide.[9] The growth of drug testing has been fueled by the fact that it deters drug use, yielding an immeasurable benefit.[10] A 2014 National Collegiate Athletic Association (NCAA) national survey of substance use habits among student-athletes indicated almost 60% believed drug testing by individual institutions and the NCAA has deterred college athletes from using drugs.[11] To fully understand today's antidoping initiatives in sport, a historical perspective of substances used to enhance performance or doping for a competitive advantage must be examined.

HISTORY

The practice of using performance-enhancing agents to gain a competitive advantage is not new to athletics. In ancient Olympic Games, athletes drank various alcohol concoctions and herbal infusions in the pursuit of victory.[6] The ancient Greeks ate sesame seeds attempting to enhance performance, and the gladiators were known to ingest plants containing stimulants to prevent the effects of fatigue.[12,13] The Berserkers, an ancient class of Nordic warriors, fought frenziedly, a "berserk" behavior attributed to a deliberate dish of wild mushrooms containing bufotenin for its stimulating effects.[14]

The reasons for anabolic steroid and stimulant doping in sport today are the same as those described in the earliest recorded history of drugs and physical activity—to increase strength and overcome fatigue. Early competitors discovered the anabolic and androgenic properties of the testes through the observation of castrating domesticated animals. Many indulged in organotherapy, the practice of eating animal and human organs to cure disease and improve vitality. As early as 1400 BC, the Susruta of India advocated consumption of testis tissue to cure impotence. During the 8th century, testicular extract was prescribed as an aphrodisiac.[13]

Early use of stimulants to enhance performance was accomplished by ingesting plants. West Africans and Andean Indians chewed the leaves of the cola plant and drank tea to increase endurance. Mexican Indians used peyote plants along with strychnine for its stimulant effects during long runs, whereas Austrian lumberjacks ingested arsenic to increase endurance.[13] The first drug-related death in sport was documented in 1886 when an English cyclist died from an overdose of trimethyl, probably a slang term for a form of ether. Prior to the 1940s, most drug use in sport consisted of ingesting a mixture of strychnine and alcohol. Strychnine taken in low doses has a stimulant effect, but higher doses are toxic.[6,13] During the late 19th and early 20th centuries, a variety of concoctions were tried, including milk-punch, champagne and brandy, belladonna, strychnine, and "morphine in hot drops" in an attempt to prolong performance efforts.[13] In the 1930s, amphetamines replaced the popular strychnine cocktail.[14] During the 1952 Winter Olympic Games, several speed skaters became ill from alleged amphetamine use.[6] As mentioned in Chapter 16, the most significant amphetamine-related tragedy occurred in the 1960 Olympic Games in Rome, Italy, when Danish cyclist Knud Jensen collapsed and died.[6,14] An autopsy revealed Jensen probably died of dehydration after taking amphetamines and cough medicine.[6]

In the mid-1930s, scientists began synthesizing the hormone testosterone. Following this discovery, oral and injectable testosterone preparations became available to the medical community.[13] It was rumored that some German athletes were given testosterone for the 1936 Olympic Games in Berlin, Germany, and that during World War II, German soldiers were given steroids before battle to enhance aggressiveness. However, the first recorded case of an athlete using testosterone was documented in the early 1940s when an 18-year-old horse named Holloway was administered testosterone in an attempt to improve his slowing performance on the track. After hormone administration and training, Holloway went on to win a number of races, establishing a trotter record at age 19.[13]

During the 1950s, it was reported that the Soviets were experimenting with hormone manipulation. At the 1956 World Games in Moscow, Russia, American physician John Ziegler witnessed the use of testosterone in highly successful Soviet athletes. During this time, CIBA Pharmaceutical Company was developing an oral anabolic steroid methandrostenolone (Dianabol). Although designed for legitimate medical uses, Dianabol was used by athletes at 10 to 20 times the therapeutic doses.[6,13] There seemed to be no widespread problem with athletes using anabolic steroids during the 1960 Olympic Games because only a few Soviet strength athletes and a few American weight lifters were suspected of using.

By the 1960s, the startling success of a number of strength athletes, known to be using anabolic steroids, created an epidemic of use. Weight lifters, track and field throwers, sprinters, and others were using steroids and breaking world records at a phenomenal pace. It was estimated that one-third of the US track-and-field team used steroids at the 1968 pre-Olympic training camp. This was at a time when steroid use was not banned and users were actually boasting of the enhanced performance effects from anabolic steroids.[13]

In response to Knud Jensen's untimely death in 1960, the sports world began exploring ways to control the use of drugs in athletics. Pharmacist Arnold Beckett introduced the first documented antidoping initiatives.[14] Beckett and some of his colleagues developed procedures capable of detecting several different stimulants and began drug testing cyclists participating in Tour of Britain races.[15] However, it was not until the death of British cyclist Tommy Simpson during the 1967 Tour de France that official antidoping programs were implemented, banning amphetamines from sport internationally. Simpson died while under the influence of amphetamines.[14,15] In 1963, in response to the widespread use of potentially life-threatening drugs in sports, the Council of Europe established the following definition of doping:

> *The administering or use of substances in any form alien to the body or of physiological substances in abnormal amounts and with abnormal methods by healthy persons with the exclusive aim of attaining an artificial and unfair increase in performance in competition. Furthermore, various psychological measures to increase performance in sports must be regarded as doping. Where treatment with a medicine must be undergone, which as a result of its nature or dosage is capable of raising physiological capability beyond normal level, such treatment must be considered doping and shall rule out eligibility for competition.*

The Council of Europe also published the first list of banned substances, which included narcotics, amine stimulants, alkaloids, analeptic agents, respiratory tonics, and certain hormones.[5]

Finally, the international sports world recognized that using performance-enhancing drugs was not only immoral but also posed significant health risks. By 1965, gas chromatography (GC) was introduced and implemented in laboratories for specimen analysis. During the 1964 and 1968 Olympic Games, small-scale testing for stimulants was introduced. In 1968, the IOC appointed a Medical Commission, adopted a Medical Code, and developed its first list of banned drugs. The IOC conducted drug testing using GC for stimulants and narcotics during the 1972 Olympic Games in Munich, Germany. Comprehensive testing with anabolic steroid analysis did not begin until the 1976 Olympic Games in Montreal, Canada.[6,14-16] Other sports-governing bodies quickly established rules against doping. During the 1980s, major athletic organizations in the United States, including the NCAA, the National Football League (NFL), USA Track and Field, and the United States Olympic Committee (USOC) implemented comprehensive drug-testing programs.[17]

In 1970, the NCAA Drug Education Committee was formed because of concern about increasing drug use and abuse among college student-athletes. Three years later, NCAA member institutions voted to establish legislation banning use of unauthorized drugs that could endanger athletes' health and safety or provide an unfair competitive advantage. More than a decade later, the NCAA Committee on Drug Testing was formed and developed a drug-testing plan, including a list of banned drugs. On November 24, 1986, the NCAA implemented its first drug-testing program during the Division I women's cross-country championships in Tucson, Arizona. During the 1986 to 1987 academic year, more than 3000 student-athletes were drug tested at NCAA championships. Two years later, the NCAA implemented out-of-competition drug testing for anabolic steroids.[18] The NCAA drug-testing program was not established without challenge, but the legal battles in the United States courts ultimately served to strengthen both the drug-testing program and its ideals. The NCAA's current drug-testing program includes both in-competition and out-of-competition drug testing of more than 13,000 student-athletes annually. In addition to the organization's drug-testing programs, the NCAA encourages member schools and offers guidelines to develop and implement institutional drug-testing programs.

Communities nationwide are adopting middle and high school drug-testing programs out of concern for the welfare of young people. State high school athletic associations are implementing state-wide drug-testing programs for both in-competition and out-of-competition athletic seasons. With the primary focus on anabolic steroid testing, other drugs of abuse are also being tested in some programs. The Supreme Court has continued to uphold the constitutionality of drug testing athletes and other student groups because of its effectiveness in preventing, deterring, and detecting drug use.[9]

Athletic performance–enhancing substances and their associated dangers are a matter of public concern today. The use of dietary supplements by athletes looking for any competitive edge is common. Organizations worldwide are constantly being challenged to develop solutions for the doping epidemic in sport. Regardless of the substance chosen in attempting to gain the competitive edge, this historical perspective demonstrates the ongoing need to confront the very fabric of the unethical and dangerous practice of using drugs in sport today.

SPORTS ORGANIZATIONS AND DRUG TESTING

Antidoping initiatives in sport are as varied and diverse as the organizations governing them. From international federations and national governing bodies to local school boards and private schools, organizations are attempting to deter drug use in sport. Although the list of banned drugs may vary, the mission is generally the same: to deter the use of drugs by athletes. There are international efforts underway to harmonize antidoping programs in an attempt to increase the effectiveness of drug detection. The United States emphasizes those same goals through its international consortium of athletic organizations and through independent amateur and professional sports groups within this country. The policies differ depending on the organization, and sometimes athletes must comply with multiple antidoping programs if they compete in more than one sports organization. It is important to be aware of the multitude of athletic organizations and their respective antidoping policies.

The IOC is an international, nongovernmental, nonprofit organization and creator of the Olympic Movement. It is an umbrella organization with primary responsibility for supervising the summer and winter Olympic Games. Over time, the IOC has designated many commissions and associations to guide it in its daily activities. The IOC Medical Commission was established to address the increasing problem of doping in sport. In the 1970s and 1980s, the IOC Medical Commission created, maintained, and circulated a list of prohibited substances and developed an accreditation process for laboratories performing doping control initiatives in sport. In the 1990s, the IOC and its doping control laboratories were pressured from the worldwide legal and laboratory community to harmonize and standardize its antidoping methods and procedures. This led to accreditation of laboratories through the International Organization for Standardization as a prerequisite to IOC.[16] For more than 40 years, the IOC Medical Commission worked in the antidoping field by establishing the Olympic Movement Anti-Doping Code, which was applicable to all constituents of the Olympic Movement. One of the Anti-Doping Code's fundamental objectives was to eliminate doping in sport. The Code applied to the Olympic Games, various championships, and all competitions to which the IOC continues to grant its patronage or support and had provisions that enabled appeals to be lodged with the Court of Arbitration for Sport (CAS).[19]

In response to the continued phenomenon of doping in sport, the IOC organized a World Conference on Doping in Sport in 1999, which resulted in the establishment of the World Anti-Doping Agency (WADA).[19] WADA is an independent body that coordinates antidoping enforcement for the Olympics and other international competitions. WADA's mission is to promote and coordinate activities against doping in sport worldwide. The purposes of WADA and the subsequent World Antidoping Code are to protect athletes' fundamental rights to participate in doping-free sport, to ensure fairness and equality for athletes worldwide, and to ensure harmonized and effective antidoping programs at the international and national level with regard to detection, deterrence, and prevention of doping. The WADA Foundation Board is composed of representatives of the Olympic Movement (IOC, National Olympic Committees [NOCs], International Association of Athletics Federations [IAAF], and athletes).[20]

As the ruling body for the Olympic Games, the IOC now delegates the responsibility for implementing doping control to the local Organizing Committee for the Olympic Games and to WADA. These groups act under the IOC's authority. The IOC Medical Commission and local Olympic organizing committee are responsible for overseeing all doping control processes on-site, which will be in full compliance with the IOC Anti-Doping Rules, the World Antidoping Code, and the International Standard for Testing (ISO9001:2000).[19]

Under the umbrella of the IOC are the NOCs. NOCs exist in various countries. Their mission is to develop, promote, and protect the Olympic Movement in their respective countries in accordance with the Olympic Charter.[21]

Also under the IOC umbrella is the IAAF. These nongovernmental organizations serve to administer one or more sports at the world level and are responsible for the integrity of their sport. While maintaining their independence and autonomy in the administration of their sports, the IAAF must ensure that their statutes, practice, and activities conform to the Olympic Charter. The IAAF administers antidoping programs under the statutes of the World Antidoping Code.[22]

The IOC also works with a variety of Olympic Movement Partners and CAS is one such partner. CAS was developed to deal with legal problems faced by athletes. Its purpose is to resolve sports-related disputes submitted through ordinary arbitration or through appeal against the decisions of sports bodies or organizations, including appeals from athletes who test positive for a WADA-banned substance.[23]

Antidoping efforts within the United States involve broader interests by including the national branches of the Olympic Movement. The USOC is one of 204 National Olympic Committees over 5 continents (http://www.olympic.org/national-olympic-committees). The USOC was established by the Amateur Sports Act in 1978 and was the first sports organization to conduct drug testing in the United States beginning in 1984.[24] In 2000, the USOC outsourced its antidoping operations to the United States Antidoping Agency (USADA), giving it full authority for testing, education, research, and adjudication for United States, Olympic, Pan Am Games, and Paralympic Games. The USADA's responsibility is to run a comprehensive national antidoping program for the Olympic Movement in the United States (www.usantidoping.org) in conjunction with the World Antidoping Code.

The NFL and the NFL Players Association have maintained policies and programs regarding substance abuse for a number of years. In the mid-1980s, the NFL began testing for illicit drugs and anabolic steroids with the primary purpose of assisting players who misuse substances of abuse. However, players who do not comply with the requirements of the drug-testing policy are subject to discipline. The league performs random drug testing of its players year-round and bases its drug-testing program on the premise that substance abuse can lead to on-the-field injuries, alienation of the fans, diminished job performance, and personal hardship. Both the NFL and NFL Players Association are committed to deterring and detecting substance abuse and to offering programs of intervention, rehabilitation, and support to players who have substance abuse problems. An important principle of this drug-testing policy is that a player will be held responsible for whatever goes into his body.[25]

In addition to the organization's substances of abuse policy, the NFL prohibits players from using anabolic steroids (including exogenous testosterone); human or animal growth hormones, whether natural or synthetic; and related or similar substances. The NFL believes these substances have no legitimate place in professional football and threaten the fairness and integrity of competition. The NFL bans performance-enhancing agents because it is concerned about the adverse health effects of steroid use, and steroid use by players sends the wrong message to young people. High school and college students use steroids with alarming frequency, and NFL players should not by their own conduct suggest that such use is either acceptable or safe.[25]

Professional sports organizations have often been divided on drug-testing issues because of the various subgroups involved (eg, players unions, owners). Following a detailed report more than 300 pages long from former Senator George Mitchell to the commissioner of baseball of an independent investigation into the illegal use of steroids and other performance enhancing substances by players in

Major League Baseball, professional sport has been scrutinized by the federal government for its weak antidoping programs and transparency of existing programs.[26] Many other professional sports organizations have implemented or strengthened their antidoping programs including Major League Baseball, National Basketball Association, Women's National Basketball Association, Professional Golf Association, and Ladies Professional Golf Association. Professional athletes, like it or not, are role models for young athletes today. Allowing or endorsing dangerous supplements and drugs sends the wrong message: "drug use is not only permissible, but desirable if an individual wants to perform at his or her best."[27]

The NCAA is a nonprofit athletic association comprising more than 1200 colleges and universities, athletic conferences, and sports organizations. Membership is voluntary. NCAA member schools strive to maintain intercollegiate athletics as an integral part of the educational program and its athletes as an integral part of the student body. Among the NCAA's goals is the protection of student-athletes through standards of fairness and integrity. The NCAA Committee on Competitive Safeguards and Medical Aspects of Sports (CSMAS) provides the NCAA with leadership and expertise on student-athlete health and safety issues. The CSMAS provides oversight for NCAA's drug education and drug-testing programs, making recommendations on drug-testing policies, procedures, and banned substances.[28] In addition, the Drug Education and Drug Testing Subcommittee of the CSMAS adjudicates appeals from institutions and student-athletes related to positive drug tests. The NCAA outsources its drug-testing program to The National Center for Drug Free Sport (Drug Free Sport). Drug Free Sport administers the NCAA in-competition and out-of-competition drug-testing programs (www.drugfreesport.com).

The NCAA's drug-testing programs were created to protect the health and safety of student-athletes and to ensure that no one participant might have an artificially induced advantage or be pressured to use chemical substances. The program involves urine collection on specific occasions and laboratory analysis of substances listed on the NCAA's banned drug classes list. The list, which was developed by the NCAA Executive Committee, consists of substances generally purported to be performance enhancing and/or potentially harmful to the health and safety of student-athletes. The drug classes specifically include stimulants and anabolic steroids, as well as street drugs. Under the direction of the CSMAS, the NCAA surveys student-athletes at all member institutions every 4 years regarding substance use and abuse habits. The committee uses this information and other scientifically researched data to maintain a sound drug-testing program that accurately addresses drug use concerns among its student-athletes.

The NCAA encourages, but does not require, its member institutions to provide in-house drug-testing programs independent of the NCAA's program. Of Division I Football Bowl Subdivision institutions recently surveyed (2009 survey), 94% reported operating independent drug-testing programs for their student-athletes.[29] In addition to the NCAA's drug-testing program, select collegiate athletic conferences have implemented both in-competition and out-of-competition drug-testing programs as an additional deterrent layer for their student-athletes.

Since the early 1990s, high school administrators have been attempting to address the alarming increase in drug use by children and adolescents by implementing random drug-testing programs. National drug use studies indicate substance abuse contributes to thousands of deaths annually, having an economic impact in the billions of dollars. Half of the nation's youth use illegal drugs before completing high school.[30] Due to Constitutional restraints, public schools cannot require the general student body to participate in random testing because it is an unreasonable invasion of one's privacy. However, landmark Supreme Court decisions now permit schools to randomly drug test participants in athletics and other extracurricular activities. With courts deciding that drug testing of athletes is constitutional, school boards nationwide have and are implementing drug-testing programs because of legitimate concerns in preventing, deterring, and detecting drug use by high school students. The national problem of adolescent substance abuse is compelling enough to justify random drug testing of America's youth, at least for those participating in sport and extracurricular activities. In addition to individual school programs, several state athletic associations have implemented statewide drug-testing programs.

In the United States, the drug-testing programs of many sports organizations have been compared with workplace drug testing implemented during the 1980s by the Substance Abuse and Mental Health Services Administration (SAMHSA) of the US government. Although the 2 programs have some similarities, the purpose and implementation of the programs are different. Administrative cut-off concentrations or detection levels have been imposed for each of the 5 analytes for the purpose of identifying individuals who have a drug abuse problem that affects the work environment. In contrast, the number of compounds included on a full sports drug-testing panel exceeds 125, with an average of 5 compounds added each year. Sports drug-testing programs involve testing at both competitive events and during out-of-competition times to assess drug use at the time that the drug is most beneficial to performance. For example, anabolic steroids may be beneficial in off-season or pre-season training, whereas a β-blocker would be more beneficial during competition.[17] In reality, workplace drug testing addresses concerns about safety and productivity in the workplace and must confront societal drug use trends. Sports organizations choose to address performance-enhancing substances but also include testing for drugs athletes may use that are dangerous to their health although nonenhancing.

TABLE 17-1

ORGANIZATION CONTACT INFORMATION

ORGANIZATION	CONTACT INFORMATION	MISSION
World Anti-Doping Agency (WADA)	Stock Exchange Tower 800 Place Victoria, Suite 1700 P.O. Box 120 Montreal, Quebec H4Z 1B7 Canada Phone: 514-904-9232 www.wada-ama.org	The WADA is the international independent organization created in 1999 to promote, coordinate, and monitor the fight against doping in sport in all its forms. WADA coordinates with IOC, ISFs, NOCs, and athletes.
United States Anti-Doping Agency (USADA)	5555 Tech Center Drive, Suite 200 Colorado Springs, CO 80919 Phone: 719-785-2000 www.usantidoping.org	USADA is dedicated to preserving the well-being of Olympic sport and the integrity of competition and ensuring the health of athletes.
International Olympic Committee (IOC)	Chateau de Vidy Case postale 356 1007 Lausanne Switzerland Phone: (41.21) 621 61 11 www.olympic.org/ioc	The IOC is the supreme authority of the Olympic Movement. Its role is to promote top-level sport as well as sport for all in accordance with the Olympic Charter. It ensures the regular celebration of the Olympic Games and strongly encourages, by appropriate means, the promotion of women in sport, that of sports ethics, and the protection of athletes.
National Collegiate Athletic Association (NCAA)	700 W. Washington Street P.O. Box 6222 Indianapolis, IN 46206-6222 Phone: 317-917-6222 www.ncaa.org	To protect the health and safety of student-athletes and to ensure that no one participant has an artificially induced advantage or is pressured to use chemical substances.
International Athletics Foundation (IAF)	6-8, Quai Antoine 1er BP 359 MC 98007 Monaco Cedex Phone: (377) 93 10 88 88 www.iaaf.org	The IAF's primary mission is to charitably assist the world governing body for track and field athletics—the International Association of Athletics Federations—and its affiliated national governing bodies in perpetuating the development and promotion of athletics worldwide.

Regardless of the organization and its antidoping policies and procedures, due to their competitive nature, athletes will continue to search for substances or methods to enhance performance whether legal or not and whether safe or not. Although diverse and broad, organizations must continually focus on antidoping in sport. Former IOC President Juan Antonio Samaranch was quoted as he relinquished his position, "In doping, the war is never won."[31] A listing of sports drug-testing organizations and appropriate contact information is found in Table 17-1.

LEGAL CONSIDERATIONS

Courts are frequently called upon to decide issues involving competing interests that are both fundamental and important to society. Drug testing is certainly an issue involving 2 competing fundamental interests and one that has been argued in the legal system numerous times.[32] In amateur sports, drug testing has raised many legal issues, including concerns about an athlete's constitutional right to due process, equal protection, and privacy, as well as protection against illegal search and seizure and self-incrimination.[33] Although the legal implications of sports drug testing vary from jurisdiction to jurisdiction, case law historically supports the reasonableness of drug testing athletes. It is important to understand the protections guaranteed by the Constitution of the United States when developing and implementing a sports drug-testing program.[34] In addition, it is prudent for administrators of such programs to be familiar with case law relevant to drug testing in sport.

One of the first legal principles to consider is state action. If an athlete is attempting to invoke constitutional law protection in a drug-testing challenge, he or she must be able to prove the school, association, or other amateur governing body is a state actor. The organization administering drug testing must be shown to be part of the federal government, state government, or an agency of state government. As a general rule, public colleges and universities are state actors, as are public high schools. Private organizations, such as the NCAA, are not subject to constitutional challenges.[35] In *Barbay v. NCAA* (1987), a Louisiana State University football player tested positive for steroids as part of the NCAA drug-testing program. He sought to prevent the NCAA from enforcing a penalty based on a violation of his Fourteenth Amendment right to due process. The Federal District Court of Louisiana held that the NCAA was not a state actor, thus the athlete had no constitutional claim against the NCAA. The State of Florida trial court reached a similar decision in *Mira v. NCAA* (1988).[33]

Athletes opposed to drug testing oftentimes bring due process claims against their institutions or athletic organizations. Due process arguments in drug testing have included objecting to the consent forms that athletes are asked to read and sign as a condition of athletic eligibility, not being afforded an adequate hearing following a positive drug test, or an unreasonable penalty based on an unreliable test. Under the due process clause of the Fourteenth Amendment, the athlete must show he or she was deprived of a significant liberty or property interest before due process requirements are applied. Case precedent generally finds that athletes have neither liberty nor property interest in athletics.[33] As a result, the general requirement of notice and a hearing need not be met. Due process was challenged in *Bally v. Northeastern University and NCAA* (1989). The Superior Court of Massachusetts ruled that the NCAA consent form did not infringe upon any due process rights. The case was dismissed.[33]

The Fourteenth Amendment of the US Constitution prevents any state from depriving any person of life, liberty, or property without due process of law, nor deny any person equal protection of the law. The Fourth Amendment of the US Constitution protects any person from unreasonable searches and seizure without warrant of the probable cause.

Athletes also have argued, albeit unsuccessfully, that they are being discriminated against and will use an equal protection argument as their legal defense. Institutions or organizations are precluded from discriminating against any one group, such as requiring athletes to submit to drug testing, unless the institution or organization establishes a rational basis justifying such.[33] Often, the rational basis for drug testing is stated in the very purpose of the program: to protect the health and safety of the participants from the increased risks associated with drug use, to uphold the integrity of sport, and to prevent or deter use.

The unreasonable invasion of privacy has been a concern in drug-testing programs as well. Courts have heard several arguments related to excessive or unjustified intrusion that drug testing causes. Does a college or school infringe upon an athlete's constitutional right to privacy to obtain a biological specimen for drug analysis? In the area of invasion of privacy, many courts have held that athletes have a diminished expectation of privacy. Courts generally cite physical examinations and athletes disrobing in front of one another in locker rooms as examples of the lower expectation of privacy.[33] One of the most prominent cases challenging drug testing as an unconstitutional invasion of privacy was *Hill v. NCAA* (1993). In 1987, a Stanford University diver challenged a requirement that she submit to drug testing to participate in NCAA diving championships. A California Superior Court granted an injunction barring the NCAA from testing her at the competition. The suit alleged an unreasonable invasion of privacy under the state constitution. A trial court found the NCAA program to be an unconstitutional invasion of privacy. The NCAA appealed, and in 1994, the California Supreme Court reversed the lower court decision, reasoning that student-athletes had diminished expectations of privacy. Additionally, the court found the NCAA's performance-enhancing drug-testing program was beneficial because it allowed them to concentrate on competition without worrying about losing a competitive edge.[34]

High school drug-testing programs also have been challenged as an unreasonable search and seizure under the Fourteenth Amendment. The Fourth Amendment of the US Constitution provides for people to be secure in their persons, houses, papers, and effects against unreasonable searches and seizures. Before requiring athletes to provide biologic specimens for drug analysis, the drug test must be deemed "reasonable."[33] In *Schaill v. Tippecanoe* (1988), the Seventh Circuit Court of Appeals held that a drug-testing program was not an unreasonable search and seizure if it did not require observation of the student-athlete during specimen collection. Monitored specimen collections are considered less intrusive than observed collections but are not as effective in deterring manipulation or substitution of donated specimens. In *O'Halloran v. University of Washington and NCAA* (1988), O'Halloran claimed the drug-testing process was an unreasonable invasion of privacy and unreasonable search and seizure. The Ninth Circuit

Court held that the interests of the university and the NCAA were compelling and outweighed the hardships placed on the student-athlete. The court ruled in favor of the university, upholding that the drug-testing program was constitutional. However, in 1993, the Colorado Supreme Court ruled differently. In *Derdeyn v. University of Colorado* (1993), the Colorado Supreme Court found the university's drug-testing program to be unconstitutional because observed specimen collections were an unreasonable search and seizure and that the consent form signed by its student-athletes was not voluntary. The Colorado court found that although promoting fair competition had value, it did not rise to a level of compelling government interest as required by the Constitution.[36]

Acton v. Vernonia (1994) and *Pottawatomie County v. Earls* (2002) are 2 landmark US Supreme Court cases supporting suspicionless random drug testing of high school student-athletes and other students involved in school-related extracurricular activities. Both Vernonia and Earls allege Fourth Amendment and due process violations.

In *Acton v. Vernonia*, a seventh grader intended to participate in grade school football. He was not allowed to participate because his parents refused to sign the district's drug-testing consent form, which was a condition of his eligibility. The US Supreme Court ruled in favor of Vernonia School District, recognizing an exception to the Fourth Amendment's search and seizure requirement in cases where a special need exists. The Court balanced the student's privacy rights against the school's interest in providing a safe athletic environment for all participants and found the search for potential drug use through urine specimen collection was reasonable.[37]

In *Pottawatomie County v. Earls*, students involved in extracurricular activities including athletics in the Tecumseh, Oklahoma, school district were required to consent to urinalysis testing for drugs. Parents of the students brought suit against the school district, citing violation of the Fourth Amendment. The Court held the school district's drug-testing policy to be a reasonable means of preventing and deterring drug use among schoolchildren and did not violate the Fourth Amendment. The health and safety risks identified in the Vernonia case were found to apply with equal force to the Tecumseh school district.[38]

Although courts have upheld sports drug testing to be constitutional, any institution or athletic organization developing a drug-testing program must involve its legal counsel throughout the development process to draft policy and recommend laws specific to the organization's jurisdiction.

The law as it applies to drug testing is still evolving. Courts are still struggling with how to balance the interests of society against the privacy rights of individuals.[39] Athletes have legally challenged drug-testing procedures on various constitutional grounds. In response to those challenges, the courts have consistently upheld legally sound programs.[39]

Another legal dilemma sports drug-testing programs face is the legalization of marijuana and how local, state, and federal laws apply. A number of states have passed laws legalizing the use of marijuana for medical reasons. "In 2012 voters in Colorado and Washington also passed initiatives legalizing marijuana for adults 21 and older under state law."[40] However, marijuana continues to be a federal offense. Regardless of state or federal law regarding marijuana use, school athletic programs and other sports organizations continue to ban the use of marijuana. Based on the premise that sports participation is a privilege and not a right, law generally allows organizations to ban substances accordingly; however, legal consult is important in developing and reviewing programs to ensure compliance with local, state, and federal statutes.

COMPONENTS OF A DRUG-TESTING PROGRAM

There are 5 elements necessary for a successful anti-doping program to function[2]:

1. Adequate analytical capacity

2. Smart sampling strategies

3. A trustworthy adjudication process

4. Research

5. A foundation of clear principles and transparent processes

The primary components for developing a drug-testing program that reflects these essential elements include a detailed written policy, educational opportunities for athletes, drug-testing procedures, and consequences for positive drug tests, including a consistent adjudication process and provisions for substance use and abuse treatment for athletes. The ultimate goal of any drug-testing program is to influence change in human behavior. To create change in behavior, all of these components must be carefully observed and practiced.[41] Designing and implementing an effective drug-testing program is often a knee-jerk response to incidents of athlete drug use. Drug testing is a complicated process, demanding research and resources and a well-prepared plan before implementation.[42]

Policy

Before any type of drug testing can occur, a specific written policy must be developed, distributed to all participants, and publicized. Sports drug-testing policies must include several elements:

- A clear explanation of the purposes for the drug-testing program

- A description of who will be tested and by what methods

- The banned drug list

- A description of the types of testing athletes will be subjected to
- The consequences for positive drug tests
- A description of the appeal process
- Any therapeutic use or medical exceptions or safe harbor programs

Organizations should also include a process for addressing substance abuse by providing a systematic approach for athlete treatment and rehabilitation. All athletes must be provided with these policies in advance of implementing a drug-testing program. Athletes must provide written consent to the administering organization indicating that he or she has received, read, and agrees to the policy as it applies to participation within the organization.[43] The very foundation of any drug-testing program is the document that states the program's goals, regulations, and procedures.[41] Written drug-testing policies should be carefully developed. In addition, drug use in sports is a constantly changing landscape demanding constant attention to emerging trends and regulations.[42] Programs should be regularly reviewed to maintain effectiveness and legal compliance.

Purpose

The purpose of drug testing must be clearly explained in the introduction of any adopted policy. These purposes are generally considered benefits, and the benefits of drug testing athletes are many and varied. Opponents of drug testing will argue vehemently against these benefits; thus, any individual or group appointed to the task of developing a drug-testing program should consider opponents' views when tackling this issue. Opposing arguments include the idea that drug testing sends mixed messages, violates a person's rights, is viewed as a punitive measure, can be divisive, and is costly.[44]

Drug testing in athletics is basically intended to check for substances that could either provide an unfair advantage over those not using them or contribute to problems in the individual's life, including impaired athletic performance.[44] The misuse of drugs and other substances in the world of sport has been recognized as a significant problem for more than 30 years, with the 2 major concerns being ethics and health. These concerns are not independent of one another. Misuse of performance-enhancing drugs in sport is a health risk given the types of drugs abused, the large doses usually taken, and the stress that is already present in the body under competitive conditions. The all-encompassing purpose of drug testing in sport is to promote fair and equitable competition while protecting the health and safety of athletes. By subjecting athletes to drug testing, no one participant will have an artificially induced advantage, will be pressured to use chemical substances in attempting to remain competitive, or will be exposed to the health risks associated with using potentially dangerous drugs and other substances.[29] The goals of all drug-testing programs should be to deter the use of banned substances, identify individuals who have substance abuse problems, and provide access to treatment for such problems.[41]

In addition to ethical and health reasons for drug testing, organizations may also include detecting drug use, enforcing banned drug lists, punishing those found to be using banned substances, and deterring drug dependency as additional purposes for drug testing. Other reasons include protecting athletes from injury, enhancing the role model perceptions of athletes, and minimizing criminality. Properly conceived and implemented, a drug-testing program can also serve as an educational vehicle.[9]

Because athletes are usually healthy individuals, signs and symptoms of drug use may not be apparent upon observation, even to the trained eye. Drug testing provides a very definitive method of detecting use of controlled or illegal substances. In addition, the threat of a positive drug test and the resulting consequences may deter or prevent athletes from using these substances.[44] This deterrent effect has perhaps been the most important contribution of drug testing to societal well-being. Testing and fear of detection forces a person to make the affirmative decision not to use drugs in an uncontrolled or illegal manner.[45] Of course, the deterrent effect is only present if policies are consistently enforced. The only thing worse than not drug testing is having a drug-testing program and not enforcing it.

Banned Substances

Any sports organization adopting a drug-testing program must develop a list of drugs for which athletes will be tested. In sport, there are 2 areas of drug use that must be deterred: performance-enhancing substances and other illicit drugs found to be detrimental to the health and well-being of athletes. Performance-enhancing substances (see Chapter 16) are banned because of their coercive nature and their potential adverse effects. "A performance-enhancing substance is any substance taken in nonpharmacologic doses specifically for the purposes of improving sports performance."[3] Substances included in this definition include pharmacologic agents taken in doses that exceed recommended dosages or when taken nontherapeutically, agents used for weight control (eg, stimulants, diuretics), agents for weight gain or increased muscle mass (eg, anabolic agents, testosterone, peptide hormones), physiologic agents or methods to enhance oxygen-carrying capacity (eg, erythropoietin [EPO]), any substance used to mask adverse effects or ability to detect use, or dietary supplements taken at supraphysiologic doses.[3] Timing and purpose of performance-enhancing substances should be considered to effectively deter use through drug testing. For example, drug testing during competition may not adequately identify users of anabolic agents. These substances are more likely to be used during out-of-competition training for their long-term performance-enhancing goals, whereas stimulants are more likely to be used during competition to enhance performance on the day of an event.

For this reason, athletes must be subjected to drug testing year-round for the total deterrent effect.

In addition to performance-enhancing substances, most athletic programs include testing for other drugs found to be potentially dangerous to an athlete's health. These drug categories include stimulants (eg, cocaine, methamphetamines, and Ecstasy), depressants (eg, marijuana, alcohol, and barbiturates), hallucinogens (eg, LSD and psilocybin mushrooms), and opiates (eg, morphine, codeine, and heroin).[44] Most athletic organizations choose to adopt an all-inclusive banned drug list providing the ability to test for any drug deemed performance enhancing and/or dangerous to the health of its athletes. Banned drug lists should be included in any drug-testing policy, readily available to participants, and updated regularly to adequately address drug use issues in sport. Banned drug lists are available from respective athletic organizations.

Testing Types and Methods

Organizations implementing drug-testing programs must consider a number of logistical and technical issues that will ultimately define the types of testing and the methods used. These types and methods must be described in the drug-testing policy. There are several types of testing available for sports drug testing with distinct reasons for each (Box 17-1). Random drug testing is the most popular type of testing used and is applied year-round to deter drug use and identify users.

Random drug testing involves maintaining a complete and accurate list of athletes and randomly selecting athletes for periodic drug testing. Effective random drug testing should be frequent, unpredictable, and unannounced. The random selection process should be completely objective, assuring nondiscriminatory identification of participating athletes to be tested. Athletes should be notified and required to report for testing at the designated collection site within preset parameters. Random testing is effective in deterring and identifying performance-enhancing drugs for training such as anabolic agents and "social/designer" drugs such as marijuana or Ecstasy. The notification of the athlete should be as short as logistically possible. The maximum time should be 24 hours prior to test time, and the ideal would be testing immediately after being notified. Testing athletes should not interfere with academic schedules or practices.[41]

Reasonable suspicion testing provides organizations with another option for drug testing athletes. Organizations can selectively test an athlete based on specific objective facts and reasonable inferences drawn from those facts in light of documented experiences related to drug use. Reasonable suspicion testing must be based on physical symptoms or manifestations of being under the influence such as behavior or appearance consistent with prohibited use (eg, odor of alcohol); direct observation of prohibited use; a report of prohibited use from a reliable source; or evidence of use,

Box 17-1

TYPES OF DRUG TESTING

- Random testing
- Reasonable suspicion testing
- Pre-participation testing to identify at-risk athletes
- Follow-up testing on athletes with previous positive drug tests
- Monitoring of athletes following drug use interventions
- Pre-competition drug testing
- Event testing

possession, or sale of prohibited drugs. An athlete notified of reasonable suspicion testing must immediately submit to a drug test.

Other types of drug testing to consider including in a sports drug-testing program include pre-participation testing to identify at-risk athletes, follow-up testing on athletes with previous positive drug tests, monitoring of athletes following drug use interventions, and pre-competition drug testing on athletes who have qualified for events where they will be subject to drug testing by other sports organizations. Sports organizations often perform event testing to ensure a level playing field for drugs taken on competition day. The NCAA, US Anti-Doping Agency, IOC, sports conferences, and even some state high school athletic associations now perform event drug testing in an effort to deter performance-enhancing drug use and to identify users of such. Stimulants, relaxants, and oxygenation enhancers are classes of drugs athletes are tempted to use in an effort to enhance performance during a specific competitive time.

Testing methods and procedures should also be described in the written drug-testing policy. Specifically the type(s) of specimens to be used for testing should be identified as well as the collection protocol that will be followed in collecting specimens from athletes. Chain of custody procedures, laboratory procedures, and methods of specimen analysis must also be described in the policy.

Consequences

The drug-testing policy should specifically describe the procedures for reporting results:

- Who receives results
- Who notifies the athletes
- Who the athlete is referred to for evaluation
- Who is granted knowledge of a positive drug test

Box 17-2

SUMMARY OF ENTITIES INVOLVED IN A COMPLETE DRUG-TESTING PROGRAM

- Donor (athlete)
- Drug-testing administrator
- Third-party administrators
- Collectors
- Laboratories
- Medical review officer (results recipient)

- What disciplinary action is imposed for a positive drug test

Confidentiality is of primary concern when communicating a positive drug test. Once positive drug test results are reported, these results must be reviewed to determine if there is an acceptable explanation for the test result. A medical review of these results is essential prior to labeling an athlete as testing positive under the program's policies. Once the result is deemed positive under the definition of the program policy, administrators must implement procedures for handling a positive drug test. Generally, the program director will meet with the athlete to discuss the nature and extent of drug use and to apply sanctions for policy violations as described. Sanctions for a positive drug test often include immediate suspension from sport participation until the athlete can be evaluated by medical and substance abuse specialists to determine the risks associated with physical exercise and prohibited drug use and a treatment plan for the athlete is implemented. Consequences for any refusal to comply with procedures or repeated positive drug test results must also be described in the written policy.

> *Chain of custody refers to the ability to completely document the handling of a specimen from the moment the donor provides a sample until it is finished being processed by the laboratory and a result is reported.*

Appeal

All drug-testing programs must include an opportunity for the athlete to appeal the decision and subsequent consequences associated with a positive drug test or noncompliance to procedures. The appeal process should include a designated committee made up of representatives from various relevant professions (eg, medicine, athletics) who meet to hear the athlete's reasons for testing positive. Technical experts, third-party administrators (TPAs), and collectors may also serve as consultants to the committee

when such matters are involved in the nature of the appeal. Unlike criminal litigation, civil cases require only that the preponderance of evidence support the finding of doping activity.[3] Following a hearing, the committee's decision will ultimately be accepted and any subsequent sanctions applied. The goal of effectively modifying behavior can only occur when the consequences are widely believed to impose accurate and even-handed results.[46]

Treatment

Following a positive drug test and subsequent evaluation by medical professionals regarding the nature and extent of drug use, an appropriate treatment plan must be implemented. At the very least, treatment should provide accurate and current information on the health hazards of drug abuse; help users overcome drug dependence; be directed based on age, interests, and special problems of athletes; emphasize immediate negative effects from drug use; and hold the athlete accountable for his or her actions.[12] Most athletes' evaluations following a positive test show a drug use problem, not dependency. Drug use is a behavioral problem, not a disease. These individuals respond well to counseling on decision making and instruction on the potential hazards of drug use. If dependency or repetitive drug use occurs, more intensive treatment is indicated.[41] Appropriate substance abuse professionals must supervise any treatment or rehabilitation program.

Before any type of drug testing can be implemented, a detailed written policy must be adopted and presented to all participants. This policy must include purpose, banned drug list, testing methods, consequences, due process, and recommended treatment opportunities. Once policies and procedures are reviewed, participants must consent to drug testing as described and a signed consent form should remain on file throughout the effective date of the policy.

Participants

Developing, implementing, and administering an effective drug-testing program involves a number of people with a variety of responsibilities. Early in the process when examining the need for program development, legal counsel should be recruited to review local, state, and federal statutes that apply. The legal aspects involved with each organization should be clarified. The development process should also involve representatives from various relevant academic departments and disciplines (eg, pharmacology, chemistry, and psychology), athletic administrators, athletes, athletic trainers, and medical doctors. Ultimately, the administration of a complete drug-prevention program will involve a number of entities (Box 17-2).

Donor (Athlete)

A donor is any person who is designated in the organization's drug-testing policies as subject to drug and/or alcohol testing. As applied to sports drug testing, the term includes any athlete who is currently listed as a participant in sport within the organization. The term *donor* is a drug-testing industry standard identifying the individual subjected to drug testing who is required to provide a biological specimen for analysis of drugs.[47] The donors in an institutional athletic drug-testing program may include student-athletes, cheerleaders, and managers. Drug testing may also include all participants of competitive extracurricular programs (eg, club sports, debate, band). The organization's drug-testing policies must identify and define all donors subject to drug testing. All donors must be provided with the drug-testing policies, and administrators of the program should describe drug testing in detail. Once all donors have been provided accurate information about the program, each donor must read and sign a drug-testing consent form, and if underage, parents of the donor must sign the consent form prior to specimen collection and testing. Once a donor has consented to participating in the drug-testing program, he or she will be expected to follow policies and procedures accordingly. Failure to abide by the policies usually have consequences similar to those of a positive drug test. These consequences should also be included in the written policy.

Drug-Testing Administrator

Each organization with a drug-testing policy should have an individual responsible for administering the program. Often, many people are involved in program administration, but one individual is identified as the program administrator. It is the drug-testing administrator's responsibility to financially manage and oversee compliance with the entire program. Often this individual coordinates annual review and dissemination of policies to all participants, collects signed consent forms from donors, schedules required drug education programs and testing events for participants, and coordinates other individuals or entities with responsibilities related to drug testing. The drug-testing administrator may have additional duties associated with actual drug testing and results handling. Athletic trainers are often responsible for administering sports drug-testing programs, but sometimes find these responsibilities place them in conflict with athlete relationships, especially if duties include specimen collection and results handling. The program administrator can effectively oversee the entire drug-testing program and maintain strong, trustworthy relationships with athletes by delegating or outsourcing specific components of program administration, including collections, results reporting, and applying sanctions.

Third-Party Administrators

Sports organizations have the option of contracting with outside agencies to provide or coordinate a variety of drug-testing services. TPAs offer organizations industry expertise and objectivity in administering drug-testing programs and allow athletic organization personnel the ability to focus on day-to-day responsibilities associated with athletics management. TPAs provide trained specimen collectors, laboratory discounts through consortium efforts, independently administered random selection services, and Medical Review Officer (MRO) expertise. When determining cost factors for considering outside agencies, organizations must include the value of time expended by the internal staff to perform these duties. In addition, using experts with extensive and detailed training further supports the effectiveness and ultimately the success of a drug-testing program.

Collectors

The collection of biologic specimens from selected donors (athletes) is crucial to the effectiveness of any drug-testing program. The collector must be trusted to perform his or her job professionally and provide for privacy while ensuring integrity and security of the specimen throughout the entire collection process. Collectors must be knowledgeable in sports drug-testing issues and maintain the skills necessary to perform specimen collections in a consistent manner. Collectors should be adequately trained and required to maintain proficiency in collection services according to industry standards and organizational diversity. Trained collectors eliminate costly and legally challenging chain of custody errors with regard to specimen handling and transfer to appropriate laboratories. In addition, collectors deter specimen adulteration, substitution, and manipulation attempts by donors at the collection site. Specimen adulteration is any attempt to change the outcome of an anticipated positive drug test by altering the biologic specimen prior to analysis. Adulterated specimens significantly compromise drug-testing programs by causing false-negative results. If a drug-testing program does not adequately deter specimen adulteration through on-site collection procedures, athletes will attempt to and successfully beat a drug test, ultimately creating a mockery of an organization's drug-testing program.

Care should be taken when determining who will be responsible for the collection process if an organization elects to perform its own collections. For example, athletic trainers may be compromising their relationship with athletes by performing collections or other judicial processes in a drug-testing program. Athletes often approach the athletic trainer in confidence when concerned about health issues, including drug use, and may no longer trust or feel comfortable disclosing such issues if the athletic trainer performs these drug-testing duties. In addition, if an organization chooses to use its own personnel because of budgetary constraints, it is important to consider the time costs this task imposes on already taxed employees.

Pharmacists are excellent candidates for drug-testing collectors because they can develop and conduct drug-testing protocols; educate athletes, coaches, and athletic trainers about drug use and abuse; and help ensure the safe and effective use of medications. Other medical professionals such as nurses, paramedics, emergency medical technicians, firefighters, athletic trainers (when conflict of interest does not exist), or medical technologists are also strong candidates. TPAs and collection companies can also provide specimen collections. There are also unacceptable candidates for specimen collections. An athlete cannot serve as a collector for his or her own specimen; neither is it appropriate for athletic training students to perform collections. Employees of any participating laboratory should not perform specimen collections, and collectors of the opposite sex should not perform direct observation collections due to the sensitivity of the process and the increased risk of litigation based on an unreasonable invasion of privacy. If a same-sex validator cannot be provided, the test should either not be performed or a monitored collection should be used, depending on the organization's policy and procedures.

Laboratories

Credentialed laboratories are vital to the ultimate success of a drug-deterrence program. Organizations must be confident that results generated by the laboratory are accurate and scientifically measured. There are a variety of credentialing entities responsible for certifying laboratories. Laboratory accreditation is an important criterion to consider when selecting a laboratory for specimen analysis. Accreditation and certification demonstrate reliability and quality assurance.[36] Before using a laboratory, the organization should request verification of the laboratory's standards of accreditation.

In 2004, WADA replaced the IOC as the official accrediting body for laboratories performing specimen analysis in sport. The World Antidoping Code International Standard for Laboratories outlines the specific requirements for WADA's accreditation process. Requirements include providing an official letter of support from the relevant national public authority responsible for the national antidoping program, signing and complying with WADA's Code of Ethics, proficiency testing of samples, sharing of knowledge with other accredited laboratories, and a strong commitment to research. Goals of the WADA accreditation program include promoting scientific excellence, harmonization of methodology, reliable scientific information, and fostering good will and cooperation. WADA's Code of Ethics forbids testing samples unless they are from a bona fide sports program. Thus, WADA-accredited laboratories are prohibited from testing to aid or abet athletes attempting to learn how to evade detection of drug use.[48]

Laboratories engaged in urine drug testing for federal agencies must be SAMHSA certified. This certification sets strict standards that laboratories must meet to conduct urine drug testing for federal agencies. To become certified, an applicant laboratory must undergo 3 rounds of performance testing plus on-site inspection. To maintain certification, a laboratory must participate in a quarterly performance testing program and periodic on-site inspections.[49]

Medical Review Officer (Results Recipient)

In workplace drug-testing programs, an MRO is used to review positive drug test results to determine if there is a legitimate reason for the positive result. The MRO is defined in federal regulations as a licensed physician with a working knowledge of substance abuse disorders who has appropriate medical training to interpret and evaluate positive drug test results.[45] In sports drug-testing programs, the team physician is often designated to receive positive drug tests. Team physicians often function as educators, MROs, and provide medical exceptions or therapeutic use exceptions (TUEs) with regard to positive drug test cases.[42] Results may be handled as part of an athlete's medical record and protected from disclosure by the laws protecting confidentiality of medical documents. Drug test results are not encompassed by the Health Insurance Portability and Accountability Act of 1996; however, drug-testing policies and consent forms athletes are required to sign should include language on exactly who has access to drug-testing results. Regardless of the individual designated to receive results, the process must be administered with the utmost confidentiality. It is important for the laboratory to be blind with respect to the donor's identity, thus laboratory personnel cannot serve as review officers for their own work.[17] Laboratories are capable of providing results to the designated individual via a number of secure methods, such as certified mail, secure facsimile, or secure Internet access. The recipient of the results must maintain these confidential records, assure adequate medical review of positive results, and present the verified positive results to the individual responsible for meeting with the athlete and other designated parties to disclose the result, apply consequences, facilitate the appeal process if requested, and/or refer for necessary counseling and/or treatment.

There are a number of responsibilities involved in administering a sound sports drug-testing program. A team of individuals generally completes these tasks, but the program administrator should play a leadership role in coordinating all aspects of drug testing.

Methodology

Before administering a sports drug-testing program, an organization should review industry-adopted procedures and scientific methodologies currently being practiced. Often there are options available and the organization should select those options that best meet its needs in addressing drug use in sport. From the specimen type that will be analyzed to the actual method of analysis, these decisions must be made based on current and accurate information.

Specimen Types

Because of many advances in analytical technology, drugs and their metabolites can be detected in a variety of tissues and biological fluids. Chemical testing of biological fluids is the most objective means of diagnosis of drug use.[50,51] A wide variety of specimens are available today, each providing valuable information concerning prior and current drug use (Box 17-3).[52] The standard for drug testing in toxicology is the immunoassay screen, a quick method of determining the presence or absence of a drug or metabolite in a urine specimen. A positive screen is followed by confirmation using GC with mass spectrometry (GC/MS), a very specialized procedure that specifically identifies the metabolite qualitatively. Although initial research in alternative specimen testing used radioimmunoassay, newer nonisotopic commercial immunoassays are now widely available for screening of drugs and drug metabolites. Enzyme-linked immunosorbent assay, a specific type of immunoassay screening, has been adapted for detection of analytes in extracts/digests of hair, oral fluid, and sweat patches. Enzyme-linked immunosorbent assays are semiquantitative, cost-effective, highly sensitive, and especially applicable to alternative specimens because of their increased specificity to parent drugs such as cocaine, rather than drug metabolites such as benzoylecgonine, a major metabolite of cocaine. The selection of a specific biological specimen for drug analysis is influenced by a variety of factors, principally ease of specimen collection, analytical and testing considerations, and interpretation of results. Interest has shifted from urine toward other specimens that can provide distinct advantages. The introduction of several laboratory-based drug test systems and on-site devices has expanded drug-testing capabilities.[52] Today there are a number of specimens other than urine, such as saliva, sweat, meconium, or hair, demonstrating viable biological options for drug detection.[50,52]

Urine

Since the 1970s, urine has been the most common biological specimen used in detecting drugs of abuse. Although other biologic matrices are now available for drug testing, urine continues to be the specimen of choice. The collection of urine is noninvasive, and large volumes can be collected

easily. Drugs and their metabolites are generally present in higher concentrations in urine than in other matrices because of the concentrating function of the kidneys. Urine is easier to analyze than other biological specimens because of less protein, and cellular constituents and drugs (and their metabolites) are usually stable in frozen urine, which allows for long-term storage of positive samples.[12] Although widely used, problems with urine testing have been identified (Box 17-4). Regardless of its limitations or the complications it imposes, urine remains the specimen standard in sports drug testing. Laboratories have extensive scientific basis for the testing methodology and scientists have developed extremely sophisticated instruments and procedures using urine specimens to effectively detect many of the more common substances currently being abused by athletes.

Blood

Compared with urine, the use of blood or plasma provides better correlations between the concentrations of the drug and its effects on performance. However, the use of blood as a specimen for analysis of drugs presents several limitations, including religious beliefs. It is an invasive technique requiring technical proficiency in collecting from the donor, analyses are expensive and more complex, specimens are smaller, and drugs (and their metabolites) are found at significantly lower concentrations than in urine.[12] Because of the invasiveness of collecting a blood sample and the inherent risks associated with such, athletic organizations have been reluctant to incorporate blood collections; however, newer methodologies being developed and implemented in today's antidoping initiatives may require blood for detecting newer performance-enhancing tactics (eg, gene manipulation, recombinant human growth hormone [hGH] detection) in sport.

Oral Fluid

Saliva, or the preferred term *oral fluid*, was originally introduced to monitor therapeutic drugs and for insurance testing; however, it has been increasingly used as an analytic tool in the detection of environmental chemicals, illicit drugs, and many endogenous substances.[51,52] Saliva is the fluid secretion of the salivary glands, whereas oral fluid contains saliva, mucosal transudate, and crevicular fluid.[51] Advantages of oral fluid over other traditional fluids are the collection is almost noninvasive, is relatively easy to perform, and, in forensic situations, can be achieved under close supervision to prevent adulteration or substitution of samples.[2] It seems the concentrations of many drugs in oral fluid correlate well with blood concentrations, which suggest that quantitative measurements in oral fluid may be a valuable technique to determine the current degree of exposure to a definite drug at the time of sampling.[53] Caution must be taken when collecting oral fluid samples. Substances containing citric acid (eg, citrus fruits, fruit juices, and certain candies) cause an overstimulation of saliva and can skew concentration levels of certain substances. In addition, certain oral fluid–collecting devices produce significantly different concentrations of marijuana after recent use. Devices placed between the gum and cheek for oral fluid collection demonstrated much higher concentrations of tetrahydrocannabinol than those with collecting procedures requiring the donor to spit oral fluid into a collection device.[50]

Perhaps the most effective use of oral fluid screening is the measurement of ethanol in saliva. Ethanol is a small molecule, is highly water soluble, and is not bound to plasma protein. Because of these characteristics, plus the rich blood flow to the oral cavity, the concentration of alcohol in the saliva should reflect the concentration in arterial blood.

Currently on-site or point-of-collection oral fluid testing devices are not considered reliable, and screening sensitivity inconsistencies exist. Laboratory-based oral fluid testing services provide a potentially viable alternative to urine testing on certain drugs. Screening is performed with an instrumental laboratory enzyme immunoassay providing less interference from endogenous compounds than when using blood or urine samples. This technique allows for the detection of cocaine, methamphetamine, morphine, cannabinoids, and phencyclidine (PCP). Because of the smaller sample volume of oral fluid, confirmed quantitative analytic procedures using MS in the chemical ionization mode, liquid chromatography (LC)-MS, and tandem MS-MS confirmation are being developed.[51,54] Overall, oral fluid testing demonstrates promise in detecting drugs of abuse, but science does not currently exist to support using oral fluid specimens for analyzing many of the drugs and substances listed as banned by many sports organizations.

Hair

Hair testing was originally used for metal detection and nutritional evaluation.[9] More recently, there are reported applications in forensic toxicology, clinical toxicology, occupational medicine, and doping control. The major practical advantage of hair for testing drugs, compared with urine and blood, is its larger detection window. Hair analysis extends the ability to provide historical detail of an individual's exposure to drugs following chronic use or a single exposure and is most commonly used in criminal investigations and in monitoring drug use of convicted felons.[55] The detection window is weeks to months, depending on the length of hair shaft analyzed. The average length of the hair sample to be tested should be 3.9 cm or 1.5 in, and because hair grows about 0.5 inch a month, the period represents approximately 90 days. It is interesting to note that hair and urine testing are complementary. Urinalysis provides short-term information on drug use, whereas long-term histories are accessible through hair analysis. The greatest use of hair testing may be in identifying a false-negative result from other biologic specimen analysis. Urine does not indicate the frequency of drug use in subjects who might deliberately abstain for several days before screening. Hair analysis is a potentially fail-safe procedure in contrast to urine testing because an identical urine specimen cannot be obtained at a later date. However, there are still concerns about the qualitative results from hair due to the influences of external contamination or cosmetic treatment and results may vary due to race.[50,56]

To date, the scientific knowledge of hair biology in attempting to detect performance-enhancing substances in sport is not available. Analytical methods do not exist for several doping compounds, such as diuretics. Peptide hormones are not extractable. Hair washing, discoloring, tinting, and hair color (resulting in potential ethnic differences) appear to influence drug concentrations in hair.[50,51] Scientists have been able to detect endogenous steroids in hair using GC/MS, and physiologic concentrations of both testosterone and dehydroepiandrosterone are distinguishable in hair between male and female subjects. Hair analysis can be used to identify the exact nature of the parent compound (eg, nandrolone, norandrostenediol, or norandrostenedione (all anabolic steroids), in the case of a urine sample positive for norandrosterone), allowing discrimination between nandrolone abuse from over-the-counter (OTC) preparations containing 19-norsteroids. Although hair is not yet a valid specimen option for the IOC, courts in Europe, Japan, and the United States have accepted drug test results from hair analysis. Recently, some conflicting results have occurred in athletes who tested positive in urine samples submitted to accredited IOC laboratories but negative in hair samples sent to certified forensic laboratories. Since 2001, hair analysis has been allowed in France to document doping practices.[50,51] Certainly the question to be asked in considering whether to use hair testing is whether the drug-testing program's purpose is to detect or to deter.

Sweat

Using the sweat patch as a detection vehicle is fairly simple. The patch contains an absorbent pad sandwiched between the skin and an outer protective membrane. A tamper-evident adhesive backing on the membrane of the patch allows easy adherence to the donor's skin. The outer membrane allows vapors from the sweat to pass through it. Thus, the donor's sweat moistens the pad, the water in the sweat eventually evaporates through the membrane, and any drugs or metabolites found in the sweat remain in the absorbent pad. Once the sweat patch is removed, it is returned to the laboratory for analysis. The sweat patch has been successful in the criminal justice system due to its reliability. It is a rugged and tamper-evident device; however, questions exist regarding possible external environmental contamination through the sweat patch membrane.[57] Profuse sweating can contribute to the susceptibility of environmental contamination by allowing external influences, such as cocaine powder, to penetrate the membrane of the patch and contribute to the ineffectiveness of its use in sports drug testing.

The value of alternative specimen analysis for the identification of drug users appears to be steadily gaining recognition.[51] Adding state-of-the-art techniques such as LC-MS and MS-MS technology will enable forensic toxicologists to facilitate the use of these additional matrices. In the future, testing of alternative specimens will expand the ability to understand the patterns of drug use and will become routine in forensic toxicology.[52] Alternative specimens, such as hair, appear to provide potential in the analysis of anabolic agents. At the very least, alternative specimens may complement traditional urine testing to further document results (Table 17-2).

Banned Drugs

In sport, substances are prohibited or banned because of performance-enhancing properties and/or the potential health risks associated with their use. The most significant difference between workplace drug testing and sports drug testing is the list of prohibited drugs and levels of detection or cut-offs used for analysis. Workplace drug testing is designed to identify prospective or current workers who have a drug problem, particularly with any of the 5 illegal substances: amphetamines, cocaine, heroin, marijuana, and PCP.[5] The cut-off levels are the values chosen for the determination of a positive or negative in a drug screen and adopted in workplace testing to identify individuals with substance abuse problems. The SAMHSA levels are recommended as the most appropriate established and legally defensible standards for workplace drug testing and have been set to avoid false-positive results.[40,42] It is often argued that these cut-offs are too high to effectively identify many substance abusers. In contrast, the purpose of sports drug testing is to detect the presence of substances identified as banned by testing organizations. Most high schools, college, and universities that drug test athletes continue to include testing for illegal substances because of the potential health risks and legal implications associated with their use but tend to use detection levels lower than the workplace model. The IOC follows the WADA Code of prohibited substances, and the NCAA and most professional sports organizations have similar banned substance

lists. Most substances on these lists have no administrative cut-off concentrations in attempting to identify the presence of such drugs. Banned substances are determined by athletic organizations, published, and updated regularly. In general, WADA, NCAA, and most professional sports associations prohibit classes of compounds rather than publishing a list of individual compounds. The lists include examples within each class to act as a guide and also to ensure that new drugs and designer substances are covered and include the words "and related substances," to describe drugs that are related to the class by their pharmacologic actions and/or chemical structure.[58] Complete and current banned drug lists are available by contacting individual athletic organizations (see Table 17-1 for organization contact information).

There are many drugs and dietary supplements extensively marketed to and used by athletes of all ages and levels of competition to enhance performance.[59] The typical testing menu in sports drug testing encompasses 5 classes of prohibited compounds: stimulants, narcotic analgesics, diuretics, anabolic agents, and peptide hormones. There are restrictions in selected circumstances on a number of other substances including alcohol, marijuana, local anesthetics, corticosteroids, and β-blockers. Blood doping procedures and agents that could mask drug detection or manipulate urinary excretion are also prohibited.[5]

Street drugs such as marijuana and newer synthetic substances such as synthetic cannabinoids, K2 or Spice, and synthetic cathinones (manmade chemicals related to amphetamines and commonly known as *bath salts,*)[60] are popular recreational drugs. Although not considered performance-enhancing drugs, most sports organizations have adopted a street drug category of banned substances due to their potential health risks and to protect the integrity of sport. Synthetic drugs have been marketed as safe, legal alternatives and sold under a variety of names. Synthetic cannabinoids are manmade chemicals often applied onto plant material. Spice has a chemical makeup known to have a high potential for abuse. The US Drug Enforcement Administration has designated 5 of the most frequently used chemicals used to make Spice as Schedule I controlled substances.[61] Bath salts products consist of methylenedioxypyrovalerone, mephedrone, and methylone. Early indications are that synthetic cathinones also have a high abuse and addiction potential[62] and the same health risks associated with stimulant use.

A short description of the classes of drugs banned by most sports organizations because of their performance-enhancing qualities follows.

Stimulants

Stimulants (see Chapter 13) have been used in sport for their performance-enhancing properties for over 2 centuries. Some of these prohibited performance-enhancing compounds include amphetamines, β-agonists, caffeine, cocaine, and ephedrine. These compounds have been used to improve concentration, increase aggressiveness, and to relieve the

TABLE 17-2

SPECIMEN COMPARISON CHART

MATRIX COMPARABLE FACTORS	LAB URINALYSIS (INDUSTRY STANDARD)	ON-SITE URINALYSIS	ORAL FLUID	HAIR	SWEAT	BLOOD
Applicability	Used to detect all types of drug use	Up to 9-drug panel	Up to 9-drug panel, including alcohol	Wide variety of drugs detected—typical 5 panel most common	Wide variety of drugs detected, including alcohol	Drugs detectable, but not applicable
Collection procedure	Procedurally strong and legally defensible May be embarrassing or uncomfortable	Similar to lab urinalysis Do not need scientific personnel to determine result	Foam absorption pad inserted in mouth for 2 minutes. Pad then pressed into reagent device for on-site result with package to send positive screen specimen to lab for confirm	Cut 1.5-inch sample of hair from back of head along scalp, package, and send to lab for testing	Use a sweat patch that is adhesively applied to skin and worn over days to weeks and then sent to lab for testing	Collecting sample is invasive and high risk, use of needles requires highly trained medical personnel
Performance criteria	Extensive research Controlled and accurate Extensive quality control testing Accurate cut-off levels	Lacks quality control Variation in cut-off concentrations No performance testing done	Limited proficiency testing has been done Not widely used Fair amount of scientific acceptability	No proficiency testing programs exist Scientifically acceptable, but controversy exists (interpretation does, time relationships)	No performance testing has been done	Accepted and widely utilized in the scientific community for therapeutic drug monitoring and for postmortem assessments
Government approval	Yes—all levels; considered standard operating	Some kits are FDA approved	Not approved by FDA	Approved by FDA for 5 panel testing (Psychemedics Corp)	Patch is approved by FDA	Yes, primarily for medical use
Sample adulteration or manipulation probability	Dilution is factor Observed collection controls	Dilution is factor Observed collection controls	None if collection procedure followed correctly	Products sold that claim to "cleanse" hair of drugs	Patch removal or contamination	None

(continued)

TABLE 17-2 (CONTINUED)

SPECIMEN COMPARISON CHART

MATRIX COMPARABLE FACTORS	LAB URINALYSIS (INDUSTRY STANDARD)	ON-SITE URINALYSIS	ORAL FLUID	HAIR	SWEAT	BLOOD
Advantages	Sufficient specimen volume Known testing accuracy/reliability Known analytes and cut-offs Extensive clinical studies Easily automated Less expensive		Observed, noninvasive More difficult to adulterate Sex-neutral specimen collection Reflects more recent drug use	Large window of detection (90 days) Ease of collection, handling, storage Retesting is possible Difficult to adulterate the sample	Convenient and less invasive way to monitor drug use Detection window greater than urine Difficult to adulterate	
Disadvantages	Need for same-sex collector Invasion of privacy Shy bladder issues Measures exposure only		Low specimen volumes collected Drug absorption to collection device Limited detection window for THC Limited number of drugs available for testing	Possibility of environmental contamination Recent drug use not detected Limited drugs tested in panel Limited number of labs performing this test Least sensitive matrix for cannabis detection	Variation in sweat production Occasional skin sensitivity to adhesive Patch is expensive No lab proficiency program Limited drug panel	

Data collected from presentation given by Marilyn Huestis, PhD, Chief, Chemistry & Drug Metabolism, IRP. National Institute on Drug Abuse/National Institutes of Health, August 2010.

Additional information provided by Dr. David Kuntz, Clinical Reference Laboratory, January 2013.

perception of fatigue during competition.[59] As examples of sympathomimetic amines, amphetamines are believed to improve physical performance by increasing strength and endurance and by improving reaction times while masking pain and fatigue.[59] Amphetamines and amphetamine analogues seem to improve mental performance by creating euphoria, boosting confidence, and intensifying aggression. Physiological effects include increased respiratory rate, heart rate, blood pressure, and metabolism. Caffeine is a socially acceptable drug, but probably the most widely abused drug in the world. Caffeine is commonly used by athletes as a performance enhancer in training and competitions and is a key ingredient in energy drinks and a plethora of dietary supplements.[59] Its use is restricted by the NCAA with urinary levels > 15 µg/mL constituting a positive drug test in sport.[63] Ephedrine is another stimulant classified as a sympathomimetic drug. It has been found to be an effective bronchodilator due to its stimulation of β_2-receptors in the lungs, but because ephedrine is nonselective for β_1- and β_2-receptors, it causes unwanted adverse effects such as increased heart rate and blood pressure. After numerous cases of documented deaths and severe side effects, the FDA banned ephedrine as an ingredient in dietary supplements, but it is still legally acceptable to include ephedrine in OTC drugs.

Narcotic Analgesics

Narcotic analgesics (opioids) (see Chapter 7) are included on banned drug lists because they potentially increase performance and because of the vulnerability of the athletes to serious injury as a result of the analgesia.[3] Prohibiting opioids is based more on their reputation and dangers when used as illegal drugs than their performance-enhancing potential. Narcotics are more likely to reduce performance than improve it.

Diuretics

Diuretics (see Chapter 12) are used to mask the presence of other substances by diluting or altering the pH of the urine. They are also used to achieve rapid weight loss through water excretion for sports such as wrestling or bodybuilding. Complications from diuretic use include fluid and electrolyte imbalances and dehydration and can lead to heat-related illnesses. Both the NCAA and WADA ban use of diuretics.[59]

Anabolic Agents

Anabolic agents (see Chapter 16) are used to achieve increases in muscle mass, strength, and speed; improve recovery from training; and increase mental aggressiveness.[5] Athletes choose to use both endogenous (eg, testosterone, dehydroepiandrosterone) or exogenous (eg, nandrolone, stanozolol, mesterolone) anabolic steroids because of claims that they increase lean body mass, increase strength, increase aggressiveness, and lead to a shorter recovery time between workouts.[50] β_2-agonists are also considered to provide ana-

bolic properties when taken in higher dosages.[51] There is a high risk of adverse effects associated with continuous use of anabolic agents especially in women and adolescents. Highly toxic effects on the liver, growth disorders in youth, and female fertility disorders are common adverse effects. Other potential risks associated with anabolic steroid use include cholesterol and lipid disorders, hypertension, heart attacks, stroke, and a variety of psychoses.[59] Prior to congressional changes made in the Anabolic Steroid Act that became effective in January 2005, it was legal for dietary supplement companies to include steroid precursors or pro-hormones as ingredients in supplement products designed to increase athletic performance. The Anabolic Steroid Act of 2004 redefined anabolic steroids to include precursors as Schedule III controlled substances (see Table 1-7). In addition to making it illegal to sell anabolic agents in dietary supplements, the strengthened law also made it easier for the US Drug Enforcement Administration to add newly detected precursors without changing the laws.

Peptide Hormones

Peptide hormones (see Chapter 16) are typically large polypeptides (eg, hGH, insulin, insulin-like growth factor 1 [IGF-1]), but may also be glycosylated (eg, human chorionic gonadotropin, EPO). Many of these are now readily available as pharmaceutical products produced through genetic manipulation. Metabolism of the substances is rapid and the detection window of the parent molecules in blood is very short. The natural levels are often low, but in some cases, they are released in a manner that causes enormous variations in blood levels. These factors make it difficult to confirm the presence of the substances.[5,58]

hGH is a hormone naturally produced by the body, synthesized and secreted by cells in the anterior pituitary gland. hGH stimulates many metabolic processes in cells, but its major role in the body is to stimulate the liver to secrete insulin-like growth factor 1 (IGF-1). IGF-1 stimulates projection of cartilage cells, resulting in growth. hGH is known to reduce body fat and increase muscle mass and strength, as well as improve tissue-repairing effects (recovery) on the musculoskeletal system. Detection of hGH involves collecting blood samples for analysis.[64] The Partnership for Drug-Free Kids, an organization dedicated to reducing teen substance abuse, surveys high-school–aged youth measuring substance abuse attitudes and behaviors. The 2013 survey found a dramatic year-to-year increase in teens' reported use of synthetic hGH, increasing from 5% to 11% in 1 year.[65] Major League Baseball and the NFL have adopted blood serum testing for hGH.

β-Blockers

β-blockers (see Chapters 12 and 16) are used in sport to improve performance in anaerobic events that require steadiness and control.[66] The use of β-blockers was first reported in the sport of rifle where the twitch caused by blood pumping from the heart was thought to be sufficient to adversely affect aim. Studies found a 13% improvement in shooting related to decreased hand tremor when β-blockers were used. Testing for β-blockers is generally limited to sports requiring fine motor skill, such as diving, shooting, or archery.[5] Golfers also may experience performance benefits through the use of β-blockers. Adverse effects include fatigue, bradycardia, hypotension, impotence, and bronchospasm.[59]

Other Prohibited Substances and Manipulators

Substances used for performance enhancement are generally divided into 2 types of compounds: those that function during competition and those that are used during training for enhancement or have a delayed effect on performance during competition. In addition, there are substances used to mask the detection of banned substances.

Organizations amend banned drug lists as needed to address the use of new compounds and methods introduced in sport to artificially enhance performance or mask drug use. The term *related compounds* will be consistently found throughout these lists because it would be extremely difficult, if not impossible, to maintain a complete and accurate listing of substances in each of the banned categories. Related compounds include any substances similar to a drug class by pharmacological action or chemical structure. In addition, because dietary supplements are not strictly regulated, most athletic organizations warn athletes of the risk involved from using any product and encourage abstinence.

Sample Collection and Chain of Custody

Collecting biological specimens for sports drug testing is an important and integral part of a total drug-testing program, yet poses a significant legal risk. Specimen collections carry a great deal of responsibility for the collector, and he/she is not immune from legal liability. There is undue risk of having a poorly managed process. Negligent collection processes by employers who choose to perform collections in-house instead of outsourcing to a third party have been challenged in the courts. In *Mission Petroleum Carriers v. Roy Solomon*, the Court of Appeals of Texas found Mission created a danger when it chose to use its own employees to collect urine specimens rather than use an outside industry source. Furthermore, the court found Mission did not properly train its employees in urine collections and the process was routinely mishandled.[53] By following industry-adopted standard operating procedures and specimen collection protocols specific to the client and using trained collectors, liability can be almost completely managed, reduced, or eliminated. The Drug and Alcohol Testing Industry Association is a workplace association that represents the industry on legislative and regulatory issues in the workplace drug-testing environment. Among

its many membership benefits, the organization promotes industry standards by offering comprehensive collector training.[67] The National Center for Drug Free Sport (Drug Free Sport) also trains and certifies sports drug-testing specimen collectors specifically for sports drug-testing programs (www.drugfreesport.com). An organization's drug-testing policies should specifically describe the specimen collection process or reference any adopted protocol from another drug-testing entity. Often colleges or universities adopt the NCAA's specimen collection protocol as standard operating procedure. By implementing a procedure, many athletes are already familiar with the consistency of the process; this familiarity facilitates compliance. Other essentials for minimizing risk include assuring collector proficiency and good collection site management.

The collection site may be a temporary or permanent facility. Any facility may require special attention to ensure that it meets requirements. The term *collection* site refers to the entire facility used to collect the urine specimen (eg, the rest room or toilet stall and the work area used by the collector). In all cases, the collection site must allow for an adequate amount of privacy and respect for the athlete while providing the urine specimen. It is appropriate for the collection site to have a source of water for rinsing hands prior to and washing hands following a specimen collection. The source of water should be separate from the immediate area where urination occurs. The use of personal hygiene is acceptable after the specimen has been provided. The collection site must have a suitable clean surface for writing so that the collector and the athlete can complete the required paperwork. The collection site must prevent unauthorized access that could compromise the integrity of the collection process or the specimen. Unauthorized access includes not only unauthorized personnel but also any unauthorized access to collection materials or supplies. The collection site must not allow the athlete access to any items that could be used to dilute or adulterate the specimen. A representative from the sports organization should ensure the security of the room(s) during the actual time of specimen collection.

The specimen collection area should be fully equipped with male and/or female restrooms adjacent to the quiet waiting area. Individuals who suffer from an inability to urinate in public restrooms or during an observed drug test, commonly referred to as *shy bladder syndrome*, sometimes find it helpful to take a warm shower to encourage urination.[68]

Paruresis or shy bladder syndrome manifests itself as an inability to urinate in public restroom followed by a considerable avoidance behavior. Although considered a phobia, some athletes attempt to use shy bladder as an excuse to avoid drug testing. Sports drug-testing protocols do not allow for exceptions based on shy bladder claims.

The specimen should remain under the direct control of the athlete and observed by the collector until it is enclosed in the sample vials. Once it is sealed for shipment, it should be immediately shipped or maintained in secure storage or remain under the personal control of the collector until shipped. Although most athletes provide a specimen in less than 20 minutes, adequate time should be given for reservation of the facility in the event that testing takes longer than expected.

When athletes arrive for testing, the collector must positively identify the athlete. If the athlete cannot be positively identified, the collection should be discontinued. Acceptable methods of identification include photo identification issued to the athlete from the institution, his or her driver's license, or a positive identification by the client representative or site coordinator. The athlete should arrive at the collection site by the predesignated time. If the athlete is delayed, the collector must inform the client representative or site coordinator to determine the appropriate measures for locating the athlete or when to consider the athlete as a no-show based on the client's policies and procedures.

All specimens collected are accompanied by a Custody and Control Form (CCF) (Figure 17-1) or a digital CCF may be submitted electronically to the laboratory and other designated parties.[69] Electronic CCF systems are currently used in sport and in non-regulated work-place testing. *Custody* refers to a *chain of custody*, which is the term used to describe the process of documenting the handling of a specimen from the time an athlete provides a specimen and the collector processes the specimen, through shipping to the laboratory, during the testing at the laboratory, and until the results are reported by the laboratory. The CCF documents all information pertinent to the collection and testing of the specimen. It is important to note that the CCF must be filled out completely and that any unusual occurrences in the collection process should be noted in the collector's final report. Any error on the CCF is considered a fatal flaw, and, if caught during the information-gathering process, the collector must have the athlete select another CCF for the collector to complete correctly. This documentation becomes an official statement of evidence that documents the possession of the specimen at all times. The collector must maintain the integrity and security of the specimen. Perhaps the most important aspect of this responsibility is maintaining absolute control of the specimen from the moment the collector receives the specimen until the specimen is transferred to the shipping agent. After the specimen is prepared for shipment, there is no requirement for couriers, express carriers, or postal service personnel to sign any custody documentation because they do not have access to the specimen or any CCF.

Other considerations for urine specimen collection include whether to perform observed or monitored collections and the decision whether to package single or split specimens. Direct observed urine collections involve having an observer accompany the athlete into the toilet area to observe the act of urination. Monitored collections involve having a monitor accompany the athlete into the toilet area but allowing the athlete to urinate in the privacy of a closed stall. An observer of the same sex as the athlete must conduct a direct observed collection. Both types of collections provide deterrence from attempted adulteration, substitution, or manipulation during the actual urinating process, but the direct observed collection process is the most effective means of verifying urine validity at the collection site.

Split specimen testing involves splitting a single urine void into 2 separate vials labeled A and B. Both are securely sealed and shipped to the laboratory. The laboratory will analyze the A sample but will freeze and store the B sample in the event additional testing is indicated. Generally, the B sample is made available if the athlete challenges the initial drug test result and requests a second analysis. Some athletic organizations require B sample analysis on all positive results.[29,45] Single specimen collections are easier; however, providing laboratories with split samples allows for testing in rare cases when a vial may have leaked or a security seal became damaged during shipping.

In the United States, the federal government regulates drug testing through the Department of Transportation (DOT). The DOT requires agencies, transportation employers, and self-employed individuals to participate in drug and alcohol testing following very specific procedures. Non-DOT–regulated companies and other organizations can adopt the DOT's collection procedures as an industry standard.[45]

Specimen Adulteration

Specimen adulteration is a potential problem in urine drug testing. There are a variety of substances and methods used to interfere with testing procedures that can lead to an unwarranted negative result. Any attempt to circumvent the identification of a drug in the donor's system can invalidate the process and compromise the very purpose of a drug-testing program.[67] Specimen adulteration can be categorized as in vivo or in vitro. In vivo adulteration refers to the process of self-administering a substance for the purpose of altering drug test results. Athletes may attempt to mask the presence of a drug in the urine or flush the drug out of the body prior to the drug test collection. The most common method of in vivo adulteration is simple overhydration. These actions occur prior to arrival at the specimen collection site, making detection of the adulterating activity practically impossible.[67] Of course, by not notifying athletes prior to specimen collection, in vivo adulteration opportunities are virtually eliminated.

There are a number of substances reputed to interfere with the drug-testing process when taken by the donor. Some potential adulterants include vitamin C, vinegar, a variety of acidic fruit juices, ibuprofen, aspirin, and golden seal root. Golden seal root is particularly popular, gaining

Drug Free Sport

THE NATIONAL CENTER FOR DRUG FREE SPORT, INC.
2537 Madison Avenue   Kansas City, Missouri 64108-2334

**DRUG TESTING
CUSTODY AND CONTROL
FORM**

SDT A-3

CLIENT ACCT #:_____

SPECIMEN ID: ||||||||||||||||||||||
C143336

TEST CODES:

☐ Basic Sports Panel with Ephedrine **BSPE W132**   ☐ UCLA Drug Free Sport Anabolic Steroid

☐ Other: ☐ UCLA Full Anabolic Steroid

COLLECTOR: _____   TEST DATE: _____

DONOR: _____   SOC. SEC. NO.: _____

SPORT/ACTIVITY: _____   ☐ Male   ☐ Female

<u>Optional On-Site Specimen Assessment:</u>   Specific Gravity: 1.0_____   pH: _____

☐ Temperature read within 4 minutes and within range of 90.5-99.8 degrees F.
☐ Temperature is not in range. Temp: _____

<u>Validator Affidavit *(If Applicable)*:</u>
I certify that I witnessed the donor during the voiding process. The collection beaker and specimen remained in control of the donor throughout this process and remained in constant view of the donor and me.

_____
   Validator's Signature

<u>Donor Affidavit:</u>
I certify that I provided this specimen. The specimen was in my control until the collector packaged the specimen in the vials and applied the security seal(s). The security seal(s) is/are numbered with the same Specimen ID number on this form.

_____   _____
   Donor's Signature   (Date)

<u>Witness Affidavit *(If Applicable)*:</u>
I certify that I witnessed this donor and the collector package and seal this donor's specimen for transport to the laboratory.

_____   _____
   Witness' Signature   (Date)

<u>Collector Affidavit:</u>
I certify that the donor provided the specimen on this date in accordance with specified collection procedures. I further certify the specimen was given to me by the donor and was packaged and sealed and will be released to the courier identified below.

_____   _____   _____ am/pm
   Collector's Signature   (Date)   (Time)

Specimen To Be Released To: ☐ Commercial Shipper   ☐ Lab Courier   ☐ Other: _____
                                                     (Name of delivery service)

Received at Laboratory: _____
           (Accessioner's Signature)   (Accessioner PRINT Name)

Specimen Vial Seals Intact: ☐ YES   ☐ NO   Comments: _____

Specimen Vial(s) Released To: _____

NCDFS 05/05

COPY 1: RETURN TO NCDFS WITH ALL UNUSED SEALS

Figure 17-1. Custody and control form.

its reputation as an adulterant because alkaloids in the plant material interfere with thin-layer chromatography (TLC) tests for opiates. However, current methodologies are no longer subject to this interference.[67] Golden seal products marketed as drug-testing adulterants typically involve adding large amounts of water prior to ingesting. This will create a dilute specimen. Dilution is another method of manipulating a drug test and is discussed later in this section. Diuretics do not typically interfere with a drug test, but they can dilute the concentration of a drug to an

	TABLE 17-3	
	ADULTERANTS	
CLASS	**EXAMPLE**	**ACTION ON URINE SPECIMEN**
Chlorine	Clorox	Oxidizer
Nitrites	Klear	Oxidizer
Peroxidase	Stealth, Stealth II	Oxidizer
Pyridinium chlorochromate	UrineLuck	Oxidizer
Acids	Amber-13	Interference
Glutaraldehydes	UrinAid, Clear Choice	Interference
Soaps	Dish detergent	Interference
Substitution: Placing clean urine (from another person or processed human powdered urine) in collection beaker or putting another look-alike liquid in collection beaker for processing in an attempt to produce a negative test result.		
Dilution: Either adding water to a urine specimen in the collection beaker or ingesting copious amounts of water/fluid, forcing the urine specimen to be dilute upon voiding.		

undetectable level. Including diuretic testing as part of the complete drug-testing panel can circumvent this type of masking.

In vitro adulteration involves modifying samples to prevent the proper identification of a drug. This type of adulteration is accomplished directly on the sample and does not involve influencing the biological system like in vivo methods.[67] By adding a foreign substance to a urine sample, the testing process is disrupted or the actual drug present in the urine is destroyed. There are many products available that claim to guarantee a negative test result when used according to directions. These products are easily available and often sold over the Internet. Glutaraldehydes are chemical additives in products like UrinAid, Klear, Whizzies, or UrineLuck used to attempt interfering with specimen analysis but are generally detectable during the analysis process. Other substances range from diesel fuel, which is easily detected, to Visine, which is extremely difficult to detect in urine samples with the intention of producing false-negative results. Other items include alcohol, ammonia, ascorbic acid, bleach, blood, soap or detergent, Dran-o, golden seal root, lemon juice, Lime-A-Way, peroxide, salt, Vanish, and vinegar. Of course, the ideal adulterant is one that can easily be introduced into the sample, interferes with the testing process causing a negative result, and will not be detected.[67] Most contain commonly used chemicals that laboratories can now detect by performing adulteration testing on all samples as part of standard operating procedures.

Nitrites added to urine oxidize drugs and their metabolites into undetectable by-products. Although nitrites are normally present in urine, laboratories now screen samples for nitrite levels and determine a level >500 mg/mL to be

adulterated.[6] Products containing glutaraldehyde will also cause abnormal immunoassay screens; however, glutaraldehyde does not normally occur in urine and is detectable (Table 17-3).[45]

Perhaps the most common method of attempting to adulterate a urine sample is dilution. Dilution refers to the process of providing a sample for testing in which the relative concentrations of drugs or drug metabolites are below applicable cut-off levels, preventing laboratories from detecting drugs present in the specimen. Donors either externally add fluids to the sample at the collection site (in vitro) or consume copious amounts of fluids prior to providing a sample (in vivo), which results in a dilute urine specimen. To prevent dilution, individuals responsible for administering specimen collections must control athlete fluid consumption from the time of notification until an adequate sample is obtained. Fluids are provided to athletes in single-serving, individually sealed containers to control fluid consumption for proper hydration purposes and to protect athletes from ingesting fluids possibly contaminated with banned drugs.

When setting up testing parameters with laboratories, organizations should request that laboratories report samples as dilute if creatinine is <20 mg/dL and the specific gravity is <1.003 so that drug-testing administrators can obtain recollection from athletes providing dilute samples. Of course, this loophole allows athletes who are intentionally diluting samples because of drug use additional time to rid their bodies of the prohibited substance. By the time another sample is collected, the drug in question may not be detectable. A more effective method of preventing dilution involves measuring samples at the collection site for specific gravity. If specific gravity is too low, collectors can withhold fluids from the donor until a concentrated sample is collected, packaged, and sent to the laboratory.

Specific gravity can be measured on site using a digital refractometer (Figure 17-2). The refractometer is a device intended to determine the amount of solute in a solution by measuring the index of refraction (ratio of the velocity of light in a vacuum to the velocity of light in the solution). A few drops of urine are dripped on the prism with the light refracted from the boundary of sample and prism projected on a scale. The urine specific gravity between healthy men and women tends to fluctuate in range from 1.010 to 1.030.[70] A laboratory's analytical methods become challenged in detecting drugs present in the specimen if specific gravity is < 1.003. Collection procedures recommend rejecting any sample < 1.005.

Substituting urine is another form of adulteration that can be accomplished in vitro or, in more extreme cases, through in vivo methods. In vitro methods of urine substitution involve concealing clean urine somewhere on the body and, once in the restroom facility, placing the clean urine in the specimen container for drug testing. This complicated procedure is difficult, if not impossible, when performing an observed collection. However, those drug-tainted donors desperate to conceal use will go to any extreme. The process involves choosing from any number of marketed contraptions or homemade devices, including the use of condoms or something as sophisticated as The Whizzinator, a prosthetic urinating device, to carry clean urine into the collection site unnoticed. Not only is concealing a device problematic, but obtaining clean urine is yet another step to this masquerade. The donor may ask a trusting nondrug user to provide him or her with drug-free urine or may choose to purchase clean urine from any number of marketing suppliers. Collectors who witness attempts to adulterate a drug test are obligated to report such activities to drug-testing administrators because in many programs an adulterated drug test is considered a positive drug test.

Specimen Analysis

Laboratory Analysis

Forensic drug testing is the process of analyzing biological specimens for illicit drugs.[71] Sports drug testing expands on this principle to include not only illicit drugs but also many other compounds, including a variety of performance-enhancing substances. Most testing for drugs of abuse is done using urine specimens and involves 2 procedures: screening and confirmation. Screening tests have high sensitivity (low rate of false-negative results), are fast, and are less expensive, whereas confirmatory tests have high specificity (low rate of false-positive results).[6] A false-negative result refers to a negative report when a sought-after substance is actually present in a concentration greater than a predetermined cut-off level yet not detected

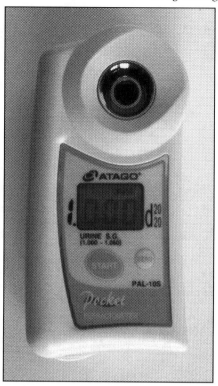

Figure 17-2. Digital refractometer.

through the analytical method used. As an example, one might falsely conclude that cocaine was not used 24 hours ago when examining urine using TLC as opposed to a more sensitive method.[12]

False negative: The laboratory reports a negative result when the specimen actually contains a substance that is being tested for but for whatever reason is not reported as being found present in the specimen.

False positive: The laboratory reports a positive result when the specimen does not actually contain the substance the laboratory reported.

Toxicologists involved with drug testing have identified several compounds that may possibly interfere with initial absorbance readings on immunoassay screenings. Glutaraldehyde is an adulterant that can cause a false-negative result.[45] Laboratories now include screening for a number of adulterants that contribute to false-negative results and observed specimen collections virtually eliminate adulteration of samples.

A false-positive result means that a positive result is produced when the substance being sought is not present, is not confirmable as present, or is present at a concentration below the cut-off value.[12] A sample may screen positive but must be considered as presumptive positive until confirmation specifically indicates the presence of a banned substance. Screening methods do not merely test for presence or absence of a drug but provide a quantitative

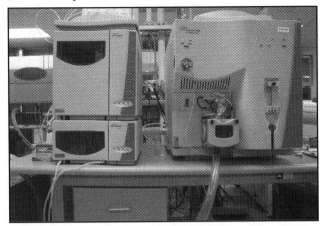

Figure 17-3. Gas chromatography.

or semiquantitative result based on the specific cut-off values previously established. If a sample screens positive, it is important for a laboratory to use highly specific methods of testing for confirmation.[6]

Current standard operating procedures for federally regulated drug-testing programs require laboratories to screen using immunoassay and confirm presumptive positives using GC/MS.[72] Federal and state courts have supported the legal reliability of immunoassay urine drug tests either used singly or a double immunoassay test and/or confirmation by an alternate method. Immunoassays have over 25 years of successful legal history.[39]

During screening, specimens are subjected to nonspecific assays for the presence of drugs, metabolites, and related compounds.[4] Before testing, samples must be prepared for analytical techniques. Pretreatment of biological specimens is done to release drugs from the biological matrix; remove interfering particles; and adjust the pH, ionic strength, and concentration of the sample to allow optimum extraction.[73] Immunochemical assays are popular for screening of the more typical drugs of abuse because these assays are very sensitive, detecting nanogram quantities of drug metabolites in urine and techniques that have been extensively developed through high-volume workplace drug testing. They are rapid tests producing results in minutes. Perhaps the greatest disadvantage is the cross-reactions that occur with loosely related endogenous or exogenous substances, thus the need for specific confirmatory tests.

There are a number of different immunochemical methods available. One of the most popular immunoassay procedures is the enzyme immunoassay. The enzyme immunoassay is based on an enzyme bound to the drug that can also bind to a specific antibody. A newer method is fluorescent polarization immunoassay. It is also very sensitive and rapid. Less specimen manipulation is required, but the testing procedure is more expensive. Latex agglutination testing is another screening method that is easy to use and appears to be as accurate as other immunoassay techniques.[6] If the screening process does not detect any

banned substances, the test result is reported as negative. If the screening assay detects a compound that is consistent with a banned substance, a confirmation assay is conducted. A positive screen is confirmed or refuted by using a different assay technique. The confirmation process identifies the specific compound, minimizing a false-positive result. Although liquid and GC can be used for confirmation, GC/MS is the standard.[10] As an alternative to GC, which involves heat to separate compounds, LC allows compound separation without heat, allowing thermolabile compounds to survive the LC process for better detection.[16]

GC can be used for screening or for confirmation (Figure 17-3). It requires expensive equipment and personnel with specific training. A small amount of an extract from the specimen is injected into a heated chamber that immediately volatilizes the liquid and sweeps it into a column by a carrier gas. Compounds are then absorbed to a stationary phase (column). Each compound has its own retention time, the time of emergence of the compound from the column, and thus separates individual components in a mixture. A detector and recorder at the end of the column records height and area of the peak that correlates with the quantity of each compound present.[6] This procedure is generally joined by a MS (see Figure 17-3). MS uses an electron beam to ionize each compound. These ions are filtered and separated electromagnetically and identified according to their mass/charge ratio. A detection system then detects the amount of each ion present as a result for the electron beam. Each substance has a unique pattern (mass spectrum) or fingerprint. MS is often combined with GC to produce a sensitive and specific detection system. GC/MS is the gold standard in small molecule identification for confirmation of positive screens. Testing methods have become extremely sensitive, which provides organizations the opportunity to work with laboratories to determine levels of detection when testing for specific drugs.[6,16]

Testing for typical drugs of abuse is relatively straightforward and similar to other areas of forensic toxicology. Sport drug testing is a unique area within the field of toxicology. Both the scope of testing provided and the analytical techniques applied are among the most sophisticated in the field. A unique challenge in sport drug testing is identifying whether performance-enhancing substances occur naturally or are exogenous (eg, peptide hormones and testosterone).[17] When testing for these types of substances, analysis must be performed at highly specialized laboratories. Anabolic steroid testing requires a minimum of one GC/MS and one technician devoted entirely to anabolic steroid testing. In addition, interpretation of results requires a certifying scientist knowledgeable in steroid metabolism and pharmacology.

Until 1984, samples were initially screened using radioimmunoassay and presumptive positive samples were confirmed using GC/MS techniques. It was during the 1984 Olympic Games in Los Angeles, California, that

GC/MS was adopted for both screening and confirmation for anabolic steroid analysis.[15,16] Detection of testosterone using GC/MS was developed involving the measurement of both testosterone (T) and epitestosterone (E). The normal ratio of T to E is approximately 1:1 for both males and females. Use of T raises this ratio appreciably. A ratio of 6:1 or greater is considered evidence of T administration and classified as a positive drug test.[17] However, limitations to the T/E ratio test, including microbial degradation, excessive alcohol consumption, and genetic and pathologic conditions, complicate the interpretation of T/E results.[17] Testosterone has been the most commonly used endogenous steroid, and lately its OTC precursors, such as androstenedione (anabolic steroid) and dehydroepiandrosterone, have become very popular. These substances occur naturally in the body; therefore, a process that distinguishes natural from administered substances was needed. The introduction of carbon isotope ratio < S as a complementary means of performing a single measurement on a suspect sample with a T/E > 6:1 or 4:1, depending on the sport organization policies, has helped resolve the issue of endogenous production.[51] GC/combustion/isotope ratio MS is another method that has been developed for detecting the use of exogenous testosterone. The premise of this approach is that the relative amount of the naturally occurring carbon-13 isotope in a pharmaceutical preparation of testosterone is different than that produced from dietary precursors, thus providing the ability to distinguish between endogenous and exogenous testosterone. Although successful at identifying the carbon difference, GC/combustion/isotope ratio MS is extremely expensive and time consuming. Carbon isotope ratio values for a urinary steroid can determine if a steroid is natural or synthetic.[16]

Another analytical advancement was the introduction of high-resolution MS (HRMS) at the 1996 Olympic Games in Atlanta, Georgia. Prior to the availability of HRMS, the main technique used was the GC/MS. The detection levels by GC/MS for anabolic steroids has a limit of about 10 µg/mL but with HRMS levels of detection are lowered to <1 ng/mL. These capabilities extended the detection period from last ingestion of the anabolic agent.[16,58] Although detection of a limited list of substances is possible using several techniques, the only technique presently available for detecting the full list of prohibited anabolic agents is the HRMS.[5,16,58]

With the introduction of recombinant human EPO (rHuEPO) for therapeutic use of disease, the sports world quickly recognized the performance-enhancing effects from misuse of rHuEPO. Early attempts at detection of EPO in athletes involved indirect tests on blood prior to endurance-demanding sports competitions by measuring hematocrit or hemoglobin. Increased levels of 47% to 50% were considered positive. More recent methodologies include direct tests for rHuEPO itself. Research has found the family of isoforms is different for recombinant EPO and natural EPO. The isoform pattern of urinary endogenous EPO differs from the pattern of urinary rHuEPO, leading to successful testing of rHuEPO in urine.[16] Work continues on an ongoing basis on all detection methods to refine sensitivity and interpretation of results.[65]

Efforts to develop methods for detecting recombinant hGH have been underway for years. Most experts agree the blood matrix is the most reliable matrix in detecting hGH. Blood serum is stable frozen, allowing samples to be tested in the future. Storing serum for future testing has a significant deterrent effect. There are currently 2 methods of testing for hGH in blood matrices: the isoform differential immunoassay and the hGH biomarker test. The biomarker is an indirect test based on a medley of markers. hGH affects the expression of different proteins that may serve as biological markers of hGH activity. Measuring IGF-1 and N-terminal peptide of procollagen type III (P-III-NP), 2 hGH markers in blood serum, may uncover manipulation of hGH/IGF-1 as doping substances used to increase circulating hGH. The isoform differential immunoassay (isoforms approach) is designed to measure the naturally constant proportions between the different isoforms of hGH in blood. An individual doping with recombinant hGH alters the natural constant proportion of isoforms. The hGH isoform differential immunoassay detects these changes in proportions. The current isoforms test has been found robust and scientifically reliable. The hGH biomarker approach has been documented in several scientific publications for years, but these markers have also been influenced by confounding factors including age, sex, ethnicity, and exercise. Further studies are indicated.[65]

On-Site Screening Devices

On-site urine testing, also referred to as *point-of-collection urine testing*, has recently been adopted in the drug-testing industry. On-site testing includes both benchtop screening instruments, which are less expensive and easy to use analytical devices for non-experts, and immunoassay kits at the collection site. Point-of-collection testing is an initial test conducted at the collection site for either the presence of drugs or to determine specimen validity. This type of testing can be done for both urine and oral fluid. Any on-site screening device being considered for use should be approved by the FDA and supported by validation studies. In addition, collectors using on-site testing devices must be adequately trained and certified to administer these testing devices.[74] On-site tests produce rapid results using simple procedures and do not require sending a specimen to a laboratory. Results are available within minutes, eliminating uncertainty and substantially reducing the administrative burden posed by chain of custody. Point-of-collection testing is perceived as a strong deterrent to drug use because it decreases the time between results and consequences, providing an opportunity to promptly and positively reinforce drug-free behavior. On-site testing has other advantages, including flexibility as to where testing is conducted.[39] However, on-site testing products are manufactured for workplace drug-testing panels (eg, marijuana, cocaine, and amphetamines) and use SAMHSA cut-offs. These products do not include testing opportunities for most of the drugs found on sports organizations' banned drug lists. When considering on-site devices or alternative specimens for drug testing, procedures and products must have scientific acceptance and be able to withstand legal challenges. The level of services available from the supplier, including litigation support, is essential. Use of these products or procedures must be specifically described in written drug-testing policies and procedures and the specimen collection and chain of custody procedures must be clearly defined.[39]

Today's technology provides many options for drug testing. It is important to remember the relationships that exist between the various methodologies. For example, the banned drug list should be considered before the type of specimen to be analyzed is selected. There are limitations to what drugs can be identified in certain specimens. In addition, the collection procedures should be carefully considered to prevent specimen adulteration challenges. Ultimately, the ability to detect drug use will only be as strong as the scientific methodologies and industry-adopted procedures being used.

Results Verification and Applying Sanctions

After receipt of drug-testing results from the laboratory, it is critical to review all reports carefully for any inconsistencies and to compare these reports with chain of custody forms, ultimately matching an athlete to his or her result via specimen identification numbers. Positive results must then be reported to the athlete and discussed. Interviewing the athlete is imperative to determine whether there is an alternative medical explanation for the positive result. In many cases, a team physician or another designated medical review officer best completes this process. Ultimately, this verification process must be carried out on all positive drug tests before classifying the result as positive and applying sanctions.

An unintentional positive result may occur when an athlete is prescribed a medication or elects to take an OTC substance without knowing the medication was banned or contained a banned substance. The difficulty exists in trying to accurately determine whether the ingestion was unintentional or not. Many sports organizations support the position that any substance an athlete places into his or her body is intentional; ignorance is no excuse. This is a perfect example of how a drug-testing program without education is problematic. It is critical to provide all athletes with policies, procedures, and a list of prohibited substances. In addition, all athletes should have access to resources designed to assist in determining if a medication or OTC product contains banned substances. Some organizations

allow athletes to take a banned substance (eg, stimulant, β-blocker) for legitimate medical reasons. The WADA Code provides for TUEs. This exemption program enables athletes to be treated by a physician with a prohibited substance and still compete, safeguarding the health of the athlete and the integrity of antidoping efforts.[16] The NCAA may grant a medical exception for certain classes of banned drugs. These exceptions to the consequences of a positive drug test result must be fully documented by the attending physician and usually reviewed by a medical review board for the sports organization either before or after testing occurs depending on the organization.

Most positive drug tests are reviewed by adjudicating bodies such as committees of administrators, medical doctors, and athletes. When dealing with OTC drugs, athletes will often accept the result but ask for leniency based on inadvertent use or lack of understanding of a product. Contentious cases may lead to appeals, hearings, and arbitration at the national and international level.[10] The path to final adjudication depends on the type of organization and its existing policies and procedures. The arbitration process in sports is unlike criminal or civil proceedings in a variety of ways. One area of controversy is the shift in burden of proof from the national governing body or international governing body to the athlete.[17] Once a positive result has been reported and confirmed positive through interpretation and due process, appropriate sanctions must be applied. Drug testing in sport has been criticized for alleged inefficiencies, for unfairness in testing methods, and for the way sanctions have been levied. It is vital to apply appropriate sanctions consistently.

There should be a detailed description of the sanctions applied for policy violations. Penalties are generally imposed for athletes who refuse to sign a consent form, athletes who engage in criminal misconduct (eg, drug trafficking), athletes who refuse to submit to a required drug test, and athletes who have positive test results. Institutional penalty structures generally involve a 3-tiered system of sanctions:

- First offenses involve suspension from participation until the nature and extent of the involvement with prohibited drugs can be determined. Athletes are usually referred to a substance abuse specialist for appropriate counseling and treatment, if necessary. Athletes are then allowed to return to participation but will be required to undergo unannounced follow-up testing.

- A second offense requires immediate suspension, reevaluation for substance abuse and/or addiction, and a predetermined period of nonparticipation. Return to participation will include evaluation by a medical doctor to determine that reentry would not pose a health risk to the athlete.

- Third offenses result in permanently suspending the athlete from athletic participation at that institution.

Sanctions should also be included for athletes who voluntarily disclose drug use, but penalties for first offenses should be graded to encourage athletes with drug-use problems to seek help.

Regardless of the drug-testing entity, a process for interpreting the result of a positive drug test result must be described in the written policy, completely followed, and documented. Once a drug test result is deemed positive, athletes must be given the opportunity to appeal the interpretation of the positive result. The penalties or consequences must be explicitly defined in the policy and fully applied once any appeal process concludes the positive result to be final.

DEVELOPMENT OF A DRUG TESTING PROGRAM

In developing any type of program or service, the first step is to determine if a need exists. The need to drug test in sport may seem obvious because it deters athletes from using potentially dangerous substances and because it creates a level playing field; however, a needs analysis is encouraged to further support the implementation of an often-controversial program. In determining this need, athletic organizations should define the nature and the extent of any drug use problem. There are numerous national surveys and studies that have examined drug use in sport at various levels of competition, but local applicability must also be considered. Athletic organizations, such as the NCAA, survey student-athletes at member institutions periodically and provide information on drug use trends. Other methods of determining the need for drug testing include reviewing reports from staff members and campus security, engaging in focus group discussions, examining current institutional data and referral trends, and discovering evidence indicating drug use (eg, finding drug paraphernalia).

Once a needs assessment is complete, a committee or task force comprising an attorney, physician, athletics administrator, athletic trainer, toxicologist, and possibly a coach and student-athlete should be formed. The organization's legal counsel should be involved with program development from the onset, particularly with regard to right-to-privacy statutes, which may vary from state to state.[43] The committee should submit a proposal for implementing a drug-testing program to decision makers and be prepared to discuss a number of issues, including constitutionality, effective methodology, confidentiality, administrative impact, and budgeting. There may be outside resources available for schools eligible for federal funding, including assistance from the United States Department of Education, Department of Health and Human Services, Partnership for Drug-Free America, and National Institute on Drug Abuse. Private schools may be exempt from federally funded programs but may find funding opportunities through other corporations and nonprofit groups.

Once approval for drug testing is accomplished, a detailed written policy must be developed before any testing can occur. The policy should include a clear explanation of the purposes of the program, who will be tested and by what methods, which drugs will be tested for and under what conditions (eg, announced, reasonable suspicion), and what actions will be taken against those who test positive. A copy of the policy should be given to each athlete, along with a written consent form that each athlete should read and sign, confirming receipt and understanding of the policy and agreement to participate in the drug-testing program.[43] A list of banned substances must be developed and should be included in the policy. Athletic organizations should consider including performance-enhancing substances and illicit drugs in the banned list. The NCAA list of banned drug classes may be used if an institution wishes to adopt it for its own drug-testing program (http://www.ncaa.org/health-and-safety/policy/2014-15-ncaa-banned-drugs).

There are numerous logistical, technical, and economic issues to consider for proper administration of a drug-testing program. Administrators must determine how and when samples will be collected, secured, and transported. The appropriate personnel responsible for these duties must have a clear understanding of procedures. If the institution elects to outsource the collection of specimens to a third party, a complete description of each party's responsibilities and a description of the services being provided should be agreed upon prior to testing. If a TPA is used, typically the TPA contracts with certified laboratories for specimen analysis. Often this relationship provides the institution with discounted laboratory costs because the service provider can negotiate lower pricing due to a higher testing volume. If the institution chooses to contract directly with a laboratory, there are a number of issues that need to be considered. The institution should request documentation supporting the laboratory's accreditation and certification along with staff qualifications. Depending on the credentialing agency, laboratories are required to complete proficiency programs and to maintain quality control programs. The laboratory should also provide the institution with a description of what analytical methods are available for testing samples, concentration levels of drug detection available, and how specimens are handled within the laboratory from receiving and processing to storage. The chain of custody of samples should be described, along with a list of the certified scientists who will review and approve results for processing. Turnaround times for drug test results can be crucial depending on the reason for testing. Usually laboratories will provide a quote for turnaround times on negative results and another quote for turnaround times on positive results because of confirmation testing.

Results reporting and maintaining confidentiality of results is critical. Laboratory pricing is usually quoted on a per-sample basis and should include screening and confirmation testing, necessary supplies, and shipping of samples to the laboratory, with pick-up from the collection site and delivery to the laboratory within 24 hours of collection.

Programs should be reassessed annually to maintain effectiveness. Surveying athletes who participate in drug-testing programs, obtaining current national drug use trends and research, encouraging substance abuse counselor feedback, and gathering other anecdotal information will be helpful in evaluating a drug-testing program. Building a consortium to fully address drug use and improve the deterrent effect strengthens the effectiveness of a program. Athletic organizations are encouraged to include the medical community, local law enforcement and municipal alliances, and other related businesses to assist in these efforts.

Drug testing cannot be the only element in an effective antidoping program. Educating athletes about the potential dangers of drug and dietary supplement use is critical, and all participants must be made aware of their respective responsibilities. A drug-testing program is designed to create awareness and evoke sound decision making with regard to drug use in sport. Integrity is an obvious ingredient in drug testing; it is an active process that cannot be taken for granted. Implementing a drug-testing program requires the courage to draw a line between acceptable and unacceptable behavior.[10] Developing a drug-testing program based on a solid, purposeful foundation and a commitment from informed and courageous individuals will produce an effective deterrent to drug use in sport and promote ethical behavior by the athletes it serves.

CURRENT AND FUTURE CHALLENGES IN DRUG TESTING IN SPORT

Performance-enhancing substances have been used since ancient times. Athletes today use a wide range of substances from anabolic steroids and stimulants to hGH, EPO, and genetic material transfer. Technical advancements have inadvertently led to new delivery of "old" drugs such as testosterone administration through nasal mists or skin patches.[31] Doping has developed into a widespread problem in competitive sport because of increased financial incentives from professional opportunities and commercialism. It is possible to earn more money as a highly paid top athlete in a short time than over an entire conventional career.[75] Doping in sport has grown in scientific and ethical complexity. The future limits to athletic performance will be determined more by technological advances than innate physiology of the athlete. Where do we draw the line between what is natural and what is artificially enhanced?[73] Some of the new and emerging technologies challenging the ethical fiber of sport today include stem cell transplantation, red blood cell substitutes, and genetic enhancement.[76] Invariably, athletes will turn to these and other unknown doping agents in search of the competitive edge. Every time a new drug or technology is developed, an athlete determined to gain an athletic advantage finds a way to misuse or abuse that drug or technology, perverting its original intent.[17]

Controversy surrounding blood doping has been evident for more than 30 years. Following the 1984 Olympic Games, the IOC banned all forms of blood doping. In 1990, the organization added recombinant human EPO to the banned list. The definition of doping was modified in the WADA Code to account for the developments in biotechnology. The definition of blood doping now includes the administration of blood, RBCs, artificial oxygen carriers, and related blood products to an athlete. International testing protocol now includes both blood and urine testing to determine recombinant human EPO use.[77] The 1996 Olympic Games in Atlanta, Georgia, were rumored to have so many athletes using hGH that the games were informally referred to as the Growth Hormone Games. Elite athletes from around the world have been caught with possession of large doses of recombinant hGH, and professional sports figures and even actors have even admitted to growth hormone use. Over 3% of college athletes and 5% of male high school students have reported use of growth hormone. Athletes are choosing to use hGH despite lack of evidence supporting any significant performance-enhancement effects, the potential adverse effects, and the expense of obtaining the hormone. Today's technological advances allow laboratories to adequately store blood and urine samples, only to analyze them for banned substances at a later date when more reliable analytical methods have been developed.[65]

The current use of anabolic steroids and EPO is being replaced by injecting genes to enhance performance and appearance. Within the next decade, genetic engineering will probably change the course of competitive sport.[31,78] The IOC Medical Commission and WADA are currently developing high-tech, anti-abuse tests that analyze blood and saliva for antibodies produced as a result of taking gene medications and are working on the creation of gene footprint detection.[2,31] As medical research continues to develop methods of human gene therapy in the treatment of disease, athletes will obtain these same methods to enhance human traits desired in sport. Today's anti-doping entities are studying athlete biological passports to monitor selected biomarkers of doping over time. This indirectly reveals the effect of doping as opposed to direct detection of a banned substance.[65] As we question the moral fiber of such activity, we are forced to look at the role of sport in society. "...The very concept of a sport, and its apparent evolution from a rule-based noble and romantic striving for individual achievement to potentially grotesque uncontrolled biotechnology."[79]

Despite the development of advanced drug-testing systems, doping, both deliberate and inadvertent, continues to plague sport today. A particular problem is the risk posed by today's dietary supplement culture. An effective antidoping program must incorporate educational components in addition to testing, and these educational initiatives need to be collaborative and proactive. Athletes, coaches, managers, governing bodies, and athletic trainers and other health care professionals must come together in these efforts. Technological advances cannot address what is essentially a behavioral problem.[14] Leaders of the antidoping movement are using biological passports to profile athletes biological specimens. This biological profiling assesses significant variations in the biological system throughout time to identify doping activities without directly detecting substances. Another revolutionary concept is a volunteer program consisting of just the opposite goal of the current antidoping movement: athletes volunteering for testing to demonstrate nonuse would be rewarded as drug free through public recognition that they are drug free.[16] Doping leads to major health problems, including death, and violates the basic principles of equal opportunity and fair play. More frequent testing and more severe punishments for doping violations by the sports associations themselves may be one way of fighting doping in sports. More thorough education of athletes on the negative effects of uncontrolled drug use may also help.[75] Educational efforts designed to encourage informed, responsible, and healthy decisions can supplement athletes' understanding and perceptions of the effectiveness of drug testing and can encourage athletes to develop decision-making skills that are internally motivated, rather than externally driven.[80] Manufacturers and suppliers of dietary supplement products containing banned substances must be confronted and held accountable if a victim-blaming approach is to be avoided.

Role of the Athletic Trainer

The athletic trainer plays an intricate role in sport antidoping campaigns. Whether working with youth groups or professional athletes, the athletic trainer is positioned to provide participants with direct and immediate feedback regarding the risks of using drugs regardless of their intent. It is critical for athletic trainers to become and remain knowledgeable about all types of drugs and the implications of substance use in sport. Likewise, it is extremely important for the athletic trainer to understand the application of drug education and testing programs and to be prepared to contribute in the ongoing commitment to athlete health and welfare, as well as fair play.

Case Study 1

As an athletic trainer working at an NCAA Division II university, Kent is meeting with the athletics director to discuss developing and implementing a student-athlete drug-testing program at their school. In preparation for this meeting, Kent needs to outline the primary components for developing a drug-testing program. What components should he include for discussion?

Case Study 2

As an athletic trainer at a NCAA Division I university, Beth has just been designated as the drug-testing administrator for their student-athletes' anti-doping program. The university's student health clinic has been performing urine specimen collections and sending samples to an US Department of Health and Human Services–certified laboratory. Beth has recently noticed an increase in samples being received at the laboratory that are deemed untestable due to being too dilute and some being identified as non-human biological specimens. Perplexed, Beth meets with the director of the student health clinic to evaluate the collection process and she reviews the program's policy and protocols. Her findings reveal that protocol does not include determining specimen adequacy prior to sending the sample to the laboratory and vaguely describes the actual collection of urine from the student-athlete. What recommendations should Beth provide to the athletics director to prevent unacceptable samples from being sent to the laboratory?

References

1. Shorter F, Bowers LD. Foreword. In: Bahrke MS, Yesalis CE, ed. *Performance-enhancing substances in sport and exercise.* Champaign, IL: Human Kinetics; 2002:v-vi.
2. Murray FH. Doping in sports: challenges for medicine, science and ethics. *J Intern Med.* 2008;264:95-98.
3. Committee of Sports Medicine and Fitness. Use of performance-enhancing substances. *Peadiatrics.* 2005;115:1103-1106.
4. Ambrose PJ. Doping control in sports—a perspective from the 1996 Olympic Games. *Am J Health Syst Pharm.* 1997;54:1053-1057.
5. Bowers LD. Athletic drug testing. *Clin Sport Med.* 1998;17:299-318.
6. Landry GL, Lokotailo PK. Drug screening in the athletic setting. *Curr Probl Pediatr.* 1994;24:344-359.
7. Green GA, Uryasz FD, Petr TA, Bray CD. NCAA study of substance use and abuse habits of college student-athletes. *Clin Sport Med.* 2001;11:51-56.
8. Wadler G. Science and research. Paper presented at First Meeting of the White House Task Force on Drug use in Sports Proceedings, December 7, 2000; Salt Lake City, UT.

9. Walters JP. *What You Need to Know About Drug Testing in Schools.* Washington, DC: Office of National Drug Control Policy; 2002:i-16.

10. Shults TF. The intangible elements of successful drug testing programs. *MROAlert.* 2002;131-132.

11. National Collegiate Athletic Association Research Staff. NCAA National Study of Substance Use Habits of College Student-Athletes. Indianapolis, IN: National Collegiate Athletic Association; 2014:1-101.

12. Wadler GI, Hainline B. *Drugs and the Athlete.* Philadelphia, PA: FA Davis Co; 1989:197-212.

13. Yesalis CE. History of doping in sports. In: Bahrke MS, Yesalis CE, ed. *Performance-Enhancing Substances in Sport and Exercise.* Champaign, IL: Human Kinetics; 2002:1-20.

14. Sheehan O, Quinn B. Doping in sports—a deadly game. *Irish Pharm J.* 2002;80(6):256-262.

15. Kammerer RC. Drug testing in sport and exercise. In: Bahrke MS, Yesalis CE, eds. *Performance-Enhancing Substances in Sport and Exercise.* Champaign, IL: Human Kinetics; 2002:323-339.

16. Catlin DH, Fitch KD, Ljungqvist A. Medicine and science in the fight against doping in sport. *J Intern Med.* 2008;264:99-114.

17. Bowers LD, Black R, Borts DJ. Athletic drug testing: an anylyst's view of science and the law. *Ther Drug Monit.* 2000;22:98-102.

18. Uryasz FD. Historical review of NCAA involvement with drug education and drug testing: Addendum for NCAA Committee on Competitive Safeguards and Medical Aspects of Sport; March 1994.

19. International Olympic Committee. The Medical Commission. www.olympic.org/medical-commission. Accessed November 2, 2014.

20. World Anti-Doping Agency. A brief history of anti-doping. https://www.wada-ama.org/en/who-we-are/a-brief-history-of-anti-doping Accessed November 2, 2014.

21. International Olympic Committee. National Olympic Committees. http://www.olympic.org/national-olympic-committees. Accessed November 2, 2014.

22. International Olympic Committee. International Sports Federations. http://www.olympic.org/content/the-ioc/governance/international-federations. Accessed November 2, 2014.

23. Court of Arbitration 20 Questions About The CAS. http://www.tas-cas.org/en/20questions.asp/4-3-217-1010-4-1-1/5-0-1010-13-0-0/. Accessed November 2, 2014.

24. Catlin DH, Kammerer RC, Hatton CK, Sekera MH, Merdink JL. Analytical chemistry at the games of the XXIIIrd Olympiad in Los Angeles. *Clin Chem.* 1987;33:319-327.

25. National Football League Players Association. SOA Drug Policy. https://images.nflplayers.com/mediaResources/lyris/pdfs/PlayerAffairsMailers/FINAL%20SOA%20Policy%209%2029%2014%20%282%29.pdf. Accessed November 2, 2014.

26. Major League Baseball. MLB News. Report to the commissioner of baseball of an inependent investigation into the illegal use of steroids and other performance enhancing substances by players in Major League Baseball. http://files.mlb.com/mitchrpt.pdf. Accessed November 2, 2014.

27. House of Representatives Resolution 496. House passes resolution supporting mandatory testing in Major League Baseball players for steroids. *MROAlert.* 2002;13:10-11.

28. National Collegiate Athletic Association. Committee on Competitive Safeguards on Medical Aspects of Sports. http://www.ncaa.org/governance/committees/committee-competitive-safeguards-and-medical-aspects-sports. Accessed November 2, 2014.

29. National Collegiate Athletic Association. NCAA Drug Testing Program. http://www.ncaa.org/sites/default/files/16.%20INstitutional%20DrugEducation%20and%20TestingSurvey2009.pdf. Accessed November 2, 2014.

30. Johnston LD, O'Malley PM, Bachman JG. *Monitoring the Future National Results on Adolescent Drug Use Overview of Key Findings, 2001.* Bethesda, MD: National Institute on Drug Abuse; 2002:3-5.

31. Bahrke MS, Yesalis CE. Issues, concerns, and the future of performance-enhancing substances in sport and exercise. In: Bahrke MS, Yesalis CE, eds. *Performance-Enhancing Substances in Sport and Exercise.* Champaign, IL: Human Kinetics; 2002:351-355.

32. Curtis R. What are the issues surrounding drug testing privacy? *Workplace Substance Abuse Advisor.* 1999;13:3.

33. Wong GM. Drug testing in amateur athletics. In: Wong GM, ed. *Essentials of Amateur Sports Law.* Westport, CT: Praeger Publishing; 1994:711-731.

34. Niccolai FR. Legal considerations of drug testing. In: Banks R, ed. *Substance Abuse in Sport: The Realities.* Dubuque, IA: Kendall/Hunt Publishing Co; 1990:77-88.

35. Wong GM, Barr CA. Passing the test NCAA drug testing program gets ok from California high court. *Athletic Business.* 1994;10:13.

36. Barr CA. Busted in Boulder. *Athletic Business.* 1994;18:10,16.

37. Vernonia School District 47J v. Action, 515 US 646 (1995). http://caselaw.findlaw.com/us-9th-circuit/1034778.html. Accessed November 2, 2014.

38. Board of Education of Independent School District No. 92 of Pottawatomie County et al v. Earls et al (2002). http://www.law.cornell.edu/supremecourt/text/536/822. Accessed November 2, 2014.

39. Evans D. *Drug Courts and On-Site Drug Testing: Effective Weapons in the War on Drugs.* Indianapolis, IN: Roche Diagnostics; 1995-1997.

40. Marijuana Resource Center: State Laws Related to Marijuana. http://www.whitehouse.gov/ondcp/state-laws-related-to-marijuana. Accessed November 9, 2014.

41. Lombardo JA. Drug programs. *Clin Sport Med.* 1998;(17):319-326.

42. Green GA. Doping control for the team physician. *Am J Sport Med.* 2006;34:1690-1698.

43. NCAA Drug-Testing Program 2014-15. http://www.ncaa.org/sites/default/files/DT%20Book%202014-15.pdf. Accessed November 9, 2014.

44. Ringhofer KR, Harding ME. *Coaches Guide to Drugs in Sports.* Champaign, IL: Humana Kinetics; 1995.

45. Shults TF. *The medical review officer handbook.* Research Triangle Park, NC: Quadrangle Research, LLC; 1999:XXI-XXIV, 3-26, 65-89, 223-237.

46. Petit GE. Form over substances: the legal context of performance-enhancing substances. In: Bahrke MS, Yesalis CE, eds. *Performance-Enhancing Substances in Sport and Exercise.* Champaign, IL: Human Kinetics; 2002:341-350.

47. Procedures for transportation workplace drug and alcohol testing programs. http://www.dot.gov/odapc/part40. Accessed November 9, 2014.

48. World Anti-Doping Code International Standard Laboratories January 2015. https://wada-main-prod.s3.amazonaws.com/resources/files/WADA-ISL-2015-Final-v8.0-EN.pdf. Accessed November 9, 2014.

49. National Laboratory Certification Program. http://www.samhsa.gov/sites/default/files/workplace/SAMHSA_NLCPdoc_updated_Mar2013.pdf. Accessed November 8, 2014.

50. Substance Abuse and Mental Health Services Web Page. http://www.drugfreeworkplace.gov/DrugTesting/Files_Drug_Testing/Labs/Natl_Lab_Cert_Prog_Background1007.pdf. Accessed February 8, 2009.

51. Kintz P, Cirimele V, Sachs H, Jeanneau T, Ludes B. Testing for anabolic steroids in hair from two bodybuilders. *Forensic Sci Int.* 1999;101:209-216.

52. Kintz P, Samyn N. Use of alternative specimens: drugs of abuse in saliva and doping agents in hair. *Ther Drug Monit.* 2002;24:239-246.

53. Caplan YH, Goldberger BA. Alternative specimens for workplace drug testing. *J Anal Toxicol.* 2001;25:396-399.

54. *Mission Petroleum Carriers Inc v. Soloman.* The risks of employer collecting urine specimens for its employees. *MROAlert.* 2001;12:8-11.

55. Pil K, Verstraete A. Current developments in drug testing in oral fluid. *Ther Drug Monit.* 2008;30:196-202.

56. Cooper G, Manfred M, Kronstrand R. Current status of accreditation for drug testing in hair. *Forensic Sci Int.* 2008;176:9-12.

57. Hair test confirmation, interpretation face DTAB as major issues. *Workplace Substance Abuse Advisor.* 1999;1:9-10.

58. Update on the war on adulterants and substitution. *MROAlert.* 2002;13:8.

59. Ambrose PJ. Drug use in sports: a veritable arena for pharmacists. *J Am Pharm Assoc.* 2004;44:501-516.

60. Synthetic Drugs (a.k.a. K2, Spice, Bath Salts, etc.). http://www.whitehouse.gov/ondcp/ondcp-fact-sheets/synthetic-drugs-k2-spice-bath-salts. Accessed November 9. 2014.

61. DrugFacts: Spice ("Synthetic Marijuana"). http://www.drugabuse.gov/publications/drugfacts/spice-synthetic-marijuana. Accessed November 9, 2014.

62. DrugFacts: Synthetic Cathinones ("Bath Salts"). http://www.drugabuse.gov/publications/drugfacts/synthetic-cathinones-bath-salts. Accessed November 9, 2014.

63. Spriet LL. Caffeine. In: Bahrke MS, Yesalis CE, ed. *Performance-Enhancing Substances in Sport and Exercise.* Champaign, IL: Human Kinetics; 2002:267-278.

64. The Partnership Attitude Tracking Study Teens & Parents 2013. http://www.drugfree.org/newsroom/pats-2013-full-report-key-findings. Accessed November 9, 2014.

65. Questions & Answers. https://www.wada-ama.org/en/questions-answers. Accessed November 9, 2014.

66. Kazlauskas R, Trout G. Drugs in sports: analytical trends. *Ther Drug Monit.* 2000;22:103-109.

67. *DATIA Certified Professional Collector Trainer Manual of the Drug & Alcohol Testing Industry Association.* Washington, DC: DATIA. February 2012:7-94.

68. Hammelstein P, Soifer S. Is "shy bladder syndrome" (paruresis) correctly classified as social phobia? *J Anxiety Disorder.* 2006;20(3):296-311.

69. Federal eCCF: HHS/NLCP Oversight and Requirements. http://www.samhsa.gov/sites/default/files/eccf_oversight-requirements.pdf. Accessed November 9, 2014.

70. Atago Co Ltd. *Clinical Refractometer Instruction Manual.* Tokyo, Japan: Author.

71. New Jersey latest state to pass drug test anti-fraud statute. *MROAlert.* 2002;13:8-9.

72. Jenkins AJ. Forensic drug testing. In: Levine B, ed. *Principles of Forensic Toxicology.* Washington, DC: American Association for Clinical Chemistry; 1999:31-35.

73. Chen XH, Franke J-P, de Zeeuw RA. Principles of solid-phase extraction. In: Liu RH, Goldberger BA, ed. *Handbook of Workplace Drug Testing.* Washington, DC: American Association for Clinical Chemistry; 1995:1-21.

74. Proposed revisions to federal drug testing procedures. *MROAlert.* 2000;11:4-9.

75. Striegel H, Vollkommer G, Dickhuth HH. Combating drug use in competitive sports: an analysis from the athletes' perspective. *J Sport Med Phy Fitness.* 2002;42:354-359.

76. Wadler G. Future and designer drugs: emerging science and technologies. In: Bahrke MS, Yesalis CE, ed. *Performance-Enhancing Substances in Sport and Exercise.* Champaign, IL: Human Kinetics; 2002:305-321.

77. Mendoza J. The war on drugs in sport: a perspective from the front-line. *Clin J Sport Med.* 2002;12:254-258.

78. Corrigan B. Beyond EPO. *Clin J Sport Med.* 2002;12:242-244.

79. Friedmann S. Gene transfer in sports: an opening scenario for genetic enhancement of normal "human traits." *Adv Genet.* 2006;51:37-49.

80. Tricker R, Connolly D. Drugs and the college athlete: an analysis of the attitudes of student athletes at risk. *J Drug Educ.* 1997;27:105-119.

BIBLIOGRAPHY

Karch SB. Amphetamines. In: Bahrke MS, Yesalis CE, eds. *Performance-Enhancing Substances in Sport and Exercise.* Champaign, IL: Human Kinetics; 2002:257-265.

Pharmacological Abbreviations

ā, a	before	CV	cardiovascular
aa, āā, āa	of each	d	day
a.c.	before meals	d/c	discontinue
ad	to, up to	D₅W	5% glucose in distilled water
a.d.	right ear	dil.	dilute
ad lib	as desired, freely	disp.	dispense
ACE	angiotensin-converting enzyme	dist.	distilled
ADH	antidiuretic hormone	DC	discontinue
a.l.	left ear	DX	diagnosis
ALT	alanine aminotransferase	D.W.	dextrose water; distilled water
alt. h.	alternate hours	ECG	electrocardiogram (EKG)
AM	in the morning, before noon	EEG	electroencephalogram
amp	ampul	EENT	ear, eye, nose, and throat
amt	amount	elix.	elixir
aq.	water	F	Fahrenheit
aq. dest.	distilled water	FBS	fasting blood sugar
A.S.A.	acetylsalicylic acid (aspirin)	FDA	Food and Drug Administration
ASAP	as soon as possible	fl., fld.	fluid
AST	aspartate aminotransferase (SGOT)	g, gm	gram
a.u.	each ear	gal	gallon
AV	artrioventricular	GI	gastrointestinal
b.i.d.	twice per day	gr	grain
b.i.n.	twice per night	gtt	drop
BM	bowel movement	h., hr	hour
B/P	blood pressure	H₂	histamine₂
BS	beats per minute	Hgb	hemoglobin
BSA	body surface area	HR	heart rate
BUN	blood urea nitrogen	hs	at bedtime
C	Celsius	ID	intradermal
c̄	with	IgG	immunoglobulin G
CAD	coronary artery disease	IM	intramuscular
cal	calorie	INF	infusion
cap., caps	capsule	INH	inhalation
CBC	complete blood cell count	inj.	injection
cc	cubic centimeter	K	potassium
CHF	congestive heart failure	kcal	kilocalorie
cm	centimeter	kg	kilogram
CNS	central nervous system	IV	intravenous
CO₂	carbon dioxide	L	liter
comp.	compound	LA	long acting
cont.	continue	lb.	pound
COPD	chronic obstructive pulmonary disease	LDH	lactic dehydrogenase
CPK	creatine phosphokinase	LE	lupus erythematosus
CPR	cardiopulmonary resuscitation	LFT	liver function test
CrCl	creatinine clearance	liq.	liquid
CSF	cerebrospinal fluid	LLQ	left lower quadrant

LOC	level of consciousness	q.6h	every 6 hours
LT	leukotriene	q12h	every 12 hours
LUQ	left upper quadrant	q.i.d.	4 times per day
M	meter	q.o.d.	every other day
m²	square meter	q.o.h.	every other hour
MAOI	monoamine oxidase inhibitor	qPM	every night
MI	myocardial infarction	q.s.	quantity sufficient; as much as needed
min	minute	qt	quart
mcg, μg	microgram	RBC	red blood cell count or red blood cell
mEq.	milliequivalent	rep.	repeat
mg	milligram	Rx.	a medical prescription
ml	milliliter	s̄	without
Na	sodium	sc	subcutaneous
neg	negative	sig	label, or let it be printed
ng	nanogram	sl	sublingual
non rep	do not repeat, no refills	sol., soln.	solution
NPO	nothing by mouth	solv	dissolve
NS	normal saline	SQ, sq. or sub q̄	subcutaneous(ly)
O₂	oxygen	SR	slow release
OD	right eye	ss, s̄s̄	one half
o.n.	every night	STAT, stat	immediately
OR	operating room	subq.	subcutaneous
os	left eye	supp	suppository
OU	both eyes	syr.	syrup
oz	ounce	tab.	tablet
p	*per*	tbs., tbsp., T	tablespoon
p̄	after	t.i.d.	3 times per day
pc	after meals	tinct., tr.	tincture
per	by	tsp.	teaspoon
pH	hydrogen ion concentration	U	unit supplied
PM	afternoon; evening	u	unit ordered
PO	by mouth	u.d., ut dict	as directed
p.r.	by rectum	μg	microgram; one-millionth of a gram
p.r.n.	as needed, when necessary	ung	ointment
pt	pint	USP	United States Pharmacopeia
pulv	a powder	UTI	urinary tract infection
PVC	premature ventricular contraction	UV	ultraviolet
pwd	powder	vol	volume
q.	each, very	WBC	white blood cell count
qAM	every morning	wk	week
q.d.	every day	wt	weight
q.h.	every hour	yr	year
q.2h	every 2 hours	>	greater than
q.3h	every 3 hours	<	less than
q.4h	every 4 hours		

Glossary

5-lipoxygenase: A human enzyme that transforms essential fatty acids into leukotrienes and is a current target for pharmaceutical intervention in a number of diseases.

α-adrenergic agonists: Drugs that combine with the α-adrenergic receptor and initiate the biological response.

α-cells: Endocrine cells in the pancreas that are responsible for synthesizing and secreting glucagon, which elevates the glucose levels in the blood.

α-receptors: A type of adrenergic receptor. Activation by adrenergic agonists cause constriction of peripheral blood vessels, constriction of urinary sphincter, pupil dilation, and increased glycogenolysis in the liver.

α₁-receptor: A subtype of α-adrenergic receptor; when stimulated it results in peripheral vasoconstriction, pupil dilation, and contraction of urinary sphincter.

α₂-receptor: A subtype of α-adrenergic receptor located on peripheral nerve terminals; activation of these receptors inhibits the release of additional norepinephrine.

Abortifacient: Produces abortion.

Absorption: Refers to getting the drug into the bloodstream.

ACE: See *angiotensin-converting enzyme.*

ACE inhibitors: A drug that relaxes blood vessel walls and lowers blood pressure by blocking ACE.

Acetylcholine: A neurotransmitter released by several types of nerve fibers; notably by the parasympathetic postganglionic nerve fiber.

Acetylsalicylic acid (ASA): Chemical name for aspirin.

Acid: A proton donor; a molecule capable of releasing hydrogen ions (ie, protons, H+) in solution. Also refers to a solution with a hydrogen ion concentration high enough to give a pH < 7.

Acid secretion transporter: An active transport mechanism in the renal tubule cells that moves acid compounds from the blood into the renal tubule for excretion.

Acneiform eruptions: Resembling acne.

Active drug: The chemical structure of a drug that combines with the receptor to produce the response.

Active transport: A mechanism for the transport of substances across membranes. The compound being transported attaches itself to a particular binding site of a protein transporter. The mechanism can transport against the concentration gradient but requires cellular energy.

Addiction: A behavioral disorder that is characterized by obsessive drug use typically accompanied by extreme measures to obtain the drug. The driving force that causes addiction is the desire for the euphoria from the drug.

Additive effects: When the response obtained from 2 or more drugs is equal to the sum of the responses obtained when the drugs are used individually.

Adenosine receptors: Receptors to which the chemical mediator adenosine combines and may contribute to bronchoconstriction. Inhibition of adenosine receptors may be part of the mechanism of theophylline action.

Adrenaline: See *epinephrine.*

Adrenergic: Relating to nerve cells or fibers of the autonomic nervous system that use norepinephrine as their neurotransmitter; relating to drugs that mimic the actions of the sympathetic nervous system.

Adrenergic receptor: Receptors to which epinephrine and norepinephrine combine to initiate a sympathetic response. Drugs that combine with the same receptors either mimic (agonist) or inhibit (antagonist) the sympathetic response.

Adulteration: The alteration of any substance by the deliberate addition of a component not ordinarily part of the substance.

Adverse drug reaction (ADR): Any undesirable response from a drug. These reactions can range from dry mouth to life-threatening organ damage. Some ADRs are not dose related. A broader term than *side effect.*

Affinity component: The first phase of the drug-receptor interaction; refers to the strength of the chemical binding interaction between the drug and the receptor. The second phase of this interaction causes the biological response (see *efficacy component*).

Agonist: A drug capable of combining with a receptor and activating the transduction mechanism to initiate the biological response.

Agranulocytosis: An acute disease in which the white blood cell count drops to extremely low levels.

Akathisia: Inability to sit down because the thought of doing so causes severe anxiety.

Albumin: The plasma protein with the largest concentration in the blood. Many drugs bind to albumin, which increases the drug's volume of distribution.

Aldosterone: A mineral corticosteroid hormone that causes reabsorption of sodium and water by the renal tubule and increases potassium excretion.

Aldosterone antagonism: The physiological effect of an aldosterone antagonist.

Aldosterone antagonist: A drug that blocks the effects of aldosterone to cause a response that is opposite of the effects of aldosterone, such as increased sodium excretion and potassium retention.

Alkaloids: Naturally occurring chemical compounds containing nitrogen atoms that are bases. Occur especially in seed plants and are typically physiologically active.

Alkylation: Substitution of an alkyl radical for a hydrogen atom.

Allergic reaction: An exaggerated immune response initiated by the exposure to certain drugs or other chemicals and causing effects ranging from skin rash to life-threatening anaphylaxis. Typically not dose-related effects.

Allergic rhinitis: Hypersensitivity reaction in response to inhaled allergens.

Alliin: Natural constituent of fresh garlic.

Allyl isothiocyanate: A compound used as a counterirritant.

Alopecia: Absence or loss of hair, especially on the head.

Amino acid: Organic compounds containing nitrogen, carbon, hydrogen, and oxygen; building blocks of protein.

Amylin: A peptide hormone and is co-secreted with insulin by the pancreatic β-cells. It decreases gastrointestinal motility, thereby slowing the rate of glucose absorption. It reduces the release of glucagon, thus decreasing the glycemic-enhancing effects that glucagon has on the liver.

Anabolism: Energy requiring reactions whereby small molecules are built up into larger ones.

Analgesic: A drug that is used to alleviate pain without causing the loss of consciousness.

Analyte: A substance whose chemical constituents are being identified and measured.

ANC: Abbreviation for *acid-neutralizing capacity.*

Androgen: A general term for male sex hormones that produce male sex characteristics; testosterone is a specific example and is the major androgen produced in the body.

Androgenic: Having a masculinizing effect (see *androgen*).

Androgenic-anabolic steroids (AAS): Derivatives of the male hormone testosterone, which produce both masculinizing (androgenic) and tissue-building (anabolic) effects.

Angina: A type of coronary heart disease in which the coronary arteries are not able to supply sufficient oxygen to the heart muscle.

Angioneurotic edema: A rare condition in which rapid swelling in the nose, throat, and larynx may lead to death if not treated; it occurs more frequently in Blacks than in Whites.

Angiotensin: Either of 2 forms of a peptide (angiotensin I or angiotensin II) associated with regulation of blood pressure.

Angiotensin I: A peptide produced by the action of renin on angiotensinogen and is converted to angiotensin II.

Angiotensin II: A peptide hormone produced from the action of angiotensin-converting enzyme on angiotensin I; produces vasoconstriction and triggers the release of aldosterone to increase blood pressure.

Angiotensin II receptor blockers: Drugs that combine with the angiotensin II receptor to prevent the response of angiotensin II.

Angiotensin-converting enzyme (ACE): An enzyme that catalyzes the conversion of angiotensin I to angiotensin II and also the inactivation of bradykinin. Angiotensin-converting enzyme is present in cells of blood vessels and is therefore readily available to catalyze the formation of angiotensin II.

Angiotensinogen: A glycoprotein that is continuously produced by the liver; converted by renin to angiotensin I.

Antacid: A pharmacologic agent used to neutralize the acidity of hydrochloride acid released by the stomach. Common agents include sodium bicarbonate, magnesium hydroxide, aluminum hydroxide, and calcium carbonate.

Antagonist: A drug that reduces the effect of another drug.

Antagonistic effect: When the use of a second drug reduces the effect of another drug.

Antibiotic: A drug used to treat bacterial infections, although the origin of the term is broader and sometimes refers to any antimicrobial agent.

Antibody: A protein produced by certain cells in the body in response to a specific antigen; the antibody combines with the antigen to neutralize, inhibit, or destroy it. Also called an immunoglobulin.

Anticholinergic: Generally refers to antagonistic to the action of parasympathetic nerve fibers although broadly may also refer to antagonism of other cholinergic nerve fibers.

Anticholinergic effects: Refers to a group of adverse effects that are similar to the effects from drugs in the pharmacological category called anticholinergic drugs, which inhibit the parasympathetic nervous system. Anticholinergic effects include blurred vision, constipation, dry mouth, decreased sweating, urinary retention, and increased heart rate.

Antiemetic: A pharmacological agent used to treat nausea or vomiting.

Antigen: A substance that is recognized as foreign by the immune system, activates the immune system by inducing the production of antibodies, and reacts with immune cells or their products.

Antihistamine: A pharmacologic agent used to treat allergic reactions by inhibiting the effects of histamine.

Antihyperuricemic: A pharmacological agent that reduces the enhanced blood concentration of uric acid.

Antileukotriene: See *leukotriene modifiers.*

Antimicrobial: Any drug used to treat any microorganism, bacteria, fungi, or virus.

Antipyretic: A pharmacological agent used to reduce fever.

Antiseptics: Products applied to tissue such as hands or a site of injection or incision to kill or inhibit the growth of microorganisms.

Antitussive: Drug that suppresses a cough.

Anxiolytic: Drug that relieves anxiety.

Aplastic anemia: Anemia caused by deficient red cell production due to disorders of bone marrow.

Arachidonic acid: Unsaturated fatty acid that is the starting point (substrate) for the biosynthesis of several groups of compounds (eicosanoids). These compounds are metabolites of arachidonic acid, which contribute to the inflammatory response.

Assay: To examine; to subject to analysis to determine purity.

Asthma: A chronic inflammatory disease of the airways. The inflammation results in obstruction of the airways from bronchoconstriction, edema, and excessive mucus production.

Autoimmune disease: Arise from an overactive immune response of the body against substances and tissues normally present in the body.

Autonomic neuropathy: Occurs when there is damage to nerves that regulate blood pressure, heart rate, bowel and bladder emptying, digestion, and other body functions.

β-adrenergic agonists: Drugs that combine with the β-adrenergic receptor and initiate a biological response.

β-adrenergic antagonists: See *β-blocker.*

β-adrenergic receptors: Receptors through which the sympathetic nervous system is activated along with β-receptors. Principal subtypes are β_1 and β_2.

β-agonist: Drug or hormone that combines with the β-adrenergic receptors to activate a transduction mechanism to initiate a response.

β-blocker: Drug that combines with the β-adrenergic receptor but does not initiate a transduction mechanism and therefore prevents the corresponding agonist response; examples of primary effects include decreased heart rate and force of contraction.

β-cells: Cells in the pancreas that secrete insulin.

β-lactam: A class of broad-spectrum antibiotics that are structurally and pharmacologically related to the penicillins and cephalosporins.

β-lactamases: A group of enzymes that inactivate some penicillins and cephalosporins by breaking apart a key chemical structure of these antibiotics.

β_1-adrenergic receptors: The subtype of β-adrenergic receptor found principally in the heart.

β_1-blockers: Drugs that combine with β_1-receptors but do not initiate a transduction mechanism and therefore prevent the corresponding agonist response; primary effects include decreased heart rate and force of contraction.

β_1-receptors: Another name for β_1-adrenergic receptor.

β_2-agonists: Drugs that combine with the β_2-receptor and mimic certain sympathetic responses such as bronchodilation. The most effective drugs for treatment of an acute asthma attack are the short-acting β_2-agonists administered by inhalation. Short-acting refers to the duration of action, but these drugs also have a short onset of action. Long-acting β_2-agonists are used for long-term control but not for quick relief.

β_2-receptors: A type of adrenergic receptor that is predominant in the skeletal muscle, liver, and bronchial smooth muscle.

Bacteremia: Presence of viable bacteria in the circulating blood.

Bactericidal: Drug that kills bacteria.

Bacteriostatic: Drug that slows the normal growth rate of the bacteria so that the patient's immune system has a better opportunity to eliminate the infecting organisms.

Banned substance: Any substance foreign to the body or any physiological substance prohibited from use by an athletic or sport-governing body during competition and/or training, and if present in a urine and/or blood sample, would result in some form of penalty.

Baroreceptors: Receptors that are stimulated by changes in blood pressure and initiate the baroreceptor reflex as a compensation mechanism; specifically found in the wall of the auricles of the heart, vena cava, aortic arch, and carotid sinus.

Baroreceptor reflex: An automatic response stimulated by baroreceptors in an attempt to maintain blood pressure. Causes constriction of arterioles and veins and increases heart rate in response to a drop in blood pressure; the opposite responses occur when blood pressure rises sharply.

Barrett's esophagus: A premalignant change in epithelial cells of the esophagus, which significantly increases the risk of esophageal cancer.

Base: A proton acceptor; a molecule capable of binding with hydrogen ions. Also refers to a solution with a hydrogen ion concentration low enough to give a pH >7.

Basophil: Type of white blood cell.

Benign prostatic hyperplasia (BPH): Refers to the increase in size of the prostate in middle-aged and elderly men.

Benzodiazepine: Compounds that as a group have many uses, such as to treat insomnia, anxiety, alcohol withdrawal syndrome, various seizures, as well as muscle spasm; some drugs in this group are significantly more effective for one or more of these therapeutic uses than others; all benzodiazepines have an abuse potential and thus are controlled substances (Schedule IV) and all cause central nervous system depression and thus produce drowsiness.

Beta-blocker: See *β-blocker.*

Bioavailability: The portion of a drug dose that reaches the systemic circulation and thus has an opportunity to produce a biological effect.

Bioequivalent: When the amount and rate of a drug entering the blood stream is approximately the same for 2 or more formulations of the drug.

Biotransformation: See *drug metabolism.*

Bismuth: A trivalent metallic element in which several of its salts are used in medicine, such as bismuth subsalicylate (Pepto-Bismol) used to treat diarrhea and as a component in the drug regimen for *Helicobacter pylori*–induced peptic ulcers.

Bisphosphonate drugs: Drugs with a particular phosphate structure; used to treat and prevent osteoporosis.

Blood-brain barrier: A term used to describe the inability of most ions and large molecules to pass from the blood to the central nervous system. This selectivity occurs in part because of the tight junction between the endothelial cells of the capillaries that supply the brain.

Bradykinin: A peptide hormone that is formed during inflammation. It contributes to the pain response but also has vasodilation properties, which contribute to reducing blood pressure.

Breath-actuated metered dose inhaler: Used in asthma treatment. The technique to operate this inhaler is somewhat of a cross between MDI and dry powder inhaler; a propellant is used to expel the drug but it is not activated until the patient inhales.

Calcium channel blockers: Drugs that inhibit the influx of calcium into the cells of arterial smooth muscle and cardiac muscle, resulting in peripheral vasodilation, decreased heart rate and force of contraction, and dilation of arterioles of the heart.

Camphor: A compound used as a stimulant, carminative, expectorant, and diaphoretic.

Capsicum: A compound used as a gastric stimulant and counterirritant.

Capsules: Two-piece gelatin containers that are oblong or bullet shaped. The drug and inactive ingredients are placed in one piece of the container and the second piece acts as the cap.

Cardiac remodeling: Process that changes the shape, size, and effectiveness of the heart because of cardiac injury.

Catabolic: The breaking down in the body of complex chemical compounds into simpler ones.

Catecholamine: Any of several compounds occurring naturally in the body, including dopamine, epinephrine, and norepinephrine, that function as hormones or as neurotransmitters in the sympathetic nervous system. They are derived from the amino acid tyrosine and resemble one another chemically in having an aromatic portion (catechol) to which an amine or nitrogen-containing group is attached. They have a marked effect on the nervous and cardiovascular systems, metabolic rate, temperature, and smooth muscle.

Central nervous system (CNS): Composed of brain and spinal cord.

Chain of custody: Used to describe the process of documenting the handling of a specimen from the time an athlete provides a specimen and the collector processes the specimen, through shipping to the laboratory, during the testing at the laboratory, and until the results are reported by the laboratory.

Chemical mediators: Compounds that are released by one cell type, attach to the receptor of a second cell type, and affect the response of that second cell.

Chemotactic mediator: Chemical compound that causes movement of selected cells to the site of inflammation.

Chemotaxis: Attraction of phagocytes by a chemical stimuli as a result of an inflammatory or immune response.

Cholinesterase: An enzyme that inactivates acetylcholine.

Cholesterol: Steroid found in animal fats as well as in most body tissues, made by the liver. Located in cell membranes and used in the synthesis of steroid hormones and bile salts.

Cholestyramine: A drug used to decrease blood cholesterol. It is taken prior to meals, is not absorbed from the gastrointestinal tract, and increases the excretion of bile acids, which are made from cholesterol.

Cholinergic: Relating to nerve cells or fibers that use acetylcholine as their neurotransmitter; denoting an agent that mimics the action of acetylcholine.

Cholinergic receptor: Receptor to which acetylcholine binds.

Chromatography: A process in which a chemical mixture carried by a liquid or gas is separated into components as a result of differential distribution of the solutes as they flow around or over a stationary liquid or solid phase.

Chronotropic: Affecting the rate of rhythmic movements such as the heart beat.

Churg-Strauss syndrome: Rare but has also been noted with the use of leukotriene-receptor antagonist. This syndrome involves vasculitis, which primarily affects the respiratory tract during its early stages and can progress to become life threatening.

Clearance rate: A measure of the efficiency of the metabolism and excretion of a drug to terminate the action of the drug.

Comorbidity: Presence of one or more additional disorders or diseases co-occurring with a primary disease or disorder.

Competitive antagonist: A drug that combines with the same receptor as the agonist but does not activate the transduction mechanism. When the competitive antagonist is binding to the receptor, it prevents the agonist from binding to that receptor, thus reducing the effect of the agonist.

Complement system: A group of blood-borne proteins that, when activated, enhances the inflammatory and immune responses and can lead to the lysis of invading microorganisms.

Conjugation: The addition of another molecule (eg, glucuronic or sulfuric acid) to a drug (primarily in the liver) to terminate the biological activity of the drug and prepare it for excretion.

Controlled substance: Any drug or other substance, or immediate precursor, included in Schedule I, II, III, IV, or V as defined by the Controlled Substance Act. These include narcotics analgesics, stimulants, depressants, hallucinogens, anabolic steroids, and chemicals used in the illicit production of these drugs. The term does not include distilled spirits, wine, malt beverages, or tobacco.

Coronaviruses: A category of RNA viruses that can cause the symptoms of the common cold.

Corticosteroids: Steroid hormones released by the adrenal cortex; synthetic corticosteroids are used for their anti-inflammatory effect.

COX: See *cyclooxygenase.*

COX-1: A form of the cyclooxygenase enzyme that is produced in most tissues. It catalyzes the synthesis of several arachidonic acid metabolites (ie, eicosanoids), which are important to the normal physiology in those tissues.

COX-2: A form of the cyclooxygenase enzyme that is primarily activated at the site of inflammation and tissue injury. It catalyzes the synthesis of several arachidonic acid metabolites (ie, eicosanoids), which contribute to the pain and inflammation.

Crohn's disease: An inflammatory disease usually affecting the small and large intestines but can affect any part of the digestive tract. Ulcerative lesions affect all layers of the intestinal wall. Treatment includes antibiotics, immunosuppressive drugs, and in some cases, removal of the affected part of the intestine.

Cross-reactivity: When patients who experience a hypersensitivity reaction from drugs in one category are also likely to experience a similar adverse response from drugs in another category because the drug categories share a common chemical characteristic.

Cross-tolerance: The development of diminished therapeutic and/or adverse effects (tolerance) to additional drugs as a result of tolerance from another drug.

Cushing syndrome: Condition caused by a hypersecretion of glucocorticoids characterized by spindly legs, moon face, buffalo hump, pendulous abdomen, flushed facial skin, poor wound healing, hyperglycemia, osteoporosis, weakness, hypertension, and increased susceptibility to disease.

Cyclooxygenase (COX): An enzyme found in virtually all cells and uses arachidonic acid as substrate to initiate the production of several chemical mediators. Isoforms are COX-1 and COX-2.

Cytochrome P450 (CYP 450): A family of isozymes responsible for the biotransformation of several drugs.

Cysteine: An amino acid that is a component of many proteins but is also a component of some leukotrienes referred to as cysteinyl leukotrienes.

Cytokine: Generic term for nonantibody proteins, such as interleukins and tumor necrosis factor, released by a certain cell population on contact with a specific antigen; they act as intercellular chemical mediators, as in the generation of immune response.

DEA: Abbreviation for US Drug Enforcement Administration; a federal agency.

Decongestant: Having the property of reducing nasal congestion by constriction of blood vessels and decreasing mucosal edema in the nasal passage through β-adrenergic agonist activity.

Dehydroepiandrosterone (DHEA): Hormone that is naturally made in the human body and secreted by the adrenal gland. In sports used to increase muscle mass, strength, and energy.

Dependence: Occurs because of cellular changes within the body in response to continual exposure to the drug.

Digoxin: A drug used to treat congestive heart failure; it increases the force of contraction without increasing heart rate.

Disease-modifying antirheumatic drugs (DMARDs): Drugs that delay or stop the progression of rheumatoid arthritis, but it takes weeks to months for the effects of DMARDs to develop.

Disinfectants: Products applied to inanimate objects, such as surgical areas or instruments, to kill or inhibit the growth of microorganisms.

Dissolution: The process of dissolving.

Distribution: Refers to the movement of the drug throughout the body to the various compartments. Besides blood, these compartments include the central nervous system, cells (eg, muscle, adipose, liver, kidney), excretory fluids (eg, urine, bile, sweat), and plasma proteins (primarily albumin).

Diuresis: Excretion of urine; commonly denotes production of large quantities of urine.

Diuretic: A pharmacologic agent designed to increase the amount of water in the urine thereby removing excess water from the body; commonly used to treat fluid retention and hypertension.

DNA (deoxyribonucleic acid): A nucleic acid in the shape of a double helix found in all living cells; carries the organism's hereditary information.

DNA recombinant (rDNA): Form of DNA that does not exist naturally, which is created by combining DNA sequences that would not normally occur together.

Dopamine: Neurotransmitter in the brain.

Dosage form: Physical form in which the drug exists for administration, such as tablet, capsule, solution for injection.

Dose-response curve: See *dose-response principle*.

Dose-response effect: When the magnitude of the effect being measured increases as the dose increases.

Dose-response principle: As the concentration of drug increases, more receptors are occupied by the drug, producing a greater effect until the dose is high enough that all of the receptors are occupied and therefore additional drug does not produce additional effect; maximal response is achieved.

Dosing interval: The time period between doses.

Drug: A chemical that has demonstrated to be effective for the prevention or treatment of a disease.

Drug interaction: Occurs when one drug increases or decreases the effect of another drug.

Drug metabolism: The chemical alteration of the drug by one or more enzymes in the body with an associated change in pharmacological activity (see *biotransformation*).

Drug resistance: A change in the susceptibility of the organism to a particular drug or group of drugs so that drugs that were once effective against the microorganism are no longer effective.

Dry powder inhaler (DPI): A device used to administer drugs by inhalation. The drug exists as a dry powder, and a controlled amount is released when the patient inhales deeply from the device. Used for delivery of asthma medications to the lungs. DPIs provide an alternative to the use of pressurized gases. As the patient inhales deeply, the process of inhalation through the inhaler draws the powdered drug into the lungs. The drug is contained in a capsule or other package form that the inhaler breaks open during use to allow the powder to be inhaled.

Duration of action: The time between onset and termination of action, and represents the length of time the drug produces its effect.

Dynorphins: A family of endogenous peptides found in the central nervous system that act as a painkiller (see *endorphins*).

Dyslipidemia: Elevated blood lipid beyond normal range; most commonly as elevated cholesterol or triglycerides.

Dysphoria: A feeling of unpleasantness or discomfort.

Dysrhythmia: Abnormal, disordered, or disturbed rhythm and typically referring to the heart.

Dystonia: Defect in voluntary movement.

ED$_{50}$ (effective dose): The dose of drug that is effective in producing 50% of a specified response.

Efficacy component: The second phase of the drug-receptor interaction and the phase that produces the biological response. The first phase of this interaction is the ability of the drug to chemically bind to the receptor (see *affinity component*).

EIB: Exercise-induced bronchoconstriction.

Eicosanoids: Physiologically active substances derived from arachidonic acid (ie, the prostaglandins, leukotrienes, prostacyclin, and thromboxanes).

Elixirs: Sweetened and flavored solutions of ethanol and water containing one or more drugs.

Emulsions: Liquids usually consisting of small droplets of oil dispersed in water. The oil may be the drug or may be used to dissolve a lipid-soluble drug.

Endogenous: Arising from inside of the body.

Endorphins: As β-endorphins, a family of peptides in the central nervous system that act as a pain killer. Also used as a broader term to collectively refer to β-endorphins, enkephalins, and dynorphins.

Enkephalins: A family of peptides found in the central nervous system that act as a painkiller (see *endorphins*).

Enteric coating: Coating on the outside of a solid dosage form that prevents it from dissolving in the acidity of the stomach and is intended to delay the release of the drug until it reaches the small intestine.

Enterohepatic: Blood circulation from small intestine directly to the liver.

Eosinophils: Type of white blood cell.

Epinephrine: Also known as adrenaline, a hormone secreted by the adrenal glands in response to stress or fear. Stimulates α and β-adrenergic receptors, resulting in increased heart rate, increased metabolism, and improved breathing.

Equipotent dose: The dose of one drug adjusted so that it gives the same response as the dose of a similar drug. If 20 mg of one drug gives the same response as 10 mg of a similar drug, these 2 doses are equipotent.

Erythema: Redness of the skin.

Erythropoietin (EPO): A hormone secreted by the kidneys to increase the rate of production of red blood cells in response to falling levels of oxygen in the tissues.

Ester: A chemical component of a molecule usually formed by the reaction between an acid and an alcohol with elimination of water.

Estrogen: A female hormone produced by the ovaries.

Euphoria: An exaggerated feeling of well-being.

Excretion: Process whereby the drug and metabolites of metabolism are eliminated from the body.

Exogenous: Arising or produced outside of the body.

Expectorants: A drug that decreases the viscosity of lower respiratory tract secretions so that they can be moved out of the respiratory tract more efficiently by coughing.

Extrapyramidal: Outside the pyramidal tracts of the central nervous system.

Facilitated diffusion: A membrane transport mechanism that combines the characteristics of passive diffusion and active transport. It requires a carrier protein but it does not use energy.

Fasciculation: Small, local, involuntary muscle contraction (twitching) visible under the skin arising from the spontaneous discharge of a bundle of skeletal muscle fibers.

Fatty acids: Acids produced when fats stored as triglycerides are broken down.

First-pass effect: The inactivation of drugs by enzymes in the intestinal cells or liver before the drug enters the general circulation, thus decreasing the bioavailability of the drug.

Flavonoids: Antioxidants found naturally in plants.

Flora: Various bacteria and other microorganisms that normally inhabit an individual without causing disease.

Formulation: The total composition of a drug product and nature of the dosage form, including the inactive ingredients and the means by which the ingredients are put together.

Free drug: Drug that is not bound to albumin and is free to bind at its site of action.

Gamma aminobutyric acid (GABA): A neurotransmitter that is widely distributed in the central nervous system and involved in inhibiting responses that would otherwise cause pain, depression, and convulsions.

Ganglion: Collection of nerve cell bodies outside the central nervous system.

Gas chromatography (GC): Chromatography in which a sample mixture is vaporized and injected into a stream of carrier gas moving through a column containing a stationary phase composed of a liquid or particulate solid and is separated into its component compounds according to their affinity for the stationary phase.

Gastrin: A hormone produced in the pyloric regions of the stomach that stimulates the production of gastric acid.

Gastroesophageal reflux disease (GERD): A chronic condition that exists when heartburn occurs regularly (ie, more than twice a week).

Ginkgolic acid: Toxic compound found in ginkgo leaves.

Glinides: Drugs that stimulate the pancreas to release insulin.

Glomerulus: A tuft of capillaries surrounded by the Bowman's capsule forming part of the nephron and aids in filtration of the blood by the kidney.

Glucagon: Hormone secreted by the pancreas and is released when blood glucose levels start to fall too low, raising blood glucose levels and preventing the development of hypoglycemia.

Gluconeogenesis: The process by which glucose is made from amino acids or lactic acid.

Glycemia: Sugar or glucose in the blood.

Glycogenolysis: The process of converting glycogen to glucose.

Glycoproteins: A molecule that consists of a carbohydrate plus a protein and play essential roles in the body.

Glycoside: A drug that contains a sugar and a nonsugar component bonded together (eg, digoxin).

Glycosylated hemoglobin: See *hemoglobin A1C.*

Gout: Inflammation and joint pain because of elevated uric acid blood concentration.

Gram-negative: Bacteria that do not retain dye from a Gram stain laboratory test.

Gram-positive: Bacteria that retain dye from a Gram stain laboratory test.

Gynecomastia: Development of abnormally large mammary glands in the male.

H₁-receptors: One of the 3 types of histamine receptors; found in the respiratory tract and near peripheral blood vessels. Antihistamines that block the H_1-receptor were on the market for decades prior to H_2-blockers and thus, historically, any reference to antihistamines without specifying the receptor type is generally understood to be referring to antihistamines that block the H_1-receptor.

H₂-blocker: See *histamine (H₂)-receptor antagonists.*

H₂-receptors: One of the 3 types of histamine receptors; located primarily on stomach cells; activation causes an increased production of stomach acid.

H₃-receptors: One of the 3 types of histamine receptors; located in the central nervous system. Their function is not clearly understood and there are no drugs clinically available that are known to specifically block these receptors.

Half-life (t½): The time required for the amount of drug in the body (as measured in the blood, serum, or plasma) to be reduced by one-half.

HDL (high-density lipoprotein) cholesterol: Considered to be the "good cholesterol"; a specific lipoprotein in the blood that removes cholesterol from the blood, thereby protecting against heart disease. The HDL cholesterol is considered good because cholesterol in the blood is captured by the HDL particles and thus the cholesterol is no longer able to deposit in unwanted places such as the interior of blood vessels.

Heart block: A condition in which the impulse from the atria to the ventricles is partially or totally prevented. If untreated, the ventricles fail to contract.

Heartburn: Also called acid indigestion, results from the contact of gastric acid, and to some extent bile and pepsin, with the esophageal mucosa.

Heart failure: Also known as congestive heart failure. With this condition the heart cannot pump with enough force to adequately supply blood to the tissues.

Helicobacter pylori (H. pylori): A gram-negative bacteria that promotes peptic ulcer disease and is the most common cause of gastric and duodenal ulcers.

Hemoglobin A1C: Form of hemoglobin in which glucose has become attached to the hemoglobin. The level of A1C is based on the glucose concentration in the blood and thus the A1C value is used primarily to identify the average plasma glucose concentration over prolonged periods. Used to determine how well diabetes is being controlled. Also called glycosylated hemoglobin.

Hgh: Abbreviation for *human growth hormone.*

Hiatal hernia: This condition exists when the stomach partially sits in the chest cavity because of a weakness in the diaphragm. Can also be the cause of GERD.

Hirsutism: Excessive growth of body and facial hair, especially in women.

Histamine: Substance found in many cells, especially mast cell, basophils, and platelets released during inflammatory and immune responses or tissue injury and causes vasodilation and increased vascular permeability.

Histamine (H₂)-receptor antagonists (H₂RAs): Also known as H_2-blockers; competitive antagonists to histamine receptors on the stomach parietal cells. These drugs suppress gastric acid secretion and are effective in treating mild heartburn, GERD, and peptic ulcer disease.

Hydrolyzed: Process by which water is used to split a substance into smaller molecules.

Hydrophilic: Means "love water." Drugs that are more water soluble in an aqueous environment, such as blood or urine, because the polar and ionized chemical groups form bonds with water molecules. They do not dissolve readily in lipid environments such as membranes.

Hydrophobic: Means "fear water." Drugs that have more nonpolar than polar chemical characteristics. They have low water solubility, but dissolve more readily in the lipid environments of membranes (see *lipophilic*).

Hyperforin: A phytochemical produced by some of the members of the plant genus *Hypericum*, notably *Hypericum perforatum* (St. John's wort):

Hypericin: One of the principal active constituents of St. John's wort and believed to act as an antibiotic and non-specific kinase inhibitor.

Hyperkalemia: Too much potassium in the blood.

Hypokalemia: Deficiency of potassium in the blood.

Hypothalamic-pituitary-adrenal (HPA) axis: A physiological control mechanism in which the amount of cortisol produced by the adrenal gland is regulated based on the amount of cortisol the hypothalamus detects in the blood. If there is a sufficient amount in the blood, the hypothalamus sends a hormone signal to the pituitary, which sends a hormone signal to the adrenal gland to decrease cortisol production. Excessive inhibition of cortisol production occurs (adrenal suppression) when corticosteroid therapy lasts for more than several days. If adrenal suppression occurs, the corticosteroid dosage must be gradually decreased to give the adrenal gland time to begin making cortisol, otherwise fatal deficiency of corticosteroid may result.

Idiopathic: Unknown cause.

Immunoglobulin E (IgE): Antibodies located on the surface of mast cells in the airways.

IgE antibodies: A type of immunoglobulin located on mast cells and basophils. When ige antibodies combine with specific antigens, they initiate an allergic response by causing the release of chemical mediators from these cells.

IGF-1: Abbreviation for insulin-like growth factor 1.

Immune cells: Any type of cell that contributes to the immune response by synthesizing antibodies, releasing chemical mediators, or removing foreign substances.

Immunoassay: An analytical method used for the detection and analysis of the presence of hormones or other substances.

Incretins: Hormones that increase insulin secretion.

Induce: To initiate, cause, or bring about.

Inflammatory bowel disease (IBD): A term that refers to 2 similar diseases: Crohn's disease and ulcerative colitis.

Inotropic: Influencing the contractility of muscular tissue.

Insulin secretagogues: Drugs that increase the secretion of insulin.

Interferon beta-2: Antiviral agent that can fight tumors.

Interleukin-1: Substance from monocytes and macrophages important in the acute phase response that includes fever, initiation of immune response, and immobilization of amino acids from muscle tissue.

Intrinsic efficacy: The ability of the drug to cause a response due to interacting with the receptor.

In vitro: Taking place outside a living organism (ie, test tube, culture dish, etc)

In vivo: Taking place in a living organism.

Ion: Any positively or negatively charged particle; usually formed when a substance, such as a salt, dissolves and dissociates.

Ionization: Dissociation into ions with a positive and negative charge.

Irritable bowel syndrome (IBS): A common disorder in which the colon, for no apparent reason, is more sensitive to stimuli than normal.

Isoenzymes: See *isozymes*.

Isoform: Different forms of an enzyme that vary slightly in chemical structure but catalyze the same reaction. Also called isoenzymes or isozymes.

Isomer: One of 2 or more chemical substances that have the same molecular formula but different chemical and physical properties due to different arrangement of the atoms in the molecule.

Isozymes: Two or more enzymes that catalyze the same reaction, but may be differentiated by variations in physical properties.

Ketoacidosis: A serious condition that can lead to diabetic coma or even death. Occurs when sugar (glucose) is not available as a fuel source by the body and therefore fatty acids are used excessively.

Ketone bodies: Chemicals (ketones) that the body makes when there is not enough insulin in the blood and therefore the body must break down fat extensively without sufficient availability of glucose for energy.

Ketosis: Ketone bodies in the blood.

Kinase: An enzyme that catalyzes the transfer of phosphate from ATP to an acceptor.

Kinin system: A group of blood proteins that when activated, enhance the inflammatory and immune responses, increase vascular permeability, and contribute to the pain response.

Lactic acidosis: Accumulation of lactic acid in the blood without respect to the etiology.

Lactose: A disaccharide found in dairy milk.

LD$_{50}$ (lethal dose): The dose that will cause death in 50% of the population as extrapolated from animal data.

LDL (low-density lipoprotein) cholesterol: Considered the "bad cholesterol"; a specific lipoprotein that carries cholesterol in the blood and deposits it at tissues. The LDL cholesterol is considered bad because high levels of LDL cause the deposit of cholesterol in unwanted places, such as the interior of blood vessels, and is associated with heart disease and atherosclerosis.

Leukopenia: Abnormal decrease in white blood cells.

Leukotriene modifiers: Also called antileukotrienes, a group of long-term control medications used to treat asthma. They can be subdivided into drugs that block the leukotriene receptor (leukotriene-receptor antagonists) and drugs that decrease the synthesis of leukotrienes (leukotriene-synthesis inhibitors).

Leukotrienes (LTs): Products of arachidonic acid metabolism by the lipoxygenase pathway. They serve as chemical mediators of inflammation, allergic reactions, and asthma.

Lipase: A fat-splitting enzyme; it releases fatty acids from triglyceride molecules.

Lipoxygenase: Family of iron-containing enzymes that catalyse the deoxygenation of polyunsaturated fatty acids in lipids.

Lipolysis: The breakdown of fat (triglyceride) to form fatty acids and glycerol products.

Lipophilic: Means "love lipid." Drugs that have more non-polar than polar chemical characteristics. They have low water solubility, but dissolve readily in the lipid environments of membranes (see *hydrophobic*).

Liquid chromatography (LC): Chromatographic technique that is useful for separating ions or molecules that are dissolved in a solvent.

Loading dose: One or more doses that are higher than the maintenance dose and administered at the beginning of therapy for achieving the desirable therapeutic concentration quicker.

Luteinizing hormone: Hormone produced by the anterior pituitary gland and in the female triggers ovulation.

Macrophages: Phagocytic cells that phagocytize tissue cells, bacteria, and other foreign debris.

Maintenance dose: Repetitive use of the same dose of a drug at the same dosing interval.

Mania: Mental disorder characterized by excessive excitement.

Mast cells: Cells found in connective tissue along blood vessels that produce a variety of chemical mediators during inflammation. Chemical mediators include arachidonic acid metabolites that cause vessel dilation and increased permeability, and chemotactic factors that attract phagocytic cells to the site of inflammation.

Mass spectrometry (MS): An instrumental method for identifying the chemical constitution of a substance by means of the separation of gaseous ions according to their differing mass and charge.

Mast cell stabilizers: Pharmacological agents used to treat asthma by inhibiting the release of inflammatory mediators for mast cells.

Mechanism of action: The biochemical changes that occur to cause the observed effects from a drug.

Menthol: An alcohol obtained from peppermint oil or other mint oils; used as an antipruritic and topical anesthetic.

Metabolic alkalosis: An increase in blood pH resulting in a pH more basic compared with normal due to an imbalance in one or more biochemical processes.

Metabolites: Product of the reaction of a parent drug or substrate interacting with a metabolizing enzyme.

Metered dose inhaler (MDI): Used for delivery of asthma medications to the lungs. The drug is contained in a pressurized container with a metering valve to control the amount of drug released as a mist during each use. A propellant is used to force the metered amount of drug from the inhaler each time the device is actuated.

Methylxanthine: A group of compounds such as caffeine, theophylline, and theobromine that have varying degrees of effects on cardiac muscle, the CNS, and bronchial and other smooth muscle.

Mimetic: Imitative.

Molecular weight: The weight of a molecule determined by adding the atomic weight of each atom that comprises the molecule; the larger the molecular weight, the larger the size of the molecule. Most drugs have a molecular weight 100 to 1000; drugs that are proteins being the primary exception.

Monoamine oxidase (MAO): An enzyme that inactivates norepinephrine and epinephrine.

Monoamine oxidase inhibitors (MAOIs): A group of drugs that are categorized therapeutically as antidepressant drugs, although they also have some other uses. MAOIs have a significant drug interaction with sympathomimetics; MAOIs inhibit the inactivation of sympathomimetics, enhancing their activity and causing a potentially dangerous exaggerated hypertensive response. They also exhibit anticholinergic adverse effects.

Monomer: Any molecule that can be bound to similar molecules to form a polymer. Amino acids are monomer units of proteins; glucose and other monosaccharides are monomer units of polysaccharides.

Mononuclear cells: Phagocytic cells having only one nucleus and include macrophages and monocytes. They engulf and remove debris from the site of inflammation, injury, and immune response.

Muscarinic receptor: Another name for cholinergic receptor at the site where the parasympathetic nerve innervates the tissue.

Myocardial infarction: An ischemic heart disease. Occlusion of a coronary artery prevents sufficient blood from reaching a portion of the heart muscle, thus causing death of some heart cells.

Nandrolone: Anabolic steriod.

Narcotic: Used in a legal context to refer to any controlled substance.

Narcotic analgesic: Another term used to refer to opioids. They can produce a state of narcosis (drowsiness or sleep) and relieve pain.

Nebulizer: A device used to deliver liquid medication as an extremely fine cloud; useful in delivering medication to the deep part of the respiratory tract. These devices are larger than mdis or dpis and are used primarily in hospitals and clinics, or in homes if the patient is unable to use inhalers.

Nephron: The active filtering unit of the kidney that consists of the glomerulus and renal tubule.

Nephropathy: Disease of the kidney.

Neuropathy: Any disease of the nerves.

Neutrophils: Most common type of white blood cell and ingests bacteria.

Nociceptors: Afferent nerves responsible for sensing pain.

Nonsteroidal anti-inflammatory drugs (NSAIDs): A group of anti-inflammatory drugs that is not from the steroid family; used to reduce inflammation and pain.

Noradrenaline: See *norepinephrine*.

Norandrosterone: Metabolite of the anabolic steroid nandrolone.

Norepinephrine: A hormone secreted by the adrenal medulla that produces actions similar to those that result from sympathetic stimulation.

Nucleic acid: Class of organic molecules that include DNA and RNA.

Onset of action: The time it takes for the concentration of drug molecules at the site of action to become large enough to cause a noticeable biological response.

Opiates: Drugs that are obtained from the opium poppy, opium being the extract from the plant. Morphine and codeine are 2 of the components of opium and thus are opiates.

Opioids: A broader term than *opiates* and refers to drugs that have effects similar to the opiates. Oxycodone (oxycontin) and meperidine (Demerol) are examples.

Organelle: Small cellular structures that perform specific metabolic functions for the cellular functions (eg, ribosomes, mitochondria).

Orthostatic hypotension: Also called postural hypotension. A decrease in blood pressure upon standing from a sitting or supine position due to an insufficient automatic baroreceptor reflex.

OTC: Abbreviation for over-the-counter medications; medications that do not require a prescription.

Oxidation: Addition of oxygen to or removal of hydrogen from a molecule.

P450 enzymes: A group of proteins that are important in catalyzing the metabolism of steroid hormones and fatty acids and in the detoxification of a variety of chemical substances. Also called cytochrome P450. There are several subcategories of P450 enzymes.

Parasympathetic: Division of the autonomic nervous system that oversees digestion, elimination, and glandular function.

Parasympathomimetics: Drugs that mimic the parasympathetic nervous system.

Parent drug: The drug reacting with a metabolizing enzyme and converted to metabolites (see *substrate*).

Parenteral route: The use of an intravenous, intramuscular, or subcutaneous injection to administer a drug.

Parietal cells: Cells of the stomach that produce hydrochloric acid.

Passive diffusion: Refers to the drug penetrating through the membrane due to the solubility of the drug in the membrane and is the transport mechanism of greatest impact for most drugs; does not require cellular energy.

PCP: Abbreviation for the drug phencyclidine. Drug used as an anesthetic by veterinarians; illicitly taken for its effects as a hallucinogen.

Peak expiratory flow (PEF): A pulmonary function test that determines the maximum flow rate of forced expiration that the patient can achieve at that time.

Peak flow meter (PFM): Hand-held device used to determine peak expiratory flow.

Pepsin: The principal digestive enzyme of the gastric juice.

Pepsinogen: The inactive form of pepsin; it is produced by stomach cells and released in the stomach in response to autonomic regulation. The acid pH of the stomach catalyzes the conversion of pepsinogen to pepsin.

Peptide: Any sequence of amino acids joined by peptide bonds. Proteins are larger peptides.

Perforation: An abnormal opening in an organ or body tissue from disease or injury.

Perioral dermatitis: A rash that occurs around the mouth.

Peripheral neuropathy: Problem with the nerves that carry information to and from the brain and spinal cord.

Peristalsis: Progressive, wavelike contractions that move foodstuffs through the gastrointestinal tract.

Phagocytosis: Engulfing of foreign debris by phagocytic cells.

Pharmacodynamics: The study of the impact of drugs on the body. The primary focus of pharmacodynamics is on the molecular mechanism by which drugs exert their therapeutic and adverse effects.

Pharmacogenetics: Study of how the actions of and reactions to drugs vary based on variations of genetic composition.

Pharmacokinetics: The study of the impact of the body on drugs. The primary focus of pharmacokinetics is on the rate and extent to which drugs are absorbed into the bloodstream, distributed throughout the body, metabolized, and finally excreted.

Pharmacology: The effect of drugs on the body and the effect of the body on drugs.

Phosphodiesterases: An enzyme that inactivates second messengers such as cyclic AMP.

Phospholipase A2: An enzyme that catalyzes the intracellular release of arachidonic acid from the membrane-bound phospholipid.

Phospholipid: Modified lipid-containing phosphorous.

Pills: Small, spherical, solid dosage forms that are rarely used any more. The drug and inactive ingredients are rolled together rather than being compressed.

Placebo: A dosage form that contains no active ingredient (eg, capsules filled with lactose).

Placebo effect: Either a therapeutic or adverse response that can not be attributed to the pharmacological effect of the drug.

Plasma protein systems: Biochemical sequences that produce several proteins with specific important functions in the inflammatory response; blood clotting, kinin, and complement systems.

Platelet-activating factor (PAF): A phospholipid chemical mediator produced by a variety of cells including platelets, neutrophils, mast cells, and vascular endothelial cells. Platelet-activating factor causes vasodilation, increases vascular permeability, and platelet aggregation.

Polar compounds: Drugs or other chemical compounds that have predominately polar characteristics, which increase their solubility in water.

Polar conjugated metabolites: Drugs that have been made more polar by a conjugation reaction as part of the drug metabolism process. Conjugation with sugar molecules, for example.

Polarity: A chemical characteristic of a molecule that increases the water solubility of the molecule.

Polydipsia: Increased thirst.

Polypeptide: A peptide formed by the union of an indefinite number of amino acids.

Polyphagia: Increased appetite.

Polysaccharides: Any of a class of carbohydrates, such as starch and cellulose, consisting of a number of monosaccharides (sugars) linked together to form a polymer of sugar molecules.

Polyuria: The excessive passage of urine (at least 2.5 L per day for an adult) resulting in profuse urination and urinary frequency (the need to urinate frequently). A classic sign of diabetes mellitus that is under poor control or is not yet under treatment.

Postprandial: Following a meal.

Potency: Compares the dose of a drug required to produce a particular effect relative to the dose of another drug that acts by a similar mechanism to produce that same effect.

Preprandial: Before a meal.

Probenecid: A synthetic compound that promotes increased excretion of uric acid and is used to treat gout.

Prodrug: The inactive form of a drug that is administered with the intent of a metabolic reaction converting the drug (biotransformation) to a form that has pharmacologic action (ie, active form).

Progestin: A general term for female hormones that produce some or all of the biological changes produced by progesterone.

Prostacyclin (PGI$_2$): A derivative of prostaglandin that is a natural inhibitor of platelet aggregation and is also a vasodilator.

Prostaglandins (PGs): A group of lipid-based chemical messenger synthesized from arachidonic acid (ie, eicosanoids) by most tissue cells, which acts locally as a hormone-like substance.

Proton pump: Actively transports hydrogen ions (protons = H+) into the stomach to combine with chloride ions to form hydrochloric acid (HCl).

Proton-pump inhibitor (PPI): Drugs that inhibit the production of gastric acid by inhibiting the H+, K+ ATPase mechanism that releases the acid into the gastric lumen.

Protozoa: A eukaryotic microorganism, characteristically unicellular and motile. Many are parasites of animals.

Pruritus: Itching.

Pseudoparkinsonism: A reversible syndrome resembling Parkinsonism that may result from the dopamine-blocking action of antipsychotic drugs.

PUD: Abbreviation for *peptic ulcer disease.*

Radioimmunoassay (RIA): Immunoassay of a substance that has been radioactively labeled.

Rate of solubility: Rate that a drug becomes dissolved; it impacts the rate of absorption as drugs must be dissolved to be absorbed.

rDNA: See *DNA recombinant.*

Receptor: Any macromolecule that has specific chemical characteristics allowing it to selectively bind to drugs or hormones. Typically receptors, when activated by an agonist, have the ability to initiate a signaling mechanism (see *transduction mechanism*), which ultimately produces a biological response.

Receptor antagonist: See *competitive antagonist.*

Recombinant: A microbe, or strain, that has received chromosomal parts from different parental strains.

Renal tubule: Part of the nephron into which filtered fluid passes.

Renin: An enzyme released by the kidney into the plasma where it produces angiotensin from angiotensinogen (angiotensinogen $\longrightarrow$ angiotensin I); also referred to as angiotensinogenase.

Renin-angiotensin-aldosterone system: See *renin-angiotensin system.*

Renin-angiotensin system: A series of enzyme reactions initiated by renin and resulting in the production of angiotensin II, which causes the release of aldosterone. Plays an important role in regulating blood pressure.

Retinopathy: General term that refers to some form of noninflammatory damage to the retina of the eye.

Reye's syndrome: A rare but potentially fatal disorder mainly affecting children and teens, characterized by vomiting, disorientation, lethargy, and liver damage following a viral infection. May be linked to the use of aspirin in the treatment of viral infection.

Rheumatoid arthritis: A common systemic inflammatory disease caused by an autoimmune response, possibly initiated as a result of a bacterial or viral infection.

Rhinorrhea: Runny nose.

Rhinoviruses: Category of viruses for which more than 100 specific viruses have been identified and are associated with the common cold in human beings.

Rhizomes: A horizontal stem of a plant that is usually found underground, often sending out roots and shoots from its nodes.

Ribosomes: Cytoplasmic organelles at which proteins are synthesized.

RNA (ribonucleic acid): Nucleic acid that contains ribose rather than deoxyribose; acts in protein synthesis.

Rubefacient: Causing redness of the skin due to cutaneous vasodilation; a counterirritant that produces erythema when applied to the skin surface.

SAMHSA: Abbreviation for Substance Abuse and Mental Health Services Administration.

Sarcolemma: Membrane of a muscle fiber.

Second messenger system: An example of a transduction mechanism; a series of reactions initiated inside a cell in response to a receptor being activated on the cell surface by a drug or hormone (the first messenger). The series of reactions is the messenger system that allows the drug or hormone to cause a biological response inside the cell without entering the cell.

Secretagogue: An agent that causes secretion.

Selective serotonin re-uptake inhibitors (SSRIs): A class of compounds typically used as antidepressants in the treatment of depression, anxiety disorders, and some personality disorders.

Serotonin: Also called 5-hydroxytryptamine (5-HT). A neurotransmitter important for regulating many functions including sleep, mood, pain, appetite, gastrointestinal motility, and as a chemical mediator affecting inflammation.

Serotonin syndrome: A potentially life-threatening drug reaction that causes the body to have too much serotonin, a chemical produced by nerve cells. The adverse drug reaction that may occur following therapeutic drug use, inadvertent interactions between drugs, overdose of particular drugs, or the recreational use of certain drugs.

Side effects: Expected undesirable responses based on the pharmacologic action of the drug. Dose-related effects (ie, larger doses will increase the frequency of the undesirable effects). A type of adverse drug reaction.

Site of action: The molecular site where the drug has a significant chemical interaction to produce a biological effect.

Sitz bath: A shallow bath of warm water, usually for therapy, which allows for immersion of buttocks and hips. The tub is usually shaped to allow the legs to be out of water.

Spirometer: A gasometer that measures respiratory gases; device to measure lung capacity by measuring the volume of air exhaled.

Steady-state concentration: The concentration of drug in the blood that is reached when a dose of drug is given at regular dosing intervals and the clearance rate is equal to the rate of absorption. Steady-state is reached after the drug has been given for a time equivalent to 4 to 5 half-lives of the drug.

Streptococcal: Gram-positive bacteria that cause a variety of diseases, including scarlet fever, pneumonia, and strep throat.

Substance P: A neurotransmitter that is thought to be involved in pain sensation at peripheral sites.

Substrate: The compound that reacts with and is chemically changed by an enzyme. A broader term than parent drug. Encompasses all substances that are converted to product by an enzyme.

Sulfonylureas: A class of antidiabetic drugs that are used in the management of type 2 diabetes. They act by increasing insulin release from the beta cells in the pancreas.

Superinfection: A second infection that develops during the treatment of an initial infection as a result of the antibiotic used to treat the initial infection but also kills a sufficient number of normal flora in the gastrointestinal, respiratory, or urinary tract, allowing for the increased growth of resistant microorganisms that cause the second infection.

Suspension: Liquid dosage form in which a solid (the drug) is dispersed (not dissolved) throughout the liquid.

Sympathetic: Division of the autonomic nervous system that activates the body to cope with some stressor (eg, danger, excitement, etc); the fight, fright, and flight responses.

Sympathomimetics: Drugs that mimic the sympathetic nervous system.

Synergistic effect: When the response obtained from 2 or more drugs is greater than what would be expected by adding the responses obtained when the drugs are used individually.

Syrups: Sweetened and flavored aqueous solutions containing one or more drugs. They contain little or no alcohol and thus are particularly suitable for children, as well as for adults who have difficulty swallowing tablets or capsules.

t½: See *half-life*.

T lymphocytes: Also called T cells. A lymphocyte that becomes immunocompetent in the thymus gland and differentiates into one of several kinds of effector cells that function in cell-mediated immunity.

Tablets: Solid dosage forms, most of which are prepared by compressing the powders into the desired shape.

Tardive dyskinesia: A disorder that causes involuntary movements, especially of the lower face. Tardive means "delayed" and dyskinesia means "abnormal movement." Also a side effect of long-term or high-dose use of dopamine antagonists, usually antipsychotics.

TD$_{50}$ (toxic dose): The dose that will produce a specific toxic effect in 50% of the population.

Tetrahydrocannabinol (THC): Active component in cannabis preparation (marijuana, hashish, etc).

Therapeutic drug monitoring: Measuring the blood (or serum or plasma) concentration of a drug; usually done with drugs that have a low therapeutic index.

Therapeutic index (TI): The ratio of the dose that causes a specified toxic effect compared to the dose that causes a specified therapeutic effect. The larger the TI, the greater the margin of safety.

Therapeutic range: The range between the lowest and the highest desired concentration of a drug in the blood (or serum or plasma). The range of a drug concentration that will produce the desired effects without the unwanted side effects.

Therapeutic window: See *therapeutic range*.

Therapeutics: The study of the parameters that determine the most appropriate therapy for a patient. It considers the parameters necessary to individualize treatment for the specific patient, including all of the patient's diseases, all of the drugs the patient may be using, the dosage regimen of each drug, and the impact of potential adverse effects.

Therapeutic use exceptions: Special permission to use a prohibited substance for medical reasons based on substantial medical documentation.

Thermogenic: Producing heat in the body as a result of increased metabolic reactions.

Thin-layer chromatography: A chromatographic technique that is useful for separating organic compounds. The compounds are separated on a thin layer of adsorbent material, typically a coating of silica gel on a glass plate or plastic sheet.

Thrombocytopenia: Abnormal decrease in the number of blood platelets.

Thromboxanes (TX): Formed from arachidonic acid (ie, eicosanoids) and cause platelet aggregation and vasoconstriction.

Thyroxine: Hormone produced by the thyroid gland. Used in the treatment of hypothyroidism.

Tolerance: The diminished response to a drug as a result of continued use.

TPA: Abbreviation for *third-party administrators*.

Transdermal: A type of dosage form in which the drug is placed on the surface of the skin and the drug passes into the bloodstream to produce a systemic effect.

Transduction mechanism: Any of several mechanisms that allow a drug or hormone on the outside of the cell to have an effect on the inside of the cell, ultimately causing the biological response. Usually a series of reactions inside the cell are initiated when a receptor is activated by the drug or hormone.

Tricyclic antidepressants (TCAs): A group of drugs characterized chemically by a specific 3-ring structure and pharmacologically by their ability to relieve depression. Besides their therapeutic use as antidepressants, they are noted for anticholinergic and sedative adverse effects.

Triterpene: A class of compounds that are numerous and widely distributed in nature, occurring principally in plant resins and sap.

Triturate: To accomplish trituration, which is reducing a substance to a fine power.

Tumor necrosis factor (TNF): Protein cytokine chemical mediators produced by macrophages, T lymphocytes, and other cells. Two necrosis factors are TNF-α and TNF-β. Tumor necrosis factor contributes to the inflammatory and immune response, especially against bacteria, by promoting neutrophil infiltration, activating several cell types, including the production of other cytokines, and activating the complement and blood coagulation systems.

Type 1 diabetes mellitus: A chronic (lifelong) disease that occurs when the pancreas does not produce enough insulin to properly control blood sugar levels.

Type 2 diabetes mellitus: A chronic (lifelong) disease marked by high levels of sugar in the blood. It begins when the body does not respond correctly to insulin, a hormone released by the pancreas. Type 2 diabetes mellitus is the most common form of diabetes.

Tyramine: Naturally occurring compound found in some foods that acts as a catecholamine-releasing agent.

Ulcerative colitis: An inflammatory bowel disease of the colon and rectum.

Ulcerogenic effect: Anything that contributes to ulcer formation.

Valepotriates: A class of alkaloids from *Valeriana* sp. and *Kentranthus* sp.

Vasculitis: Inflammation of a blood vessel of a lymphatic vessel.

Volume of distribution: The apparent space in the body that is available to the drug; the more extensive distribution, the larger the volume of distribution.

Financial Disclosures

Mr. Nathan Burns has no financial or proprietary interest in the materials presented herein.

Mr. Alan D. Freedman has no financial or proprietary interest in the materials presented herein.

Dr. Gary L. Harrelson has no financial or proprietary interest in the materials presented herein.

Dr. Joel E. Houglum has no financial or proprietary interest in the materials presented herein.

Dr. Michael Powers has no financial or proprietary interest in the materials presented herein.

Dr. Teresa M. Seefeldt has no financial or proprietary interest in the materials presented herein.

Ms. Cindy Thomas has no financial or proprietary interest in the materials presented herein.

Index

absorption, 19–20, 21, 22, 25, 26–30

absorption effects, 51, 52

ACE (angiotensin-converting enzyme) inhibitors, 7, 50, 215–216, 220, 224–226, 231, 232–233, 234, 256

acetaminophen, 21
  adverse effects, 54, 129–130, 137, 153, 165
    drug combinations, 5, 129–130, 131, 133, 134, 135, 175–176, 182
    drug interactions, 50, 128, 129–130
    NSAIDs, compared with, 43, 106, 110, 128, 130, 137
    pain, treatment of, 5, 43, 128–130, 133, 134, 135, 137

acid indigestion. *See* heartburn

active transport mechanisms, 23–24, 32

addiction, 131–132, 134

additive effect, 38–39, 40

ADHD (attention deficit/hyperactivity disorder), 244, 246, 261–263, 266, 310, 315–316

administered dose, 63–64

adrenergic drugs, 179, 213

adrenergic nervous system, 212–215

adverse drug reactions (ADRs), 52–56

affinity, 40, 41, 42

agonists, 39, 40–42, 51, 52, 132

alanine aminotransferase (ALT), 43, 130, 162

albumin, 20–21

alcohol, 49, 50, 93, 110, 130, 140, 143, 230, 259, 282, 314, 318, 342, 362

aldosterone antagonists, 223–224, 225, 234

allergic reactions, drug-induced, 53–54, 81, 82, 94, 108–109, 164

allergic rhinitis. *See* antihistamines; cold and allergy treatments

α-adrenergic agonists, 173, 179, 230, 316, 326

α-adrenergic receptors, 179, 213–214, 230, 261

α-glucosidase inhibitors, 284, 285–286, 287

ALT (alanine aminotransferase), 43, 130, 162

aminoglycoside antibiotics, 25, 45, 77, 86–87, 88

amphetamines, 40, 127, 253, 261–262, 263, 310, 315–317, 328, 349, 366

ampicillin, 47, 50

amylin-like compounds, 283, 284, 287

anabolic agents, 311, 318, 328–338, 366

anabolic steroids, 8, 22, 311, 328–331, 337, 349, 350, 366, 372–373

analgesics. *See* pain, treatment of

anaphylaxis, 53, 54, 109, 164

angina pectoris, 219–221, 226–227, 229–230, 233–234

angiotensin II receptor blockers (ARBs), 215–216, 220, 225, 226, 231, 232–233, 234

angiotensin-converting enzyme (ACE) inhibitors, 7, 50, 215–216, 220, 224–226, 231, 232–233, 234, 256

anorexia nervosa (AN), 245, 265

antacids, 39, 50, 107, 189, 199–200, 206, 226

antagonists, 39, 40–42, 49, 51, 132

antianxiety drugs, 39, 50, 141, 258–261, 296

antibacterial agents, 76–88, 91, 92–93, 170

antibiotics, 27, 45, 47, 76–88, 94. *See also* resistant microorganisms; *specific type of antibiotic*
  categories of, 6–7, 76, 77, 80–88
    definition of, 76
    drug and food interactions, 27, 50, 52, 55, 83–84, 257
    foundational concepts, 76–80
    gastrointestinal disorders, 78, 80, 84, 198, 199, 206
    sexually transmitted diseases, 92–93
    unnecessary use of, 78, 79, 92, 94, 170, 183

anticholinergic adverse effects, 140, 142, 143, 144, 159, 173, 178, 184, 203, 247, 248, 249, 252, 253

anticholinergic drugs, 142, 159, 179, 213, 247

anticoagulants, 20, 55, 106, 109–110, 232, 294, 299, 300. *See also* warfarin

anticonvulsants, 20, 45, 141, 257, 296

antidepressants, 141, 142, 203, 241, 250–255, 257, 260, 263, 265, 295, 296. *See also* monoamine oxidase inhibitors (MAOIs)

antidiarrheal agents, 132, 202–203, 204, 206

antifungal agents, 50, 76, 78, 89–92, 94, 257

antihistamines, 27, 39, 50, 141, 142, 173, 174–178, 183, 184, 264, 265

anti-LTs. *See* LT (leukotriene) modifiers

antimicrobial, definition of, 76

antimuscarinic drugs, 140, 213

antiplatelet activity, 106, 109–110, 191, 232, 234, 300

antipsychotic drugs, 28, 141, 142, 246–250, 258, 261

antipyretics, 106–107, 121, 128

antiseptics, 91, 92

antitussive agents, 27, 132, 133, 175–176, 182

antiviral agents, 76, 79, 91, 92, 170. *See also* cold and allergy treatments

anxiety disorders, 242–244, 245–246, 258–261

arachidonic acid metabolites, 101–103, 104, 110–111, 149–150

Printed in the United States
by Baker & Taylor Publisher Services